The
Portable
Pediatrician

Sears Parenting Library

The Autism Book
The N.D.D. Book
The Vaccine Book
The Healthiest Kid in the Neighborhood
The Baby Sleep Book
The Premature Baby Book
The Pregnancy Book
The Baby Book
The Birth Book
The Attachment Parenting Book
The Breastfeeding Book
The Fussy Baby Book
The Discipline Book
The Family Nutrition Book
The A.D.D. Book
The Successful Child

Parenting.com FAQ Books

The First Three Months
How to Get Your Baby to Sleep
Keeping Your Baby Healthy
Feeding the Picky Eater

Sears Children's Library

Baby on the Way
What Baby Needs
Eat Healthy, Feel Great
You Can Go to the Potty

Also by Dr. Robert W. Sears

HappyBaby: The Organic Guide to Baby's First 24 Months

The Portable Pediatrician

Everything You Need to Know
About Your Child's Health

**William Sears, MD, Martha Sears, RN, Robert Sears, MD,
James Sears, MD, and Peter Sears, MD**

LITTLE, BROWN AND COMPANY
New York • Boston • London

Little, Brown and Company
Hachette Book Group
237 Park Avenue, New York, NY 10017
www.hachettebookgroup.com

First Edition: February 2011

Little, Brown and Company is a division of Hachette Book Group, Inc. The Little, Brown name and logo are trademarks of Hachette Book Group, Inc.

The publisher is not responsible for websites (or their content) that are not owned by the publisher.

Drawings by Deborah Maze

Library of Congress Cataloging-in-Publication Data
The portable pediatrician : everything you need to know about your child's health / by William Sears ... [et al.].
  p. cm.
 Includes index.
 ISBN 978-0-316-01748-0
 1. Children — Health and hygiene — Popular works. 2. Pediatrics — Popular works. 3. Children — Diseases — Popular works. I. Sears, William, M.D.
 RJ61.P685 2011
 618.92 — dc22   2010006987

10 9 8 7 6 5 4 3 2 1

RRD-IN

Printed in the United States of America

To all the Sears children and grandchildren:

James
Robert
Peter
Hayden
Erin
Matthew
Stephen
Lauren
Lea
Jonathan
Andrew
Alex
Joshua
Ashton
Morgan
Landon
Thomas

Contents

Part III: Pediatric Concerns and Illnesses: A to Z   115

How to Use This Book

Every parent desires to give a child the best possible start in life — to provide love, shelter, clothes, food, education, fun, and everything else a child wants and needs. But there's one thing that many parents forget to add to this list — the gift of health. *The Portable Pediatrician* will give you the tools you need to provide this precious gift to your children and grandchildren.

Many of our children aren't getting the level of health care that they deserve. Children are getting sicker, sadder, and fatter. Dissatisfaction with the medical insurance system is at an all-time high. How often have you left the doctor's office wanting *more:* more time with the doctor, more understanding of your child's illness, and more information about what you can *do* in addition to what your child can *take?* This book gives you the "more" you need.

The Portable Pediatrician was literally written on the job. When parents brought their children in for sick or well visits, we kept a log of the most common worries parents had and the most common illnesses children get. When you, our trusting readers, want to know how to keep your children from getting sick,

we want you to feel that you are sitting in our office and talking with one of us.

This book represents our combined experience: more than sixty years in total. We have put ourselves behind the eyes of parents and asked: "What do I need to know to keep my child healthy and if my child gets sick, what do I need to know to help her get better?" We intend this book to be a helpful addition to your present parent-pediatrician partnership. We want to help parents become wise consumers of medical care.

Throughout this book we present each pediatric problem and illness in a parent-helpful way that teaches *you* how to be watchful. This is how we practice medicine, helping parents do what they do best. We educate you about a particular illness, believing that the more thoroughly parents understand the nature of their child's illness, the less they will worry and the more effective they will be. We'll teach you what you, as your child's "home doctor," can do with time-tested home remedies. This book will enable you to solve many common pediatric problems. We will also tell you when to enlist help from your own doctor.

This is not a textbook cluttered with worrisome statistics about what may happen in 0.1 percent of cases. Your child is a person, not a case. We give you the most important points of each illness, especially those that you can do something about, either through prevention or treatment. Consider each topic a handout that we would give you as you were leaving our office, summarizing the office visit as well as providing more detail.

How to find a topic. We have arranged the topics alphabetically according to the most common medical name. But parents often use other terms to refer to the same topic. Go to the index first. Medical names and parent terms for the same concern are listed in the index. For example, *halitosis* will be discussed in the "H" section, yet the index at the back of the book will contain terms such as *breath, stinky* and *bad breath* — all referring you to the same page.

How each topic is organized. You will notice that each medical topic has a heading to make it easy to get information at a glance. Subheadings generally include what causes the behavior or illness, what the symptoms are, when to worry, and what to do.

For each topic we have included the most important information for parents. In case you need to learn more, we have included extra reading and website resources for many of the topics. We have purposely omitted prescription drug dosages, because such information

changes from time to time and should be determined by your medical provider.

SHOW ME THE SCIENCE!

We assure you that, as much as possible, all the medical advice we offer in this book is based upon solid science, the best medical references we could find, and the most current information on the subject. Children are too precious for medical advice not to be scientifically based.

Prevention is the best medicine. Perhaps the most important part of this book is the very first section where we give you four tools to keep your child healthy. By developing your own health-maintenance plan for your family, you may not even need the rest of the book very often. Wouldn't that be nice?

Guidance as your child grows. In the second section of this book, we provide a guide to each of your child's checkups, from birth through eighteen years, sharing the physical, medical, and developmental aspects of each checkup, along with all of the advice we pass on to our own patients at these visits. Of course, nothing can replace the personal care your child will receive from your own pediatrician. Our advice is simply a supplement to your medical care.

Use this book as a companion to our other books. Some other books in The Sears Parenting Library cover particular illnesses or issues in full or in part, especially development, discipline, and behavioral concerns. In this book, we might refer you to a particular section of one of our other books for more detailed information while at the same time giving you a bullet-point summary of the topic that concerns you. We will often direct you to other resources as well.

Use this book as a companion to our website www.AskDrSears.com. Because medical science is rapidly changing, go to our website for continual updates. Simply click on www.AskDrSears.com/PortablePediatrician/ updates for new medical advice on a particular subject. On this site, you will also find photos of rashes and other illnesses.

We hope that when someone asks you, "Who is your child's primary health-care provider?" you can boast: "I am." Our joy as pediatricians is to know that your family is a bit happier and healthier because of our book.

Your Portable Pediatricians,
The Drs. Sears and Nurse Sears

PUBLISHER'S NOTE

The information and advice provided by the authors in this book is not intended to replace the services of a physician or the medical care or advice you receive from your physician, nor does it constitute a doctor-patient relationship. Information in this book is provided for informational purposes only. You should consult your physician or health-care professional regarding the care of your child and, in particular, any symptoms that may require diagnosis or medical attention. You should also follow your physician's advice in the event of any conflict with any information contained in this book. This book was current as of November 2010, and as new information becomes available through research, experience, or changes to product contents, some of the data in this book may become invalid. You should seek the most up-to-date information on medical care and treatment from your physician or health-care professional. Any action on your part in response to the information provided in this book is at your discretion. The publisher makes no representations or warranties with respect to any information contained in this book and is not liable for any direct or indirect claim, loss, or damage resulting from the use of information contained in this book.

I

Four Things All Parents Must Do to Keep Their Children Healthy

In this section you will learn four important things you should do to keep your children healthy. By doing these, you can maximize the parent-pediatrician partnership:

1. Find Dr. Right for your child.

2. Get the most out of your child's checkups and office visits.

3. Practice the pills-skills approach to medical care.

4. Follow the Dr. Sears head-to-toe guide to keeping your child healthy with good nutrition and a balanced lifestyle.

1. FIND DR. RIGHT FOR YOUR CHILD: CHOOSING A PEDIATRICIAN

Thirty-five years ago when I (Dr. Bill) was finishing my pediatric training and was about to hang out my shingle and open a practice, one of my professors advised me that there are three qualities parents look for in a pediatrician — the three A's: affability, ability, and availability. Picking the best pediatrician for you and your child is one of your most important long-term investments. Medical care is a partnership between parents and pediatrician. You owe it to your child to find a good partner.

Depending on the health-care needs of your child, expect to be in your pediatrician's office at least fifteen times during the first five years of your child's life. You might as well get the most out of it. Over my years in practice I have been grilled by many parents as they begin to search for Dr. Right for their child. Most parents do their search wisely, but some don't. I have learned the following tips on how to search for Dr. Right from parents who have made the right match of health-care provider for themselves and their child, along with a few tricks of the trade for extracting the best from your child's doctor. Here is a step-by-step plan, along with some insider tips on how to choose and use your child's pediatrician.

1. Interview yourself. Before you interview prospective health-care providers, do some soul searching. What qualities do you need in your child's doctor? Are you a new parent without a lot of experience with the usual childhood developmental quirks and the common childhood illnesses? Do you lack confidence (as some new parents do) and believe you need a pediatrician who will be very involved in your family, will help you understand normal growth and development, and will competently manage your child's health care? Are you a worrier (as nearly all first-time parents are) who needs an empathetic listener to seriously address your concerns? Are you evaluating various parenting styles and need a doctor who will help you formulate a parenting philosophy? Or are you a veteran parent already firmly rooted in your parenting philosophy and style who simply needs a like-minded pediatrician? Does distance matter? Are you willing to drive farther for higher quality, or do you rely on public transportation and therefore need a doctor's office close to your home or workplace and easily accessible by bus or subway?

Do you or your child have special needs? For example, if your child has a chronic illness, such as diabetes, naturally you would want to choose a pediatrician with expertise in that illness. If you are a first-time mother and are adamant about breastfeeding your baby, obviously you want to choose a breastfeeding-friendly pediatric practice. Or do you or your child have special communication needs? One of my favorite parents is blind, and I have learned so much from her about the power of mother's intuition. I have learned to communicate by voice and touch.

3

During an exam I guide her hands over her baby's body to help her develop the feel for normal skin and normal muscle tone and to help her appreciate the marvels of her baby's developing body. One time she brought her infant in for consultation about a rash, but I couldn't see it. The next day she returned to the office with her obviously spotted child. Nancy could feel the rash the day before I could see it.

Another mother in my practice is deaf and "listens" primarily by lipreading. Initially, we had a communication problem because I did not move my lips expressively enough when I talked for her to understand me. She politely informed me that I was difficult to lip-read, which encouraged me to hone my communication skills by being more expressive with my facial language. Years ago, one of my favorite pediatric professors, Dr. Richard Van Praagh, professor of pediatrics at Harvard Medical School, gave me some valuable advice: "Surround yourself with wise and interesting parents and have the humility to learn from them."

2. Get references. Interview friends who share your parenting philosophy. Pick out the most experienced and like-minded mothers in your neighborhood and get references about the doctors they use. Ask them specific questions: "What do you like most about Dr. Susan?" "Is Dr. Tom available when you need him?" "Does Dr. Laura give you the time you need?" "Are his partners just as good?" Pick out at least three names before continuing your search. If you are choosing a pediatrician toward the end of your pregnancy, consult your obstetrician, who likely has a feel for your specific needs. Your pediatrician should be right for you and your child.

Insider's tip. Suppose the doctor you have chosen to be your child's pediatrician is not taking new patients. Write a brief letter personally asking the doctor to accept your child as a new patient, and follow up the letter with a phone call. This extra effort impresses doctors that you sincerely care and it may motivate them to actually want to open the practice to you. As I tell my receptionist, "There's always room in our practice for nice patients."

3. Do your insurance homework. It's disappointing to have chosen Dr. Right only to find out you have the wrong insurance. Once you have a list of prospective doctors, check your insurance plan booklet to see which are participating members. After you have narrowed down the list to a few finalists, check with these doctors' offices to be sure they are still members of the plan and are still accepting new patients from that plan. If you absolutely want to go to a certain doctor who is not a member of your current insurance plan, check your options with your insurance carrier. The best insurance carriers offer a "point of service" (POS) option that allows you to see health-care providers outside the plan, usually for an additional charge.

4. Check out the office. Arrive early for your interview appointment and browse around the office a bit. Chat with others in the waiting room and ask what they like, or dislike, about the office and the doctor's practice. Notice and ask the staff about how children with potentially contagious illnesses are handled. Many first-time interviewers ask whether there are separate waiting rooms for well and sick children, a question they obviously got from their childbirth class or a book written by someone who has never run a pediatric office. Most doctors who have tried separate sick and well waiting rooms found this system does not work. Nobody wants to use the "sick" waiting room. The more practical solution to minimizing the spread of illnesses is to reserve the waiting room for well children only and to usher potentially contagious children into examining rooms immediately and if possible through a separate entrance. (One comforting fact of germ spreading is that by the time many children come to the doctor's office, they are no longer contagious.)

Besides looking around the office, find out some basic information and compare it with what you know about other offices:

- What are the office hours?

- Are there any evening or weekend hours?

- Is there a doctor on call after hours and overnight, or is it an advice nurse?

- How much are checkups and sick visits (if you don't have insurance)?

5. Interview the office staff. Introduce yourself to the office staff. Are they friendly and accommodating? You're likely to be having as much contact with the office staff as you will with the doctor. During doctor-shopping interviews, I love to hear new parents say, "Your staff is so helpful." To maximize the time you have with your doctor, get as many questions answered and facts you need to know from the office staff before meeting the doctor: hospital affiliations, after-hours coverage, appointment scheduling, and anything else that is important to you.

6. Interview the doctor. Remember, the goal of your interview is to decide whether this pediatrician is the right match for your family. Try these interviewing tips:

- Be brief. Since most doctors do not charge for these interviews, expect the doctor to give you about five minutes. This is usually enough to make a doctor assessment. If you or your child have many special needs and you feel you need more time, schedule a regular doctor's appointment for a checkup rather than for an interview.

- Be concise. Bring a short list of your most pressing parenting issues. If your baby is one year old, this is not the time to ramble on about future behavior worries, such as bedwetting or learning problems.

- Be positive. Avoid opening the interview with an "I don't want" list, such as "I don't want my baby to have shots…" I remember parents who once opened their interview with "We don't want to give our baby eyedrops, vitamin K, newborn shots, newborn blood tests, immunizations…" While it's good to do your homework and formulate opinions about certain routine medical practices, it's better to phrase your question positively, such as "Doctor, what is your custom about routine immunizations?" This allows you to learn the doctor's perspective and opens the door to factors you may not have previously considered. You owe it to your child to keep an open mind. Negative openers put doctors on the defensive, as they recognize the mismatch between the parents' desires and their professional beliefs.

- Be impressive. Once, when a couple of first-time expectant parents were checking me out as a prospective doctor for their baby, they opened their interview with the impressive line: "This is a well-researched baby." I immediately warmed to these parents because this statement impressed upon me that they had done their home-work thoroughly. Both parents were in their mid thirties, well established in their careers, and were now ready to settle down and begin their parenting career and "do everything right." These parents had care-fully chosen their obstetrician and explored their birthing options, and now I was on their list of pediatric finalists. They con-veyed that the choice of a pediatrician was high priority for them. Because these par-ents expressed that they expected a higher level of medical care, I was motivated to be a more attentive doctor to them. I always advise parents about the law of supply and demand: you will get the level of medical care that you demand. Attend the doctor interview with as many family members as possible, preferably with both parents. A new family recently moved to our area and was interviewing our practice. Grand-mother came along. She sat quietly across the room while the parents grilled me. I took cues from Grandmother's nods as to whether or not I was a Grandma-approved pediatrician.

- Avoid doctor turnoffs. Remember, doctors take a lot of pride in being chosen by selec-tive parents. Don't reveal that you chose this practice "because I found you in the yellow pages" or "because you're on my insurance plan." These openers do not make good first impressions.

- Be intuitive. Within a few minutes you should get a gut feeling about whether or not this doctor is Dr. Right for your family. While this may sound subjective, try to get a feel for whether the doctor really cares about kids and enjoys his or her practice. When our two sons Dr. Bob and Dr. Jim

joined the Sears Family Pediatrics practice, I (Dr. Bill) advised the young Drs. Sears, "Run your practice the way you do your family. As you developed a parenting style to help you enjoy your children, develop a style of pediatric practice that you enjoy, because you're going to be doing it for a very long time."

- Discover the doctor's basic parenting phi-losophy. It's important to pick a pediatri-cian who either agrees with or at least supports your basic parenting philosophy. Ask a few leading questions to get a feel for the type of parenting advice the doctor will likely give you in the coming years, such as "I'm worried I won't succeed at breastfeed-ing. Is it really that important?" or "My sis-ter used the cry-it-out method to help her baby learn to sleep well. How will I know this will work on my baby?" or "My neigh-bor uses spanking as a form of discipline, and they swear by it. Do you think it works on children?" While these types of ques-tions may not really have right or wrong answers, you will get a sense if this doctor's advice will fit well with what you feel is right for your baby.

- Uncover the doctor's basic approach to medicine. You may prefer a doctor who practices straightforward standard medi-cine. On the other hand, you may enjoy one who likes to think outside the box and pro-vides some alternative approaches to treat-ment and prevention, or is at least open to your doing so on your own. Ask the doctor what his or her feelings are about antibiot-ics and other prescription medications, about adjusting your baby's vaccination schedule to suit your preferences, and about how to treat ear infections.

- Bring your child along. If you have recently moved to the area or are switching pediatric practices, take cues from your child. Watch how the doctor approaches your child and how your child reacts. Children are amazingly perceptive about their caregivers, including health-care providers.

It's important to pick a doctor who gives you the impression of really wanting to make a difference in your life and your child's life. Among the joys of pediatrics is watching patients grow from infancy through childhood. I (Dr. Bill) once attended the wedding of one of my patients whom I had first cared for twenty-two years earlier when he was a four-pound premature newborn. During the wedding, my mind filled with memories of Mark's life from incubator to altar. I was so happy that Mark's parents had chosen me as their child's pediatrician. Most doctors go into pediatrics because they can truly make a difference in the lives of young people. When our two oldest sons, Dr. Jim and Dr. Bob, joined the Sears Family Pediatrics practice, I gave them another bit of doctorly and fatherly advice: "Jim and Bob, your success in life will be measured not by how much money you make but by how many of these little lives are better because of what you did. Be successful pediatricians."

2. GET THE MOST OUT OF YOUR CHILD'S CHECKUPS AND OFFICE VISITS

Now that you've made an informed choice about your child's doctor, here's how to get the most out of the professional you have so carefully chosen. Remember, medical care of your child is a partnership between parents and pediatrician. The parent's role is to be a *keen observer* and *accurate reporter,* and the doctor's role is to take the clues provided by the parents and arrive at the right diagnosis and plan of treatment. The more you value this partnership and the better you do your job, the better you can expect the doctors to do theirs. Mothers often confide in me, "I worry too much." I reassure them, "It's your job to worry. My job is to assess the situation and tell you whether or not you need to worry. In fact, I worry about mothers who don't worry."

Periodic checkups (also called well-baby and well-child exams) are wise preventive medicine for children and their parents. Checkups are scheduled to match developmental stages; they give parents opportunities to learn about normal childhood development and their child's own individual developmental quirks, as well as to identify problems early so that they can intervene before these problems escalate. After thirty-five years in pediatric practice, I (Dr. Bill) have come to regard checkups as *growing together.* As I watch the child grow from infancy to adolescence, I also observe and counsel parents about how to expand their knowledge of their child and improve their parenting skills. I also grow in my knowledge of the whole family. Examining children when they are well gives me a frame of reference to better evaluate them when they are ill.

Over the years, I have noticed that some parents and children get more out of their checkups than others. Often I'll finish a checkup thinking, "Wow! We really accomplished a lot in fifteen minutes!" Here are eleven tips on how you and your child can get the most out of your child's checkups and sick visits:

1. Keep personal medical records. As your part of the partnership, keep a "what works" list, recording the advice and treatment that previously worked with your child. This is especially helpful if you have a child with a chronic illness and are changing doctors. Your new doctor will appreciate knowing this valuable part of your child's medical history. For example, when your doctor is prescribing an antibiotic, you may volunteer, "That antibiotic gave her terrible diarrhea, but the one you prescribed last time seemed to be easier on her intestines." Your medical records are also helpful for after-hours over-the-phone advice when your doctor, or a substitute pediatrician, may not have access to your medical records.

2. Do your homework. Before scheduling your appointment, formulate a plan, asking yourself, "What do I want to get out of the checkup?" and "What do I want my child to learn?" Write a list and prioritize your main concerns. If your concerns are minimal and your list is short, then the usual allotted time should be enough. But if you have concerns that you believe will require more time, such as behavioral or learning problems, request a "long appointment."

3. Play doctor. Before calling your doctor for advice about whether to bring your child in, do some role-playing. Imagine you are your child's doctor. What would you want to know about the illness? Think about when and how it began, whether it's getting better or worse, and what home treatments you've tried. Do your own home checkup. A wise parent's eyes and touch can often provide the doctor with valuable clues for a child's diagnosis. I (Dr. Bill) tell my patients, "Our relationship is like a partnership with both of us doing our best for the benefit of your child. Your job is to be a keen observer and an accurate reporter. My job is to take what you observe and help make the right diagnosis." The day of your child's checkup, examine your child from head to toe. Look for unusual spots, rashes, bumps, or areas of growth that concern you. Ask your school-age child, "Are there parts of your body or any aches and pains that you would like to ask the doctor about?"

4. Book the best time. The best behavior time for examining infants and toddlers is the mornings. The worst time for tired toddlers is late afternoons. The best time for school-age children is either on a school holiday in the morning or immediately after school. Mothers often apologize for a baby's upsetting behavior by saying, "It's naptime." Be sure your school-age child doesn't miss a fun activity because of the checkup; this makes for an unfriendly patient.

Insider's tip. Your best odds for the doctor being on time and avoiding a long wait is to pick the *first* appointment of the morning or the afternoon. The worst time for long appointments to discuss behavior or discipline problems is in the late afternoon when the parents, the child, and the doctor are tired.

5. Feed your child before the checkup. Feed your child before the office visit, preferably not in the office. If you bring along snacks, avoid the crumbly type so the doctor and staff do not have to clean up after your child and you don't spend your valuable office-visit time picking up crumbs. Bring juice in nonspill cups and have office-appropriate snacks, such as yogurt and apple slices.

DR. SEARS TIP
Inspect Your Insurance

Here's a way to makc points with your doctor. Before your office visit, call your insurance company and inquire: (1) Have I met my deductible? and (2) What services (e.g., immunizations and well-child visits) are covered by my policy? If you come into your doctor's office with this information (or ask your insurance company to fax your doctor's office a printout), you merit a sticker and perhaps a place on your doctor's preferred-patient list. Doing your insurance homework tells your doctor that you care enough about your doctor to save the staff and the doctor time. The less paperwork the staff and the doctor have to do, the more time they have for you.

6. Be happy to be there! Consider these two scenarios at the beginning of the exam: "He's fine, it's just a routine checkup and here's the required school form." Or, "Erin and I have been looking forward to her checkup. She wants to learn more about how her body works and I have a few concerns..." Which of these two openers do you think gets the doctor enthusiastic about routine checkups?

7. Respect private time with each child. One child per checkup, please. Even though bringing two or more children for their checkups may seem like smart parental time management, this may dilute the checkup for each of your children. When you're frazzled chasing a toddler while talking about your teen, neither child will feel special. If the luxury of separate checkups is not possible for you, bring along a friend who can care for your infant or toddler so you and your doctor can focus on the older child's checkup. The toddler then can have a checkup before or after the older child. Private time is especially important if one of the children has a complicated and time-consuming problem. A six-year-old child may be reluctant to bring up his bedwetting in front of his four-year-old sister. The older children get, the more necessary it is to separate their checkups. If there are things you feel you want to discuss with your doctor privately before your child's checkup, tell the nurse ahead of time so you can talk to the doctor in one room while your child is being weighed and measured in the other room. If a sensitive issue comes up during the exam, and you want some private time with the doctor, give the doctor a cue, such as: "Erin, perhaps you could go out and have the nurse check your vision." The doctor will pick up on your cue.

8. Play show-and-tell. If you have concerns about quirky behavior your child is showing at home, in addition to describing the behavior, bring along a video recording. A parent once brought in her two-week-old infant for a checkup and was concerned about the child's colic. To convince me (Dr. Bill) of the severity of the problem and the toll it was taking on the family, she videotaped her baby during an evening blast. When I saw how much the baby — and the parents — were hurting, I immediately gave them more time and attention than they would have gotten without this visual aid. Occasionally, a parent records our conversation during the checkups in order to play it back for the parent who wasn't able to attend.

During one recent checkup, parents asked me about their five-year-old's restless sleep. I asked them to videotape a few minutes of the unusual noises and restlessness they were concerned about. When I watched the tape on their return appointment I realized that their child suffered from sleep apnea and needed his tonsils removed.

I love to see parents whip out a written list of their concerns prior to a checkup. Sometimes they will hand me a copy of this list (please prioritize your concerns), which helps me be sure I've addressed all their concerns. A written list also helps with the doctor's time management. If I see a particularly complicated problem on the list, such as a behavior or school issue, I may address the more immediate problems first and ask the parents to schedule a longer appointment for these more time-consuming issues.

9. Respect your child's quirks. After you and your child have gone through a few checkups, note what works and what doesn't. If your toddler has previously gotten spooked on the scale, ask the nurse to save the weighing and measuring until the *end* of the exam. One day while I (Dr. Bill) was examining a toddler, I attempted to remove her shoes.

DR. SEARS TIP
Thank Your Doctor

Write thank-you notes. If you have had a particularly rewarding experience at your doctor's office or a member of the staff has gone out of his or her way to make your visit more comfortable, let the doctor know. A box of mommy-made muffins once arrived in my office to apologize for the midnight wake-up call the night before. Also, if you have had a problem, let the doctor know. Doctors have no way of evaluating their office staff unless you tell them.

She got nervous, threw a tantrum, and the exam went downhill from there. I noted this on her chart, and the mother also made a mental note. On her next checkup, the child toddled in barefoot.

10. No surprises, please. "My doctor is often in a hurry and is always running late" seems to be one of the most common parent peeves. In defense of Dr. Rush, the system of managed care has forced doctors into a "more for less" operation — seeing more patients in less time. The main reason doctors get behind schedule is that one or two routine checkups turn out to be complex problem-solving half-hour consultations. Yet the patients had scheduled only ten-minute regular checkups. If you know you don't really have many questions and your child is basically healthy, a quick checkup will usually suffice. But if you feel you need more time to address some complex issues, the best thing to do is ask for a longer visit when you book your appointment. If you demand (politely, of course) quality and quantity time with your doctor, you'll get it. But it is not fair to the child or the doctor to surprise the doctor toward the end of a regular checkup by mentioning, "By the way, the school thinks my child has ADD . . ."

11. If you and your doctor disagree. It's important that you and your pediatrician agree on major topics of child-rearing. You want to look forward to your well-baby and well-child visits and not have to feel that you're on the defensive. Disagreements between parents and pediatricians are usually more about parenting styles than medical care. The main example we see among parents who have transferred to our practice is that the former pediatrician does not support the chosen parenting style of the parents. For example, you may prefer the high-touch and highly responsive style of parenting called attachment parenting, which means feeding your baby on cue, carrying your baby a lot, and even sleeping close to your baby. Your pediatrician, on the other hand, may prefer a more scheduled and distant style of parenting — one that could be based on his or her own personal experience rather than any medical school training. Yes, you can respectfully disagree with your doctor if it's a parenting-style issue. We often hear parents complain, "My doctor is very good and is very medically competent, yet we disagree on parenting styles." Often, there is a trade-off. If your child has special needs and you are happy with your doctor's medical care, then avoid getting into the parenting-style issue. Simply tell your doctor that you are confident about what you are doing and that it is working for you and your child. Suppose you enjoy wearing your baby in a sling for several hours a day, yet your pediatrician believes that this fosters an unhealthy dependence. While you should be open to his or her viewpoint, it's appropriate to challenge your doctor and request reasons for your doctor's difference of opinion. That way, your doctor learns other viewpoints and so do you. After all, you know your child best.

Eventually, the development and behavior of your child will be your best advertisement. Once your doctor sees the result of your parenting style and witnesses that what you are doing is working, he or she is likely to compli-ment you rather than criticize your way of parenting. Many parent-doctor relationships work quite well, even though they may start out with differences of opinion. For the relationship to thrive, there must eventually be a blending of opinions. After all, both you and your doctor share the same goal: to help your child stay happy and healthy.

There is great joy and pride in being a pediatrician. After all, his or her name is at the top of the babysitter's phone list when the parents go out. One of the hallmarks of a close and long-lasting doctor/patient relationship is the "remember when" reminders that we sometimes hear from patients. Once when I (Dr. Bill) was examining Jonathan, a teenager already taller than I was, his mother reminisced about the time I had to insert a tube down baby Jonathan's windpipe to relieve his severe croup. In another instance, Dr. Bob was giving a ten-year-old girl a physical and noticed a small scar on her belly where the appendix would be, and the mom reminded him of the time he had sent her to the emergency room, certain she had appendicitis. "You were right, and the surgeon said if we had waited another hour or so it would have ruptured." Although we often forget about many of these occurrences, parents and children sure don't. It's rewarding to find a pediatrician you love and to stick with him or her until your child goes off to college. That's the kind of doctor you and your children deserve to have.

EASING EXAM ANXIETY

Exam time can be scary for little people, who may have flashbacks of the needle sticks from previous exams. Here's how you can help everyone enjoy the checkups.

Prepare your child ahead of time. Do a pretend exam at home where you show and tell the child what the doctor may do during the checkup. Keep up a running commentary: "The doctor will count your teeth, look into your ears, pat your tummy, and listen to your heart…" If your child has a history of being less than enthusiastic about being medically examined, get him or her a play doctor kit and go through a mock exam first: "Check Mommy's ears," "Look at Mommy's throat," "Listen to my heart," and so on. End with: "That's what Dr. Susan will do when she examines you." Have your child bring the doctor kit along to "examine the doctor" before his or her own exam.

Dress your child for success. Some toddlers get spooked when I (Dr. Bill) try to undress them. Dress your child for easy access, such as in a shirt that opens from the front rather than in one that needs to be pulled over the child's head.

Read all about it. Go through a picture book about getting a checkup, such as *The Berenstain Bears Go to the Doctor* by Stan and Jan Berenstain, for kids four to eight.

Bribery is okay. If your child's behavior during medical checkups has been less than ideal, entice your child by saying, "After your checkup, we'll go for a treat"— implying that you expect him to cooperate with the doctor. If bribery offends the moralist in you, call it an "incentive."

Be happy about the checkup yourself. Mothers are mirrors of anxiety and calmness. When I begin to examine a toddler, I notice the child usually reacts toward me the way the mother does. If the child clings to the mother, and the mother clings back adding an anxious "he won't hurt you," she reinforces the anxiety, and the toddler clings harder. But if the mother relaxes her grip and clicks right into a happy-to-be-here dialogue with me, often the toddler clings less to the mother. If you sense your child is anxious, greet the doctor cheerfully and carry on a happy dialogue before the exam. I watch children observing this dialogue. They feel that if I'm okay to Mommy, I must be okay. Once the child concludes I'm a mom-approved person, the exam takes on a friendlier tone.

Bring along a "friend" for the checkup. To lessen checkup anxiety, encourage your child to bring along her favorite doll or bear for a checkup, too. Pediatricians welcome these props. I often do a checkup on whatever fuzzy character is currently popular in order to win over an anxious young patient. If the doctor doesn't take the cue, ask him if he could check the doll first. I often do a brief pretend exam on an older sibling in order to win over the younger one, or let the older child hold the stethoscope or otoscope and give him a title, such as "Dr. Johnny." The younger child will often willingly join in this game and let me examine her.

Use the lap of security. If your child seems anxious, ask the doctor if your child could be examined on your lap instead of on the exam table. I rarely use exam tables for preschool children, who are much more secure and trusting while lounging on a parent's lap.

3. PRACTICE THE PILLS-SKILLS APPROACH TO MEDICAL CARE

Pediatric care is a partnership between parents and doctor. You are your child's "home doctor." We will now show you how. One of the most important concepts for parents to appreciate is one we call the pills-skills model of medical care. Nowadays, many children and adults are developing a "take a pill" mind-set. Children take pills to calm them down and perk them up, bring down a fever, or help a cold. Adults take pills for the diseases we call the "highs" — high blood pressure, high blood cholesterol, and high blood sugar. Rather than make changes in their lifestyle and diet, they feel it's easier to pop a pill. This is an unhealthy attitude that we want to change.

The pills-skills approach means the doctor is first of all the teacher, which is what the word *doctor* originally meant. The doctor prescribes a pill but also teaches the parents and child self-help skills that help the child's body muster up its own internal medicine. With the pills-skills model, you go into the doctor's office and ask the doctor not only "What can we *take?*" but also "What can we *do?*" When health-care providers see that the parents have the pills-skills mind-set, they also adopt a healthier attitude: "Here's what I *prescribe,* and here's what I *advise.*"

The pills-skills model, one that we will use with most illnesses in this book, is best explained by the following example:

Mrs. Smith brings her eight-year-old daughter, Suzy, into my (Dr. Bill's) office for consultation about her chronic asthma. Suzy has been on multiple medications, and Mrs. Smith is worried about two things: the continuation of Suzy's asthma and the possible side effects of chronic medications. After listening to these concerns, I whip out my sketch pad and draw a graph of the pills-skills model (see below). I explain to the mother that all chronic illnesses — asthma, ADD, GERD, chronic diarrhea, recurrent fevers, and all the "-itis" diseases — must follow this pills-skills model. This is, or should be, the current medical mind-set. Meanwhile, I notice Mrs. Smith's body language: "Finally, a doctor who gets it!"

PILLS PLUS SKILLS

As skill power increases, the need for pills decreases.

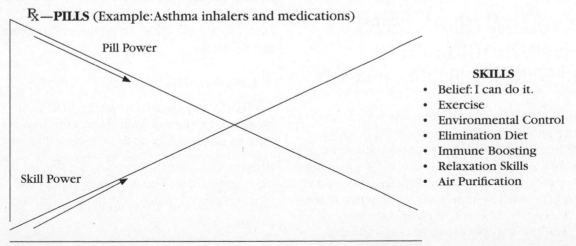

R_X—**PILLS** (Example: Asthma inhalers and medications)

Pill Power

Skill Power

SKILLS
• Belief: I can do it.
• Exercise
• Environmental Control
• Elimination Diet
• Immune Boosting
• Relaxation Skills
• Air Purification

3 Months

I go on to explain: "Our goal is to slowly wean Suzy off dependence on the medication. When and whether she will ever be completely off the medication is an unknown, but it's likely we can at least drastically lower her dosage." I tell her that we can teach Suzy self-help skills that, in effect, will help her body *muster up its own internal medicine* — medicine that is customized for her own body, and I list therapeutic things Suzy can do.

Many children have quirks — parts or systems of the body that just don't work as well as they should. We all have them; some are more major than others. In order to deal with these quirks, make a project out of your problem, study it, and become an expert on it. Then you build your own toolbox, a set of doctor-designed skills. You carry this toolbox around. We're going to help you build your toolbox with your own tools and show you when and how to use them. For example, if your child is on anti-inflammatory medicine, we'll show you how to help his body make its own anti-inflammatories. If your child is on antihistamine medication, we'll show you how to help her body make its own antihistamines. We'll help you and your child learn to rely on skills rather than pills.

4. FOLLOW THE DR. SEARS HEAD-TO-TOE GUIDE TO KEEPING YOUR CHILD HEALTHY

In this section we provide advice for using the pills-skills approach to staying healthy. When your child has a particular illness or problem associated with any of the following systems, here are practical things you can do to keep each system healthy and, when these systems do become ill, to help them heal. We give you a brief health plan for the brain, eyes, nose, heart, lungs, gut, skin, immune system, and endocrine system.

Growing a Healthy Brain

Here are some brain facts you should know:

- A child's brain grows most rapidly in the first five years, tripling in volume during the first two years and reaching 90 percent of adult growth by age five.

- The brain, above all other organs, is affected — for better or worse — by nutrition.

- Infants and toddlers use around 60 percent of their food energy for brain growth.

- In school-age children, around 25 percent of food energy goes into brain growth and function.

- For many children you can replace the term *ADD* (attention deficit disorder) with *NDD* (nutrition deficit disorder).

Nutrition and lifestyle choices dramatically affect the brain. Properly feeding your child's mind is perhaps the most important first step to get your child off to a healthy start in life. Here are seven ways to help your child's brain grow smart:

1. Eat smart foods

Go fish! Seafoods and/or omega-3 DHA supplements are the top smart food. (See page 34 for why seafood is good brain food.)

Blueberries. Help your children grow a berry good brain. The deep blue skin of the blueberry is full of phytonutrients called flavonoids. These are antioxidants or "phytos" (see explanation of phytos, page 34) that keep your child's blood/brain barrier (BBB) healthy. The BBB is a thin membrane between the brain cells and the blood supply that acts like a filter, keeping harmful substances from entering the brain and healthful substances in. Blueberries also improve neurotransmitter function, or the way nerves "talk" to each other. Also, blueberries reduce inflammation to keep your child's brain from becoming part of an iBod body (see page 35).

Greens. Not only should your children "eat blue," they should also "eat green." Many of the brain-health properties mentioned above for blueberries are also true for green veggies such as spinach, bok choy, collard greens, asparagus, and green, leafy lettuce like romaine and arugula.

Nuts. Go nuts with your children! Walnuts are the top brain nut because they're the richest in omega 3s. For toddlers and preschoolers (an age when nuts can be a choking hazard), nut butters are a great choice. Most nut butters can be offered starting at age one. Peanut butter, however, should be delayed until age two in order to help prevent peanut allergies.

Smart carbs. The child's brain is a "carbo hog" — it needs lots of sugar to function. But your child needs a right-carb diet. Two quirks make the brain particularly sensitive to carbs: first, the brain can use sugar without insulin, whereas other tissues need the hormone insulin to usher sugar into the cells for energy, and second, the brain, unlike other tissues, does not store glucose, so it needs a steady supply for brain function.

What's a "right carb" and "wrong carb," or "good carb" and "bad carb"? Here's how you can explain it to your kids: "Smart carbs have

---

SMART FOODS VS. DUMB FOODS

It just so happens that the foods that are good for the whole body are also best for the brain.

Smart Foods	Dumb Foods
• Blueberries	• Aspartame
• Dark greens	• BHT and other preservatives
• Nuts	• Fiber-poor carbs
• Right carbs	• Food colorings
• Salmon	• Hydrogenated oils
	• Hydrolyzed vegetable protein
	• "Liquid candy" — sweetened beverages
	• MSG (monosodium glutamate)

---

two friends, protein and fiber. They never play alone. These two friends keep the carb from rushing into the brain too fast and getting it too excited. Bad carbs, or dumb carbs, have no friends. They play alone. When you eat dumb carbs the friends can't hold the sugar back, so it rushes into the blood and brain and excites the brain too much. Smart carbs are found in nature: fruits, veggies, and whole grains. Dumb carbs are found in packages and bottles. The dumbest carbs are sweetened beverages."

Calcium. Calcium is an important nutrient not only for growing bones but also for growing brains. Dairy products, fortified cereals, dark green veggies, and fortified orange juice are good sources of calcium.

The Dr. Sears Smoothie. Many years ago we learned that a protein- and nutrient-rich smoothie is one of the best ways to start the day. Many of our children also join in this morning ritual. Here are the base ingredients (experiment with varying amounts to taste):

- ground flaxseeds, flaxseed meal, or flax oil
- frozen fruits: blueberries, strawberries, mango, papaya, pineapple, banana, kiwi
- organic milk (cow or others), juice (pomegranate, carrot, other veggies)
- Greek-style organic yogurt
- multivitamin/multimineral protein powder

Use varying amounts of the following special add-ins according to taste:

- cinnamon
- dates
- honey (not earlier than one year of age)
- pomegranate seeds
- peanut butter
- raisins
- spinach leaves
- tofu
- wheat germ
- whey protein powder

Pick and choose various ingredients and try some ideas of your own. Keep it simple at first so your kids won't suspect you are trying to sneak something healthy into them. As your children get into the habit, include the healthier add-ins.

2. Eat often

Grazing is good for your child's brain. Because the brain cannot store glucose, it relies on a steady supply of healthy sugar — not too much, not too little. Steady blood sugar means steady nerve function and mood. Nibbling on nutritious mini-meals throughout the day is more brain-friendly than eating fewer but bigger meals. Let's delve a little deeper into the food/mood connection. The key health-food phrase to remember is *stable insulin levels*. Throughout your child's body, many hormones play together like pieces in a symphony orchestra. Insulin is the master hormone, like the conductor in your child's hormonal orchestra. When insulin is stable, the rest of your child's body chemistry is in balance, or hormonal harmony, and the beautiful music of health occurs.

The top tip for keeping insulin stable is the rule of twos: Eat *twice* as often, *half* as much, and chew *twice* as long. This is one of the simplest and most practical of our nutri-tips, and one you will see repeated throughout this book. It is especially valuable for stabilizing moods, improving concentration and learning, and maintaining weight.

3. Eat breakfast

Feed your child a brainy breakfast. Like Grandmother said, "Breakfast is the most important meal of the day." Studies show that children who eat a nutritious breakfast, one high in protein and with fiber-filled carbs (whole grains, fruit, yogurt, oatmeal, and eggs), get higher grades, are more attentive and behave better in class, and miss fewer school days because of illness.

READ MORE ABOUT IT

Our book *The Healthiest Kid in the Neighborhood* is an easy-to-read health plan for the whole family. There you will find an entire chapter on feeding the brain as well as menus for brainy breakfasts.

4. Eat "pure"

Parents, your child's growing brain cannot handle the junk that is added to many processed foods. A simple fact of brain function is that if you put junk food into your child's brain, you get back junk learning and junk behavior. Many chemical food additives, such as those listed under "Dumb Foods" on page 15, can damage the part of the brain cell called mitochondria, the tiny packets in the center of the cell that act like batteries to give the cell energy. Dumb foods are also called excitotoxins; they can throw neurotransmitter activity (the brain's information processing system) out of balance. In our opinion, food additives have never been proven safe for adults, let alone the more sensitive brains of growing children. Even the Food and Drug Administration (FDA) gives them "GRAS" status, meaning "generally regarded as safe." Do you want to put stuff in your child's growing body and brain that is only "generally regarded as safe"?

One day a mother in our office who was holding a four-dollar cup of Starbucks coffee asked, "Is buying organic food for my children worth the extra price?" Our reply: "What's your child's brain worth?" You would do better to save money on much of the useless plastic stuff children get that they don't need. Children's growing bodies and brains are harmed by pesticides. Environmental pollutants are particularly toxic to the brain. Pesticides and other environmental pollutants are stored in fat. The brain is primarily fat. You draw the conclusion. Additionally, infants and toddlers have proportionally more body fat than do adults and are therefore more bothered by the harmful effects of pesticides. As an added perk, new studies reveal that the vitamin and mineral content of organic foods is higher. Spending more money on better food will ultimately save you much more in medical costs. (Dr. Bob is an adviser to HappyBaby organic baby foods, promoting the importance of eating organic foods.)

5. Move

Movement is one of your best brain foods for several reasons:

Movement improves blood flow to the brain. Improving blood flow to any organ, especially the brain, is like watering and fertilizing a garden. More blood means more nutrients. When you move your muscles, especially the large muscles in your arms and legs through vigorous exercise, your heart works harder to pump blood up into your brain.

Movement helps the brain grow. Exercise stimulates the release of nerve growth factors (NGF). NGF is like fertilizer to a plant. Every time your child moves, he is fertilizing one of the most important "plants" in his growing body: his brain.

Movement mellows the mind. The increase in blood flow to the brain secretes "feel good" biochemicals that have a natural calming effect.

Movement keeps insulin stable. Stable insulin means stable blood sugar, which means enough brain fuel.

DR. SEARS TIP
Walk Therapy

When your child seems tense or anxious, go for a brisk walk together. This will help her brain relax and help her sit still awhile to do her homework.

6. Keep calm

By an unfortunate quirk of biology, the organ that creates the most stress, the brain, is the very one that can handle it the least. At both ends of the life span — the first five years of the growing brain and the last few decades of the aging brain — central nervous system tissue has the most trouble handling the effects of high and prolonged blood levels of stress hormones, which can actually damage brain tissue. The effect of chronic, unresolved stress on growing brains is called glucocorticoid neurotoxicity (GCN). Although this term is a

DR. SEARS TIP
Laughter Is the
Best Medicine

Surround your children with friends and family who perk them up rather than pull them down. As much as possible, fill your child's mind with positive and happy thoughts. You may be happy to know that PET scans of the brain show that central nervous system pathways can actually change in response to positive and negative attitudes and thoughts. Let the refrain "Don't worry, be happy" permeate your home. Negative thoughts are like pollution to the mind. In our homes we have found that music mellows the mind of everyone.

mouthful, it basically means that high levels of stress hormones damage sensitive brain tissue, in addition to slowing down the ability of glucose to enter the brain cells and slowing the speed of information processing by causing a drop in the brain's neurotransmitters. This translates into less mental energy and more unstable moods, resulting in difficulty with impulse control and focusing.

7. "Exercise" the brain

The "use it or lose it" biological principle applies not only to muscle but also to brain growth. A child's brain growth is like millions of electrical wires trying to form connections. The "smart foods" listed above help insulate the wires to speed the transmission and help these wires grow branches that connect with other wires. "Dumb foods" cause the electrical wires to be frayed, and short circuits occur. But you have to do more than just provide the brain with healthy nutrition; you have to exercise your child's mind to really maximize his intellectual development. Nothing stimulates nerve growth and connectivity better than face-to-face interaction between a parent and child. Read to your child. Play interactive and hands-on games. Tell stories and play make-believe. Laugh and sing together. Draw and color pictures. And perhaps the most important advice is to keep the television off during the first two years of life. Studies have shown that the more TV or videos young children watch, the more learning and behavioral problems they may have later on. Some supposedly stimulating infant videos have been shown to actually slow down brain development. If you must use TV as the occasional babysitter, keep it limited to thirty minutes and choose shows with music.

DR. SEARS TIP
Discover Your Child's
Special Something

The earlier you can discover your child's special intellectual talents and run with them, the more lasting effect they will have on your child's developing brain. Think of your child's brain as a giant file cabinet. What files do you want your child's brain to store? The more files your child can store, the more he has in reserve to replay later in life. He can click into his cerebral DVD library and replay a scene when the situation arises. If your child has music talents, get him started early. Any time you hear that off-key or screeching sound, keep in mind that it's building another brain pathway.

Improving Your Child's Eye-Q

Since the retinal tissue of the eye is part of the brain, what's good for the growing brain is also good for growing eyes. Here are four ways that you can help your child's visual development:

1. Feed growing eyes

Like the brain, visual development is affected for better or worse by what your child eats.

Seafood is "see" food. Half of the retinal tissue is made up of DHA, the main omega-3 fat in coldwater fish such as wild salmon. Be sure your child averages at least 300 milligrams of DHA per day, preferably from coldwater seafood. An alternative would be an omega-3 DHA supplement. (See supplements, page 94.) There is a pink perk in wild salmon, called astaxanthin, that is also good eye food. It is a potent antioxidant that helps prevent wear and tear on the sensitive retinal tissue. Astaxanthin also protects the retina from the damaging effects of excessive sunlight. Think of astaxanthin as internal sunglasses for the eyes.

"Berry" good eyes. The purple pigment in berries such as blueberries is called anthocyanin, which helps the eyes adapt to changing intensities of light.

Go green. Carotenoids (nutrients that are found in vegetables, primarily green ones) also act like nature's sunglasses. The carotenoids lutein and zeaxanthin filter the UV light, preventing damage to the sensitive tissues of the eye. The best foods for carotenoid eye sunglasses are kale, collard greens, Swiss chard, spinach, and broccoli. These greens in a salad are particularly helpful because the fats in olive oil dressing can help the carotenoids be better absorbed. Tell your children to keep their eyes on their greens.

DR. SEARS TIP
Try an Eye Salad

Put all the top eye foods together, such as spinach, arugula, blueberries, walnuts, and olive oil, with a fillet of wild salmon on top. Start feeding your toddler such foods early on, and she will develop a taste for them.

2. Shade little eyes

Ever notice how fair-skinned children who go hatless and don't wear sunglasses often have squinty eyes? That's because over the years their eyes have tried to protect themselves from sun damage by squinting to let less light in. As a result, over time the bones of the orbit of the eyes actually look like they're growing over the eyes as a sort of shade, leading to a permanent squint. Growing eyes are particularly sensitive to excess sunlight exposure. During the summer months we often see reddened, swollen eyes that resemble conjunctivitis. This "sun-induced conjunctivitis" is due to the reaction of the lining of the whites of the eyes to excessive sunlight. Eye specialists recommend avoiding toy sunglasses because they simply shade the eyes, which causes a baby's pupils to enlarge and allow more damaging UV rays to reach inside the eye. Instead, use baby and child sunglasses that are labeled for UVA and UVB protection. See page 507 for more on sunglasses. Wearing a hat is also important.

3. Rest little eyes

Staring too long at a computer screen can lead to nearsightedness. Tell your children to take frequent eye breaks by simply resting their eyes when they seem tired.

4. Light little eyes

Improper lighting eventually tires out and wears out eyes. Don't let your child zone out on a light computer screen surrounded by a dark room or read in a dim light. Be sure there is adequate ambient light around the screen.

Keeping Little Noses Clear

We cannot overemphasize the importance of good nasal hygiene. Keeping little noses clear is one of the most important and one of the simplest — yet most often overlooked — ways to keep your child healthy. Babies prefer to breathe through their noses rather than their mouths, so when their noses are clogged, it throws their whole breathing mechanism off.

Also, those little nostrils are the "doors" where most germs enter the body. Here are the time-tested ways of keeping little noses clear that we use most often in our medical practice:

The Dr. Sears Clean-Nose Regimen: A "Nose Hose" and a "Steam Clean"

Remember those two phrases in the section title, as you will hear them often throughout this book. We advise parents to try all of the following techniques, select the ones that work the best, and put together their own "nose-hose" and "steam-clean" regimen:

1. Hose little noses with salt water. Make your own saltwater nose drops (one half tablespoon of salt to eight ounces of water) or buy at your local pharmacy or supermarket a prepared saltwater (saline) solution in a squirt bottle. Spritz a few drops of the solution into your child's clogged nasal passage and gently suction out the loosened secretions using a nasal aspirator, available at your local pharmacy. Veteran nose-cleaners dub this handy gadget a "snot snatcher." Older children can learn to blow their noses themselves. Nose hosing is becoming big business, and it's about time, since for years this has been one of the most overlooked and most needed "medicines." There are a variety of nasal washers that squirt water, saline solution, or a mist up into the nose under various degrees of pressure, similar to a water pick for cleaning teeth. A neti pot is another nice way to go. Our little patients call this handy snot snatcher "Aladdin's lamp" because that's what it looks like. For over a decade in our pediatric practice we have recommended a neti pot as the most effective way to irrigate nasal passages and drain clogged sinuses for children

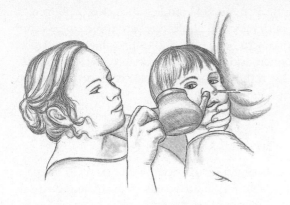

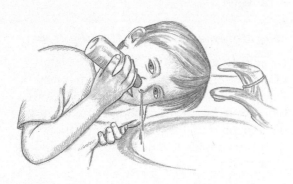

over eight, especially those with chronic nasal discharge and sinus infections. The directions come in the pot package. Basically, put warm salt water in the pot, tilt your child's head to one side, and put the spout of the pot in the upright nostril. The water then flows through one nostril and out the other, meanwhile flushing the nose and pulling gunk out of the sinuses. To some children it may initially seem scary, but once they've tried it, after a bit of parental coaxing, and see how much better they feel and breathe, they will be willing participants.

 **DR. SEARS TIP
Sit Up for Nose Hosing**

Instead of laying Baby on her back, which she will find threatening, sit her *upright* on your lap while doing the "nose hose."

2. "Steam clean" the airways. Make a home steam bath by turning on a hot shower in the bathroom with the door closed. Fifteen minutes of concentrated steam while your baby is nursing or playing will help keep her nose clear. Facial steamers are also very useful. These are not only the best way to steam clean the nasal passages and sinuses but can also be the most fun, or at least they are marketed as such. First, get your child used to seeing you use the facial steamer, even if you don't have a medical reason to use it. Many women use a facial steamer for home facials. After using the facial steamer, let your child see you cheerfully boast, "Oh, it makes my face feel so good." Let your child try it. Sit her on the couch in front of the TV. Put the steamer on the table in front of her and prop it up with a few books so the child can comfortably

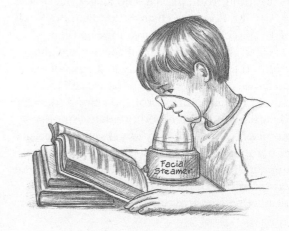

sit on the couch and bend over with her face in the steamer, while at the same time keeping her eyes riveted on the TV to distract her from what's going on in her nose.

3. Vaporizers are very good. Children's noses and central heating are not a match. When the heat goes on, so should a vaporizer. Besides humidifying the air and the breathing passages, warm-mist vaporizers have a double benefit: steam sterilizes the water, and when the steam condenses, it releases heat to the bedroom, allowing you to turn off or turn down the drying central heat. Steam can pose a burn hazard, so be sure to keep the vaporizer and cords out of reach of infants and toddlers. Try for a relative humidity of around 50 percent in your child's bedroom. (An inexpensive humidity-measuring device, called a *hygrometer,* is available at hardware stores.) Excessive humidity in a bedroom can foster allergens and mold growth, while low humidity dries out the skin, especially during the winter months.

Raising a Healthy Heart

While you may think of cardiovascular disease as an adult problem, that's no longer necessarily so. The Bogalusa Heart Study, a famous study of 14,000 children ages five to seventeen, revealed that around half of the overweight children in the study already had signs of early cardiovascular disease, or what we call the "highs"— high cholesterol, high blood triglyceride levels, and high blood pressure. Autopsy studies have shown fatty streaks and early signs of coronary artery disease even in preschool-age children. Because nowadays many children eat too much of the wrong foods and sit too much, they are growing up with early cases of

"heart overload." Studies show that children with elevated cholesterol are three times more likely to have high cholesterol, high blood sugar, and high blood pressure levels as adults. Even though heart disease strikes in adulthood, it begins in childhood.

The two best preventive medicines for cardiovascular disease and raising healthy hearts are

- Eating a heart-friendly diet (see Go Fish! page 34; Smart Foods, page 15; and anti-inflammatory foods, page 36).

- Moving!

Why Movement Grows a Healthy Heart

Growing bodies are only as healthy as the blood vessels that supply them. A fun health exercise is to take a trip through a fictitious blood vessel with your children. Here's how we explain it to our curious older patients (you can simplify this description for children under ten):

You may think that your blood vessels are like rubber hoses. The heart pumps blood in one end of the hose, and it comes out the other end of lots of little hoses to nourish all the tissues.

There is a lot more to the cardiovascular system than a bunch of hoses. One of the newest and most exciting discoveries is that the endothelium (the lining of the blood vessels) is the largest endocrine organ of the body. The billions of cells that line your arteries don't just sit there — they do something. When you exercise, the blood flows faster across the surface of your blood vessels like traffic across a highway after rush hour ends.

What's in your arteries?

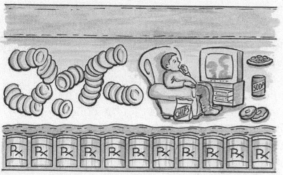

Sticky stuff, rough edges, endothelial <u>dysfunction</u>

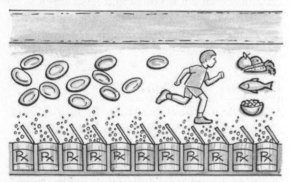

Easy blood flow, smooth edges, healthy endothelium

Special glands inside the lining of your blood vessels function like a giant pharmacy within your body. When the blood flows fast across these glands, these little medicine bottles open up and release custom-made medicine into your bloodstream according to your body's needs. These glands especially make medicines to lower the highs — high blood pressure, high cholesterol, and high blood sugar — the three main causes of cardiovascular disease.

Movement helps the lining of your blood vessels repair itself, just as the maintenance crew of a highway repairs the wear and tear of lots of traffic. If your blood vessels get rusty, they build up clots and gradually shut off the blood supply. Then your organs can't grow and function right. When you exercise a lot, the maintenance crew inside your blood vessels repairs them and keeps them open so you get lots of blood to your brain, your heart, your muscles, and all over your body to help you learn, grow, and play well.

But if you just sit around and eat junk food all day, the inside of your blood vessels gets rough like Velcro instead of smooth like Teflon. This is what happened to Uncle Johnny [or whoever in your family has had a heart attack]. He didn't take care of his blood vessels, so they clogged up and his heart stopped working right.

DR. SEARS TIP
Check Your Child's Cholesterol

According to the American Academy of Pediatrics, routine cholesterol testing is not necessary until puberty. But you should have your child's cholesterol checked in the pre-school years if

- you or your parents have a history of cardiovascular disease or developed cardiovascular disease before turning fifty-five.

- you have a family history of *hypercholesterolemia*, a metabolic quirk in cholesterol metabolism that leads to fatty deposits in the skin and arteries, even at an early age.

Five Ways to Cut Your Child's Cholesterol

1. Move! Exercise raises good cholesterol (HDL) and may reduce the so-called bad cholesterol (LDL). Exercise is one of the most effective cholesterol-lowering "drugs" and doesn't have unpleasant side effects.

2. Graze! Grazers (eating frequent mini-meals throughout the day) tend to have lower cholesterol than gorgers (eating three big meals a day). (See why grazing is good for you, page 37; and the rule of twos, page 97).

3. Stay lean! Trimming excess body fat trims excess cholesterol.

4. Eat a right-fat diet, not necessarily a low-fat diet. (See Fats, page 94.)

5. Eat cholesterol-lowering foods. The following foods have been shown to help lower cholesterol:

- soy protein

- fiber-filled foods, such as bran, prunes, and legumes

- nuts

New insights have revealed that cholesterol may not be the main cardiovascular culprit that it's made out to be. Growing kids need some cholesterol. In fact, breast milk, the gold standard of infant nutrition, is a medium-cholesterol diet. Certainly, do not put your child on a low-cholesterol diet unless your doctor advises you to.

Growing Healthy Little Lungs

The quality of air your children breathe affects how healthy they are. The two most important lung-health tips are: breathe healthy air and grow healthy respiratory passages.

Help Your Children Breathe Clean Air

Just as you take special care to help your children ingest clean food, do your best to help them inhale clean air. Little breaths add up. For example, you're doing carpool and there is a bus or a big truck ahead of you spewing out polluted exhaust. The light goes on in your head: "I can't let my children breathe this." So you pass the truck, take an alternative route, or roll up the windows. Avoid daycare and preschools that are downwind from pollution, such as near freeway interchanges. Make a list of all the daily changes you can make to help your children breathe clean air. If your child has allergies, use an air purifier, especially in the child's bedroom. (See Allergy-Proof Your Home, page 154.)

Humidify Your Child's Air

As a guide for the winter, turn the heat down and put the hot-steam vaporizer on. During naptime and nighttime run a vaporizer in Baby's bedroom. The dry winter air of central heating can thicken nasal and bronchial secretions, further compromising Baby's tiny airways. Also, like water in a stagnant pond, mucus that sits too long gets infected. Besides adding nasal-friendly humidity to dry winter air, as we've already mentioned, a vaporizer acts as a healthy and stable heat source at night. A word of caution: Vaporizers can pose a burn hazard. Be sure you keep them, and the cords, out of reaching distance of little hands.

Breathe to Relax!

You've probably heard Grandmother say "Take a deep breath." Grandmother was physiologically correct. Deep, relaxed breathing mellows stress by turning on the part of the nervous system that relaxes you and turning

NO SMOKING AROUND CHILDREN, PLEASE!

Everyone knows that smoking is hazardous to children's health, but here's a reminder:

Suppose you're about to take your child into a room when you notice a sign that reads: *Warning! This room contains poisonous gases, containing more than 4,000 chemicals, some of which have been linked to cancer, asthma, lung damage, and Sudden Infant Death Syndrome (SIDS).* You certainly wouldn't take your child in there, would you? Yet that's exactly what happens when you take your child into a room frequented by smokers. Even sitting in "non-smoking" areas of restaurants, while helpful, is not enough. Having a non-smoking area is like chlorinating half a swimming pool. Pollutants travel through the air. If a restaurant allows smoking anywhere, don't patronize it. It's not family-friendly. The risk of just about every disease you don't want your children to get goes up in proportion to the amount of cigarette smoke they're around.

Children of smoking parents have over twice as many doctors' visits because of respiratory infections. Here's why: Your child's breathing passages are lined with tiny filaments called cilia that wave back and forth like sea plants under the ocean and function to clear mucus from the airway passages. When a germ, irritant, or pollutant gets into the airway, these cilia, and the mucus around them, act like a miniature conveyor belt to move the harmful stuff up into the airway where the child can cough or sneeze it out. Smoke paralyzes these cilia, so the conveyor belt stops and the mucus and germs clog and infect the lungs. (See Smoking, page 482.)

DON'T ALLOW SMOKING AROUND CHILDREN!

down the part of the nervous system that revs you up. Deep, slow, relaxed breathing lowers the levels of circulating stress hormones. The younger your child learns this very simple mood mellower, the better.

Helping Your Child Enjoy Good Gut Health

Intestinal upsets rank second to respiratory problems as the reason for pediatrician visits. Although you may think of the intestines as simply being a long tube that helps food get from the mouth to the bloodstream, there is a lot more going on. Next to the brain, the intestines have the richest supply of nerves; hence the name *gut brain*. The intestines are the most important part of your child's immune system. The healthier the intestines, the healthier the immune system. Here are seven things your child can do to grow healthy intestines:

1. Graze. Perhaps the simplest yet scientifically proven home remedy for intestinal health is the Dr. Sears rule of twos:

- Eat *twice* as often.
- Eat *half* as much.
- Chew *twice* as long.

This simple way of eating allows more digestion to occur at the upper end of the digestive tract while the lower end is healing. (See page 37.)

2. Eat healthy. See the nutrition tips on page 420 (Traffic-Light Eating). The healthier the food that goes into the intestines, the better they perform.

3. Eat smaller bites. Children love to stuff food in their mouths, which encourages not only overeating but indigestion. Give your child a small fork and cut the food into smaller bites.

DR. SEARS TIP
The Sipping Solution for a Healthier Gut

A fruit, yogurt, and ground flaxseed smoothie (see recipe, page 15) is a recommendation we make frequently in our medical practice. The sipping solution is good for just about every intestinal ailment or pain in the gut. Blending the food increases absorption, decreases heartburn, and decreases constipation. Since the blender does much of the digestion, the gut has to work less and there is less undigested food to reach the colon. The fiber is also very friendly to the gut.

4. Play chew-chew. Hurried children wolf down their food. The more work that can be done in the mouth, the less wear and tear at the other end of the digestive system. Mom's mealtime advice to "chew your food" is biochemically correct. Digestion begins in the mouth. Chewing breaks up the fibers that hold the food together. Digestive enzymes target chewed-up food particles. Chewing stimu-

lates saliva, which lubricates the esophagus for smoother passage and also protects the lining of the esophagus against the irritating effects of stomach acids. Saliva is rich in enzymes that pre-digest food. Another reason why saliva is dubbed the body's own "health juice" is that it contains a substance called *epidermal growth factor,* which helps repair inflamed intestinal tissue. This may explain why animals lick their wounds. Play the chew-chew game. Encourage your child to chew each bite at least ten times.

5. Eat slowly. Take time to dine. Eating slowly gives the upper end of the digestive tract more time to do its work, and it also discourages overeating. Ask your child questions between bites and encourage him to talk. Children who eat too fast don't give the stomach time to signal the brain, "Enough, already. I'm full."

6. Serve smaller portions. A child's tummy is the size of her fist. Next time you serve a heaping plateful of pasta, put it next to your child's fist and notice the mismatch. Put a fistful of food at a time on the plate and refill as desired. Even better, let your child serve herself. Studies show that kids tend to self-serve smaller portions than others serve them.

DR. SEARS TIP
Smaller Portions, Happier Gut, Leaner Child

When children are served smaller portions, take smaller bites, chew longer, and eat slowly, they tend to eat just the right amount and seldom overeat and become overweight.

7. Probiotics: Put the best "bugs" in your kid's bowels. You may not realize this fact, but your child's largest immune organ is the gut, so it stands to reason that the better you feed your child's intestinal system, the better his immune system works. Also, a medical truism at all ages is: "You're only as healthy as your colon." One of the best "medicines" for colon health is putting the right bacteria in your bowels.

Let's begin with Colon Health 101. Billions of bacteria normally reside in your large intestine. And, in return for a warm place to live, they do good things for the gut. These "bowel bugs," as we like to call them, are also called *intestinal flora,* because they are the fertile soil that contributes to colon health and to the health of the whole body. Besides the healthful bacteria residing in your colon, harmful bacteria also get in from the food supply. Most of these harmful bacteria (those that cause intestinal upsets such as diarrhea or gastroenteritis) are killed by the stomach acids, but some do get into the colon. The way to keep the colon healthy is to help the good bacteria outnumber the harmful "bugs." The healthful bacteria are also known as *probiotics* because they support good health.

Here are the good things that probiotics do for your gut:

- Boost intestinal immunity. The gastrointestinal tract is the body's largest immune organ. Probiotics enhance the immune barrier of the gut lining. They help increase the immunoglobulin IgA and the thickness of intestinal mucus, which acts like a protective paint to keep harmful bacteria from getting through. Probiotics compete with the bad bacteria, thereby discouraging their growth and harmful effects.

- Promote a healthy gut environment. Probiotics produce lactic acid, which creates a more acidic environment in the gut, and this favors the growth of good bacteria and discourages the growth of harmful bacteria. Keeping the intestinal environment slightly acidic is especially necessary if you are taking antacids for heartburn.

- Reduce intestinal allergies. Probiotics promote anti-allergic processes by stimulating the production of growth factors that suppress the allergic response and generally increase food tolerance by the intestinal lining. These growth factors are helpful in reducing the severity of conditions such as gastroenteritis, colitis, and inflammatory bowel disease (IBD).

- Produce healthful nutrients. Probiotics ferment some of the fiber in food to form short-chain fatty acids (SCFAs), which nourish the cells lining the colon, stimulate healing of these cells, and reduce the likelihood of colon cancer. These short-chain fatty acids are also absorbed into the bloodstream and travel to the liver where they lessen the liver's production of cholesterol. These SCFAs also inhibit the growth of yeast and harmful bacteria in the gut.

You may also have heard the term *prebiotics*, which, like fiber, are indigestible carbohydrates that feed the probiotics. Think of prebiotics as food for the good bowel "bugs." When you eat probiotics and prebiotics, you essentially are feeding your immune system to help it work better.

Suggested gut food. Here are our recommendations for prebiotics and probiotics to nourish your intestinal health:

- Eat yogurt. Yogurt and other fermented dairy products such as kefir are the main dietary source of probiotics. The two most familiar bowel "bugs" that are added to yogurt during the culturing process are *Lactobacillus bulgaricus* and *Lactobacillus acidophilus*. Be sure to use organic yogurt.

- Eat prebiotics. Foods that contain prebiotics often list the carbohydrate/fiber combination *fructooligosaccharides (FOS)* on the label. Another cue word is *inulin,* a prebiotic that is an important ingredient in many healthy foods, such as Stonyfield Farm yogurts. Foods that contain natural prebiotics include whole grains, fruits, and vegetables (such as onions, garlic, leeks, and artichokes). You will commonly see healthier foods, such as HappyBaby organic baby foods, promoted as "containing prebiotics and/or probiotics."

- Take probiotic supplements. Besides suggesting yogurt at least several days a week, your doctor may advise you to give your child a probiotic supplement. There are many different species of probiotic supplements. The most commonly known one is called *acidophilus*, but there isn't necessarily any one that's particularly better than another. They come in liquid, powder, capsule, or pearl form and can be mixed into any cool food or drink. Follow the dosing instructions on the package. If no infant dosing is given, it is usually safe to give half of the child's dose to an infant two months and older.

What science says. Hundreds of scientific studies show that probiotics have many health benefits. The species most commonly used in medical studies has been *Lactobacillus GG (LGG)*, although most other species of probiotics probably yield many of the same benefits, including the following:

- Daycare children given LGG had fewer respiratory infections and fewer absences due to illness.

- In children with diarrheal illnesses, LGG cut the duration of the diarrhea in half.

- Hospitalized children had 80 percent less chance of acquiring acute diarrhea in the hospital if they received LGG as prevention.

- Probiotics have been shown to improve eczema.

- The *Lactobacillus reuteri* species has been shown to reduce infant colic.

- Children who were given LGG had a 47 percent lower risk of dental cavities compared with the unsupplemented group.

 DR. SEARS TIP
Give Probiotics with Antibiotics

In our pediatric practice we routinely prescribe a probiotic to be given during antibiotic courses and for at least two weeks following treatment. Antibiotics kill not only the germs that are causing the infection but also the healthful germs that normally reside in the gut, which is one reason that children routinely get diarrhea after taking antibiotics. Giving probiotics replenishes the healthful bacteria that were harmed by the antibiotics.

Keeping Your Child's Skin Healthy

That soft, smooth, adorable baby skin we all love to see and feel also gets rashy and itchy. Skin irritations are one of the top causes of night waking and one of the most frequent reasons for consulting the doctor. First, let's learn Skin 101:

The skin is the largest organ in the body, so it's important to care for it. Certain unique features of infant skin make it more prone to rashes:

- The epidermis (outer skin) is the surface layer of the skin. It's about as thick as a piece of paper, but it's composed of very tough material called *keratin,* which acts like a protective shield. The outer layer of the cells of the skin are continually rubbed or sloughed off and then replace themselves every few weeks. So, in effect, your child gets a new surface coat of skin about every month. The surface layer of baby skin is thinner because it hasn't been exposed to years of conditioning by wear and tear and environmental exposure. Because it is thinner, it is more sensitive to irritation, such as scratches and friction rubs. When this thinner protective barrier is damaged, baby skin becomes prone to infection and rashes.

- Not only is the outer layer of Baby's skin thinner and less protective, the underlying skin (the *dermis*) contains fewer melanin-producing cells, making it more prone to sunburn. (*Melanin* is the pigment that colors the skin and helps protect it against ultraviolet [UV] radiation from the sun.) As skin is exposed to sunlight, these cells churn out more melanin to darken the skin and help shield it from UV damage.

- The dermis contains a lot of materials that support skin health, including fibrous struc-

tures made of proteins called *collagen* and *elastin* that act like a spongy web to give the skin a strong padding. Unlike the weaker fibers of an adult's thinning and sagging skin, these fibers in baby skin are like springs in a mattress and give the skin a bouncy feel.

- The dermis is rich in *sebaceous glands* that secrete an oil called *sebum.* Sebum travels up the natural passageway of each hair shaft and secretes a thin, oily film on the surface of the skin. Throughout the dermis are jelly-like materials that act like sponges to absorb water so the skin has its own internal, natural moisturizers. Sweat glands are coiled throughout the dermis and worm their way to the surface of the skin, and sweat cools the skin by evaporation.

New insights into skin function and health have shown that many of the skin changes and irritation can be prevented, or at least lessened, by controlling two things: what you put *onto* the skin and what you put *into* the skin.

 DR. SEARS TIP
Teach Proper Hand Washing

Children share germs from hand to hand or nose to hands. Teach them to wash their hands thoroughly throughout the day before eating, after using the bathroom, and after they've sneezed into their own hands. Teach them to use soap and warm water and to scrub their hands thoroughly, including the backs of their hands, between fingers, and under fingernails. Teach them to wash their hands for as long as it takes to sing the ABC song twice, which takes around twenty seconds.

To keep your infant's or child's skin from becoming dry, flaky, and prone to rashes, try these general tips:

1. Moisturize your child's skin. Moisturizers contribute to healthy skin in two ways: they act as a seal to slow the loss of water from the skin and keep it from drying out, and they help bring up water from the lower layers of the skin. Moisturizers contain barrier agents, such as *petrolatum,* that seal in the moisture. They also contain substances called *humectants* that hydrate the skin from beneath by attracting water to the surface of the skin. Think of using moisturizers as dressing your child's skin in protective layers. This is especially important during the dry winter months. Dry air and sensitive skin are a recipe for a rashy winter, particularly if your child's skin is prone to eczema or allergic dermatitis. Once you turn the heat on, expect skin irritations to go up. The low humidity of central heating dries the skin. Dry skin gets flaky and itchy. The child scratches the itchy skin, further irritating the rash, and the cycle continues.

2. Seal in moisture and nutrients. We recommend what we call the *soak-and-seal* method. After giving your child a bath, gently blot the skin with a towel, then leave a thin layer of water to soak into the skin. Apply moisturizing cream, ointment, or oil to the skin to seal in the moisture.

3. Vaporize bedroom air. Put a vaporizer in your child's bedroom. As we've said, vaporizers increase the humidity in the bedroom and help prevent winter skin from drying out. A relative humidity in your child's bedroom of around 50 percent is ideal.

4. Water growing skin. Water is the primary component of skin and the underlying tissues. Dehydrated skin is more prone to get itchy and rashy, and, the more irritated the skin, the more prone it is to dehydration. Be sure your child drinks at least *an ounce of fluid per pound of body weight per day*.

5. Feed growing skin. The skin is greatly affected, for better or worse, by nutrition. Because both the skin and brain tissue develop from the same root cell, foods that are good for the brain are also good for the skin. Feed these foods for keeping skin healthy:

- Go fish! Seafood is the top skin food. We have been prescribing omega 3s for skin problems since 1999, with amazing results. Most skin irritations are due to inflammation, and omega 3s are the top anti-inflammatory food (see Keep Your Child from Having an iBod, page 35). "Oiling" your baby's skin not only decreases drying, but speeds healing from eczema or rashy illnesses. Since omega-3 fats are one of the top nutrients for healthy skin, be sure your child gets an average of 300 milligrams of DHA a day, either in the form of an omega-3 supplement or by eating around four ounces of coldwater fish, such as salmon, three times a week.

- Go nuts! Bet you never realized that a peanut butter or almond butter sandwich could be great for the skin. The healthy fats, protein, vitamins, and minerals in nuts are nutrients for the skin.

- Eat colorful! The more colorful the fruit and veggies, the more they contribute to skin health. Phytonutrients ("phytos" for short) are antioxidants (aka "anti-rust"), and they help keep the skin from becoming inflamed. Keeping high levels of phytos in your child's skin helps keep the "-itis" out.

DR. SEARS TIP
A Word for Kids

We tell our little patients, "To keep your skin from looking like a fish, eat fish!"

6. Avoid powders. We discourage sprinkling babies with powders for three reasons: Powders tend to cake in skin folds, such as the groin, and actually aggravate the rash; they do absolutely nothing for Baby's skin; and, if applied too liberally, they can be inhaled and irritate Baby's sensitive respiratory passages.

7. Clothe sensitive skin. Infants with any type of dermatitis are often sensitive to wool and synthetic materials. Use soft, breathable, cotton clothing, as well as cotton sheets and blankets. Wash new clothing before use to remove any possibly irritating chemical residues.

8. Protect growing skin. That adorable baby skin is also prone to sunburn. Avoiding sunburn in infancy and childhood helps prevent skin cancer from developing later. Dermatologists believe that repeated sunburn in childhood can increase the risk of skin cancer in adulthood. Be especially sun protective if you have a fair-skinned, blue-eyed, freckled child who is particularly sun sensitive. Don't let sunscreen give you a false sense of security and allow your child to spend excessive time in the sun unprotected. Be sun-savvy to help your child grow healthy skin. Try these sun protection tips:

- During the sunnier months, let your baby and child enjoy the healthy outdoors at the least sunny times of the day, usually before 10 a.m. and after 3 p.m. Avoid the peak hours of the day when sunrays are most intense.

- Put Baby in a wide-brimmed hat.

- To protect Baby from reflected rays off the sand at the beach, use an appropriately positioned umbrella.

- Put your child in tight-weaved fabric shirts specially designed to screen out a lot of the sun's rays.

- Apply lip balm or moisturizer with SPF to sun-exposed lips.

- Use a sunscreen with an SPF between 15 and 30 that blocks out both UVA and UVB radiation, and, if your child is going to be swimming, make sure it's waterproof. Sunblock potions that contain vitamins C and E are helpful.

- Dab a test dose on a small area of Baby's forearm to be sure the skin is not sensitive to the sunscreen.

- Apply sunblock immediately before sun exposure, but apply sunscreen thirty minutes before exposure to give it time to work into the skin and exert its sun-protective effects. Reapply every couple hours.

Sun Protection 101

Understand the difference between sunscreens and sunblocks. *Sunblocks* are simply a physical barrier to the ultraviolet sunrays — both UVA and UVB sunrays. These are usually made from zinc oxide or titanium oxide and resemble diaper rash cream. *Sunscreens* work their way into the skin and absorb the sunrays before they can do their damage. Many of them contain the active ingredient PABA (para-aminobenzoic acid), which blocks UVB radiation, but the occasional child may have a skin sensitivity to PABA. The SPF in sunscreen stands for *sun protection factor.* An SPF of 15 will block 95 percent of the radiation; an SPF of 30 will block about 97 percent. Usually an SPF between 15 and 30 is sufficient.

For babies, we prefer sunblocks instead of sunscreens. Sunblocks are okay for infants under six months because the potentially irritating chemicals are not absorbed by the skin. Because sunscreen chemicals are absorbed, parents are advised to avoid them for babies under six months. Even though sunscreen hasn't been proven harmful to infants, it hasn't been studied enough to be proven safe at that age.

Although it's important to be sun-savvy, don't let the fear of skin cancer deprive your child of the *health* benefits of sunshine. Children need vitamin D for general health, especially for strong bones, healthy skin, and a healthy immune system, and sunshine triggers vitamin D production in the body. If your child is exposed to a lot of sun during the warmer months, enough vitamin D may be stored in her body fat to tide her over during the winter months of less sun exposure. Expose your child to at least fifteen minutes of direct sunlight without sunblock on the hands, arms, and legs at least several times a week for as many months of sunshine as you can. (See vitamin D supplementation, page 34.)

SOAP SENSE FOR BABIES

Soap helps suspend oils and other stuff that collects on the skin so that they can be more easily washed off, yet too much soap applied in places that don't need it can both dry out and irritate the skin. Here's the skinny on soap cleaning your baby's skin:

• Use soap only on grungy areas that are caked with secretions, such as on the groin, in the skin folds of the neck, and on any other areas that obviously need it. Use soap sparingly on the face.

• Some babies' skin is more soap-sensitive than others'. If your baby is prone to eczema or any type of dermatitis, use soap sparingly or not at all on the most irritated areas.

• Do the soap test. Apply a dab of soap on the forearm to be sure your baby is not sensitive to it. The more additives, the more likely your baby is to be sensitive to that particular soap.

• Use soap that contains built-in moisturizing creams.

• Rinse soap off thoroughly and gently *pat* dry instead of rubbing the skin.

• Limit soap time on the skin. Wash off as soon as possible and rinse well.

• Mothers often feel that too much unnecessary soap and other fragrances camouflage a baby's naturally appealing scents.

Boosting Your Child's Immune System

As your child enters child-care settings or pre-school, he will be exposed to an increasing variety of germs. Boosting the immune system is like planting a "doctor" within your child. Here's how:

1. Have Your Child Vaccinated

Vaccinations stimulate your child's own immune system to produce antibodies against germs that cause serious childhood illnesses. (See page 43 for discussion of individual vaccines and the recommended schedule.)

2. Breastfeed for as Long as Possible

Consider breastfeeding your baby's first and most important immunization. New research has proven what mothers have long suspected: The longer babies are breastfed, the healthier and smarter they are. Here's why:

Breastfed babies are smarter. Studies of breastfed babies have shown that they tend to have a higher IQ. The reason for this intellectual advantage is that, in addition to the increased touch and maternal interaction, breastfed babies get more smart fats such as docosahexaenoic acid (DHA), from mother's milk. DHA is the prime structural component in the insulation that lines nerves, enabling messages to travel faster and more efficiently through the nervous system.

Breastfed babies are healthier. Research has shown that every system in your child's growing body is likely to be healthier if breastfed: visual development, lung function (such as preventing asthma), cardiovascular health, intestinal health, and the immune system. The incidence of just about every illness you don't want your child to get — including diabetes,

LEARN MORE ABOUT IT

Read *The Breastfeeding Book* by Martha Sears (Little, Brown, 2000). Martha is a nurse and a lactation consultant, and has logged nineteen years of breastfeeding eight children.

cancer, and cardiovascular disease — is lower in breastfed babies.

Breastfed babies are leaner. With the number one medical problem currently being the epidemic of obesity-related illnesses, breastfeeding is good preventive medicine. Long-term studies have shown that breastfed babies tend to grow up to be leaner children, and leanness is associated with increased health and well-being. As you will later learn in our section on Obesity, page 417, lean does not equate with being skinny, but rather means having the right amount of body fat for the child's individual body type.

3. Feed Your Child's Immune System

As we were preparing to write this book, we discussed why some children in our practice are healthier than others. We came to the conclusion that kids who eat healthier are healthier. We have noticed a group of mothers in our practice we call "pure moms," or what some might call "health-food nuts." These mothers seldom let a morsel of junk food enter their homes or the mouths of their children. We all notice that we don't need to see these children as often in the preschool years because they are sick less often than those who regularly ate junk food. When these "pure children" get sick, they recover sooner because their immune systems work better.

When these "pure children" go to school, we notice we don't see them as often for the D's—ADD, learning disabilities, and mood disorders. Not only are their growing bodies healthier, but so are their brains.

Consider foods your family's own *farm*acy. Here is our pick of the top "health foods," those that have been proven to boost a child's immunity:

Fruits and vegetables. Feed your family phytonutrients ("phytos" for short), which are immune-boosting substances found in fruits and vegetables. Phytos are the germ-fighting nutrients that give fruits and vegetables their color. Besides fighting germs, these phytos act as natural anti-inflammatories, meaning they help slow down the wear and tear on the tissues and help organs repair themselves. In general, the deeper the color, the better the "medicine." Foods that are rich in color—such as blueberries, bell peppers, spinach, papaya, and strawberries—are examples of top phyto foods.

Vitamin D supplementation. New studies have revealed a concerning fact: Most Americans are deficient in vitamin D. We have tested numerous kids in our practice during the writing of this book, and most were low. Vitamin D is a substance that plays an important role in many body functions and ensures a healthy immune system. For a boost up to a proper level, a child must take higher-than-normal daily doses for six months or longer. Ask your pediatrician about having your child tested and treated if her vitamin D level is low. You can also discuss treating presumptively for several months without testing, as it is fairly safe to assume most children are low. For more information on the health benefits of vitamin D and correcting deficiency, visit www.VitaminDCouncil.org.

Go fish! Seafood is the top health food, especially for growing children. Let's go head-to-toe to see why the phrase "a salmon a day can keep the doctor away" has scientific merit.

- *Eat seafood, be smart.* Seafood is your top brain food. Your child's brain grows more in the first five years than at any other time in life. Feed it well. The omega-3 fats in seafood form the structural component of cell membranes and *myelin* (the fatty layer of tissue that covers nerves, like the insulation of electrical wires), increasing the speed and efficiency of nerve messages. In light of recent studies, omega-3 DHA is now recommended for children with behavioral and mood disorders, as well as for those with attention and learning problems.

- *Eat seafood, see better.* Seafood is "see food." Half of the retinal tissue of the eye is made up of DHA, the same omega-3 seafood fat that is good for brain tissue.

- *Eat seafood, have a healthy heart.* One of the biggest medical breakthroughs in the prevention of cardiovascular disease in the past decade is the discovery that cultures where people eat the most fish have a much lower incidence of cardiovascular disease.

- *Eat seafood, have a healthy repair system.* Omega 3s are anti-inflammatories. The arteries throughout your child's heart, body, and brain are constantly bombarded with high-pressure pounding on the sensitive lining of blood vessels. With time this rough arterial lining attracts buildup of debris called *fatty deposits* or *plaque.* Alarmingly, recent studies have found that cardiovascular disease is occurring at a younger age. Many teens are now found to have fatty deposits on their arteries. Here's how omega 3s help. Your child's immune system perceives that the arteries are like a road in need of repair and sends out a repair crew to fix the damage.

Omega-3 oils feed the maintenance crew — the body's immune system, which repairs the lining of the bloodstream that can be damaged by the wear and tear.

- *Eat seafood, have less cancer.* Studies show that people who have higher levels of omega 3s in their blood have fewer intestinal cancers.

- *Eat seafood, prevent diabetes.* In addition to acting as anti-inflammatories, omega 3s help steady blood sugar and lower the risk of diabetes.

- *Eat seafood, have healthier skin.* As you will learn in the section on eczema, omega 3s are one of the best natural medicines for keeping skin smooth. (See Eczema, page 297.)

Consider omega 3s your child's best anti-inflammatory against all the "-itis" illnesses such as bronchitis, arthritis, colitis, dermatitis, otitis, and gingivitis.

HEALTH FOODS FOR A HEALTHY FAMILY

Here are the foods that boost the immune system the most:

Apples	Papaya
Beans	Pink grapefruit
Blueberries	Red grapes
Broccoli	Salmon, wild
Cantaloupe	Shiitake
Chili peppers	mushrooms
Cranberry juice	Spinach
Flax oil	Strawberries
Garlic	Sweet potatoes
Lentils	Tomatoes
Nuts	Turmeric
Olive oil	Watermelon
Onions	

---

4. Keep Your Child from Having an iBod

We coined the term iBod (or *inflamed body*) to describe a child who is prone to the "-itis" illnesses. In fact, *inflammation* has been the buzzword in adult medicine for the past decade and is now becoming equally important in childhood illnesses. Inflammation simply means that the body's immune system and repair system have gotten out of balance. When the immune system is in balance, the body's inflammatory or repair system works. Cuts, scratches, and wounds heal. Your child's immune system is like a road-repair maintenance crew. When the immune-system repair crew is healthy, the body's wear and tear on the tissues is mended. When the repair crew isn't healthy, the repair work doesn't get done, resulting in an "-itis" illness. The inflamed tissues lining the body's cavities such as joints (arthritis), intestines (colitis), breathing passages (bronchitis), ears (otitis), gums (gingivitis), and skin (dermatitis) are all the result of the inflammatory response causing the child to be an iBod. To prevent and treat childhood "-itis" illnesses, here are five things to do:

1) Encourage exercise. Exercise perks up the immune system by stimulating the body to produce more infection-fighting substances. Exercise perks up the mind. We think of anxiety and depression as adult mental problems, but, not surprisingly, mood disorders are occurring more frequently and at younger ages in children. Exercise is not only healthy for growing bodies; it's also good for the mind. Exercise increases blood flow to the brain, which increases "feel-good" and "think-right" neurochemicals.

Exercise reduces inflammation in three ways. Movement stabilizes insulin, and the more stable the blood insulin, the more stable the blood sugar. Stable blood sugar promotes a balanced immune system. Exercise burns fat.

Leanness balances the immune system. Finally, exercise stimulates the body to produce its own anti-inflammatory medicines.

2) Help your child stay lean. A phrase that we use to counsel overweight children in our practice is "reduce your waist." Once upon a time it was thought that excess abdominal fat was simply a nuisance. New studies have shown that excess abdominal fat spews out chemicals into the body that can cause all the "-itis" illnesses. These are known as pro-inflammatory chemicals. (See the Dr. Sears L.E.A.N. Kids Program, page 417, for an understanding of how being overfat can make kids oversick.)

3) Feed your family phytos. Phytonutrients (phytos) are the immune-boosting stuff that gives fruits and veggies their deep color. In fact, the deeper the color, the stronger the phytos.

4) Give your family an oil change. Feed your child more omega-3 oils (which are anti-inflammatory) and fewer omega-6 oils (which are pro-inflammatory). Oils and foods that are anti-inflammatory (promote a balanced immune system) include fish oil, flaxseed oil, olive oil, fruits and vegetables, chili peppers, coldwater fish (especially wild salmon), whole grains, nuts, and spices (such as cinnamon, ginger, and turmeric). Pro-inflammatory foods

---

HEALING FOODS VS. HURTING FOODS

Some foods boost your child's immune system; others hurt it.

Immune-system boosters	Immune-system breakers
Avocado	Animal fats
Chili peppers	Artificial sweeteners
Fish oil	Food dyes and colorings (e.g., red #40)
Flaxseed oil	High-fructose corn syrup
Flaxseeds, ground	Oils, processed: especially partially hydrogenated oils; processed foods made with these oils: salad dressing, French fries, shortening, most fast foods
Fruits	
Olive oil	
Nuts and nut butters	
Seafoods: coldwater fish, especially wild salmon	Other oils: corn oil, safflower oil, soybean oil, sunflower oil
Sesame oil	
Spices: cinnamon, turmeric, ginger	Sweetened beverages
Veggies	Trans fats
Whole grains	
Wild game meats	

Essentially, if it grows, runs, or swims, it's likely to boost your child's immune system. If the food makes a trip to the factory and gets processed, it's likely to harm your child's immune system. To help your child grow a healthy immune system, feed your family as "pure" as possible.

that promote an imbalance of the immune system include animal fats, corn oil, partially hydrogenated oils, vegetable oils (such as sunflower, safflower, and soybean oil), and high-fructose corn syrup. We call anti-inflammatory foods "healing foods" and pro-inflammatory foods "hurting foods."

5) Encourage grazing on frequent mini-meals. Grazing keeps insulin and blood sugar stable, which keeps the body in balance. One of the best eating-pattern changes you can make for maintaining optimal weight and promoting a healthy immune system is to follow Dr. Bill's rule of twos: Eat *twice* as often, *half* as much, and chew *twice* as long.

5. Boosting the Immune System During an Illness

Besides the everyday immune-building tips we offer you in this section, there are several ways to give your child an added boost during an illness. These tips can help to resolve a variety of illnesses more quickly and lessen the need for antibiotic treatments. They are generally not recommended until six months of age (not because they may cause any harm to younger infants, but because they haven't been adequately researched yet).

Vitamin C. This antioxidant can help fight off viruses and bacteria. It comes in liquid, powder, chewable, and capsule forms (chewable forms can damage tooth enamel, so follow them with tooth brushing). Start treatment at the first sign of illness and continue until your child is well, following these doses:

- six months to two years — 150 milligrams once or twice daily

- two years to five years — 250 milligrams once or twice daily

- six years to eleven years — 500 milligrams once or twice daily

- twelve years and older — 1,000 milligrams once or twice daily

Echinacea. In proper doses, this herb can give the immune system a nice boost against infections. A recent study attempted to prove it ineffective. However, infant doses were used for this adult study, so no wonder it didn't work. Echinacea comes in infant drops, chewables, or capsules. Here is our suggested dosing at the first signs of illness:

- infants six months to two years — 250 milligrams three times daily for two days, then 125 milligrams three times daily until well

- two years to five years — 500 milligrams three times daily for two days, then 250 milligrams three times daily until well

- six years to eleven years — 1,000 milligrams three times daily for two days, then 500 milligrams three times daily until well

- twelve years and older — 2,000 milligrams three times daily for two days, then 1,000 milligrams three times daily until well

Zinc. This mineral has some useful immune-boosting properties. Follow these suggested doses:

- six months to two years — 10 milligrams once or twice daily

- two years to five years — 15 milligrams once or twice daily

- six years to eleven years — 20 milligrams once or twice daily

- twelve years and older — 25 milligrams once or twice daily

Herbal remedies. Various herbal supplements are available that help boost the immune system. In our practice we've found that Sinupret (an herbal blend made in Germany) works well to support sinus and respiratory health and the immune system. Visit www.SinupretForKids .com for more information.

Minimize sugar, maximize fruits and veggies. What your child eats can have an immediate effect on the immune system. Take extra care to feed your child well during any illness.

Frequent illnesses. If your child seems to catch more than his fair share of illnesses, try giving the above supplements on a daily basis at half our suggested doses, even when he is well. Note: when using echinacea on an ongoing basis, take a two-week break every eight weeks to retain its effectiveness on the immune system.

Balancing Your Child's Endocrine System

One of the most important keys to health is to put your child's body and brain in *hormonal harmony.* Hormones are chemical messengers that travel throughout the body telling the organs how to work together optimally. They work best when they are just at the right levels — not too much and not too little. For example, hormones tell the child when he is hungry and when he has eaten enough. Hormones also tell him when he's tired and it's time to go to bed and when it's time to wake up. The body is often described as a "chemical soup." If hormones and other biochemicals are in the right balance, the body is healthy and happy. One of the reasons kids are getting sicker, sadder, and fatter is that growing bodies are out of biochemical balance more than ever before. The health program you are now learning is designed to keep your child's hormones in biochemical balance.

Think of your child's endocrine system as a symphony orchestra and all the hormones, such as growth hormone and thyroid hormone, as instruments in this orchestra. Insulin, appropriately called the "health hormone," is like the master conductor of your child's hormone orchestra. When blood insulin levels are optimal, the rest of the body and brain chemistry are in balance, or hormonal harmony, and the beautiful music of health results. One of the most important goals in keeping your child healthy is to promote hormonal harmony by keeping blood insulin levels stable. The four magic words that promote hormonal harmony are *movement, grazing, happiness,* and *leanness.*

While there are hundreds of hormones trying to work in harmony throughout your child's body, let's divide them into two groups: grow-right hormones and feel-right hormones. Growth hormone, for example, helps the cells recharge and grow by instructing them how to use nutrients in food for energy; it builds muscle by telling the muscle cells to take up the amino acids from the foods that enter the blood and assemble them together as muscle-building proteins; and it tells fat cells to release some of their stored fat for energy when the other cells need that fuel to grow. Sleep and exercise are powerful stimulators of growth hormone. Insulin is also a grow-right hormone because, as we said before, it is the master conductor of the hormonal harmony orchestra.

Think-right hormones, like serotonin and endorphins, keep the thoughts in balance. Too much of these hormones and the child can become anxious or silly; too little and the child can become sad and depressed. The body and brain get used to the right level of these mood-managing hormones, all of which are regulated by the four magic words *movement, grazing, happiness,* and *leanness.*

Move. Movement is one of the healthiest things your child can do to keep the levels of insulin and blood sugar stable. Remember, when insulin is stable the whole body is more likely to be in biochemical balance. For parents who want to understand how exercise promotes stable insulin, let's go inside one of the cells of your child's body. On the cells there are tiny "doors" called receptor sites. These doors let just the right amount of fuel, such as sugar, into the cells to provide energy. Insulin is like the doorman for these cells: it opens the door to let just the right amount of fuel into the cells — not too much, not too little. Increased blood flow past these receptor sites during exercise increases "insulin sensitivity," meaning it makes the doors more efficient to let the right amount of fuel in. When every cell in the body works more efficiently, overall health results. Movement also keeps the happy hormones of the brain more stable. This is why recent studies have shown that vigorous exercise helps children with learning and mood disorders by stabilizing their neurochemicals.

Graze on "grow" foods. Grazing on good foods (see Healthy Munching, page 422) stabilizes insulin levels. Nibbling on nutritious mini-meals throughout the day is more brain-hormone-friendly than eating fewer big meals because, unlike other organs of the body, the brain cannot store glucose. It relies on a *steady* supply of glucose — just the right amount. Steady blood sugar results in steady brain neurotransmitter function so that the child can learn and behave well. In addition, insulin and the stress hormone cortisol are interrelated. Grazing keeps insulin stable, which helps to keep stress hormones stable. When stress hormones are out of balance, the immune system is also out of balance, which makes the child more prone to illnesses. In short, grazing stabilizes insulin, and stable insulin leads to hormonal harmony. (See benefits of grazing, page 37.)

Think happy thoughts. New studies have shown that the thoughts that go into your brain can keep the mood-producing hormones in balance. If your child thinks more positive thoughts, the happy hormones are higher. If your child thinks predominantly negative thoughts, the happy hormones are lower. This isn't something you can really teach children to do. You have to model it for them. Be a positive parent. Frequent encouragement and praise will build up a child's confidence and self-esteem. Criticism and impatience will not. An uplifting mood and everyday interaction with your child can help keep the hormones in a positive balance.

Live lean. Part of your home health-maintenance program is to keep your child lean. Lean does not mean skinny, but rather just the right amount of body fat for one's body type. Your doctor can help you assess your child's body balance at checkups. Excess body fat, especially around the middle, causes hormonal disharmony, especially with insulin. Excess body fat causes the cells to become increasingly resistant to the effects of insulin, leading to conditions called *insulin resistance* or *Type-2 diabetes* — which are becoming more prevalent in children at younger ages. This is why *leanness* is one of the most important health words you can teach your child. Here's a list of illnesses whose incidence goes way up proportional to the excess fat your child lugs around:

- acne

- arthritis

- asthma

- attention deficit disorder (ADD)

- cancer
- cardiovascular disease
- dental cavities
- diabetes

- eczema
- gastroesophageal reflux disease (GERD)
- headaches
- vision problems

YOUR HOME HEALTH-MAINTENANCE PLAN CHECKLIST

Here is a summary of the home "medicines" that you have learned about in Part I of this book. This plan helps you to provide basic medical care for your child at home. If you have checked "no," try to take steps that enable you to check "yes" in every column:

	Yes	No
Have you chosen Dr. Right for your child? (See p. 3.)		
Do you take steps to get the most out of your doctor visits? (See p. 7.)		
Do you keep your own health diary and records? (See p. 8.)		
Are your child's immunizations up to date? (See p. 33.)		
Does your child have the recommended periodic checkups? (See p. 41.)		
Do you practice the pills-skills model of health care? (See p. 13.)		
Do you feed your child "brainy" foods? (See p. 14.)		
Do you routinely exercise your child's mind? (See p. 18.)		
Do you take good care of your child's eyes? (See p. 19.)		
Do you feed your child immune-boosting foods? (See p. 33.)		
Do you do the "nose-hose" and "steam-clean" techniques to keep your child's nasal passages clear? (See p. 20.)		
Do you keep the air around your child clean and clear of smoke and allergens? (See p. 25.)		
Does your child have lots of strenuous exercise? (See p. 17.)		
Do you raise a grazer by following the rule of twos? (See p. 37.)		
Do you help your child stay lean? (See p. 39.)		
Do you keep your child's skin healthy? (See p. 29.)		
Do you help your child think happy thoughts? (See p. 39.)		
Do you keep "iBod" (inflammation-producing) foods out of your child's diet? (See p. 35.)		

II

Well-Baby and Well-Child Exams:
How to Get the Most out of Your Parent-Pediatrician Partnership

In Part I, you learned the pills-skills model of medical care and all the things you can do to help keep your child healthy. You also learned how to choose and effectively utilize your health-care providers. Now, when someone asks you, "Who is your child's primary health-care provider?" you can proudly answer, "I am!"

Next, as part of your child's health-maintenance plan and an important part of preventive medical care, you will learn about the well-baby and well-child checkups recommended by us and the American Academy of Pediatrics (the AAP — we will refer to this organization often throughout this section). We will walk you through each of these age-by-age checkups as if you were sitting right in our office. Of course, nothing can replace the hands-on care and face-to-face advice of your own doctor. You may find that some of our recommendations may differ slightly from what your own doctor tells you. We urge you to make informed decisions about your child's care with your own doctor's guidance.

VACCINES

Vaccines are an important part of pediatrics health care. Parents often have many questions that are beyond the scope of this book. In *The Vaccine Book: Making the Right Decision for Your Child*, Dr. Bob has put together a comprehensive and balanced guide for parents who want to learn more. You can get a preview at www.AskDrSears.com/TheVaccineBook.

Below we provide basic information about the current recommended vaccine schedule and a brief description of each disease.

DTaP. Diphtheria, a serious and treatable infection, can cause severe respiratory illness. It is transmitted the same way as a cold. It is virtually nonexistent in the United States.

Tetanus is a bacterium that can cause serious, but usually treatable, paralysis when allowed to fester in a deep, dirty wound. This rare disease virtually never occurs in children. See page 45.

Pertussis or "whooping cough" is transmitted just like a cold, and causes one to three months of severe coughing fits. This is not a rare illness, and outbreaks do periodically occur in the United States. It is very serious in infants younger than six months, and can be fatal or cause brain damage because the severe coughing fits can deprive the brain of oxygen. Antibiotic treatment sometimes helps decrease the severity and duration of the illness. See page 540.

THE AMERICAN ACADEMY OF PEDIATRICS RECOMMENDED VACCINE SCHEDULE, 2010

Birth	Hep B
1 month	Hep B
2 months	DTaP, Hib, PCV, IPV, RV
4 months	DTaP, Hib, PCV, IPV, RV
6 months	DTaP, Hib, PCV, RV, Hep B, Influenza*
12 months	MMR, Varicella (Chicken pox), Hep A
15 months	Hib, PCV
18 months	DTaP, IPV,* Hep A, Influenza
2–3 years	Influenza each year
4–6 years	DTaP, IPV, Influenza each year, MMR, Varicella (Chicken pox)
7–10 years	Influenza each year
11–12 years	Tdap, MCV, HPV (three-dose series), Influenza each year
13–18 years	Influenza each year

*Influenza vaccine is given at the start of every flu season (October through December) for every child 6 months through 18 years. Two shots are needed the first year the vaccine is given. The third IPV can be given at any time between 6 and 18 months.

PCV (Pneumococcal disease). This shot protects against pneumococcus, the most common cause of infant and child meningitis, pneumonia, and bloodstream infections. This fairly rare disease is transmitted like a common cold and is treatable with antibiotics.

Hib (*Haemophilus influenzae* type b). This disease is now an extremely rare cause of infant meningitis. It is transmitted like a common cold and treatable with antibiotics but can be fatal.

RV (Rotavirus). This is a liquid vaccine given orally. This disease is the most common and severe cause of vomiting, diarrhea, and dehydration in infants. About 50,000 infants are hospitalized each year during the fall and winter months. See page 448.

IPV (Polio). This disease causes paralysis in about 0.5 percent of those who catch it. It is transmitted like a common cold. There have been no cases of polio in the United States for over twenty-five years, and it now occurs only in parts of Asia and Africa.

MMR. Measles is a rare disease causing fever and rash. It is usually harmless, very rarely fatal, and passed like a common cold. See page 392.

   Mumps is also rare and usually harmless, causing swollen neck and face glands, fever, and rash. Transmitted like a cold, it is virtually never fatal, but rarely can cause sterility in adults. See page 408.

   Rubella is a harmless fever and rash disease for kids. When contracted by a pregnant woman, however, it can cause birth defects. It is extremely rare and is transmitted like a cold.

Hep A (Hepatitis A). This harmless virus usually doesn't cause any noticeable symptoms in young children. Older kids and adults will experience one or two weeks of intestinal flu symptoms. The virus comes out in the stools, so an infected person can transmit it if he doesn't wash his hands after using the bathroom. Restaurant outbreaks are the most common mode of contagion. See page 361.

Chicken pox (Varicella). This fever and rash illness is uncomfortable but rarely causes any complications. It is transmitted like a cold, and is becoming less common. See page 215.

Hep B (Hepatitis B). This sexually transmitted disease causes liver failure and is only contracted through exposure to infected blood and body fluids. See page 467.

HPV (Human papillomavirus). The human papillomavirus is a sexually transmitted disease that can cause genital warts and cervical cancer. See page 469.

MCV (Meningococcal disease). This bacterial infection causes meningitis in children and adults of any age. It is commonly known as "college dorm meningitis." See Bacterial Meningitis, page 394.

Influenza (Flu). This fall and winter illness can be prevented by either a flu shot or a nasal spray vaccine. Although most people get through this illness without any trouble, some fatalities do occur every year. See page 325.

Many diseases discussed here are now rare or nonexistent in the United States. Our successful vaccination program is the cause. Keeping it going is very important.

Expected Vaccine Side Effects

Fever, fussiness, redness, swelling, and pain at the injection site are common vaccine side effects. Holding a cold compress to the area helps. Giving ibuprofen every six hours to infants three months and older (see dosing on page 553) can help if symptoms are bothersome. Acetaminophen (Tylenol) is a second choice and can be used at any age. MMR and chicken pox (varicella) shots can also cause a rash. These situations don't warrant an after-hours call to the doctor (unless the child is extremely ill), but contact the doctor during regular hours to let her know. See page 529 for more details on vaccine reactions.

Vaccines in Special Situations

Rabies vaccine. This disease is contracted through the bites of infected animals, usually bats, raccoons, coyotes, and skunks (other small animals such as pet dogs and wild rodents almost never carry rabies). If left untreated, rabies is usually fatal once symptoms (anxiety, seizures, paralysis) develop. Symptoms usually occur about two months after a bite, although they can appear as soon as five days or as late as one year. The rabies vaccine is given as five injected doses over the month following a high-risk bite. Flu-like side effects from the vaccine are common. Another type of injection, called rabies immunoglobulin, can also be given if a person is bitten by an animal known to have rabies.

Tetanus. All vaccinated children get enough tetanus shots to cover them in the event of a severe cut or bite until they are about twenty years old, so kids usually don't get an extra shot if wounded. By age twenty the last tetanus shot (given as Tdap at twelve years of age) has worn off. Any adult who has a wound that is deep and dirty enough to go to an emergency room will get a tetanus shot if it's been at least seven years since the last one. If the wound is particularly deep or dirty, five years is the cutoff. Any child who is not vaccinated

against tetanus doesn't need to worry about scrapes, scratches, and minor cuts. If the wound doesn't warrant an emergency room visit for cleansing and stitches, it probably wouldn't cause tetanus.

Travel vaccines. Vaccine requirements vary greatly for international travel, and details are beyond the scope of this book. Contact your doctor at least six months before travel to discuss what may be needed. Possible travel vaccines include yellow fever, typhoid fever, Japanese encephalitis, and hepatitis A.

YOUR NEWBORN

Congratulations! You have been blessed with life's most precious gift — a tiny, warm, cuddly bundle of joy. Here are some of the most important highlights about getting started with your newborn during the first week.

Bonding in the First Hours

Forget that you will need to learn many things about caring for a baby. Don't worry about bathing, diaper changes, feeding, sleeping, or dressing. There is absolutely only one thing you need to do with a new baby in the first few hours, and that is to hold her. You'll have to take turns with your spouse, of course. And the baby will want to spend some time feeding. But the rest of the time is all yours to just sit there and hold the baby. Right after birth is not the time for a hospital nurse to rush your baby off to the nursery for a shot, eye ointment, and bath. There will be plenty of time for this several hours later, after bonding has started. Bonding in the first hours creates physical and hormonal changes in both parents and baby that set the stage for a life-long healthy relationship.

Nutrition

Breastfeeding

There are many strategies and tips you will learn about successful breastfeeding, but for the first couple of days, there's virtually nothing special you need to do. In past years, breastfeeding experts thought that newborns needed to be taught how to breastfeed, that they needed to be put to the breast every two hours, that they needed to be positioned in a special way and taught how to latch on properly. New research, however, has revealed that as long as a normal, uninterrupted bonding experience is allowed to happen between Mother and Baby at birth, a baby will seek the breast, latch on correctly, and wake up often enough to feed in the first few days with just a little bit of guidance from the mother.

So relax. Just bond with your baby and let breastfeeding happen naturally. Don't worry about waking the baby up to eat every two hours, unless your health-care provider advises you to. Don't stress when she falls back to sleep after just a few minutes of nursing. She'll wake when she gets hungry.

This advice, however, only applies to the first few days. Some babies will need more encouragement, teaching, and guidance if breastfeeding doesn't become a nice routine by day three or four. For more detailed information on successful breastfeeding, see our breastfeeding section on page 33 or see *The Baby Book* or *The Breastfeeding Book*. If you do experience some challenges with breastfeeding, seek help from a certified lactation consultant. Virtually all hospitals either have one on staff or have referral numbers to give

DR. SEARS TIP
The Lower Lip Flip

The best way to prevent sore nipples is to make sure your baby's lower lip is "fished out," away from the nipple. Once your baby is latched on, slowly insert your finger (or your spouse's) in between Baby's chin and the breast. Pull the chin down gently. This will pull the lower lip away from the nipple and allow it to spread out further around the breast. Baby's lips should look like fish lips from the side.

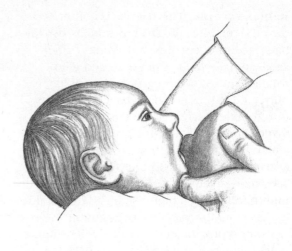

you. You can also obtain support over the phone at 1-800-LALECHE.

Bottlefeeding

Formula-feeding begins in a similar way to breastfeeding in that you don't have to worry about how much or how often in the first few days. When your baby is awake, offer her a bottle and let her take whatever amount she wants to. Most newborns won't take more than an ounce at a time on the first day. Don't worry about waking her up to feed, unless more than six hours have passed or the hospital staff feels there is a reason for more frequent feeding.

A cow's milk–based formula is the standard. You can either bring your own or use what the hospital provides. Over the next few days, you will notice your baby wanting more and more formula and settling into a somewhat predictable routine of taking about two ounces every two to four hours. For every pound a baby weighs, she should eat about two to two and a half ounces per day. So, an eight-pound newborn would start to want sixteen to twenty ounces every twenty-four hours. Most babies don't get up to this pace until around one week of age. See Formula-Feeding, page 52, for more information.

Weight Loss

Every baby will lose several ounces of weight each day for the first few days, so don't be alarmed. Babies are born with extra body fluids to sustain them while waiting for Mom's milk to start flowing.

Routine Baby Care

Hospital Procedures

During the first few hours, the hospital staff will want to give your baby a vitamin K shot, some antibiotic eye ointment, a nice thorough bath, a vaccine, and possibly a heel-prick blood test. Although all of these are important, they can interfere with the initial bonding and breastfeeding routine. We suggest delaying these until your baby is several hours old and has had a few feeding sessions. Then it won't be so disruptive. The American Academy of

Pediatrics (AAP) recommends all such procedures be postponed at least until the first feeding is finished.

Bathing

Make your baby's first bath as gentle as possible, when Baby is a few hours old and you are done with the initial bonding time. Once home, babies really only need to be bathed about once a week. They simply don't get dirty, except for around the neck and face, and the diaper area, which are easy to wipe with a moist cloth. If your baby enjoys baths (most newborns don't!), go ahead and give them more often. Until the umbilical cord falls off, you should not submerge the belly area in water. Give a sponge bath until the cord falls off and has dried out. See *The Baby Book* for more details on bathing Baby.

Umbilical Cord Care

Some research shows you don't have to do anything with the umbilical cord, but other studies suggest that alcohol can decrease the likelihood of an infection. We recommend you don't do anything at first, but if you begin to see redness or discharge around the cord, apply rubbing alcohol to the moist end of the cord and around where the cord enters the skin three times a day, using a cotton swab.

Umbilical cord blood banking. This innovative procedure is becoming more and more popular, and we believe it is a worthwhile investment. Instead of discarding the blood that drains out of the umbilical cord and placenta, the obstetrician or midwife will collect this stem-cell-rich blood and ship it to a storage facility in case it is ever needed in the future to help treat a growing list of medical conditions. Storing a portion of the umbilical cord tissue is an additional useful option. Visit www.CordBlood.com for more scientific information.

Wet Diapers

You may have heard that babies will have six (disposable), eight (cloth), or more wet diapers each day. In truth, this doesn't happen until Baby is a few days old. You should expect only two to four wet diapers each day in the beginning.

Bowel Movements

During the first few days, Baby's stools will be black and sticky. This is the old "meconium" that has been sitting inside Baby for a while. Around day three to five, the stools will transition through brown to green to yellow. Most babies have four to eight small soft, pasty yellow stools each day by one week of age. This means that your baby is getting enough milk.

Circumcision Care

If you have a boy and choose circumcision, your doctor or nurse will show you how to apply petroleum jelly (Vaseline) to the sore areas of the penis with every diaper change. Be generous with this; you can't overdo it. Keeping the circumcised area continuously moist helps with pain and healing. Some advise only using petroleum jelly for about a week. We believe a month is better. Some recommend gently wiping the petroleum jelly onto the penis tip. We've found it more useful to gently massage the jelly into the folds of skin where the circumcision was done as well as over the penis tip. This creates a better barrier between the skin and the raw head of the penis to prevent sticking during the healing process. Ask your pediatrician to give you specific instructions. Expect the penis to appear red and swollen, with some crusty discharge, for about a week. Your doctor will make sure it's healing well at your first checkup in the office.

Jaundice

Most babies will turn slightly yellow on the face and upper chest around day two or three from a natural pigment that builds up in the bloodstream. Expose your baby's bare skin to as much sunlight as possible filtered through a glass window to help minimize the jaundice. Your doctor may test the baby's jaundice level through a blood test or a newer transcutaneous method (a light shining through the skin) if your baby begins to look jaundiced in the hospital. Once home, if you see the yellow color spreading to include all of your baby's face, chest, and abdomen, see your doctor sooner than the one-week appointment. See page 381 for more details.

DR. SEARS TIP
Yeast Infection on Mom's Nipples

One of the most common challenges for new moms is yeast infection on the nipples. This most often occurs with nursing moms who receive antibiotics during labor or need to take an antibiotic for any type of illness later on. It can cause severe soreness, itching, and burning during and between feeds. If you require antibiotics, we suggest that you also take a probiotic like acidophilus for one month to prevent yeast. Make sure the doctor checks your baby's mouth for signs of yeast. See page 542 for more details.

Physical Exam

Within the first twenty-four hours, your doctor will come to examine your baby. Here is a brief overview of what your doctor is looking for with all that poking and prodding:

Head. The doctor will make sure all the skull bones have formed properly. You will notice ridges along the front, top, and back of Baby's head as well as the large soft spot. It is normal for part of the head to be swollen or bruised for several days.

Eyes. The doctor will use an eye light to make sure the pupils have formed correctly and are responding to light. It is normal to see some blood spots in the whites of Baby's eyes for a few weeks. Some mild eye drainage is also common.

Mouth. The doctor will check the tongue and palate. If you see some tiny white bumps on the roof of Baby's mouth or on the gums, don't worry. These are called "pearls" and are normal.

Face. You may notice red splotches on your baby's forehead and eyelids. Called "angel's kisses," these patches of blood vessels in the skin will fade away over the months. You may also see numerous tiny white plugged pores, called *milia*, which will resolve within months.

Ears. The doctor will look for any deformities. Don't worry if one of the ears is a bit folded over. It will move back into place over the months.

Collarbones. These are prone to breaking during a tough delivery. The doctor will check for swelling or tenderness.

Heart. The doctor will take a careful listen and check your baby's pulses.

Abdomen. It may seem to you that the doctor is pushing a little too far into your baby's tummy. This is necessary to check for enlarged organs or any abnormal masses.

Umbilical cord. Don't worry if you see a little bleeding or discharge over the next few days.

Hips. The doctor will do a bit of hip aerobics, and your baby probably won't appreciate it too much. It's important to make sure the hips are moving properly in their sockets.

Genitals. The doctor will make sure everything appears normal and that both testicles are in place. Expect the scrotum or labia to appear swollen for several weeks. You may even see some mucus or bloody discharge from the vagina. This is harmless.

Feet. A minor in-curving of the feet is expected. The doctor will make sure the feet aren't too curved. Expect some wrinkling and cracking of the skin.

Skin. You will notice numerous red blotches and some red bumps with a white center that look like bug bites. There are normal, and will fade away. The doctor will check for any abnormal birthmarks.

Spine. The doctor will check for any defects in the vertebrae. You may notice a harmless dimple in the upper part of the groove between the buttocks.

Muscles and reflexes. The doctor may test reflexes and observe your baby to make sure he is moving all four limbs symmetrically.

Unusual but Normal Newborn Signs

There are minor things newborns do that seem worrisome to new parents but are actually normal. Here's a list of them:

- excessive sneezing

- excessive hiccups

- diaper rash

- slightly blood-tinged urine or bloody vaginal discharge

- jelly-like crystals in the diaper (diaper gel)

- nasal congestion or noisy, congested breathing

- spitting up and gagging on stomach mucus

Vaccines

Most hospitals will give your baby the first vaccine for hepatitis B. Some doctors prefer to wait until the one- or two-month checkup. It is safe to delay this one vaccine. See page 43 for more details on vaccines.

ONE-WEEK CHECKUP

Congratulations! You have made it through the first week and hopefully things are settling down into a more comfortable routine. Following is our guide to your one-week-old.

Growth

Weight gain. Babies can safely lose as much as 10 percent of their birth weight during the first several days. That means an eight-pound baby could lose approximately twelve to fourteen ounces. Many babies don't gain this weight back until two weeks of age. Therefore, don't be alarmed if your baby is still below birth weight at this one-week visit. We encourage you to recheck Baby's weight at two weeks of age to ensure he is thriving.

Length. In general, babies grow about one and a half inches per month during the first three months, then a little more slowly after that. It is difficult to measure the length accurately during the first year of life, so don't be surprised if the length percentile seems to go up and down between visits.

Head circumference. Your doctor will make sure the head circumference is growing consistently within a particular percentile.

Growth percentiles. Your baby's growth will be plotted on a growth chart at each visit. *Percentile* refers to how your baby compares to all other babies of the same age. For example, if a baby's weight is at the fortieth percentile he weighs more than 40 percent of babies do and less than 60 percent of babies do at that age. Percentile is not a reflection of how healthy a baby is. A baby who is at the ninety-fifth percentile is not necessarily healthier than a baby who is at the tenth percentile.

New 2010 infant growth charts. The World Health Organization created growth charts from six industrialized countries in which breastfeeding predominates, including the United States. In 2010 the AAP recommended that all pediatricians change to these for all infants, as they reflect more accurately how a baby should be growing. The old growth charts were based primarily on formula-fed American babies, who tend to weigh more. With the new charts, slimmer breastfed babies are considered within normal range.

Physical Exam

In the Newborn Checkup section on page 49, we described this entire exam in detail. However, various ages warrant more or less attention to different parts of the exam. Here are some particular items your doctor may give special attention to at one week:

Head. The doctor will make sure the soft spots and the various parts of the skull bones feel normal, and that any swollen areas have subsided.

Eyes. The doctor will use an eye scope to make sure the pupils are reflecting light properly.

Tongue. It's important to make sure the baby's tongue is flexible and not tied down by a tight membrane attached to the floor of the mouth. This condition, called *tongue-tie,* can interfere with breastfeeding. It is easily correctable with a minor scissor cut through the membrane. See Tongue-Tie, page 521.

Collarbones. These thin, fragile bones sometimes break during delivery if the shoulders become stuck. Sometimes this isn't noticed at birth because no swelling has yet occurred. The doctor will feel for a large lump over the area, indicating a fracture. Not to worry though; these heal without any trouble.

Heart. Heart conditions, although very rare, sometimes aren't obvious in the first day or two of life. A careful listen at one week is very important.

Umbilical cord. The doctor will make sure this isn't becoming infected.

Abdomen. A careful check for masses or swollen organs is important at this age.

Circumcision. Sometimes part of the skin edge sticks to the head of the penis during healing. You can prevent this with proper care; see page 48. At the doctor's discretion, this may need to be unstuck now or in a few weeks.

 DR. SEARS TIP
How to Avoid a Flat Head

A newborn's head is very susceptible to developing flat spots on the back or sides. This happens because some babies have a preference for turning the head in the same direction when they sleep on their back, and spending night after night with only one part of the head against the mattress can create a flat spot. Babies who prefer to face straight up during sleep can develop a flat spot right in the middle of the back of the head. Be sure to alternate which way your baby faces when he sleeps (see Flat Head, page 324).

Testicles. It's important to note that both testicles are in the scrotum.

Hips. Very rarely a baby may be born with one or both hips out of joint. The doctor will check the range of motion of both hips.

Spine. The doctor will check carefully to make sure there are no spine deformities.

Nutrition

Breastfeeding

Hopefully by now Mother and Baby have gotten the hang of this. Mom's milk should have come in and her nipples should not be sore. Mom should be offering Baby the breast approximately every two hours during the day, or sooner if he shows interest, and whenever he wakes up at night. No need to wake the baby up at night to eat (unless instructed by a lactation consultant to do so if Baby isn't gaining enough weight) — he'll do that often enough on his own. Baby should be nursing for fifteen minutes or more on each side at each feeding. Some babies won't quite be up to this schedule by day seven. Some won't feed for longer than a few minutes without falling asleep. Some won't wake up to feed in a timely manner no matter what you do. Some will nurse nonstop for hours.

The bottom line is this: Feed Baby "on cue," which means as often as he shows signs of hunger, with a *minimum* of about ten feedings every twenty-four hours. This works out to about every two hours, with a couple of longer stretches at the baby's discretion.

How to determine if your milk supply is adequate. Your breast milk should have come in between days three and five after Baby was born. Here are six signs to watch for that indicate a good milk supply:

- You've gone through a period of engorgement.

- Your breasts feel fuller before feedings and emptier after.

- You can see milk pooling in Baby's mouth and leaking down his cheek.

- Baby seems satisfied after feedings (in a deep sleep or quiet and content).

- Your breasts leak milk in between feedings.

- Baby is having at least six very wet diapers (pour two tablespoons of water onto a clean diaper to see what a soaked diaper feels like) and four or more yellow, seedy stools every twenty-four hours.

If you don't see at least four of these signs by seven days of age and your baby is persistently fussy, wants to constantly nurse or suck frantically on a pacifier, and rarely seems content, see your doctor right away and contact a lactation consultant.

Vitamin D supplements for breastfeeding babies. Although breast milk is complete nutrition, if Mom's level of vitamin D is low, the breast milk will be low as well. It is standard practice to supplement breastfeeding babies with a daily oral dose of vitamin D (400 IU daily, available as drops from any drugstore or health-food store). We agree with this policy and recommend continuing it throughout childhood. A blood test will show if Mom is low.

Feeding the breastfeeding mother. A healthy diet is important for every new mom. Mom doesn't have to restrict her normal diet at all unless Baby has colic or painful gas (see page 229). Here are three more tips:

- Make sure Mom gets enough healthy omega-3 fats, such as DHA (docosahexaenoic acid), in her diet to help insure Baby's optimal brain growth and development. She should eat safe fish, such as wild salmon, twice a week, or take a fish-oil supplement at least four days per week.

- Avoid mercury fish — these include shark, swordfish, tilefish, and mackerel.

- Continue your prenatal vitamins as long as you are breastfeeding.

Formula-Feeding

A regular cow-milk formula with DHA and ARA (arachidonic acid) is the standard beginning formula. If your baby is tolerating this well, without excessive spitting up, painful gas, or colic, then continue. See page 331 if your baby's formula isn't sitting well with her.

In general, most babies will take in about two to two and a half ounces of formula for every pound of body weight. Don't purposely limit your baby to this, however; let her have more if she's not satisfied. The frequency of feeding is up to you and your baby. Some will want to eat every two hours and others won't mind longer stretches. In the first few weeks, make sure your baby gets at least one feeding during the night.

General Health and Parenting Issues

There are many challenges that occur during a baby's initial months. These are covered in great detail in *The Baby Book*. Here are the most common issues that parents ask us about:

Bowel movements. Your baby's stools should be transitioning to softer, seedy, yellow stools by this time. Some babies may have runny stools, and this is okay as long as your baby is happy and growing. Color will also vary from brown to green to yellow, and frequency can vary from two to ten times daily.

Wet diapers. Most babies will have at least six to eight soaked diapers each day. This is a good sign that she's getting enough milk. If you continuously have to look closely and feel each diaper to detect urine, she might not be getting enough milk. Talk to your doctor.

Parenting style. We know there are many different books to read, classes to take, and videos to watch to help you prepare for parenthood. Don't rely too much on these, however, because no one knows your baby the way you do. When it comes to parenting, nothing beats on-the-job training. If you take care of your baby's bodily needs, feed him, hold him, and observe him, your own intuition will guide you. Following someone else's

written guidelines can rob you of one of life's most precious experiences — learning how to become an involved, attached, empathetic, and confident parent. Put the books away. Spend the time with your baby instead. We call this approach *attachment parenting*. See page 160 to read the Seven Baby B's of Attachment Parenting.

Sleep. Most babies have their sleep schedule mixed up; they sleep all day and then want to eat and play all night. This is very normal and will only last a few weeks. One way to change this is not to let your baby sleep more than an hour and a half at a time during the day. Don't let her take those four-hour naps during daytime, although such a break is tempting for you, and she will sleep better at night.

On the other hand, some moms prefer to sleep during the day when the baby sleeps and don't mind the nighttime wakefulness and feedings in the early weeks. There's nothing wrong with just going with the flow and letting your baby gradually sort out day and night. Don't worry about how many hours your baby is or isn't sleeping. Babies don't need a certain number of hours of sleep. They'll naturally get all they need.

Be sure to have your baby sleep on her back to decrease the risk of SIDS (Sudden Infant Death Syndrome; see page 505). See *The Baby Book* or *The Baby Sleep Book* for more advice on sleep.

Safety

There are two main safety concerns to keep in mind for newborns:

- Portable car seats. These are easily knocked off tables or tipped over with a baby inside. Be very careful when using them. It's safest just to keep your baby closer to you in a baby sling rather than leaving him in a seat.

- Smoke alarms. This is a good time to make sure these are all working and that you have a fire escape plan from all upstairs bedrooms.

Unusual but Normal One-Week Signs

There are several aspects of a baby's body and health at this age that may seem unusual and worrisome but are quite normal:

- ruptured blood vessels in the whites of the eyes

- yellow eyes (only a worry if Baby's whole body is jaundiced; see page 381)

- umbilical cord oozing and minor bleeding

- swollen scrotum or labia

- vaginal mucus and bleeding

- eye discharge (this is almost always due to plugged tear ducts, page 303)

- facial rash

 DR. SEARS TIP
Baby's First "Cold"

Most babies develop some nasal congestion that lasts for a month or two. This usually isn't an actual cold or illness. Your baby's little nose is simply getting used to all the allergens in the air. You can squirt nasal saline drops or breast milk into the nose and suction it out if it is interfering with his eating or sleeping (see nose care, page 20).

- spitting up (if projectile, see gastroeso-phageal reflux disease, or GERD, page 338)

- muscle twitching

Vaccines

There usually aren't any vaccines given to a one-week-old. Some doctors will begin the hepatitis B series at one week if it wasn't started in the hospital. See page 44.

ONE-MONTH CHECKUP

Here is our guide to the exciting changes that occur in your growing baby, as well as what commonly takes place at your one-month visit to the pediatrician.

Growth

Weight gain. Babies should by now be gaining a minimum of five ounces and a maximum of about ten ounces per week. This means your baby may weigh between 1¼ to 2½ pounds above his birth weight. If your breast-fed baby is gaining more than this, don't worry. It's normal for some to gain more rapidly during the first few months. If he's gaining less, you need to see a certified lactation consultant to help assess your milk supply and your baby's feeding technique. See Breast-feeding, pages 46 and 51, for more information.

Physical Exam

Here are some particular items your doctor may pay special attention to:

Head shape. If your baby's head shape is asymmetrical, your doctor will probably show you how to better position your baby during sleep to help reshape the head.

Neck symmetry. Sometimes a baby's neck muscles will be tighter on one side, causing the head to tilt and turn more easily to one side. Your doctor can show you some head and neck stretches.

Oral thrush. Newborns are prone to yeast growth in their mouth, visible as white patches on the tongue, inside the cheeks, or on the lips. See page 542.

Circumcision. If your son was circumcised, it's very important that the doctor checks to make sure the skin edges aren't sticking to the head of the penis. This can be prevented by following the instructions on page 48.

Testicles. Newborn boys often have extra fluid within their scrotum. Your doctor will take note of this and make sure it isn't too swollen.

Curved feet. Months of cramped living quarters within the womb sometimes leave little feet with a minor curvature. If noticeable, your doctor may show you some foot stretching exercises.

Skin. One common type of skin mark is called a *hemangioma*, a red or blue growth of blood vessels in the skin. If you notice one, show it to your doctor. These harmless growths may be as small as a pinpoint or as large as a quarter. They often get bigger during the first year, then slowly fade away by age five.

Nutrition

Adequate weight gain is the surest indicator that a baby is getting enough to eat. If the weight gain is two pounds or more over birth weight, you don't have to spend more than two seconds on this issue. If the gain is between one and two pounds, everything is probably fine, but your doctor will likely ask you some more in-depth questions about your baby's nutrition. If your baby has gained less than a pound over birth weight, further evaluation is needed.

Breastfeeding

By this time, breastfeeding should be almost second nature, with your baby latching on easily and correctly, no more sore nipples, and a plentiful milk supply. If all is going well, and you've been pushing your baby to nurse every two hours or so, you can ease up a little and let your baby "feed on cue," with a general guideline of making sure he feeds every two to three hours during the day (or more often if he demands it) for ten to twenty minutes or more on each side at each feeding. Be aware that if your baby is only "asking" to be fed every three to four hours instead of every two to three hours during the day and is only nursing on one side at each feeding, you may run into problems with decreasing milk supply and inadequate weight gain. However, the proof is in the scale. If the gain is great, the feeding frequency doesn't have to match the above description.

Formula-Feeding

At this age, most babies will want about three ounces of formula per feed, with a total of about twenty to twenty-four ounces each day. The best way to determine how much to feed a baby is to simply let him decide. If your baby is vigorously sucking each bottle dry, this may mean he wants more in each feed. The ideal is to have a few teaspoons left in each bottle as Baby's feeding slows down and he loses interest. This allows Baby's own appetite to regulate how much he eats.

Formula Allergy or Food Allergies Through the Breast Milk

If Baby has colicky episodes (hours of inconsolable screaming), has frequent gas pains, spits up excessively, or has bothersome nasal and chest congestion, she may be allergic to foods Mom is eating or to the formula. See page 327 for guidance on food allergies through the breast milk, page 331 for Formula Allergy, and page 229 for colic.

Nighttime Feeding

At night, whether you are breastfeeding or formula-feeding, you no longer need to wake your baby to eat. Hunger will wake a baby up if nighttime nutrition is needed. Some will wake up three to four times a night to feed.

General Health and Parenting Issues

Bowel movements. In general, breastfed babies have yellow, seedy, soft mushy stools several times each day. Formula-fed babies tend to have bowel movements a little less frequently that may vary in color between yellow, brown, and green but are usually soft and mushy as well. If your baby's stools have a lot of mucus, this may indicate either an allergy, inadequate intake, or, if breastfeeding, taking in too much low-fat breast milk and not enough high-fat hindmilk because the feedings are too short. See *The Baby Book* or *The Breastfeeding Book* for more information.

Urine stream. Try to observe your baby boy's urine stream during a bath or diaper change. The stream should come out strong, forming a nice arc. If it only dribbles out, let your doctor know. This may indicate a blockage in the urinary system.

Sleep. Hopefully by now your baby realizes that nighttime is for sleeping and not playing. Some babies will sleep for six-hour stretches or more at night (lucky parents!), and some babies will wake up every two hours at night for feeding (blessed parents!). The amount of nap time during the day will also vary; some babies take two-hour naps, some take thirty-minute naps. There is no set number of hours

---

 ### DR. SEARS TIP
Don't Be a One-Sided Parent

This may sound like an odd statement, but many parents develop a habit of always holding a baby with a certain arm (right-handed people usually hold a baby in the left arm, and vice versa), bottlefeeding a baby on the same side, and holding a baby in one particular position in a baby sling or in arms during fussy times. This may seem harmless, but in these positions a baby's head is often turned to only one side or tilted more toward one shoulder. If a baby is spending hours each day in these one-sided positions with the head always turned in the same direction, the neck muscles on one side can become tight and the baby will develop a head tilt (called Torticollis — see page 526). Young infants who spend a lot of time sitting up in a car seat or infant seat may tilt their head to one particular side because they aren't yet strong enough to hold their head up against gravity. Be sure to alternate holding positions, bottlefeeding sides, and baby-sling positions so that the head and neck are turned and tilted in various directions evenly.

---

of sleep a baby needs. He will naturally get as much sleep as his body requires. You probably feel very sleep-deprived at this point and are wondering, "Will I ever sleep again?" Well, you can rest assured that sleep is on the way. Many babies between one and two months of age begin to sleep for much longer stretches at night, and feed for shorter periods of time at night. So hang in there!

Development

Every baby develops at his own unique pace. Don't worry if your baby doesn't meet every milestone exactly on time. Here is a brief checklist of expected developmental milestones that most (but not all) babies will have reached by one month of age:

- gross motor — some head control, limbs flexed

- fine motor — often keeps hands tightly fisted

- language — may turn toward sounds and startle from loud noises

- social — may smile spontaneously, make eye contact with you

You can help your baby continue and thrive toward the two-month milestones by:

- skin-to-skin cuddling

- face-to-face interaction with exaggerated facial expressions

- singing and talking frequently to Baby

Safety

Sleep safety. Be sure you look through our checklist on sleep safety in *The Baby Book or The Baby Sleep Book.*

Unusual but Normal One-Month Signs

There are several aspects of a baby's body and health at this age that may seem unusual and worrisome but are normal:

- nasal and chest congestion, especially during feeding

- *erythema toxicum* (or *baby acne*) — red, raised, irritated rash that appears on the face, neck, and shoulders of most babies around three weeks of age, peaks at five weeks, then gradually diminishes by two months; will resolve without treatment and is thought to be due to the baby's withdrawal from Mom's hormones

- dry patches on the body (normal reaction to daily contact with clothes, milk, sweat, and dirt)

- dry, crusty scalp — see Cradle Cap, page 247

- eye discharge — see Tear Duct, Blocked, page 303

Vaccines

Some doctors give a Hep B shot at this time. See page 43 for discussion of the complete vaccine schedule.

TWO-MONTH CHECKUP

Your newborn is changing into an interactive, smiling, and playful baby. Here is our guide to understanding your two-month-old and what you have to look forward to in the months ahead.

Growth

Weight gain. Most babies will gain another one and a half to two and a half pounds or more in the second month. Your baby may start to show a general trend toward being large, average-sized, or slim by this time.

Length. This will be measured at each checkup. Babies generally grow about one and a half inches per month for the first three months. At this early age, length isn't necessarily an accurate predictor of eventual height.

Head circumference. Your doctor will make sure the head is growing consistently — not too fast and not too slow. Infant heads grow about three-quarters to one inch in circumference each month during the first few months.

Physical Exam

Your doctor will probably perform the same thorough exam as before. Here are some particular items your doctor may pay special attention to:

Head shape. If all is nice and even now, it will likely stay that way.

Eyes. Some babies will occasionally look cross-eyed at this age. Your doctor will take note of this to make sure it isn't too severe.

Ears. Up until this age, ears are often too small to look into. From here on your doctor will take a good look inside at each visit.

Neck strength. Your doctor should check to make sure Baby is holding his head up straight. A head tilt to either side can be a sign that the neck muscles are too tight on one side (see Torticollis, page 526).

Umbilical cord. Some babies will have a little bulge left over in the belly button. This minor hernia is harmless and should go away in the next year or two.

Hips. These should always be examined carefully at each checkup until your baby is walking to make sure the hip bones are properly in joint.

Nutrition

Adequate weight gain continues to be the best indicator that a baby is getting enough to eat. If the gain is less than one and a quarter pounds in the past month, your doctor will likely ask you some more in-depth questions about your baby's nutrition.

Breastfeeding. If the doctor says your baby is gaining plenty of weight, then whatever the frequency and duration of your baby's feeding must be just right for you and her. If the doctor tells you the baby may not have gained enough weight, you should try to figure out why and correct the situation instead of simply adding formula. Contact La Leche League, a breastfeeding support organization with trained personnel who can offer you guidance over the phone or at group meetings. Visit www.LLLI.org to find a group near you. You can also seek out a certified lactation consultant.

Formula-feeding. At this age, you can feed your baby on demand or on a schedule, whichever you prefer. Most babies will want formula every three to four hours. Remember to make sure your baby is getting at least two to two and a half ounces per pound of body weight per twenty-four hours (a twelve-pound baby should get around twenty-four to thirty ounces per day).

General Health and Parenting Issues

Sleep (or lack thereof). By this time you will have figured out whether or not you've been blessed with a good sleeper. If so, one to five months is usually what we call the "honeymoon" period, when many babies sleep long stretches at night. However, some babies have more nighttime needs: They need to be fed or rocked to sleep, they waken every few hours, they need to sleep in close proximity to you in order to stay asleep, or all of the above. These high-need babies can learn to be great sleepers, too, but handling these sleep challenges is beyond the scope of this book. *The Baby Sleep Book* explains how to help your baby learn to be a good sleeper. But there are a few important things to know right now:

- *Watch for gastroesophageal reflux disease (GERD) as a medical cause of night waking*. Some babies will wake up frequently due to this or to food allergies. See pages 327 and 333.

- *Don't give in to cry-it-out sleep training*. Some parents try this method at two months. We believe it is too traumatic for most babies, especially those with more nighttime needs. See page 252 for a more detailed discussion.

- *Try a variety of sleeping arrangements*. Some babies sleep well alone while others sleep best when nestled against Mom in bed. If your baby isn't sleeping well, try changing where he sleeps. You might be pleasantly surprised.

Car-seat screaming. Some babies simply hate to be in the car seat and will scream whenever you have to drive somewhere. This is very common, so don't worry that there may be something wrong with your baby. Unfortunately, some babies don't outgrow this until later in this first year. Mom can sit in the backseat with the baby and lean over to nurse, or try giving the baby a bottle or pacifier. Place a large mirror above your baby's seat so that he can see you. Pull over to give your baby a break as often as you need to. Here are two family scream-stopping tricks to help your noisy little traveler: Bring along one of your baby's favorite CDs that you reserve only for car travel. Or make up some fun songs that your baby will come to recognize as "car-seat songs."

Prevent labial adhesions. The inner labia of the vagina of infants have a tendency to stick together during the first few years of life in some children. You can prevent this by very gently opening the labia once a day during a diaper change. Your pediatrician will also check the labia at checkups to make sure they are remaining unstuck. See page 534 for more information.

Development

Here is a checklist of developmental milestones for this age. Although we don't expect all babies to meet all guidelines at every stage, mention any delays to your pediatrician.

- gross motor — limbs more relaxed, lifts head slightly when on tummy, some head control when sitting

- fine motor — hands partially unfolded, grasps your finger, eyes follow you from side to side

- language — cooing sounds, holds eye contact

- social — smiles responsively; may laugh out loud, show emotions (happy, sad)

Here are some ways you can help your baby develop over the next month:

- Hang a black-and-white mobile or picture so she can study patterns.

- Encourage her to play with her hands; prop her semi-upright for playtime.

- Play music (music box, mobile, CDs); let her shake toys and rattles.

- Give her infant massage; use the facing-forward position in a baby sling or soft carrier.

- Let her lie on your chest; play on the floor together.

Safety

Chokeable objects. It's not to early to develop awareness. Make sure Baby's play area is free of tiny objects that might tempt her little fingers.

Beware of rolling over. Although most babies don't roll over until four months, some will do it early. Be sure not to leave your baby alone on a counter, changing table, or couch.

Most Common Two-Month Illnesses

Many minor ailments can affect babies as they grow. Here are the most common at this age:

The common cold. If you have older children, or your baby is frequently exposed to other infants, expect colds and coughs to start. See page 222 for details on how to get your young infant through.

Diaper rash. This is par for the course for almost all babies. See page 275 for treatment and prevention ideas.

RSV (respiratory syncytial virus). This particularly tough fall and winter cold virus can be quite severe for young infants. See page 451 for details on how to handle it if your infant has a cough with wheezing.

Eczema. If your baby is going to be prone to food allergies and eczema, now is the time it may start, since he is exposed to a variety of foods through breast milk. See page 297.

Vaccines

At two months, the first big round of shots begins. There are five vaccines usually given at this age: DTaP, Hib, PCV, IPV, and RV. Some doctors may also give a Hep B vaccine here if the birth or one-month dose was missed. See page 43. For a complete discussion and information on alternative vaccine schedules, see *The Vaccine Book*.

FOUR-MONTH CHECKUP

Here is our guide to help you understand the many changes that come at this age and to help your baby grow and develop through these months.

Growth

Weight gain. Most babies will gain one and a quarter to two pounds per month at this age, or two and a half to four pounds since the two-month checkup. Babies will usually have doubled their birth weight by this time. As usual, your doctor will assess how your baby is growing. Overall, the average weight for a four-month-old boy is fifteen pounds, give or take two pounds. For girls, the average is about fourteen pounds, give or take two pounds.

Length and head circumference. Your doctor will continue to check these to make sure growth is consistent.

Physical Exam

While your doctor should perform a complete physical exam at each checkup, here are some of the items she may pay extra attention to at this age:

Eyes. By now any cross-eyed episodes you may have seen previously should no longer be happening. Let your pediatrician know if you still notice a problem.

Mouth. Your doctor may check for teething just to satisfy parental curiosity.

Neck strength and symmetry. Your baby should be able to hold his head up straight and strong and easily turn the head from side to side.

Abdomen. It's important to press deep on both sides to check for masses or enlarged organs.

Genitals. The inner labia of infant girls will sometimes begin to stick together. Your doctor will check to make sure this isn't occurring. It can be prevented by gently spreading the labia apart about twice a week during a diaper change.

Muscle tone and strength. Your baby should be able to support his weight on his legs and push his upper body up with his arms when lying on his tummy.

Skin. Rashes tend to begin around this age or older. Your doctor will look around and ask you if you've noticed anything anywhere on your baby's skin.

Nutrition

Don't be too eager to start your baby on solid foods. Virtually all pediatric experts agree that babies should only get breast milk or formula for the first six months of life. Starting foods sooner can trigger allergies that may have otherwise not occurred. Giving your baby water is fine at this age.

Breastfeeding

Most babies will begin to have shorter feeds. They aren't as patient as they used to be and are more easily distracted. Don't worry. Babies become more efficient nursers and will get as much out of a short feeding as they used to get with a longer feed. The proof is in the weight gain and whether your baby appears happy and satisfied after nursing and has good muscle tone and body fat. Your pediatrician will assess all of this.

Heading back to work outside the home? If you are breastfeeding and planning to go back to a career or job outside the home, we encourage you to continue breastfeeding. Studies have shown that mothers who continue breastfeeding after returning to work outside the home are happier and report more satisfaction in their job. Their babies also get sick less often, which means less missed work for either parent. In *The Baby Book* and *The Breastfeeding Book*, you will find many tips on how to pump, store, and manage your milk supply in your dual career.

Formula-Feeding

You can continue to give your baby as much as he seems to want to take at each feeding. Most babies won't want more than thirty-two ounces a day.

Overfeeding

If your baby is taking in more than thirty-six ounces of formula, and his weight percentile is accelerating higher and higher up the growth curve, you may be overfeeding him. Try giving him an eight-ounce bottle of water spread out throughout the day in between feedings. This may curb his thirst without giving him too many calories. If your breastfed baby is "off the charts," don't worry. It is generally believed that you can't over-*breast*feed a baby and that such weight gain from breast milk is okay.

General Health and Parenting Issues

Teething. Teething is probably the number one cause of night waking and daytime fussiness for infants from this age until two years. Although most babies won't show teeth until about six months, pain usually starts around four or five months. Signs of teething include excess drooling, chewing on everything, constant gnawing on fingers (both yours and Baby's), and long periods of unusual crankiness and night waking. See page 509 for tips on how to minimize your baby's discomfort.

**DR. SEARS TIP
The Five-Month
"Ear Infection"**

Almost all parents will bring their baby in to see the doctor at around five months to have her ears checked because the baby is fussy, sleeping poorly, and pulling on her ears constantly. Parents are naturally worried that their baby might have an ear infection. If your baby has cold symptoms (stuffy or runny nose and cough), fever, and the above symptoms, then an ear infection is possible. But if your baby has *no* cold symptoms, then the ear pulling and fussing are probably just related to teething. Understanding this distinction may save you an unnecessary trip to the doctor.

Drool cough. A common symptom at this age is the ever-present "drool cough" from teething. Parents will often state that their baby has a choking, junky-sounding cough numerous times a day. If your baby seems otherwise healthy, with no nasal drainage or congestion, and shows all the signs of teething, then this cough is probably just part of teething, and not a chest cold.

Constipation. This is a common occurrence at this age for both formula-fed and breastfed infants. The easiest fix is to try to incorporate water into the daily routine. If this doesn't help, you can try some diluted prune juice (half water) through a bottle or sippy cup. If necessary, you can try baby-food prunes if Baby is close to six months. See page 240 for more tips on treating infant constipation.

Development

Here are the developmental milestones that most babies will achieve by this age:

- gross motor — rolls over, good head control, pushes up on arms while on tummy, stands supported

- fine motor — reaches out and grabs on to objects, holds and shakes rattle

- language — will consistently turn toward sounds, makes variety of baby sounds such as "ah-oh"

- social — laughs heartily, variety of different cries for different needs, uses arms and body to indicate wants and needs

You can promote your baby's development in the coming months by:

- standing her on your lap, letting her grab your nose and hair

- letting her play while propped upright

- encouraging her to grab and chew on her toes

- giving her rattles and squeaky toys

- playing peek-a-boo and mirror games with her

Safety

Walkers. We discourage using the kind of walkers on wheels in which babies sit and use their legs to push themselves around the room. These toys are responsible for head injuries and broken bones from rolling down stairs. They may also interfere with proper leg development because they use muscles to "walk" in a sitting position, which is much different from walking upright. Stationary exersaucers are fine, but wait until six months.

Small, chokeable objects. Now that your baby is or will be rolling over, it's even more important that you scan the floor daily and pick up anything that is a choking hazard.

Sun protection. Be sure to use hats and shade to protect your baby during long hours of sun exposure. Use sunscreen on the arms and legs when a day in the sun is planned. There are some sunblocks that are labeled safe for infants from three months of age on. See page 19 for eye safety in the sun.

Hot-water temperature. Lower the temperature on your hot-water heater to 120 degrees or lower. This will avoid accidental burns if you or your infant inadvertently turns on the hot water while in the bath.

Most Common Four-Month Illnesses

Illnesses at this age are similar to those we discussed in the two-month checkup (see page 57). Rashes become more common as your baby grows. If you notice anything unusual on the skin, see page 443 to help you identify it.

Vaccines

At four months, most of the same shots that were given at two months are repeated: DTaP, Hib, PCV, IPV, and RV. There may or may not be a Hep B vaccine at this visit, depending on what schedule your doctor follows. See page 43 for more details.

Notify your doctor if your baby had any bad reaction to the first round of shots, such as fever and extreme fussiness. See page 529.

SIX-MONTH CHECKUP

So much has happened over the last six months, and the next six months will bring even more exciting changes. Here is our guide to helping you understand the most important details of this wonderful age.

Growth

Weight gain. Babies will gain anywhere from two to three pounds between four and six months.

Length. Most babies will continue to gain length at a rate of three quarters to one inch per month. The average length for boys at this age is twenty-six and a half inches and for girls is about twenty-six. The normal range can vary by one and a half inches above or below this. Length percentiles at this age are not a good predictor of eventual height as growth patterns can change significantly over the next few years. Track your baby's growth on the charts on pages 107–110.

Physical Exam

As your doctor performs a complete physical exam, here are some of the highlights she may focus on at this age:

Eyes. Your doctor will closely check Baby's eyes to make sure they are both looking straight ahead. Occasional crossed eyes can be normal in the first several months of life, but should be resolved by now. See crossed eyes on page 304 for more details.

Mouth. The bottom front teeth are usually the first to come in, but sometimes the top ones come first.

Ears. Ears are often stuffy with mucus when a baby is sick. When your baby is healthy, it's useful to confirm that the ears are clear of mucus to be sure your baby is hearing well.

Lymph nodes. Most infants have pea-sized or smaller glands that can be felt on the sides of the neck, behind the ears, or on the back of the skull.

Legs. Most babies' legs are quite curved. Your doctor will make sure the legs and feet aren't more curved than they should be.

Spine. The doctor will take a good look at your baby's spine in the sitting position to check for abnormal curvature or unusual vertebrae.

Nutrition

Solid Foods

The long-awaited moment has arrived; you can now introduce solid foods to your baby. Common starter foods include banana, applesauce, pear, sweet potato, avocado, and rice cereal. But not all babies will be ready or interested just yet. Signs that Baby is ready to start solids include:

- eagerly watching you eat

- reaching for your food

- able to sit up in a high chair

- disappearance of the tongue-thrust reflex (the tongue doesn't automatically stick out whenever something gets into the mouth)

It's important to know that just because your baby is old enough to start solids doesn't mean it's the right time for her. If your baby keeps turning her head away or pushing the spoon away, then she is clearly not ready. Trying to coax a baby to eat when she is not yet interested is a sure way to create a picky eater.

Remember, foods at this age are mainly for social and motor development. They aren't yet needed for nutrition. Breast milk and formula provide complete nutrition for the entire first year of life. So don't worry how much or how often your baby eats at this age, because it doesn't matter in the long run. Just follow your baby's cues and have fun.

For more detailed information on starting solids and moving on to more foods over the next few months, see *The Baby Book* or *The Healthiest Kid in the Neighborhood*.

DR. SEARS TIP
Go Organic!

It's best to feed your baby as organically as possible. Pesticides and hormones in foods are bad news for a baby's growing brain. When using store-bought baby food, frozen organic baby food is best. For more information on organic baby food, visit www.HappyBaby Food.com.

Shaping young tastes. When starting Baby on solid foods, make your own. Besides giving your baby extra nutrition, solid foods shape your baby's tastes. If you make your own baby food (e.g., mashed avocado, cooked squash, mashed bananas), you shape your baby's tastes toward appreciating real food, and you do this at a time when Baby's developing taste buds are most shapeable. In our medical practice, we have noticed that babies who are fed natural food early on are more likely to stick with these natural tastes on into adulthood.

On the other hand, babies who start off with bland jarred or canned food believe that this is what real food is supposed to taste like. Their tastes are shaped in a less healthy direction. Babies who start out on natural food are more likely to shun the taste of junk food later on.

Watch for constipation. Babies often become constipated when foods are started. Bananas and rice cereal can be especially constipating. If this happens, stop the foods and give baby some pureed prunes or peaches until he is more regular. Continue giving these while you slowly reintroduce the other foods again. Diluted prune juice is also very effective. If your baby was already having a difficult time passing stools before you even began foods, start with prunes and peaches before beginning any others.

Breastfeeding

The American Academy of Pediatrics recommends breastfeeding for a minimum of one year, and this should be the main source of your baby's diet until age one. Do not let your baby's interest in foods cause the breastfeeding to slow down too much. As for the timing of breastfeeds and food, it doesn't really matter. Simply offer your baby food whenever you are eating and breastfeed whenever your baby asks.

Formula

As babies begin foods, their formula intake may decrease. A baby needs formula to be the main part of her nutrition until age one, so don't let her formula intake slow down too much as the food increases. A baby needs between twenty-four and thirty-two ounces of formula a day, even when food comes into play.

Water

This is a good age to get your baby used to sippy cups of water. Juice should be avoided; it's better to forgo the extra sugar. Let your baby drink as much water as she wants. Then she won't come to expect juice as her beverage.

What About Vitamins?

Giving your baby a liquid multivitamin is generally not necessary. Babies get all the vitamins they need from breast milk (except for vitamin D; see page 52) or formula. However, using a multivitamin won't hurt, and it may provide a little vitamin insurance for your baby. Liquid vitamins are available from any drugstore, or visit www.DrSearsFamilyEssen tials.com. Follow the dosing on the bottle.

General Health and Parenting Issues

Teeth. Many babies get their first teeth by this age. Don't worry if yours hasn't just yet. Babies have been known to go without teeth even until age one. You don't have to begin brushing or using toothpaste until your baby gets some molars at around eighteen months. For now, it's prudent to simply wipe your baby's teeth and/or gums with a thin washcloth on your finger once or twice each day.

Sleep. Still searching for that magical pill that will make your baby sleep through the night? You're in good company. Although some babies do sleep through the night by this age, most babies wake up at least once, if not more. We encourage you to read *The Baby Sleep Book* for tips on how to help your baby sleep better, but here are a couple of ideas specifically for six-month-olds:

- *A bedtime snack.* If your baby is eating foods, you can try an evening meal close to bedtime. Though studies show otherwise, this may help *your* baby sleep a longer stretch, at least for the first half of the night.

- *Middle-of-the-night teething-pain reliever.* Keep some teething-pain reliever by the bed so you can give a dose during the night as needed to (hopefully) buy you a four-hour stretch of sleep. See page 552.

Stranger anxiety. Between six and nine months of age, stranger anxiety may set in. This very normal stage may last for only one or two months or for as long as a year or more. One way to help your baby mature through this anxiety is to spend time with more adults and other families with children. Surrounding your baby with more of a "village" atmosphere increases her social skills and comfort level with others.

Development

Here are the developmental milestones that most babies will achieve by this age:

- gross motor — rolls over easily both ways, may stand briefly holding on to furniture, may sit briefly by self or may use arms for balance, squirms forward on tummy

- fine motor — reaches out precisely; grabs objects with palm, fingers, and thumb; may point to objects

- language — babbles (ba-ba-ba-ba, ma-ma-ma-ma), experiments with different sounds

- social — mimics facial expressions and sounds, interacts with self in mirror

TV AND VIDEOS: HOW MUCH IS TOO MUCH?

Research has shown a possible correlation between screen time and behavioral/learning disorders such as attention deficit disorder (ADD). It is generally believed by most medical experts that the best approach is to completely avoid TV (even educational or developmental videos) for the first two years of life while a baby's brain is developing the most. Real interactive stimulation with real people and real toys is better for a baby's intellectual and emotional development. From a practical standpoint, most parents don't follow this advice. We will admit to allowing our infants and toddlers a half-hour video on many days. However, in a perfect world a no-TV policy under two years is probably best.

You can promote your baby's development in the coming months by:

- letting him play with blocks, bang toys, roll balls

- having floor play, placing toys just out of reach, propping him up to sit

- playing peek-a-boo, pat-a-cake

- letting him catch bubbles, pick up small objects (supervised)

- encouraging him to bounce to music

Safety

Babyproofing

Although your baby's mobility is limited to rolling and squirming, crawling is just around the corner. It is prudent to begin the babyproofing process now. Here is a brief checklist of the most important measures you should take at this age. As your baby gets older and more mobile, you'll have to expand your efforts:

- Install safe electrical outlet covers.

- Anchor bookshelves to the wall so they can't be pulled over.

- Tie window-shade cords up high so your baby can't get tangled, especially near the crib.

- Vacuum twice weekly to remove small, chokeable objects.

- Stop using tablecloths and other decorations that your baby could pull down on himself.

- Place household cleaners and medications in a cabinet with a babyproof latch and up high, out of reach of Baby's hands.

- Install safety gates at the top and bottom of stairs.

Poison control hotline. Get the local number for your area and tape it to your kitchen cabinet and near the phone. You can also use the nationwide number: 1-800-222-1222.

Lose the coffee table. Although this is a convenient tool for babies to learn how to pull themselves up to standing, it's also a big source of head bumps, chipped teeth, and facial cuts as babies stumble and fall into them. If you can live without it, put your coffee table away for a year until your baby is an expert walker and runner. Dr. Bill and Martha have a fabric-covered ottoman that doubles as a safe coffee table.

Most Common Six-Month Illnesses

Here are the most common ailments your baby may come across over the next few months:

Ear infections. This is the age when common colds and coughs begin turning into ear infections. Next time your child catches a cold, watch for fever, unusual fussiness, pulling on the ears, and poor sleep. See page 285 for more details.

Roseola. This very common but harmless virus causes three days of high fever. The fever then breaks, and a red, pimply, and lacy rash appears around the upper chest, back, and neck. There's no treatment except fever control. See page 319 for more information.

Croup. This cold virus is unique in that it causes a cough that sounds like a seal barking and creates raspy, labored breathing. If your baby catches this type of cough, see page 250 for treatment ideas.

Drool rash on the face. This harmless condition accompanies teething. You can limit the redness with lanolin ointment (like what you use to soothe your nipples after breastfeeding), but it will continue on and off over the next year.

Vaccines

Most of the same shots are given as at two and four months: DTaP, Hep B, Hib, PCV, IPV, and RV. Depending on what brand of Hib vaccine your doctor uses, there may or may not be a Hib shot at this visit. Some doctors give the third dose of IPV (polio vaccine) at this age; others wait until eighteen months. See page 43 for more details.

The influenza shot can also be given starting at six months of age if your baby turns six months during flu season (October through April).

NINE-MONTH CHECKUP

You have now entered a brand-new stage in your baby's life — *mobility!* This is a very exciting age for babies, as mobility gives them much more independence. Here is our guide to your nine-month-old.

Growth

Weight gain. Babies will gain from two and a half to three and a half pounds between six and nine months of age. If your baby has been crawling for the past two months, or is even beginning to walk early, do not be surprised if he has gained less weight than this and is now at a lower percentile on the weight curve. Most babies go through a "slimming down" phase during the second six months because your suddenly exercising baby is burning off his baby fat.

Physical Exam

While your doctor should perform a complete physical exam at each checkup, here are some of the items she may pay extra attention to at this age:

Head. The soft spot may be gone by this time.

Eye color. Although eye color tends to change over the first several months of life, whatever it ends up being by this time is usually final.

Heart. Heart problems can show up at any time during childhood.

Skin. It's not unusual for moles to begin showing up on your baby's skin. You can check for these and point them out to your doctor.

Nutrition

Food. Remember that foods are not nutritionally essential until one year of age, so there should be no pressure to make your child eat. There is no certain quantity or number of times each day that a baby should eat. Just do whatever fits your schedule and your baby's interest level. Some new foods that you can slowly add to Baby's diet over the next few months include salmon, poultry, egg yolk, cheese, yogurt, tofu, noodles, beans, peas, yams, and oatmeal. Foods that remain a

---

 DR. SEARS TIP
Stay Close to Nature—
Real Food, Please!

We don't mean move outdoors and live in a tent. We are referring to what you feed your child. Try to feed her foods as close to their natural origin as possible. Instead of puffed fruit or veggie snacks out of a box, give your child real food to snack on, such as bananas, rice cakes, cut-up grapes, and so on. Getting your baby hooked on convenient packaged snack foods teaches her to crave things like chips and crackers as she gets older. As a general rule, if it comes in a wrapper, it's not for your "snacker." See Shaping Young Tastes, page 65.

---

definite "no" until age one include honey, egg white, wheat, nut products, and berries. Two food groups, peanut and shellfish, shouldn't be given to kids until at least age two because of the potential for allergies.

You can start offering foods with lumpier consistency, finger foods, bite-size soft cooked foods, and melt-in-your-mouth foods. If your child continually gags on a new consistency, back off for a few weeks before you try again.

Breastfeeding. Ounce for ounce, breast milk continues to be the best source of nutrition for your baby through the first year and into the second. Don't worry about trying to get your baby to nurse any particular number of times each day or for any certain length of time. Your baby is old enough to regulate his own appetite and decide when and how long to nurse.

Formula-feeding. Continue offering four to five bottles of formula each day, including nighttime if needed. There's no need to graduate to a toddler formula; the infant one is just fine until age one.

General Health and Parenting Issues

Iron check. The iron that Baby stored in his body as a fetus typically runs out by this age. Most babies get enough iron through breast milk or formula and won't have a problem. Some, for reasons not clearly understood, become low in iron and can become slightly anemic (low red-blood-cell count) between nine and twelve months of age. Your doctor will probably test this with a small pinprick to the heel to get a drop of blood. This test is especially important for lower-weight and breastfeeding infants. If your baby has low iron, your doctor can prescribe iron supplements.

You can also focus on foods that are high in iron, including iron-fortified cereals, prune juice, beans, meat, turkey, wild salmon, lentils, and tofu.

Separation anxiety. Some babies develop separation anxiety between nine and twelve months of age. They may no longer want to be left in the nursery or with a babysitter. Some will even protest when you simply walk into the next room to get something. This is a normal and healthy stage for babies as they begin to understand social dynamics. Some parents decide to play it tough and allow some crying as the baby grows accustomed to being left. Other parents adjust their lives and expectations for several months and stay nearby, letting their baby become used to separation very gradually. Follow your intuition on this. Don't let others pressure you into one path or another. Do whatever you feel fits you and your baby the best.

Be a "yes" parent. With your baby's newfound mobility comes a desire to explore. The entire house now becomes his playground, and of course, everything he can get his hands on belongs to him! We believe that parents should encourage this sense of exploration and discovery. By allowing your baby to crawl or walk around the house picking up objects, banging on tables, opening cabinets, and dumping out containers, you give him the message that he is important, intelligent, and independent. It builds his self-esteem and confidence. Being a "no" parent and constantly pulling your baby away from "don't touch" areas can dampen his creativity and excitement. It can make him feel unsure of himself, afraid of overstepping his boundaries. Be a "yes" parent, and watch your toddler's imagination and creativity soar! See the tips below to make sure his world of exploration is safe.

Development

Here are the developmental milestones that most babies will achieve by this age:

- gross motor — crawls, pulls to standing, cruises along furniture, stands unsupported, perhaps takes some steps

- fine motor — picks up tiny objects with thumb and forefinger, may feed self with hands, drinks from cup

- language — jabbers different consonant and vowel combinations together, perhaps says "Mama" or "Dada" specifically, understands labels for objects and actions

- social — responds to own name, may wave "bye-bye," gives social signals (lifts arms to be picked up)

You can promote your baby's development by letting him:

- play with containers — filling, dumping

- bang on pots and pans

- stack large blocks

- explore your shirt pocket

- interact with himself in the mirror

- dance or bounce to music

Safety

Warning! Your job as a safety patrol officer just got a lot busier. Please take the following information very seriously. Your child's life could depend on it.

Swimming pool. If you have a pool, it is extremely important that you build a safety fence with a childproof gate around it. Do not wait until your baby is older, because he is now, or will soon be, mobile enough to go outside and into the pool.

Bathtub. Do not leave your baby unattended in the bath, even for a few seconds. She can reach up and turn on the hot water herself. You should also buy an inflatable or rubber padded cover for the water spout.

Stairs. Put baby gates at the top and bottom of the stairs so that your child doesn't take a tumble while unattended. You should also take some time to teach her how to crawl up and down the stairs safely.

Mom's purse. This is every baby's favorite thing to explore. Do *not* keep any medicine, vitamins, perfume sprays, or mace in your purse. Purses are one of the most common sources of toddler poisoning and overdoses.

Chokeable foods. Never give a child under four years old popcorn, whole grapes, hot dogs (unless cut into small pieces), nuts, seeds, hard fruit (like raw apples), hard candy, or any other small, hard, round, and firm item. Never leave a child unattended while he is eating. If a child begins to choke, the sooner you act the better.

Other babyproofing steps. Besides the measures we suggested at your six-month visit, be sure to do the following:

- Childproof locks on lower cabinets.

- Keep all medicines, even vitamins, in an upper cabinet.

- Keep all cleaners and detergents in an upper cabinet or shelf.

- Make sure you have no poisonous indoor or outdoor plants. See www.AskDrSears.com.

Most Common Nine-Month Illnesses

Besides common colds, cough, and ear infections, here are some common ailments your child may come across over the next few months:

Impetigo. This bacterial infection often occurs in the skin around the mouth, nose, or eyes. See page 378 for more information.

Hand, foot, and mouth disease. This troublesome and untreatable virus causes painful mouth sores, high fever, and sometimes tiny blisters on the hands and feet. See page 404 for more details.

Diarrhea illnesses. Toddlers become more prone to picking up intestinal infections. See page 277 if your child comes down with diarrhea and/or vomiting.

 **DR. SEARS TIP
Boost the Immune System**

Now that you and your baby are venturing out into the world more and more, it becomes important to keep your baby's immune system healthy. See page 33 for ways to boost your baby's, and your own, immune system to help avoid troublesome illnesses.

Vaccines

Depending on what schedule your doctor follows, there may be anywhere from zero to two shots at this age. See page 43 for more information on vaccines.

ONE-YEAR CHECKUP

Congratulations! Your little baby is one year old, and this coming year will hold many exciting changes. Here is our guide to caring for and understanding your growing toddler through this major milestone in your lives.

Growth

Weight gain. Most babies will have gained one to three pounds since their nine-month checkup and have tripled their birth weight by this age. Genetics really starts to play a role, and your baby will show a trend toward being slim or hefty in accordance with family body types. If your baby is programmed to be slim, no amount of food will change this. If your baby's weight is accelerating off the top of the growth chart, then it's important to shape your baby's tastes toward healthy carbs, proteins, and good fats (see page 94 in this book, *The Family Nutrition Book,* or *The Healthiest Kid in the Neighborhood*).

Length. Babies will usually have gained about one and a half inches since the nine-month appointment, with an average length of twenty-nine inches for girls and thirty for boys.

Head circumference. Your doctor will continue to make sure your baby's head is growing consistently.

Physical Exam

As your doctor performs a complete physical exam, here are some of the highlights he or she may focus on at this age:

Ears. The doctor will check for two things: mucus congestion in the ears and wax buildup, both of which can muffle the hearing.

Mouth. Since most kids don't need to see a dentist until around age three, it's important for your doctor to get a good look at the teeth to make sure there are no early signs of tooth decay or abnormal development. Most babies have about six to eight teeth by now.

Abdomen. It's important for your doctor to feel the belly for enlarged organs or masses.

Genitals. For boys, the doctor will examine the testicles for abnormal swelling or growths. For girls, she will make sure the inner labia aren't stuck together. Be sure to continue to gently spread the inner labia apart until your child is out of diapers to prevent adhesions (see page 534).

Legs and feet. The doctor will want to watch your baby move around to make sure there is no unusual limp or curved legs and feet. Now that your baby can stand, the doctor will check for flat feet and unusually curved legs.

Nutrition

Food

Now that your baby is one year old, there is really no food substance that he cannot have except for choking foods (see page 218) and shellfish and peanut products (due to the high allergic potential). You no longer have to fix something special for meals. Just give him what the rest of the family is having. You can offer your baby new foods, such as milk, cottage cheese, eggs, beef, fish, pasta, graham crackers, wheat cereal, honey, muffins, pancakes, and all fruits and vegetables (except anything chokeable). Remember to go organic.

Breastfeeding

Continuing to breastfeed beyond one year is very healthy for your baby. The specific nutrients and types of fats, proteins, and calcium in breast milk can continue to benefit her through the second and third years of life. Don't worry if your child nurses less often than she used to. Most toddlers are too distracted to settle down for serious nursing. On the other hand, some toddlers regress into a clingy phase again and want to nurse more often for a few months. Your baby does not need any cow's milk as long as you are breastfeeding at least twice a day.

Switching from Formula to Organic Cow's Milk and Yogurt

Now that your baby is one year old, he no longer needs formula. You can switch over to whole cow's milk and yogurt.

Cow's milk. A baby's brain needs the extra fat from whole milk for brain growth until age two, at which time you can switch over to low-fat milk. Babies should not get as much milk as they had formula. Limit milk to about sixteen ounces for each twenty-four-hour period. More than this can be a little rough on the intestines and may decrease the appetite for regular foods. You can either transition to milk over a couple of weeks by mixing some milk with the formula, or you can just switch straight over. It's up to you. If your baby had a suspected cow's–milk–formula allergy during infancy, you can still try to transition over to cow's milk now. Watch Baby for signs of allergy. Alternatives to cow's milk include unsweetened rice, soy, or almond "milk," which are calcium-fortified. Another good choice is goat's milk.

Yogurt. Yogurt is an excellent source of calcium, and its natural culturing process makes it less allergenic and less irritating to the gut. Most children who seem allergic to milk or lactose intolerant do very well with yogurt (we suggest organic), which has the extra benefit of probiotics. Greek yogurt has twice as much protein per bite as regular yogurt.

 DR. SEARS TIP
Rice and Almond Milk Are Not Protein Substitutes

Beverages made of rice or almonds are not, technically speaking, milk. Unlike cow's milk and soy milk, they are largely made up of carbohydrates and have little protein, fat, and other nutrients babies need. If you must rely on it due to allergies, a calcium-fortified rice or almond beverage will at least fulfill a baby's calcium requirement.

Calcium requirements. Here's a little-known secret: Once weaned off formula or breast milk, a baby doesn't technically need any other type of milk at all. The two things that milk provides, calcium and fat, can easily be obtained from cheese, yogurt, vegetables, meats, and other foods. Milk happens to be a convenient substitute for formula, but it's certainly not a necessary one. Babies need two to three servings of a calcium-rich food every day. Actually, yogurt (organic, no added sweeteners) is higher in calcium than the same amount of milk, and it is less allergenic.

Vitamin D. Remember to continue this supplement (400 IU daily) throughout childhood as directed by your pediatrician.

Slim babies. As we discussed earlier, some babies naturally slim down at this age. Your doctor will examine your baby's muscle tone, fat layers, and developmental status, and if all is well, there's nothing to worry about. To help ensure that your slim baby continues to get the calories and nutrition he needs, try to incorporate these favorite "grow foods" (the most calories, protein, vitamins, and minerals per bite) into his diet:

Avocado	Broccoli
Beans	Cottage cheese
Blueberries	Lentils
Eggs	Olive oil
Fish	Oranges
Flaxseed meal or oil	Papaya
Nut butters (not peanut)	Pink grapefruit
Oatmeal	Sweet potatoes
Spinach	Poultry
Tofu	Whole-grain bread
Tomatocs	Hummus
Yogurt	

General Health and Parenting Issues

Picky eaters. If you have been challenged with a finicky eater, don't fret. In the long run, picky eaters turn out to be just as healthy as eager eaters. See page 294 for some useful tips on feeding your picky toddler.

Weaning off the bottle. If your baby is still using bottles, it's time to begin weaning her off. The easiest way is to simply not have bottles visible anymore. Put milk or water into sippy cups and leave them conveniently placed within your child's reach. Bring them along in the car. Let your child quench her thirst this way. This "out of sight, out of mind" approach works best if you do it before your baby is old enough to walk around asking for bottles of milk by name. She may notice something is missing, but she may not be able to put her finger on it and will just move on with her day.

Some toddlers really do still need one or two bottles every day as part of a comfort routine, such as at naptime or bedtime or on waking up. After all, breastfed babies still nurse at these times, why not bottlefed babies? If you feel your child needs the bottle in certain situations, don't take it away. Enjoy those quiet baby moments together while you still can. There's no harm in part-time bottle use at this young age.

If your child refuses milk out of a cup, don't fret. As you learned above, toddlers don't actually have to drink milk at all. So don't worry if losing the bottle also means very little milk. Most kids do start taking milk in other ways. Even if they don't, there's plenty of other ways to get calcium.

Teeth. You don't need to use a toothbrush and toothpaste yet until the molars come in, which usually doesn't happen until eighteen months. Wiping the teeth with a washcloth every day is adequate.

Biting, hitting, and other undesirable behaviors. Some kids will start exploring the limits of acceptable behavior at this age. This is actually a positive thing, because it displays

 DR. SEARS TIP
"No" Is a No-No

Instead of constantly saying "no" to your toddler, personalize your directive: "Not for [your child's name]." Otherwise your toddler will start saying "no" a lot. It's an easy word for toddlers to say, and it eventually loses its impact.

a more outgoing and expressive personality. Discipline doesn't have to be too complicated or strict just yet. Simply saying, "Ow! No biting" or whatever applies to the situation, and either walking away from the scene or moving your baby away and putting him down somewhere else is enough to get your message across.

Development

Here are the developmental milestones that most babies will achieve by this age:

- gross motor — crawls well, crawls up stairs, stands without holding on, cruises around furniture. Many babies will be walking by this time, although some won't walk until fifteen months. Frequent falls are common.

- fine motor — has accurate pincer grasp (thumb and forefinger), points with index finger, stacks blocks, shows hand dominance, may be able to drink from sippy cup unassisted.

- language — many babies will know one or two words at this age, such as *Mama* or *Dada*. Some babies won't use any specific words. Your baby should be using a lot of jargon (many different consonant/vowel combinations).

- social — waves bye-bye, points, understands "no" and other simple commands. When you ask where an object is, such as "Where's doggy?" your baby should turn, look, and point.

You can promote your baby's development in the coming months by letting her:

- throw balls

- push/pull toys while walking

- play "this-little-piggy"

- learn facial parts — "Where's Mommy's nose?"

- empty cabinets and containers of toys

- learn animal sounds

Safety

The nine-month concerns continue to apply at this age and beyond. Here are a few new ideas to follow:

Car-seat safety. Before 2009, laws and safety guidelines stated that when a baby turned one year *and* weighed twenty pounds or more, parents could turn the car seat to the forward-facing position. However, research has shown that it is safer to stay rear-facing beyond this age and weight. A toddler is five times more likely to be seriously injured in an accident in a forward-facing car seat compared to the rear-facing position. New guidelines have just been developed that state a baby should remain rear-facing until at least two years of age and can continue to remain rear-facing up to the height or weight limit of the particular car seat (there is no age limit). If your baby has been using a smaller rear-facing-only car seat, you may find that you'll need to upgrade to a larger "convertible" seat that will accommodate your child's growing body up until age two in the rear-facing position. You will find weight and height limitations on the side of the seat. Once your child's height or weight exceeds the rear-facing limit specific to your car seat (regardless of age), it's time to turn the seat around. Another car-seat tip:

Don't let your child see how you unbuckle the seat strap; you don't want her learning how to unbuckle herself.

Sun protection and hat-wearing. What makes us get facial wrinkles when we get older? It is *not* the sun exposure we endure during our adult life. It is the cumulative sun damage we experienced during childhood and adolescence. Start protecting your child at an early age from sun damage to the face and eyes by having her wear a hat whenever she goes outside for extended periods. Sunblock is also a good idea when your child is going to play outside for a few hours.

Reaching up to counters and tables. Be aware that Baby will try to reach objects up on tables and countertops or pull on tablecloths. Do not leave any heavy or breakable objects near table and counter edges. Try to only use the back burners on the stovetop, especially when boiling water.

DR. SEARS TIP
A Safe Room

Some parents find the idea of babyproofing the entire house overwhelming or impractical. A nice alternative is to create just one room that is completely safe for your toddler. Block it off with furniture and a baby-gate system bolted into the wall. Choose a centrally located room, such as the family room, so that your child can play safely for hours with his toys and other objects while you move about the house doing whatever you need to do while still keeping an eye and ear on him. Of course, when your child wants to explore other parts of the house that aren't fully babyproofed, he must be supervised.

Most Common One-Year Illnesses

Besides regular colds, coughs, and ear infections, here are some common ailments your child may experience over the next few months:

Viral sore throats. The most common cause of sore throats in the first three years are viruses, not bacteria like strep. So these are usually not treatable with antibiotics. See page 514 for information.

Pink eye. During your child's early years, he is bound to have red eyes at least once. See page 307 if this occurs.

Colds and ear infections. These become more common between age one and three years. See page 222 if your child catches a cold.

Vaccines

During the first six months, your baby received three rounds of the same shots. Now it's time for three new shots your baby hasn't had before: MMR (Measles, Mumps, Rubella), Varicella (chicken pox), and Hep A. See page 43 for more details on the vaccination schedule.

Tuberculosis skin test. Some offices, especially those in large cities, will begin doing tuberculosis (TB) skin tests at this time and may repeat this every year hereafter to check to see if a toddler has been near someone with infectious tuberculosis. This serious lung infection is common among homeless persons and those who live in crowded conditions, but it can infect anybody. Kids typically don't show any signs of being sick if exposed, yet the germ will lie dormant within a child's body for many years, only to spontaneously activate and cause a very serious case of TB as an adult. The skin test will detect if your child is carrying the germ this way. If the test is positive, treatment can kill the dormant germs before they cause any harm. Some doctors who practice in suburban or rural areas, where TB is less common, may delay this test for a few years.

FIFTEEN-MONTH CHECKUP

What an exciting year this is going to be! Your baby's language and motor skills will increase dramatically, and her social interaction with you and others will mature surprisingly quickly. Your little baby will start to seem so "grown up"! Much of your time may be spent chasing her around the house to keep her from getting into trouble, but you will also enjoy your toddler's more advanced social and verbal responsiveness to you, her desire to learn new words and skills, and her ability to accurately communicate her wants and needs. Here is our guide to your fifteen-month-old.

Growth

Weight gain. Most toddlers will have gained one to two pounds since twelve months of age. More active toddlers who spend their whole day running around may have gained no weight at all, as they continue to burn off their baby fat.

Length and head size. These measurements are always checked, and your pediatrician will make sure your child is growing consistently.

Physical Exam

While your doctor should perform a complete physical exam at each checkup, here are some of the items she may pay extra attention to at this age:

Eyes. As always, the doctor will take a careful look at the eyes to make sure your child doesn't have a lazy eye that could affect long-term vision.

Tonsils. Some children will begin to have larger tonsils by this age. Although this usually has no effect on their health, it's useful to note if they are larger than normal now so that you can observe for breathing problems at night.

General. Ears, teeth, heart, lungs, abdomen, genitals, arms, legs, and back are just as important to examine as always.

Nutrition

Shape your toddler's taste buds. Back at your nine-month checkup, we encouraged you to feed your baby as naturally as possible. We would like to remind you again to "shape your child's tastes" by feeding your child only natural whole foods. Of course, such kids do grow up to enjoy treats as much as the next kid, but junk foods may not taste right to them, and they won't overdo it.

Breastfeeding. Some toddlers go through a clingy phase at this age and want to nurse more often than ever. It's almost as if they realize they're becoming independent and want to take a step back. Babies will mature through this after a few months and move out to explore the world again.

Calcium requirements. Babies need two to three servings of a calcium-rich food every day. If your child likes milk, and doesn't show any allergic signs, then a couple of cups each day are fine. If he doesn't, don't push it. Rely on other sources such as yogurt, cheese, and fortified orange juice.

Still using formula? Some parents find they are unable to get their child to drink milk or wean off the bottle. They may therefore continue using formula. That's okay. The only reason we tell parents to stop using formula at age one is the cost. There's physically nothing wrong with your child drinking formula for the rest of his life if he wants and if you want to pay for it. However, try to at least get your child off the bottle and on to sippy cups of milk or formula.

DR. SEARS TIP
Stuck on the Bottle

Some parents will allow their child to continue taking several bottles of milk or formula each day because he refuses to take a sippy cup, and parents worry that without milk or formula their child will be malnourished. This is not the case. Kids get plenty of nutrition from foods and other dairy products. So don't let your desire to get milk or formula into your child allow him to stay on the bottle through this year. It may be time for you to bite the bullet and restrict the bottles to comfort-routine times only or lose them altogether, especially at night. Nighttime bottles of milk, formula, or juice can cause tooth decay. Try a trick we call "watering down." Gradually dilute the milk or formula with water until your toddler gets all water in the bottle. Then you can "lose" the bottle and just provide water out of sippy cups.

General Health and Parenting Issues

Cow's-milk allergy. Although food allergies are fairly rare, the most common culprit is cow's milk. If your child has had more nasal congestion, cough, skin rashes, or diarrhea than normal over the past few months, consider a trial period off of cow's milk to see if these symptoms improve. See page 327 for more details on food allergy.

Kids who are allergic to milk may also get more ear infections due to the recurrent nasal congestion and frequent colds and coughs. If your child has had a recent ear infection, stop milk for several months and use an alternative milk, like soy, goat, almond, or, as a last resort, rice.

Picky eaters, part II. We mentioned this issue at your one-year checkup, and for some of you, the saga continues. If your child's finicky behavior hasn't changed, here are a couple of ideas that may help:

- Restrict milk to stimulate the appetite (don't restrict breastfeeding, though).

- Try reverse psychology by pretending you don't care if your toddler eats. This may spur his interest. See page 294 for more tips on picky eaters.

Teething. After the eight teeth in the front come in, the first molars are next. These are usually more painful and take longer to come in than other teeth. You will see the gums bulging near the back. Your baby may also begin waking up more often at night. See page 509 for tips on how to get through these particularly tough couple of months.

Tantrums. Although most people equate tantrums with "the terrible twos," you may find that your toddler begins having tantrums as early as fifteen months. At this age, there is not much you need to do about it. Alternate between consoling your child and stepping back to let her work it out on her own. It also helps to redirect her attention to something else or help her work through whatever caused the frustration. Realize that tantrums are normal behavior. Toddlers are supposed to respond this way when things don't go their way. It isn't your job to try to stop the tantrums or prevent them from happening. The goal is to help your child mature past this phase in a timely manner. You can read more about tantrums in *The Discipline Book*.

The car-seat battle. Many toddlers hate to be put in a car seat. They will kick and scream bloody murder while you struggle to buckle their arching and squirming bodies into the car seats. This is a normal phase of toddlerhood. But your child needs to learn that for this issue, there is no choice. Calmly reassure him as you gently force him into the seat. Do not get angry at him, because he is not really doing anything wrong. His brain is designed to protest this intrusion on his freedom. The calmer you remain, the sooner he will come to accept his place in the car seat. Give him a snack to distract him as you put him in.

Night-nursing. If your breastfed baby has always been somewhat of a night nurser, you may find he wants to night-nurse even more at this age. If you aren't bothered too much by this habit and aren't feeling too sleep-deprived, hang in there. This should slow down for good in a few months. If, on the other hand, you are finding yourself burned out, resentful, and dysfunctional during the day from lack of sleep, it may be time to make a change. Discouraging the all-night nurser or night weaning completely are complicated tasks. For more information, see *The Baby Sleep Book*.

Development

Here are the developmental milestones that most babies will achieve by this age:

- gross motor — walks well alone, may take running steps, able to climb out of high chair, climbs up stairs and ladders

- fine motor — feeds self with spoon, brushes hair and teeth (not well!), holds phone correctly, cooperates in dressing, can stack two small blocks, opens cabinets and containers, can hold own bottle well

- language — says approximately five intelligible words, speaks partial words ("ba" for *ball*, "do" for *dog*), says and gestures *no*, understands and follows simple directions

- social — knows your facial parts, asks for help by pointing and gesturing, recognizes and points to familiar named people and objects, laughs at funny scenes

You can promote your baby's development in the coming months by encouraging him to:

- push toy buggies and lawn mowers

- bang with toy hammer, practice stacking blocks

- learn parts of the body

- press buttons, turn knobs

- read picture books, learn animal sounds

Safety

Here are the primary safety issues that come into play as your baby matures and develops his skills and curiosity to a higher level:

Climbing safety. Babies love to climb. Be sure to anchor all bookshelves, cabinets, and dressers to the wall so that *when* (not if) your baby climbs up they won't tip over.

Kitchen. As your baby gets taller, her ability to reach up and pull things off the counter increases, so you'll need to keep an eye out.

Going outside. Your baby will soon know how to open doors, so you need to be extra vigilant about this. Use a chain lock on as many doors as you can so that you don't have to run after him when you hear the door slam.

Parking-lot safety. Toddlers love to let go of your hand and run across a parking lot. Teach your toddler the unbreakable rule that he must always hold your hand in a parking lot. If he protests, then carry him until he complies. Give him the choice to be carried or to walk holding your hand.

Most Common Fifteen-Month Illnesses

If your baby is getting sick more often than you feel is normal, there are some ways you can boost her immune system. See page 33 for more details. Besides regular colds, cough, and ear infections, your child may also experience the following:

Reactive airway disease (RAD). Has your child had several chest colds that have caused wheezing but otherwise seems very healthy? He may have a mild form of asthma called reactive airway disease (RAD). Though not true asthma, this form of wheezing during colds can be bothersome for you and your child. See page 152 for more information.

Vaccines

The shots that most doctors give at this age are boosters of two vaccines that were already given during infancy: PCV (pneumococcal) and Hib vaccines. See page 43 for more details.

EIGHTEEN-MONTH CHECKUP

Your toddler continues to amaze you! It seems as though she is saying a new word, learning a new task, or playing a new game almost every day. She seems so much more like an actual person now rather than a little baby who requires every need to be met. She has her own distinct personality, desires, moods, and abilities. Each day is going to bring new joys and challenges as your child transitions out of babyhood into toddlerhood. Here is our guide to meeting the rewards and challenges of this wonderful age:

Growth

Weight gain. Most toddlers will have gained one to one and three quarter pounds since their fifteen-month checkup. Some children won't have gained any weight, and that is okay. An active toddler burns a lot of calories, and the baby fat continues to melt away.

Length. Growth charts are designed based on height measured while the child is lying down until age two. However, some toddlers are reluctant to lie still for this, and doctors might begin measuring height standing up at this age. Toddlers measure shorter standing up than they do when lying down. This means that when your doctor begins to measure standing up, your child will appear not to have grown since the last visit. Your pediatrician will use this first standing height as a baseline for future height measurements.

Head circumference. This may be the last time your doctor measures the head size to make sure the growth is consistent.

Physical Exam

As your doctor performs a complete physical exam, here are some of the highlights she may focus on at this age:

Ears. Your doctor will check to make sure any colds, allergies, or ear infections your child has had haven't left residual ear congestion that can muffle the hearing.

Teeth. With first molars on the way or already there, your doctor will check to make sure they are healthy.

Neck. It's common for some pea-sized or larger lymph nodes to be found around your child's neck. The doctor will make sure these seem normal.

Spine. Now that your child is old enough to stand up and perhaps bend over and touch her toes, your doctor will want to take a good look at the spine in this position to make sure all is well.

Legs and feet. Your doctor will watch your child stand and walk to check for flat feet, knock-knees, and in-toeing.

What if your child doesn't comply with the exam? Many kids at eighteen months and two years of age are so fearful of the doctor's poking and prodding that they'll scream, cry, and claw their way up over your shoulder to get away. Of course, the doctor's exam isn't very

thorough under such conditions. If this describes your child, don't worry. It happens often enough for us to include it in our book, so you're in good company. The doctor will quickly check a few main things and then back off and discuss any concerns and questions you may have.

Autism screening. Autism is on the rise, and early detection and intervention can make a big difference in a child's eventual social and intellectual development. Doctors are now supposed to perform a specific autism screening test at eighteen months to look for early signs. Yet, early signs of autism can be subtle and difficult to pick up during a fifteen-minute doctor's appointment. You should be aware of what signs to watch for and share any concerns with your child's doctor. See page 167 for more on the detection of autism.

Nutrition

Slim toddlers. If your toddler is on the slim side, and you want to put a little more "meat on his bones," try to get him interested in eating more protein and healthy-fat foods such as fish, eggs, lean meats, nut butters, avocado, and legumes, and supplement with an omega-3 fish oil. Keep in mind, however, that if you or your spouse have slim body types or your other children are slim, then genetically your toddler may stay slim, and all the food in the world won't change that. Don't worry; slim kids are perfectly healthy.

Overweight toddlers. Some toddlers who really love to eat may retain much of their baby fat and put on even more, keeping their weight above the top line of the growth curve. Although this can still be healthy at this age, your doctor should assess whether or not your baby's weight trend is going in the wrong direction. If so, begin eliminating empty carbs like white breads and crackers, and limit milk to sixteen ounces per day. If Baby's weight gain doesn't slow down by age two, as we will discuss in that checkup, it will be time to read about our L.E.A.N. Kids Program on page 417.

Picky eaters, part III. Here are some ideas that might help at this age:

- Grazing. Instead of insisting your toddler sit down and eat a full meal three times a day, keep a plate of finger foods (healthy ones) on the table. Let him graze on and off throughout the day at his own pace.

- Share what's on your plate. Prepare your own plate of food to include things that your toddler can eat. Sit next to him and start eating. Give him bites off of your plate when he asks. See more picky-eater tips, page 294.

 DR. SEARS TIP
Table Manners? What's That?

You may find your toddler likes to spend more time having fun with his food than eating it at mealtime. What's more fun than making a mess? We believe it's unrealistic for you to expect your toddler to be a perfectly neat eater. Let him have fun and make a little mess, within reason. Gradually start teaching your toddler what type of behaviors are acceptable at the dinner table without starting too many battles of will.

Remember to use whole organic milk. If your child drinks milk, stay with whole milk until age two. Babies need the extra fat for brain growth at this age.

Breastfeeding. Continue breastfeeding as long as you and your baby are both enjoying this part of your relationship. Breast milk is the best source of calcium there is, and it contains some nutrients you won't find anywhere else. Don't worry that time at the breast may be taking away from the amount of "real" food your child would otherwise be eating. Breast milk is still just as nutritious as food.

Vitamins. Although children don't need these if they are generally good eaters, kids who are very slim or are still picky eaters may benefit from a little vitamin insurance. Chewable and liquid vitamins are available from any health-food or vitamin store. Choose one without artificial additives and sweeteners. You can also mix a vitamin-and-mineral-enriched protein powder into cereals or smoothies or a fruit and vegetable supplement product. See www.AskDrSears.com.

General Health and Parenting Issues

Still Haven't Lost That Bottle?

The main worries about prolonged bottle use are that it may contribute to an overbite and that falling asleep with bottles of milk can cause cavities. The closer your baby gets to age two, the harder it will be to wean her. The one thing you want to accomplish by this age is to eliminate daytime bottles. Bedtime bottles may be more challenging. Use a sippy cup, pacifier (if already using one), or other methods of calming and soothing to sleep. You may have to be your baby's "pacifier" by lying down with him while he falls asleep. Additional tricks include:

- "Losing" the bottles—You simply cannot find a bottle at bedtime and tell your baby "all gone."

- Bye-bye ceremony — You can have a little ceremony of throwing the bottles into the trash and saying "bye-bye, bottles" or "Baby is sooo big — no more bottles."

- Cut the nipple — For stubborn babies, you can try cutting the nipple hole so that he won't like it anymore.

If your baby simply refuses to go to bed without a bottle, at least try to fill it with water instead of milk. If it must be milk, don't let him fall asleep with milk in his mouth. Finish with some water to rinse the teeth off.

Brushing Teeth

Most toddlers hate to have their teeth brushed. However, those crevices in the molars are just begging for cavities. It is very important to brush twice a day. If your toddler is not yet accustomed to this, let him watch you brush your teeth in the mirror. Show him how much fun it is! Tell him every night that soon you will start brushing his teeth. After a week or two of this, Baby should be intrigued enough to let you start brushing for him. It's best not to use a fluoride toothpaste until your child is old enough to spit it out (age three or more). Natural toddler toothpastes that don't have artificial colors and sweeteners are best.

If your toddler continues to fight you on this, you have two choices. Wait a few months and then try again, or force the issue now. The longer you wait, the more you risk cavities. If you choose to force the issue now, here's how: Give your child a choice — you brush his teeth in the bathroom, lying down on the bed, or lying down on the floor. This gives him the power to choose. If he resists, then simply lay him down on the floor on his back with his head in between your knees and his arms pinned under your legs. This puts you in the "dentist" position and allows you to keep his head still. Gently insert the toothbrush between his clenched lips and brush away. It is very important for you to remain happy, positive, and calm and gently repeat such phrases as "It's okay, Mama's brushing your teeth" and "Almost done." Try not to make it seem like a battle. If your toddler senses that you are calm, he may calm down as well. After a week or two, most toddlers will learn to accept their fate.

Discipline

You may think you are months away from the "terrible twos," but most kids begin to show signs now. Does your toddler seem to do the opposite of whatever you ask him to do? Does he go around the playground hitting and pushing? Does he try to break just about every safety rule in the book? Well, of course he does! This is what he is supposed to do at this age. The key to toddler discipline isn't necessarily to change your child's behavior quickly. Rather, it's to help him mature through this stage before you go crazy. The primary discipline concept for this age is balance. On the one hand, you want to let your toddler be himself, have his way, and explore the world around him without dampening his curiosity. And you shouldn't expect perfect obedience. But you also want him to learn that there are certain lines that he can't cross. Find a balance between permissiveness and setting limits. We suggest that most of the limits that you enforce be safety violations or major issues (like hitting and biting). Use timeouts to help your toddler learn what is appropriate behavior and what is not. But don't expect him to learn quickly. It can take several months, and hundreds of timeouts, for a toddler to learn to stop an unwanted behavior, but patient persistence on your part will usually pay off. We suggest you check *The Discipline Book* for useful guidance on timeout and other ideas.

DR. SEARS TIP
Limit TV and Videos

Most parents love to be able to rely on a favorite video or TV show to keep a baby or toddler occupied when things get hectic around the house. If you must do so, keep it limited to a half hour, and try to make it something with music. As you learned on page 67, research has shown that extended TV or video watching (more than half an hour each day) can slow down a baby's intellectual development and can lead to later problems with attention deficit disorder (ADD). Even some videos that seem to be developmentally stimulating have been shown in research to be the exact opposite. It seems that the old saying "TV will rot your brain" may not be so far off, so never purposely let your baby watch the "tube" because you think it's good for him. If you need the occasional electronic babysitter, that's probably okay. Just keep it brief, and don't let it become a daily routine.

Development

Here are the developmental milestones that most toddlers will achieve by this age:

- gross motor — walks in circles and backward, runs, walks up stairs holding on to railing, bends down easily to pick up objects, climbs, rides toddler bike

- fine motor — able to stack four small blocks, feeds self with spoon without spilling much, scribbles with crayon, opens drawers and doors, cooperates with dressing

- language — typically knows at least ten words (some children may know fewer, some many more), points to and names objects, completes words ("ba" is now "ball"), understands many commands

- social — knows most body parts, feels less separation anxiety, plays hide-and-seek, dances to music

Here are some ways you can promote your baby's development in the coming months:

- Give her a wagon to pull.

- Read books to her, letting her turn pages herself.

- Assist her as she balances and walks on curbs or low walls.

- Let her "help" around the house.

- Encourage her to sing nursery songs.

- Point out colors.

Safety

Here are the primary safety issues that come into play as your baby matures and develops his skills and curiosity:

Crib safety. Your baby will soon try to climb out of the crib. When you think he is close to doing this, switch to a toddler bed.

Medicines/cleaners/poisons. The older your child gets, the stronger his curiosity grows and the more his ability to get into things increases. If you haven't already baby-proofed the areas where you keep these dangerous items, *do so now*.

Swimming pools. We have mentioned this before, but it bears repeating: You must have a safe fence and a childproof gate for your pool. Your child's ability to sneak out into the pool area is now greater than ever.

Most Common Eighteen-Month Illnesses

From this age on, children tend to catch a variety of illnesses such as fevers, sore throats, colds, ear infections, vomiting, diarrhea, the flu, rashes, and many other things. No particular illnesses are more or less common than others over the next few years, so we will no longer highlight any particular ones in each checkup.

Vaccines

The shots that most doctors give at this age are boosters of some vaccines that have already been given. These include DTaP, IPV, and Hep A. Some doctors give this third IPV shot as early as six months of age, so your child may not need any more at this point. See page 43 for more information on vaccines.

TWO-YEAR CHECKUP

This year will show remarkable advances in your child's skills, language abilities, and personality. Although the "terrible twos" have a reputation of being quite difficult, there are many things you can do to make this year a positive experience. Here is our guide to meeting the rewards and challenges of this wonderful age.

Growth

Weight gain. Most kids will have gained two to four pounds since the eighteen-month checkup. For two-year-old boys, the average weight is about twenty-seven pounds, and for girls, it is around twenty-five pounds. Normal weight ranges can be as much as four pounds above or below this. The natural slimming-down process that you may have seen between nine and eighteen months should be over; your child should be progressing along the growth curve normally.

Height. Most children will have grown about two inches since eighteen months. The average height for two-year-old is about thirty-four inches, with a normal range of two inches above or below this.

Your child's position on the percentile curve at this age is some indication of whether or not he will eventually end up being tall, average, or shorter than average. Many people believe that you can determine your child's eventual height simply by doubling his height at age two. This sometimes does turn out to be true but not in most cases. Genetics can cause kids to suddenly grow faster later on, or even to slow down.

Head circumference. This will be the last time your doctor checks head circumference (some stop at eighteen months if all is well). Most head growth occurs in the first two years of life, so if growth has been normal up to this point, you don't need to follow it anymore.

Overall body type. By now you will have an idea of what kind of body type your child has. You can determine this by comparing the weight to the height. If the weight percentile is much higher than height, your child has a heavier body type. If they are similar, whether high or low, this is a medium body type. If the weight is much lower than the height percentile, then your child will probably be slim. Of course, this isn't an exact prediction: Your child's growth pattern may alter later on because of genetics as well as nutritional habits.

Physical Exam

As your child's doctor performs a complete physical exam, here are some of the highlights she may focus on at this age:

Ears. Because good hearing is important for language development, it's useful to have your pediatrician check each year for ear wax buildup or mucus congestion in the ears.

Teeth. The two-year molars, the last of the baby teeth, typically come in around this time. Once these are in, it's time to think about seeing a dentist.

Tonsils. These tend to gradually grow larger until age six. Your pediatrician will check to see how they are doing now.

Heart and lungs. The doctor will listen to these carefully to check for problems with asthma or heart disease.

Skin. Point out any moles you've noticed so that the doctor can make note of these.

Social development. The doctor will also assess your toddler's social development and interaction to make sure there isn't any delay in this area.

Autism screening. The doctor may have performed a basic screening test at the eighteen-month checkup, but watching for proper social development doesn't end there. See page 167 for a review of how to screen for autism and how early detection and intervention can make a huge difference.

Nutrition

Nutrition 101. A basic understanding of balanced nutrition is important for every parent. We encourage you to educate yourself about healthy eating for the whole family by reading *The Healthiest Kid in the Neighborhood*. You will learn what foods to offer your children, what *not* to serve them or buy at all, and how to get them to want to grow up to be healthy and wise eaters. See page 93 for an introductory lesson on good nutrition.

Overweight kids. If your child has remained on the top of the weight growth curve or is moving higher and higher over the top, it is time to begin addressing this through nutrition and behavior modification. If you and your spouse have slim or average body types, then with some basic changes your child should follow suit. However, if your family has larger body types, then your child's genetics will be working against him, and growing up with a healthy body type will be a greater challenge. With some wise changes in nutrition and lifestyle, you can set the stage for a leaner future for your whole family. See our L.E.A.N. Kids Program section, page 417, for some guidelines to help you get started.

Switch to low-fat milk. At this age, you no longer have to use whole milk. Switch your child over to organic low-fat milk.

Calcium requirements. Remember that kids need about two to three servings of a calcium-rich food every day. Cow's milk, goat's milk, soy milk, almond milk, breast milk, yogurt, cheese, calcium-fortified orange juice, and green vegetables are all good sources of calcium.

General Health and Parenting

Dental health. Most doctors recommend that your child see the dentist as soon as all the baby teeth are in, which occurs between ages two and three. He should go sooner if your pediatrician notices any problems, or if you believe your child will be cooperative. Here are some steps to follow to insure your child's teeth stay healthy:

- Brush your child's teeth twice daily. We recommend you use a natural non-fluoride toothpaste for now. Most popular children's toothpastes from grocery or drugstores are loaded with artificial sugars (like saccharin), food coloring, and other chemicals. These are not the kinds of things you want to be grinding into your child's teeth every night.

- Floss. Young children's teeth tend to be close together, which can lead to cavities in between the teeth by age three or four. Try to floss your child's teeth a few times each week.

- Don't let your child fall asleep with a bottle of milk. The milk sugar stays on the teeth and causes decay.

Discipline. Whether your child is still right in the middle of "the terrible twos" or is just starting them, read page 83 for some useful tips on setting limits, giving timeouts, and minimizing tantrums. As your child grows older, his ability to understand guidance and instruction will mature, and your approach should grow and change with your child.

Sleep. By this age, your child has either learned to fall asleep on her own in her own bed, or she still requires you to "parent" her to sleep in her bed or yours. If you are in this second group, realize that your child will probably continue to need you for bedtime for at least another year. You can gradually begin the process of teaching your child to go to bed on her own over this year — in *The Baby Sleep Book* we show you how. However, some parents cherish their nighttime ritual with their child. If you do, then continue as you are. There's no hurry to make your child grow up and become independent.

Potty training. Most kids don't train until closer to age three, and pushing a child too early can create resistance. The best approach at this young age is to do nothing. Allow your child to watch you use the toilet, talk about it, make it seem fun, and leave it at that. Wait for your child to show that she wants to try. If it's her idea (instead of yours) she'll be much more excited. Buy some pairs of underwear and place them where your child will routinely notice them. Ask your child if she wants to try them on like a big girl. This will help prompt toilet use.

Development

Here are the developmental milestones that most children will achieve by this age:

- gross motor — runs well, jumps off a step, may pedal tricycle, walks up stairs without holding on, kicks ball without falling, opens doors, throws ball overhand

- fine motor — able to stack six small blocks, may copy a line or circle with a crayon, removes clothes, unwraps presents, does simple puzzles

- language — typically knows at least twenty words (some children may know fewer, some may know fifty words or more), talks in two- to three-word (or longer) sentences, speech is somewhat understandable to a stranger, understands much more than able to speak, answers simple questions (e.g., "What does a cat say?")

- social — washes hands, cooperates with dressing, says own name, sings

The following will help promote your child's development in the coming year:

- Gymnastics, somersaults, playgrounds

- Reading books, turning pages herself

- Using her own table and chairs

- "Helping" around the house

- Singing nursery songs

Safety

Here are the primary safety issues that come into play as your child matures and develops his skills and curiosity:

Time for a toddler bed. Most two-year-olds are capable of climbing out of a crib. If you haven't done so already, transition to a toddler bed low to the floor. Don't wait until you are woken up in the middle of the night by a loud thump as your child hits the floor after climbing over the crib rail.

Hats and sun protection. Try to get your child to be a hat lover. Whenever you are going to be outside for more than a half hour, on goes the hat. Sunscreen is also important

for outdoor day trips. Kids do need some sunlight to help generate their own natural vitamin D through the skin, so make sure your child gets three to four hours of outdoor playtime each week, without sunblock. See page 31 for more details.

Car seats. New car-seat guidelines state that a child should use a car seat in the rear-facing position until at least two years of age and that it's safer to continue in this position beyond age two until the child exceeds the upper weight or height limit for the car seat. Even though your child is now old enough to turn around to the forward position, it's best for her to remain rear-facing as long as possible. Once your child has graduated into the forward-facing position, continue to use the car seat until at least four years of age. Follow the instructions on the side of the car seat or in the instruction manual.

Vaccines

Most doctors will have given your child his last infant shot at eighteen months. Some pediatricians, however, may spread the shots out a bit more and leave some final ones for age two. Your child may also get a flu shot each year at the beginning of flu season (October or November). See page 43 for more details.

THREE-YEAR CHECKUP

You've made it through the "twos," hopefully without too many new gray hairs — but you're not out of the woods yet. The preschool years can bring even more challenges, only now your child is smarter, stronger, more talkative, and more opinionated. This age is also very rewarding for parents as they watch their child's language, abilities, curiosity, and personality soar! Here is the Dr. Sears guide to your child's three-year visit to the pediatrician.

Growth

Weight gain. Most children will have gained about three pounds since age two. Average weight for three-year-olds is thirty-one pounds, give or take about four pounds.

Height. Children will have grown approximately three and a half inches and follow a similar percentile curve since age two. Although weight gain was the main indicator of proper growth in the first two years, by age three and beyond we pay much more attention to height gain. Growing faster than usual is fine at this age, but falling lower and lower on the height percentile curve may indicate a problem. Average height for three-year-olds is thirty-eight inches for boys and thirty-seven and a half for girls, with a variation of about two inches taller or shorter. Switch to the older-child growth charts on pages 111–114 from now on.

Body mass index (BMI). This is a new measurement your doctor should begin calculating at each visit. It is an assessment of how well your child's weight matches his height. Your doctor can tell you what your child's BMI is, but you can also calculate it yourself. Simply take the weight in pounds, divide that by the height in inches, divide that number by the height again, then multiply that result by 703. The final number is the BMI:

Weight (pounds) ÷ Height (inches) ÷ Height (inches) × 703

You can chart your child's BMI on page 112 or 114. A normal range is 15–17 at this age.

Physical Exam

Yearly physical exams performed by your pediatrician are very important from now until age six, at which time every two years is adequate. There are many important physical aspects about your growing child that a doctor needs to evaluate on a regular basis. Certain medical conditions can show up at any time during a child's life, and many of these conditions can be found early by your pediatrician during a complete physical exam. Here are the important aspects of the exam at this age:

Eyes. Children can develop "lazy eye," a condition in which the eyes do not coordinate well with each other. The doctor can identify this condition early before it has a permanent effect on your child's vision.

Ears. Children can develop two problems with their ears. One is wax buildup, which can sometimes completely block the ear canal and muffle your child's hearing. The other problem your doctor will check for is ear fluid or congestion behind the eardrums, which can also lead to muffled hearing.

Teeth. Children usually begin going to the dentist by age three. Your pediatrician will look for any major problems and remind you to start taking your child to the dentist.

Tonsils. Tonsils can begin enlarging at this age; this is normal. They may continue to enlarge until age seven, then slowly shrink back down again. If too large, they can block breathing at night. Your pediatrician may ask you about nighttime snoring or breathing problems if the tonsils appear unusually large.

Neck glands. Most kids have some glands in the neck that are easy to feel, which is usually normal. Your pediatrician will check to make sure none of these glands are too large and check for any abnormal underarm glands.

Heart. Heart disease is extremely rare in children. Most childhood heart problems occur at birth or early in infancy. It is important, however, for the doctor to listen carefully for any signs of abnormal heartbeat or function.

Lungs. Your pediatrician will listen for any wheezing sounds.

Back. Scoliosis (an abnormal curving of the spine to the right or left) is not uncommon. When it does occur, it is usually during adolescence, and it will only rarely occur during infancy. It is important for your pediatrician to check each year to make sure the spine is straight.

Abdomen. Your doctor will feel your child's belly to make sure no organs are enlarged and no tumors or masses are present (these, of course, are extremely rare).

Genitals. For girls, your doctor will check to make sure the inner labia are not stuck together (a condition called *labial adhesions*). Beyond this age, most male doctors won't examine a girl's genital area because of concerns about privacy as well as because there isn't anything medical to check until puberty. For boys, your doctor will continue to check the testicles to make sure there are no tumors growing (extremely rare) and to look for *hernias* (a large bulge of intestine pushing down into the scrotal sac).

Legs and feet. The doctor will check for any unusual curvature in the legs and make sure your child isn't developing flat feet.

Skin. Almost all children develop some small moles on their skin. Your doctor will make sure none of the moles appear abnormal.

Blood pressure. Kids are now old enough to cooperate with a blood pressure cuff. The doctor (or nurse) will test blood pressure every year from now on.

Nutrition

Eating habits. By this time, it will be clear whether you have been blessed with a good eater or a picky one. Don't expect this to change much over this year. Follow our suggestions on page 294 to help get enough nourishment into your child.

A word of encouragement: keep in mind that there have been billions of picky eaters before yours. You may have been one of them. Even though your child may not get quite enough of each important vitamin and mineral, and might not get quite as much protein and fat as he should, in the long run, he will grow up just fine.

Say no to added sugar. Now that your child is going to be out and about in the world, she's sure to be offered junk food sooner or later. Hopefully you've been minimizing this at home, but should you be just as strict at parties, playgroups, and other outings? What we found worked great for us is the "one-treat-a-day" rule. As your child discovers treats, make a big deal of pointing out that this is a treat and she only gets one today. Promote a "one-treat-a-day" rule so your child grows up knowing she can't overdo it outside the home. Of course, some days will go by without even coming across any opportunities for a treat.

Restaurants. Be careful what you order when going out to eat. Most kids' menu items are high in trans fats. Order your child a healthier option off the adult menu, such as chicken or fish. Some restaurants will serve your child something like this at a kids' meal price. Avoid condiments and salad dressings, as these usually have corn syrup or chemicals like MSG (monosodium glutamate).

For more useful nutrition information, check out one of these three books in the Sears Parenting Library:

- *The N.D.D. Book: How Nutrition Deficit Disorder Affects Your Child's Learning, Behavior, and Health, and What You Can Do About It — Without Drugs*

- *The Healthiest Kid in the Neighborhood*

- *The Family Nutrition Book*

General Health and Parenting

Time for school? Some parents start their kids in preschool around age three. Others wait until four. There's no right or wrong choice here. It depends on your own child's needs, level of social development, and desire for more interaction with peers and other adult authority figures. Keep in mind that *academically* a child doesn't need school until age four or about one year before kindergarten. Starting school at age three is mainly for social development.

Boosting the immune system. When your child first begins school, you can be sure she'll catch more than her fair share of coughs and colds (unless she's been around a lot of other young children growing up and had plenty of colds already). You can help minimize these by supplementing your child with echinacea, vitamin C, zinc, probiotics, omega-3 oils, and other nutritional supplements. See page 33 for more details.

First dentist visit. By this age, your child should have all her baby teeth, and it will be time to go to the dentist. Start by having her go with you to your visit (as long as no major work is planned). Make it seem fun. Tell your child it's her turn next time, and plan a suitable reward she can look forward to (like a visit to a nearby toy store on the way home). Pediatric dentists are great, and so is your family dentist if you feel he or she is good with kids.

Discipline. If your child is like most others, the "terrible twos" may seem like nothing compared to the types of tantrums and defiance that can come out at this age. Although such behaviors are normal, it is useful to begin instructing your child regarding obedience, listening, using nice voices, and so on. Don't expect perfection, or anything even close, for another year or two. Using a combination of positive and negative reinforcement techniques such as star charts and timeouts will help your child mature through this age. See page 83 for a discussion on child behavior issues and *The Discipline Book* for more information on appropriate use of techniques.

Development

Here are the developmental milestones that most children will achieve by three years:

- gross motor — able to balance on one foot for at least one second, can jump over a sheet of paper placed on the floor, alternates feet when walking up stairs, pedals a tricycle

- fine motor — able to draw a straight line and circle, can undo buttons, wiggles thumb, can stack eight small blocks, able to undress completely and partially dress

- language — a large vocabulary (two hundred words or more), uses three- to four-word sentences, uses pronouns and plurals correctly, knows a few colors

- social — has an imagination, is potty-trained (at least for urination), knows full name and age, shares toys and takes turns, knows and names friends

 **DR. SEARS TIP
When Is Speech
Therapy Needed?**

By three years of age, about 75 percent of what a young child says should be understandable to a stranger. This means that you shouldn't often have to translate for your child when talking to other adults. Of course, you may understand everything your child is trying to say, but if others often can't, it may be time to see a speech therapist. Early intervention for unclear speech can save your child from some frustration when school starts.

Here are some ways you can promote your child's development in the coming year:

- music participation classes

- playdates

- frequent trips to a playground

- playing together with puzzles and building blocks

- imaginary role-playing or costume games together

- paper for drawing and coloring

Safety

Helmets and pads. Riding trikes and scooters typically begins at this age, and it's important to instill a proper respect for personal injury prevention. Helmets, elbow pads, and knee pads should be a must for any type of riding.

Street smarts. As outdoor play becomes more frequent, so does a child's tendency to run out into the street unaware of the danger. Teach your child to stop, to look both ways, and never to go into the street without holding a grown-up's hand.

Swimming pools. Even if you don't have a pool, we suggest swimming lessons (professional or just do-it-yourself) so your child can be more water-safe. If you have a pool, make sure it is childproofed with an appropriate fence and lock.

Car seats. Remember, your toddler must stay buckled into a car seat (using the car seat's own built-in harness) until at least four years of age. Although it is safest for her to remain in a rear-facing position as long as the car seat accommodates her height and weight (these limits vary with each car seat; see your instruction manual or information printed on the side of the car seat), most children will exceed one of these limits by age three. When this happens, turn the seat around and continue to use the car seat until she reaches at least four years of age.

Vaccines

There usually aren't any three-year shots except for a flu vaccine given during October through December. Some doctors will do a TB skin test (see page 76) at this age, others will wait until the kindergarten checkup.

FOUR- THROUGH SIX-YEAR CHECKUPS

As your toddler matures into a child, life will bring a new round of joys and challenges. Here is our guide to understanding your child's checkups during the prekindergarten and kindergarten years (we've grouped these years into one section):

Growth

Weight. Most kids will have gained about four pounds since last year, but for the next few years weight gain increases a little faster, at about five pounds per year. At age five, the average weight is about forty pounds. Slim five-year-olds can weigh as little as thirty-three pounds and heavier kids as much as forty-eight pounds and still be considered within the typical range.

Height. Height gain slows down significantly by this age, and children typically gain about two and a half inches per year for the next several years. The average height for five-year-olds is about forty-three inches. The normal variation is considered to be two and a half inches above or below.

Body mass index (BMI). Your pediatrician should be assessing this measure at each checkup. A healthy BMI for children at this age is between 14½ and 16 (see charts on pages 112 and 114). This will slowly increase during the preteen years. If his BMI is too high, your child may weigh more than what is healthy for his height, and you may need to pay closer attention to what he is eating and increase his activity level. If it is too low, some extra calories and healthy protein and fat may be in order. You can calculate BMI using the formula on page 89.

Physical Exam and Health Screening Tests

The physical exam at this age is similar to the one at the three-year checkup. By this time a child is old enough to begin cooperating with some basic health screening tests:

Vision. The nurse will likely give your child a vision test with a standard eye chart. Normal vision for four-year-olds is between 20/30 and 20/40. By age six, a child's vision should have matured to a perfect 20/20. If your child's vision falls outside of the normal range, a more thorough exam by an eye doctor is warranted.

Hearing. The nurse will also give your child a hearing test using headphones and quiet beep tones.

Urine test. Your child will pee in a cup, and this will be checked for sugar, blood, and protein to screen for diabetes and kidney disease.

Nutrition

We've written entire books on this topic, and we suggest you fully educate yourself about your family's nutrition. Here are some basic ideas to keep in mind for your family:

Doctor's pep talk. At this age it's useful to ask your pediatrician to give your child a two-minute pep talk on good nutrition. Children are usually very open to taking instruction from the doctor. Ask the doctor to address issues such as finishing dinner, eating vegetables, choosing fruit for snack, and limiting junk food. Parents can use the "Dr. Bob says..." line if kids need a reminder throughout the year. Of course, this doesn't work for everybody, but it's worth trying. Instead of referring to nutritious foods as "healthy," find more creative labels, such as "grow foods" or "run-fast foods." One preteen patient in our office asked us when he was going to start his growth spurt. We told him what "tall foods" he could start eating more of. His mom called later to thank us for getting her child to eat more fruits, vegetables, whole grains, and fish.

Nutritional supplements. Most kids who eat a well-balanced diet and are generally healthy don't need any particular supplements. But that's the problem; most kids don't eat a diet rich in fruits and veggies, omega-3 fats, and other nutrients (despite the pep talk). Here is a list of the most appropriate supplements that are worth the cost:

- omega-3 oil (fish oil) — 400 to 500 milligrams daily

- multivitamin — for extra insurance

- fruit- and vegetable-based supplements

- probiotics (see page 27)

Protein. A high-protein breakfast greatly enhances learning and attention. Kids need *at least* twenty to twenty-five grams of protein per day (or half a gram for every pound they weigh, whichever is more), which means at least two servings of the following: dairy products, fish, meats, nut butters, nuts and seeds, eggs, soy, and legumes.

Carbohydrates. Incorporate the following into your family's diet: fruits, veggies, whole-grain breads and cereals, legumes, dairy, and nut butters.

Fats. Include the following healthy fats in your meals: fish, oils (such as fish, flax, nut, olive), avocado, eggs, nuts, and seeds. Use only lean meats to limit animal fats.

Calcium. Kids need about 800 milligrams daily, which they can get from two to three servings of the following: milk (cow, goat, soy, or almond), eggs, yogurt, and dark green veggies.

As you can see, many of these foods overlap, and they should be the backbone of your family's diet.

General Health and Parenting

Sleep. Children should get eleven to twelve hours of sleep each night, and by age four most kids will have given up their naps. If your child isn't waking up easily to get ready for school, an earlier bedtime may be in order. It's common for some kids to still need you to stay nearby while they sleep. We wrote a whole chapter on how to wean your child from this gradually and without fuss in *The Baby Sleep Book*.

Discipline. By this age, your child should be maturing out of the "even more terrible threes." It's time to begin offering more guidance and direction when it comes to whining, obedience, respect, rules, and helping around the house. Without being too strict, which can dampen a child's self-esteem, appropriate discipline helps build your child's character and confidence. See *The Discipline Book* for more information.

Development

By this age, we no longer track the specific areas of motor, language, and social development, so there are no particular milestones to anticipate. The main way to know that your child is thriving in these various areas is to watch him in playgroups and classrooms. But parents aren't the most objective observers and are likely to dismiss or overlook issues that may be apparent to others. The best source of assessment is probably your child's teacher. She should let you know if she has any concerns. And the fifteen or twenty minutes your pediatrician spends with you during your yearly checkup is often long enough for him to notice any significant social or intellectual developmental delays.

Sports and classes. Even if your child isn't athletic, participation in local sports leagues is fairly important, not only for exercise but also for building social confidence and learning respect for adult authority figures like coaches. If your child doesn't seem to enjoy sports, there are plenty of classes and lessons he or she can explore, like gymnastics, dance, music, martial arts, and swimming.

Safety

Strangers. Have a talk once or twice each year about stranger safety and remind your child that genitals are private and should only be seen by Mom or Dad, or, in some cases, the doctor.

Helmets. Helmet safety becomes even more important as your child's abilities, balance, and speed increase. Be sure to ask your doctor for a mini–pep talk on this topic as well.

Car seats. Children should use a car seat (and the five-point harness that's built into it) until at least four years of age. Beyond age four, it's safest to continue using the seat and harness for as long as possible until your child's height or weight exceeds your particular car seat's and harness's upper limit. This limit varies widely among various seats, but many will accommodate a child up through eighty pounds and fifty inches. Be sure to check your car seat's limit. Once your child outgrows your current car-seat harness, you have three options: Buy a car seat designed for older children that has a five-point harness they can use for several more years; remove your current car seat's harness (if it has that option) and use the seat as a booster with the car's own seat belt; or buy a new booster seat for your child to use with the car's seat belt. The first choice is probably the safest. Regardless of what you do, continue to at least use a booster seat until your child is 4 feet 9 inches tall, which usually occurs between eight and twelve years of age. At that height, your child is tall enough to safely use the car seat belt without a booster.

Vaccines

Before kindergarten begins, your child will need boosters of four shots that she had as an infant. These are DTaP, IPV (polio), MMR, and varicella (chicken pox). A yearly flu shot is also recommended. A TB (tuberculosis) skin test is also done again. Some doctors do these all at once at the four- or five-year checkup, while others split them up over two years. See page 43 for more information.

SEVEN- THROUGH TWELVE-YEAR CHECKUPS

Children should have thorough checkups during the elementary years. If your child is very healthy, growing well, and has no ongoing medical problems, you can probably get by with a checkup every other year. Your doctor will focus on several aspects of your child's health, including height and weight gain, proper nutrition, sports health, injury prevention, and any chronic health conditions that have persisted into childhood. Here is our guide to what typically happens at a checkup at this age and how you can contribute to monitoring your child's health.

Growth

Weight. At this age, your child enjoys more access to food outside the home, and you have less control over what he eats at school, friends' houses, and parties. With any luck, your lessons on healthy eating sank in. Average weight for seven-year-olds is fifty pounds and for twelve-year-olds is about ninety pounds. Kids will typically gain four to eight pounds each year between ages seven and ten, and about six to twelve pounds yearly until age twelve. Gaining more than this in one year isn't a big deal, but two or three years of faster weight gain doesn't bode well for a healthy body type as an adult. Now is the time to intervene. See our discussion on childhood obesity, page 417.

Height. Average height at age seven is about forty-eight inches for both boys and girls. Children gain about two to two and a half inches each year until age ten or eleven. Then the pubertal growth spurts typically begin. If your child is growing less than one and a half inches each year for more than two years, this may indicate a growth hormone deficiency. On the other hand, growing too quickly (four or more inches each year before age ten) can also indicate a problem with precocious puberty, a situation in which adolescent hormones surge too early and cause accelerated growth. See page 438 for more details.

Body mass index (BMI). Be sure your doctor calculates BMI for you and shows you where your child falls on the curve. Watch your child's BMI carefully over these years so you can intervene if it gets too high. Average BMI for both boys and girls is about 15½ at age seven and increases to 18 by age twelve.

Adolescent growth spurts. Parents (and preteens) often wonder when that long-awaited growth spurt is scheduled to begin. Ladies first (literally): girls begin growing faster between age ten and eleven, and continue until about age thirteen. Growth will then begin to slow down again. For boys, the growth spurt starts between eleven and twelve, and continues until age fourteen. Children will gain about three inches each year during the spurt. The timing of growth spurts can vary; late bloomers may start a year or two behind, but the spurt should continue to a later age as well.

Physical Exam and Health Screening Tests

Physical Exam

A thorough physical exam is still important every other year. Your pediatrician should look for the following problems from head to toe:

Head. Ear wax, enlarged tonsils, and neck glands.

Heart and lungs. The doctor will listen for abnormal heart rhythms and sounds, wheezing in the lungs.

Back. The doctor will check for spinal symmetry. Scoliosis can begin to develop toward the preteen years.

Abdomen. The doctor will examine for signs of enlarged organs or masses.

Genitals. The doctor completes testicle checks for hernias and masses.

Fingertips. Swollen nail beds can be a sign of heart disease.

Legs and feet. The doctor will examine for signs of flat feet.

Skin. The doctor will look for abnormal moles, growths, or rashes.

Screening Tests

Blood pressure. As children near puberty, high blood pressure can become apparent and should be screened every couple of years.

Vision. Some children begin to lose some distance vision, especially if this runs in the family. But kids often won't report this to parents for fear of needing glasses. Be sure the nurse checks this.

Cholesterol. If anyone in your family has a genetic cholesterol disorder, be sure to ask your doctor to begin screening for this at an early age. If no such thing runs in your family, it can wait until the preteen years.

Urine. Urine should be screened for diabetes and kidney problems at each checkup.

Nutrition

We hope that by the time your child reaches this age range, good nutrition habits have set in for the whole family. Here are a few additional tips to keep in mind during the elementary-school years:

Soda. During the elementary-school years kids begin to develop a taste for carbonated beverages. We hope you are setting a good example and are keeping the "diabetes in a can" (our term for soda) out of the house. Sure, kids may grab an occasional soda when out with friends, but it should not be a custom at every restaurant or fast-food joint you hit as a family. There are two things about soda that make it particularly bad for kids: (1) The sugar really adds up and creates a risk for diabetes and obesity; and (2) the phosphoric acid carbonation in most colas sucks the calcium right out of the bones and sets children up for fractures during sports and weakened joints and bones when they are older. Don't bring it into the house!

Portion control. One of the easiest steps to take if your child is trending toward the large side is to make sure he eats reasonable portion sizes at dinner. Most kids tend to eat the same amount at breakfast and lunch (because there's usually a time limit to these meals), but dinner has the potential to be a bottomless pit. Allow your child to eat a regular helping of "firsts," then relax and chat for ten to fifteen minutes; it takes that long for a full stomach to let the brain know it's had enough. If your child still wants "seconds," make it a few bites of the main course as well as veggies again, not another plateful of the main course. It's especially important to limit the carbs at dinner (breads and pastas). Remember the Dr. Sears rule of twos:

- Eat *half* as much
- Eat *twice* as often
- Chew *twice* as long
- Take *twice* the time to dine

"Brainy" breakfasts. By this age, what your child eats for breakfast becomes more important as the expectations for better attention and focus at school increase. The three main ingredients for a "brainy" breakfast are protein, omega-3 fat, and antioxidants. Here are some good suggestions:

- veggie omelet with whole-grain toast and milk

- berries, yogurt, and granola

- nut butter on whole-grain English muffin, fruit and berries

- half of a whole-grain bagel, peanut butter, and orange juice

- breakfast burrito with veggies and cheese

- breakfast smoothie with milk, yogurt, berries, protein powder (see page 15)

- omega-3 fish oil supplement

General Health and Parenting

Discipline. You'll probably begin to experience more talking back, sassiness, and arguments as your child gets older, especially right before puberty begins. This is normal and to be expected. In fact, it's probably a good sign that your child begins to stand up for herself and think she's always right. Find a balance: Let your child stand up for herself without allowing disrespect for parents and other authority figures to set in.

Peer influences. The old saying "you become like those around you" becomes truer as your child's social life expands. Although you can't always choose your child's friends, you can steer him toward other families and children that you have a good feeling about.

Sports. Sports are a great way to keep your child in shape, build confidence, and establish friendships. If your child isn't naturally athletic (which can eventually become counterproductive to self-esteem in team sports as your child gets older), you can still keep him active in individual sports, lessons, and classes such as tennis, gymnastics, martial arts, and dance.

Music. Now is the time to begin exploring your child's musical talent. Piano lessons are a great way to learn the basics. Depending on your child's skills and interest, expand into other instruments over the years.

Safety

Helmets. As kids get older, it becomes less and less "cool" to wear head protection while riding, scooting, or skating. Ask your pediatrician to throw in a quick reminder about what it's like to suffer a brain injury from falling without a helmet.

Firearms. As you begin to allow your child to play at other houses, it's important to find out if the host family owns a gun. Tragic accidents happen every year when curious children find an improperly stored firearm. If your children are going to be regular playmates with a neighbor, insist that your acquaintance lock up any guns and store the ammunition in a separate locked place. (If you own a gun, it is extremely important that you also take these precautions.) You may want to let your child know that the family owns a gun (if you feel that's appropriate), how dangerous a gun is, and what to do if the other child suggests they go hunt for it and play around with it.

Vaccines

At the eleven- or twelve-year checkup, the American Academy of Pediatrics recommends three vaccines. One is a Tdap booster that builds on the immunity from earlier shots. The other two are new vaccines your child won't have had before. MCV (meningococcal vaccine) is given as one shot to protect against a teenage form of meningitis. HPV (human papillomavirus vaccine, given as three doses: one now, another in one month, and the third six to twelve months after the first) protects against a sexually transmitted virus that causes genital warts and cervical cancer (see page 469). A flu shot is also recommended every year in October.

ADOLESCENT PHYSICAL EXAM

Adolescence is a time of great change: changing bodies, changing behavior, changing attitudes! Here we will address the various health and behavior issues that will come into play during the teen years. Many people ask us, "How frequently does my teenager need a routine physical?" Normal, healthy teenagers usually do not need yearly physicals; we often recommend physicals every two years. However, if your teenager is on a sports team, a yearly physical exam is needed. And if your teenager has any special issues — such as short stature, behavioral or mood problems, or any other chronic medical problem — he should have an annual physical.

Key Elements of a Routine Teenage Physical Examination

There are thirteen important elements to your teen's physical examination. Your doctor should address the following:

1. Height, weight, and body mass index (BMI). Your child's height and weight should be discussed at the routine physical. This is done to ensure that the teenager is in a healthy weight range for her height. Your doctor may calculate your child's BMI (body mass index). You can also calculate this yourself (see page 89), then plot the number on the BMI charts on page 112 and 114. Although BMI charts are useful, muscular and large-boned teens will plot as "overweight" when they are often at appropriate growth. Waist size is a better indicator of obesity. (See waist measurements, page 418.)

2. Sexual development. Many years ago pediatricians devised guidelines called Tanner stages, which describe normal sexual development for boys and girls (see chart, page 439). Although these stages vary widely from teen to teen, these guides help your doctor detect signs of early or abnormally delayed sexual development. Some medical conditions can cause early or delayed puberty and can respond to treatment.

3. Menstrual history in girls. Your doctor will ask your daughter whether or not she has begun periods and how frequent these periods are. Menstruation in young women usually begins between the ages of ten and fourteen. Body type affects the timing and heaviness of menses. Very lean, athletic girls, such as gymnasts, tend to be later and lighter; plumper girls tend to be earlier. When girls first begin having their periods, they are often irregular for the first year or so. After a year of having periods, they are normally on a once-a-month cycle. Talk to your doctor if your child has irregular periods or if the periods are prolonged (more than a week) or abnormally uncomfortable, painful, or excessively heavy. Gynecological exams aren't usually needed until sexual activity begins.

4. Tobacco/drug/alcohol use. Your doctor should talk to your teenager about these issues. Normally, this is done without the parents present, which may help the teenager speak openly. This is an important part of the routine physical that can identify at-risk teens. Your doctor should also ask whether your teen has friends who use drugs, alcohol, or tobacco.

5. Sexual activity history. Your doctor will ask your teenager if she has ever been sexually active, how many partners she has had, and whether she understands "safe-sex" practices (condom use, birth-control methods, avoiding high-risk sexual behavior). Doctors can also advise teens that the only sure safe-sex practice is abstinence. Most health professionals recommend that Pap smears begin no later than three years after becoming sexually active or by age twenty-one, whichever comes first. Sexually active teens should be screened for sexually transmitted diseases (STDs) at least once a year. STDs typically screened for include chlamydia, gonorrhea, HPV, and HIV (human immunodeficiency virus). Screening is important, especially among females. Often teenage girls have very mild symptoms or none at all. This can lead to health problems and even infertility.

Discussions between a doctor and a teenager are considered confidential, and the doctor will let the teen know that nothing they discuss will be shared with the parents, even if the parents request it, without the teen's permission. There is one exception to this, however: If a teenager tells the doctor he is involved in anything that puts his life, or the life of another person, in immediate danger, the doctor is obligated to share this with the parents, and possibly the authorities.

See page 465 for tips on talking to your teen about sexual behavior and abstinence.

6. Eating habits and nutritional status. Your physician should inquire about your teenager's eating habits. Adolescents are notorious for making poor nutritional choices. Good, healthy meals are very important for the developing teenager. Your doctor should assess overall nutritional status to be sure your child is not underweight, undernourished, or overweight. Nutritional supplements, such as omega 3s, fruit- and veggie-based supplements, and vitamins, may be needed if your child has very poor nutritional habits. This is also a good opportunity for your doctor to counsel your teenager about the importance of eating well.

7. Exercise. Daily exercise is vital for young people. We usually recommend at least forty-five minutes of vigorous exercise every day for a healthy body and mind. School physical education programs may or may not meet this need, but being on a sports team certainly does. For those not in sports, we recommend after-school or before-school daily exercise. Running, swimming, biking, or using an exercise machine (such as an elliptical trainer) are all examples of high-quality exercise. Walking is usually not enough for teens.

8. School performance. This should be discussed during your teenager's physical exam. Grades are very important for teenagers now and in their future. Your doctor should inquire about your teenager's overall view of school and what her favorite subjects are. This is a good opportunity to identify any struggles with goal setting and to give encouragement. Studies show that academic high achievers (dubbed AHAs) all share a common attitude — love of learning.

9. History of depression or other mental illness. Inform your doctor if your teenager has any history of emotional problems. Discuss with your doctor any current or past medication use or past problems with depression or other mental illness. If your child does have a history of any of these problems, your doctor should inquire in private about any thoughts of or attempts at suicide or thoughts of or attempts at harming others.

10. Safety issues. A safe lifestyle should be encouraged. If your child is driving, he should always use seat belts. Helmets should always be worn if bike-riding, skateboarding, motorcycle riding, or other high-risk activity is undertaken where head injury could be involved. The leading causes of death among teenagers are car accidents and accidental injury.

11. TV and computer use. Another common problem among teenagers is too much time spent watching TV and playing video and/or computer games. Ideally, these activities should be limited to less than sixty minutes a day. The average teenager, however, usually has three hours of screen time daily. Excessive TV or computer use can lead to poor school performance, higher risk of obesity, and diminished daily exercise. A teenage checkup is a good opportunity for your doctor to give your teen a quick encouraging word about limiting screen time.

12. Sleep. For optimal growth and school performance, your teenager needs at least eight hours a night of good-quality sleep. Your physician should inquire as to whether or not this goal is being met. Going to sleep too late should be avoided, as this usually leads to problems with daily fatigue. Most teenagers do not meet the goal of eight hours a night. Insufficient quantity and quality of sleep is a common cause of academic and behavior problems.

13. Routine dentist and/or orthodontist appointments and dental hygiene habits. Your teenager should have a routine dental examination every six months and visits to the orthodontist as directed. The dentist should examine your child's teeth for any signs of decay and should remind her to brush at least twice a day as well as floss at least once a day, as both are crucial to overall dental health.

What Should I Talk to the Doctor About at My Teenager's Physical?

Of course, inform the physician if there are any ongoing problems or other concerns you might have. It is also important to discuss medical problems in your child's past (for example, a history of allergies or asthma). Tell your doctor if there are any medical problems that run in the family, for example, certain cancers, heart problems, a family history of high cholesterol, or other diseases. It is very important to be perfectly open and honest about any past or current problems so that you, your child, and your doctor can work together as a team to ensure your child's optimal health.

Will My Teenager Have Tests Done at the Physical?

It depends. Certain tests, such as blood work or urine samples, may be obtained if your child is having symptoms and the doctor wants to explore further. A cholesterol test should be performed whether or not there is a family history of high cholesterol. Young women should have a blood test to check for anemia once they begin having menstrual cycles. Sexually active teens should be screened for STDs as discussed above. Your doctor will decide what tests, if any, will be ordered as part of the routine physical.

The Routine Teenage Physical Exam

A complete head-to-toe exam is a key part of this visit. Briefly, we will explain some of the most important elements of the physical.

Heart rate and blood pressure. The doctor will check to be sure the heart isn't beating too fast or too slow and that the blood pressure is in a healthy, normal range. Ideally, blood pressure should be below 120/80.

Height and weight. It is important to make sure your child's weight is in a healthy range. Height will be checked to make sure there are no problems with growth delays.

Vision exam. Vision should be tested, generally by using a basic eye chart, to screen for vision problems. Any evidence of impaired vision should prompt a consultation with an eye doctor.

Heart and lungs. The physician will carefully listen to the heart in order to check for any irregular heartbeats or heart murmurs. Heart murmurs are occasionally not diagnosed until the teen years or even later. The presence of a heart murmur in this age group could indicate underlying structural heart problems. Any abnormality found on the heart exam should prompt a consultation with a pediatric cardiologist. The doctor will listen to the lungs and check for any abnormalities with breathing.

Teeth. The doctor will check inside the mouth to insure strong, healthy teeth.

Spine. The pediatrician should examine the spine to insure proper alignment. Scoliosis, or excess curvature of the spine, should be ruled out. The doctor will perform specific examinations in order to do this. Many schools also have scoliosis screening programs. (See Scoliosis, page 455, for more information.)

Male genitalia. The testicles should be examined by the physician. Although rare, testicular cancer is the most common cancer among teenage males. Checks for hernias will also be done at this time.

Female genitalia. This is usually not examined as part of the routine physical exam — unless, of course, there are any problems or concerns.

Sexual development. Your doctor will make an overall assessment to insure your child's sexual development is appropriate for his or her age.

Overall signs of good health. The doctor should examine for signs of malnourishment or developing obesity.

Joint flexibility. Assessing healthy flexibility of joints, especially the hips, knees, shoulders, and ankles, is very important. Less flexibility means more likelihood of injury.

Muscle strength and reflexes. Healthy muscles are important for growing bodies. Proper muscle strength and tone is a sign of good health. Normal, brisk reflexes are a good indicator of an overall healthy nervous system.

Will My Teenager Need Any Vaccinations at the Physical?

Your child's immunization history should be checked as part of the physical. If she is behind on any of her shots, your doctor may give some catch-up immunizations. Assuming she has gotten all her shots on time in the past, she may still need some booster shots. The following are common vaccines administered during routine adolescent and teenage physical examinations.

Tdap (tetanus/diphtheria/pertussis) booster. This combined vaccine is often given to children at twelve years. The tetanus booster protects them from tetanus if they should suffer a major wound or penetrating injury. Pertussis is a type of bacteria that causes whooping cough. Each year, many outbreaks of whooping cough often begin in the adolescent population because teens are often in close quarters (classrooms, locker rooms, etc.), so it is now considered routine to give this booster at this age. Diphtheria protection is mainly important for international travel.

MCV (meningitis) vaccine. This is usually given between the ages of fifteen and eighteen, often right before college, although it can be given as young as age twelve. This type of bacterial meningitis is rare, but it is a potentially devastating and often fatal disease. High-risk groups include college students living in dorms and military recruits living in barracks. This is a one-time-only vaccine.

Chicken pox (varicella) vaccine. If your teenager has not had the chicken pox, or has never received the vaccine, now is a good time to get it. Chicken pox infections are more severe in adolescents.

Hep B (hepatitis B). This vaccine is now part of the normal schedule for infants, but some teenagers may not have received it. If they haven't, now is a good time to have it. It is a three-shot series: The first shot is given at the physical; the second dose should be given one month after the first; and the third shot should be administered six months after receiving the first dose.

HPV (human papillomavirus) vaccine. This is a vaccine against certain types of human papillomavirus (see HPV, page 469) that are known to cause genital warts in men and women and cervical cancer in women. HPV is transmitted sexually and can infect cells of the female's cervix. In approximately 90 percent of cases, it naturally clears on its own. However, 10 percent of the time the virus remains in the cells of the cervix and over time the cells can become cancerous. This vaccine is considered part of a teenager's standard immunization schedule. Originally the vaccine was recommended for girls only, between the ages of nine and twenty-six. In 2009 this was expanded to include boys as well. Talk to your doctor about any update in this policy. It is a three-shot series: the first shot is given at the physical; the second is given two months after the first; and the final

 **DR. SEARS TIP
Spread the Shots Out**

Although it may be nice to get all the shots over with as quickly as possible, we prefer to limit children to two shots at any one time. We suggest you develop an approach with your doctor that provides these teen vaccines over a period of a few years, rather than grouping them together in one year.

LEARN MORE ABOUT IT

Vaccine schedules are constantly being updated and new vaccines are being developed. Discuss new changes with your doctor, or read *The Vaccine Book* by Dr. Robert Sears. For vaccine updates, consult www.AskDrSears.com/the VaccineBook.

dose is administered six months after receiving the first shot.

Hep A (hepatitis A). This vaccine was only recently added to the standard infant schedule, so many of today's teens may not have had the shots yet. Hepatitis A is a food-poisoning illness that mainly occurs during travel to developing countries; however, some outbreaks also occur in the United States. Talk to your doctor about the two-dose series if your child hasn't had it already.

Influenza (flu) shot. It is now recommended to get a flu vaccine every October through eighteen years of age.

Travel immunizations. If your teen is planning a trip to other parts of the world, talk to your doctor about whether or not other vaccines might be needed. If she is traveling to an area considered high-risk for malaria, your doctor may recommend antimalarial pills to help lessen the chance of malaria infection.

SCHOOL SPORTS PHYSICAL

If your child is going to participate in a sport, he'll need a sports physical. This must be done in order to insure that he can be cleared to safely play in a school sport.

Many aspects of the sports physical are the same as the regular physical. Your pediatrician will take a complete history and discuss any new or ongoing medical problems, and will give a complete physical exam. There are, however, some special issues that should be addressed during a sports physical. The physical examination focuses on assessing an athlete's fitness to be able to participate in his chosen sport. The following are some special items that you'll need to be aware of for the sports physical examination.

Bring the clearance form! Your pediatrician may have sports clearance forms; however, many schools require their own individual forms for the doctor to complete and sign. Talk to your school administrator regarding this.

Sports-related history. Your doctor should ask about any major past injuries related to sports. These include major fractures, sprains, concussions, among others.

DR. SEARS TIP
Cushion Growing Heels

In our practice we recommend heel cushions (available at drugstores) for all teens during sports. The foot was never designed to pound on gym floors and concrete. The heel bones are still growing and are sensitive.

History of asthma or allergies. It's important to inform your pediatrician if your child has had a history of asthma or allergies in the past. Heavy exercise is a very common trigger for asthma. If your child still suffers from asthma, discuss with the doctor about how well the symptoms are currently being controlled. Allergies can also be troublesome for young athletes. If they seem to be poorly controlled or if your child is experiencing worsening allergies while participating in a certain sport, inform the doctor.

History of chest pains, shortness of breath, palpitations, or loss of consciousness at rest or while exercising. We've all heard stories of an otherwise healthy, well-conditioned athlete collapsing on the field. This is a rare occurrence, but with proper questioning it may be preventable. Your pediatrician will ask whether or not your son or daughter has ever experienced any of these symptoms in the past. Many of these symptoms must be carefully explored with a thorough physical examination of the heart and lungs, and possibly other tests (such as an EKG or echocardiogram) if your pediatrician recommends them.

Family history of heart problems or unusual fainting spells at a young age. Inform the doctor if any parents or grandparents of the child developed such conditions before age forty. Further testing may need to be done with a cardiologist to make sure any serious, but hidden, heart conditions weren't passed down to your child.

Inform your pediatrician if your child has a history of any major surgery and/or hospitalization. The doctor will need to make sure such issues won't interfere with sports.

Safe and proper practice routines. To reduce the risk of an injury, your doctor should discuss how best to practice and train. Important points include:

- adequate stretching before and after practices and games

- safe workout techniques

- staying properly hydrated

- communicating with the coach or with the parents when the young athlete is experiencing ongoing pain

- proper use of sports equipment, especially free weights. It's best to begin with stretch bands and gradually progress to a weight machine, and then finally to free weights.

 DR. SEARS TIP
If It Hurts, Stop!

We always tell our young athletes, "Pain that doesn't get better is your body's way of telling you something is wrong." Teens should listen to what their bodies tell them and should not be afraid to communicate this to adults. Don't believe the outdated "no pain, no gain" dictum of muscle training. If it hurts, your teen is either overusing or misusing the training exercise.

Female athlete's menstrual history. I always inform female athletes that they may begin to have irregular periods when they begin training. This is very common in highly trained female athletes, and it is usually not a cause for concern. Less body fat leads to less estrogen, which can slow menses. You should talk with your child's doctor, however, if your daughter stops having periods altogether.

Physical Examination for the Sports Physical

The exam for the sports physical is very similar to the adolescent physical exam. There are certain aspects that your pediatrician will pay particular attention to. Here are some of the more important components of the sports physical examination:

Heart rate and blood pressure. Heart rate should be taken before and after activity (the doctor may have your child run around outside the office for a few minutes) to be sure there is an appropriate increase in heart rate from a resting to an active state and a decrease from an active to a resting state. Abnormally high blood pressure could indicate possible underlying cardiovascular concerns and should be remeasured one week later, before your child receives clearance. Persistently elevated blood pressures warrant consultation with a cardiologist prior to sports clearance.

Heart. Your pediatrician will listen carefully to your teen's heart for any abnormal heart sounds, heart murmurs, or irregular heartbeat. An assessment for overall heart size will also be made. Any abnormality in the heart examination warrants further consultation with a cardiologist.

Lungs. The pediatrician will listen to your child's lung sounds in order to insure good movement of air into them. She will also listen carefully for any signs of obstruction or wheezing, which may indicate underlying lung problems such as asthma.

Joints. The doctor will assess the level of flexibility and range of motion of the major joints, including shoulders, elbows, hips, knees, and ankles. Any limited range in motion or limited flexibility raises the risk for injury while playing sports.

Muscles and tendons. Tendons are parts of the muscles that attach to the joints. Your pediatrician will test to see how flexible the major muscle groups of the body are, particularly the quadriceps, hamstrings, and calf muscles of the legs. Poor muscle flexibility raises the risk for injuries, such as muscle strain, muscle pull, or muscle tears.

Spine. The doctor will check the spine for any abnormal curvatures and will test flexibility of the spine.

Eye exam. Testing to insure normal vision is important for any aspiring athlete. Any evidence of nearsightedness or farsightedness should be further evaluated by an eye doctor. Recommendations should be made with regard to safe eyewear for the particular sport.

Hernia check in males. The doctor will perform the "turn your head and cough" exam. This involves checking for any evidence of hernia in the groin area. Participation in sports can cause hernias to worsen in males.

Routine checkups are an important part of your child's health care. Some parents may wonder if they are really necessary. Truthfully, most exams we perform don't reveal any health problems. That's one of the joys of pediatrics; most children are nice and healthy! But occasionally a problem is discovered that can be corrected or treated before serious or permanent consequences develop. Even if nothing is discovered to be wrong with your child (which is what you would hope for anyway), what you and your child can learn about health, nutrition, safety, and the human body can provide some useful lessons about health maintenance.

We have now completed the preventive medicine section of the book. In fact, if we've done our job well, and if you follow most of our suggestions, you may not need the rest of this book at all. Of course, even children with the healthiest lifestyles will inevitably get sick on occasion. We hope to equip you with all the information you will need for virtually every medical situation that may arise.

Birth to 24 months: Girls
Length-for-age and Weight-for-age percentiles

NAME _____

RECORD # _____

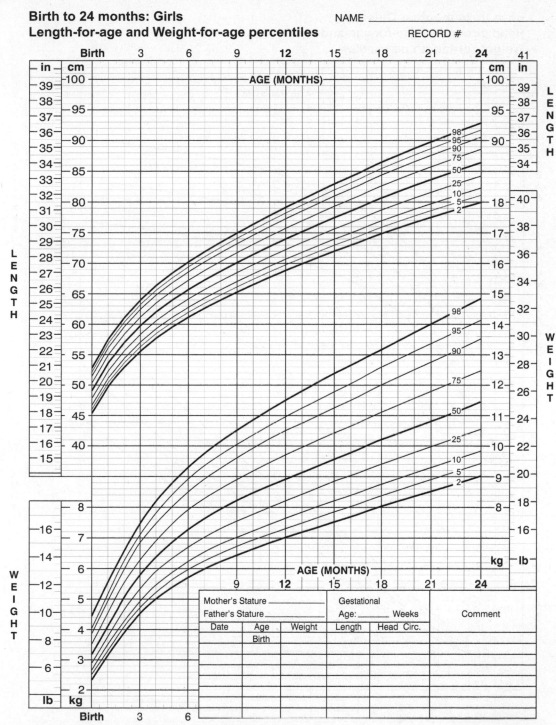

Published by the Centers for Disease Control and Prevention, November 1, 2009
SOURCE: WHO Child Growth Standards (http://www.who.int/childgrowth/en)

Birth to 24 months: Girls
Head circumference-for-age and
Weight-for-length percentiles

NAME _____

RECORD # _____

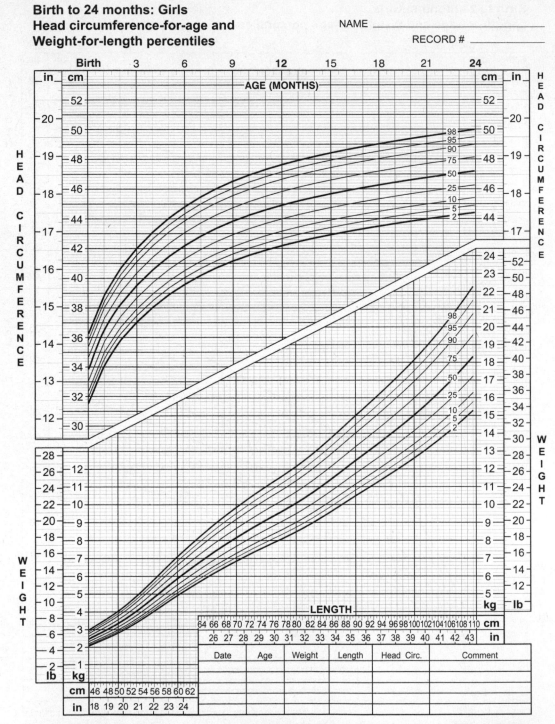

AGE (MONTHS)

Birth   3   6   9   12   15   18   21   24

HEAD CIRCUMFERENCE

98
95
90
75
50
25
10
5
2

LENGTH

| 64 66 68 70 72 74 76 78 80 82 84 86 88 90 92 94 96 98 100 102 104 106 108 110 | cm |
| 26 27 28 29 30 31 32 33 34 35 36 37 38 39 40 41 42 43 | in |

WEIGHT

Date	Age	Weight	Length	Head Circ.	Comment

cm	46 48 50 52 54 56 58 60 62
in	18 19 20 21 22 23 24

Published by the Centers for Disease Control and Prevention, November 1, 2009
SOURCE: WHO Child Growth Standards (http://www.who.int/childgrowth/en)

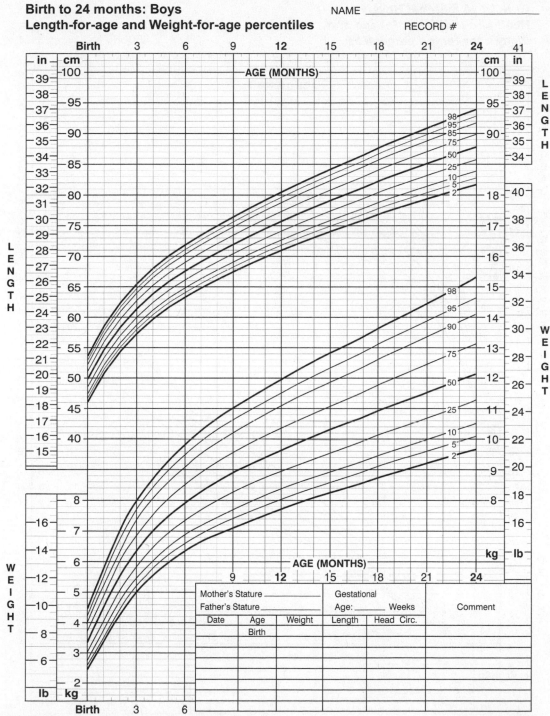

Birth to 24 months: Boys
Length-for-age and Weight-for-age percentiles

NAME _____

RECORD # _____

Published by the Centers for Disease Control and Prevention, November 1, 2009
SOURCE: WHO Child Growth Standards (http://www.who.int/childgrowth/en)

Birth to 24 months: Boys
Head circumference-for-age and
Weight-for-length percentiles

NAME _____

RECORD # _____

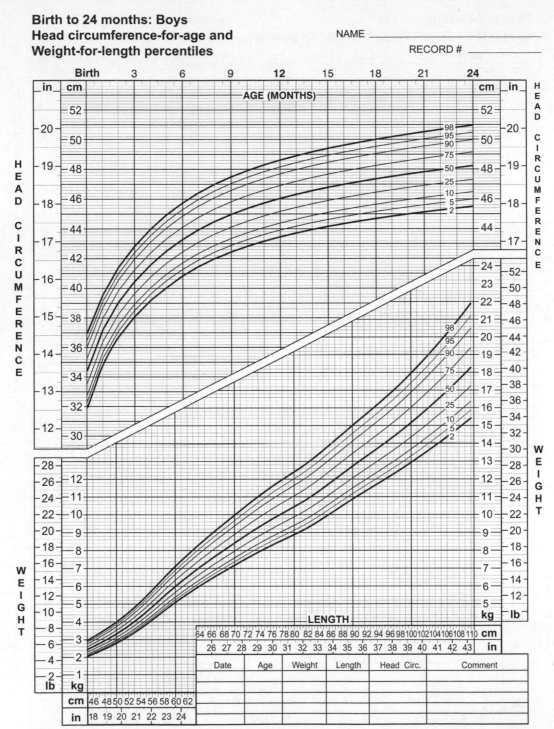

AGE (MONTHS)

Birth 3 6 9 12 15 18 21 24

HEAD CIRCUMFERENCE

98
95
90
75
50
25
10
5
2

LENGTH

Date	Age	Weight	Length	Head Circ.	Comment

cm 46 48 50 52 54 56 58 60 62
in 18 19 20 21 22 23 24

Published by the Centers for Disease Control and Prevention, November 1, 2009
SOURCE: WHO Child Growth Standards (http://www.who.int/childgrowth/en)

2 to 20 years: Girls
Stature-for-age and Weight-for-age percentiles

NAME _____

RECORD # _____

Mother's Stature		Father's Stature		
Date	Age	Weight	Stature	BMI*

*To Calculate BMI: Weight (kg) ÷ Stature (cm) ÷ Stature (cm) x 10,000
or Weight (lb) ÷ Stature (in) ÷ Stature (in) x 703

AGE (YEARS)

12 13 14 15 16 17 18 19 20

STATURE

WEIGHT

AGE (YEARS)

Published May 30, 2000 (modified 11/21/00).
SOURCE: Developed by the National Center for Health Statistics in collaboration with
the National Center for Chronic Disease Prevention and Health Promotion (2000).
http://www.cdc.gov/growthcharts

SAFER·HEALTHIER·PEOPLE™

2 to 20 years: Girls
Body mass index-for-age percentiles

NAME _____

RECORD # _____

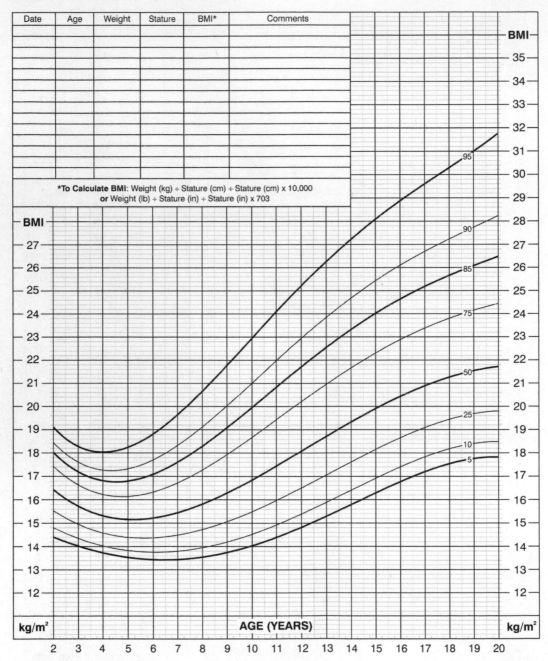

Date	Age	Weight	Stature	BMI*	Comments

*To Calculate BMI: Weight (kg) ÷ Stature (cm) ÷ Stature (cm) x 10,000
or Weight (lb) ÷ Stature (in) ÷ Stature (in) x 703

BMI

AGE (YEARS)

kg/m² ... kg/m²

Published May 30, 2000 (modified 10/16/00).
SOURCE: Developed by the National Center for Health Statistics in collaboration with
the National Center for Chronic Disease Prevention and Health Promotion (2000).
http://www.cdc.gov/growthcharts

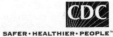

SAFER · HEALTHIER · PEOPLE™

2 to 20 years: Boys
Stature-for-age and Weight-for-age percentiles

NAME _____

RECORD # _____

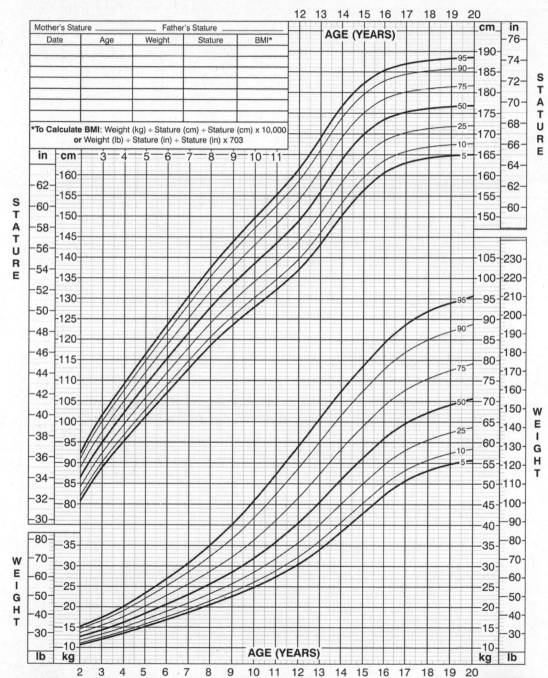

Published May 30, 2000 (modified 11/21/00).
SOURCE: Developed by the National Center for Health Statistics in collaboration with
the National Center for Chronic Disease Prevention and Health Promotion (2000).
http://www.cdc.gov/growthcharts

SAFER • HEALTHIER • PEOPLE™

2 to 20 years: Boys
Body mass index-for-age percentiles

NAME _____

RECORD # _____

Date	Age	Weight	Stature	BMI*	Comments

*To Calculate BMI: Weight (kg) ÷ Stature (cm) ÷ Stature (cm) x 10,000
or Weight (lb) ÷ Stature (in) ÷ Stature (in) x 703

BMI

AGE (YEARS)

kg/m²

kg/m²

Published May 30, 2000 (modified 10/16/00).

SOURCE: Developed by the National Center for Health Statistics in collaboration with
the National Center for Chronic Disease Prevention and Health Promotion (2000).
http://www.cdc.gov/growthcharts

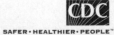

SAFER • HEALTHIER • PEOPLE™

III

Pediatric Concerns and Illnesses: A to Z

In this section of the book we will present, from A to Z, the concerns that most parents have and the illnesses that many children get. With each topic we will teach you the pills-skills model of medical care: not only what your child can take (pills), but what parents can do (self-help skills). Most of the topics are divided into what the concern or illness is, when to worry, and what to do. Our goal in presenting this information is to help parents and caregivers be more informed consumers of medical care. Also, we will teach you how to be an advocate for your children to be sure they receive the best medical care.

Note: *Even though our topics are presented in A-to-Z format, you should first consult the index for the page number of the topic you are looking for. Many topics come under different names, and we have listed all the most common names in the index.*

ABDOMINAL PAIN

Abdominal pain is one of the most confusing and worrisome situations for parents because they can't actually see what the problem is. With causes ranging from harmless gas or heartburn to life-threatening appendicitis, it is very difficult for a parent to know just how serious it might be. "Tummy aches" can come on suddenly, or they can persist on and off for months, and the various causes and treatments are many. We have divided our discussion into two parts: sudden abdominal pain and chronic pain.

Abdominal Pain: Sudden or Short Term

This section will help you understand the various causes of sudden abdominal pain, tell if your child's pain might be serious, and explain what you can do.

Abdominal Pain During the First Six Months of Life

Figuring out the cause of abdominal pain in young infants is difficult because they are unable to describe the type of pain or the exact location. In fact, they won't even be able to tell you whether the pain is in the abdomen at all. So if your baby has inconsolable periods of crying and a tense belly, pulls up his legs, and is passing gas, but the episode resolves itself after an hour or two and he falls peacefully asleep, you can be fairly sure there's nothing seriously wrong. However, you will obviously want to figure out what triggered this so you can keep it from happening again. Here are the typical causes:

Food allergies passed through breast milk. For a list of foods that can cause this and guidelines on how to investigate the cause, see page 327.

Formula intolerance. If a baby is allergic or sensitive to a certain formula, he'll let you know. See page 331 for more details on what to do.

Colic. This refers to episodes of inconsolable crying for hours. The baby seems to be crying in pain, and the source of the pain appears to be the abdominal area. As mentioned above, often this is due to something in the breast milk or a formula intolerance. If you've made those changes, and your baby still has episodes of pain, see page 229 for a complete discussion on how to solve your baby's colic.

Gas. This is by far the most common cause. Almost every baby goes through fussy, gassy periods, but they are usually much shorter than colic episodes. Gas often results from an irritating food in Mom's diet, a formula intolerance, swallowed air during excessive crying, or inadequate burping after feeds. The main difference between plain gas and colic is that gas gets better once you eliminate the cause. Colic may not. See page 337 for more details.

Serious causes. Review the information on page 120 regarding intestinal obstruction to understand signs of this serious condition in young infants. Fortunately, such situations are extremely rare.

Abdominal Pain in Older Infants and Children

Belly aches in older infants and in children are approached differently than in younger infants. The causes are different, and parents can usually deduce more clues as to what the cause may be based on the child's behavior and ability to communicate details about the pain. We will first discuss various non-serious causes of pain. The following situations, although uncomfortable, probably don't warrant an emergency room visit or an immediate doctor's appointment:

Intestinal infection. The most common cause of abdominal pain is the stomach flu. If your child has vomiting, diarrhea, and fever, then you can be fairly sure the stomach pain is simply part of an untreatable infection. See page 535 for diagnosis and treatment options.

Food poisoning. This isn't really "poisoning," as the term implies. It simply means there were some bad bacteria in something your child ate. If your child has sudden abdominal cramps, vomiting, and possibly diarrhea within one to eight hours after eating some suspicious food, then it is probably food poisoning. See pages 278 and 535 for diagnosis and treatment ideas.

Heartburn. This occurs when a child eats something that triggers an overproduction of stomach acid, which results in burning pain, usually over the stomach (the upper-middle and left side of the belly below the ribcage) or in the chest. You can distinguish this from

food poisoning or illness because of the burning nature of the pain, which starts right after eating, and because there isn't any diarrhea or fever. Typical food culprits include tomato sauce, greasy food, citrus fruit or juice, and spicy food. See page 122.

Upset stomach. This is a generic dull stomach pain that occurs right after eating, but for unknown reasons. The pain is usually over the stomach or in the middle of the belly. You can distinguish this cause from food poisoning or illness because it starts right after eating and there isn't any diarrhea or fever. It can occur after eating too much junk food or unfamiliar foods. There are no specific treatments except for general soothing with a warm bath and gentle tummy massage.

Gas. This is probably the most common cause of sudden abdominal pain in the absence of any vomiting and diarrhea. Your child will experience sharp pains on and off that may move throughout the abdomen. Older children may tell you they can feel the gas bubbles moving along as the abdomen is massaged. Unfortunately, these pains can be quite severe. Simethicone gas drops (over the counter) may help move the gas along.

Lactose intolerance or milk allergy. This pain is similar to upset stomach, but it may also take on a gassy quality, and diarrhea and cramping can occur. It usually comes on within thirty to sixty minutes after ingesting cow's milk products. See page 122 for diagnosis and treatment options.

Sore abdominal muscles. Active sports or activities involving use of the abdominal muscles can create extreme soreness of these muscles. The pain is worse when you push on the belly or when your child uses the muscles, for example in sitting up. These muscles can also become sore after prolonged vomiting. Ibuprofen can relieve this type of pain (see page 553 for dosing).

Menstrual cramps. This is the most common cause of abdominal pain in teenage girls. Once a teen has had them, subsequent episodes are no longer a mystery, especially as they are followed by menstruation. But the first episode or two can be worrisome. They feel like cramping lower abdominal pain that may radiate to the back. Menstruation, and along with it cramps, can start as young as nine or ten years of age. Ibuprofen will be your daughter's best friend (see page 553 for dosing).

Constipation. This is more often a cause of chronic abdominal pain. However, your child may have a sudden onset of constipation that can cause severe abdominal pain. The pain can occur anywhere in the belly, although it is most often right in the middle near the belly button. The pain will come and go in waves as the colon naturally contracts, trying to move the hard stool along. Reports from the child about recently hard, difficult-to-pass stools are a clue to this cause, as is a known history of constipation. See page 240 for diagnosis and treatment ideas.

Bladder infection. Lower abdominal pain, along with painful or frequent urination, can indicate a bladder infection. See page 191.

 THE DR. SEARS RULE OF TWOS
Eat Twice as Often, Eat Half as Much, and Chew Twice as Long

For any temporary intestinal illness, especially one caused by food poisoning, food intolerances, or reflux, the intestine needs to rest, like any hurting organ. Grazing causes less wear and tear on the intestine.

Diagnosing Non-Serious Sudden Abdominal Pain

For all of these harmless causes of pain, there's no way for a doctor to determine the cause by examining your child. The causes are figured out by considering the overall situation and any clues suggested in the descriptions above. What a doctor *can* do is rule out the more serious causes in the next section. Once that is done, he can help you decide which one of the less-serious causes it might be and how to go about relieving it. In the end, however, it's not critical to determine the exact cause of non-serious pain, since it will resolve over time. The relief measures discussed on page 25 can help your child through in the meantime.

When to Worry

There are two emergency situations that can cause severe pain that, if left undiagnosed and untreated, can lead to serious complications.

Appendicitis. This is probably the most worrisome cause of sudden abdominal pain for parents. The appendix is a one-inch-long piece of intestine that branches off the colon in the lower right part of the abdomen. It can become inflamed and infected for a variety of reasons. The pain most often starts as mild to moderate discomfort around the belly button. Unfortunately, this is where children feel pain for most other non-serious causes as well, so appendicitis is difficult to catch in the early stage. The pain will move down to the lower right side of the abdomen and become much more severe. Here are the classic signs of appendicitis:

• severe right lower abdominal pain

• constant pain — doesn't usually come and go

- gradually increasing pain

- fever

- refusal to eat

- vomiting — sometimes present, but not always

- refusal to walk — lying down curled up in a fetal position

 **DR. SEARS TIP
The Jump Test**

Have your child stand and jump up and down. With appendicitis, this will cause increased sharp pain. The child will refuse to jump again, or may refuse to jump in the first place. If your child can jump up and down repeatedly without much discomfort, then he probably doesn't have appendicitis (this is not a perfect test, just a tool to help decide how likely appendicitis is).

Keep in mind that many illnesses start off with vomiting, fever, and belly pain. Don't jump to the conclusion of appendicitis until you have observed your child for several hours. Appendicitis rarely has the frequent vomiting and diarrhea that is characteristic of the stomach flu. Most causes of abdominal pain don't occur in the lower right area of the belly. Unless the pain moves to the lower right abdomen and becomes increasingly severe, and your child is unusually ill, then appendicitis is unlikely. Appendicitis is also very rare in children younger than four years old.

Intestinal obstruction. This is by far the most life-threatening cause of sudden abdominal pain, but it is also the least common. It is characterized by sudden excruciating belly pain, usually in the middle, with persistent projectile vomiting. One unique aspect of the vomitus is that it is dark green. It is important to know the difference between light green stomach mucus (which is not serious) and dark green bile (the color of a dark pine tree). There are two processes that can occur in the intestines that can cause sudden obstruction:

- Intussusception. This unusual word refers to when a part of the intestine "telescopes" in upon itself, just like a telescope collapsing. This usually only occurs in children under age two. The unique aspect of this pain is that it can come and go. Your infant can be in severe pain, with his legs drawn up to his belly, for twenty minutes, and then relax and be pain-free for a half hour. This occurs because the "telescoped" intestine may intermittently open up again. An infant may act calm and quiet during the periods of relief, or may be pale and lethargic (won't respond to stimulation, won't open the eyes). The intussusception may continue to come and go for many hours.

- Volvulus. This occurs when the intestines get twisted. It is similar to when a balloon is twisted up into an animal shape. The twisted area gets closed off. This occurs mostly in children over two years. The pain is severe, and constant.

If your infant or child is experiencing these signs, you should call your doctor immediately or take your child straight to the emergency room.

The bottom line is that if your child is in severe pain, is vomiting dark green bile repeatedly (not light green mucus), and seems severely ill, you should seek immediate medical attention.

DR. SEARS TIP
When in Doubt, Check It Out

It's safest to have your pediatrician, in partnership with you, make a decision on whether or not the abdominal pain is serious.

Abdominal Pain: Chronic or Recurrent

If your child's pain has persisted on and off for more than two weeks, it's time to take a more detailed look at what might be going on. Here is our guide to solving the mystery of chronic abdominal pain.

Why Little Intestines Are So Sensitive: The Stages of Gut Growth

Two anatomical quirks make the intestines the most sensitive organ in the body. First, except for the brain, the intestines contain more nerves than any other organ, hence the term *gut brain.* It stands to reason that if there are a lot of pain fibers and emotion-sensitive nerves in the gut, the child will experience frequent bouts of gut sensations. Next, infant intestines contain a larger surface area than any other system, including the skin. Anatomists estimate that if you stretched out all the linings of the intestines, they would have a surface area larger than a tennis court.

Growing children go through stages when they have frequent growing pains in the gut. In the first year, the immature intestines are getting used to processing and digesting all sorts of different foods, so *food intolerances* top the list of gut pains during infancy. Once the gut learns to digest all the usual foods, those "still-learning" intestines need to master elimination of the leftovers. *Constipation*

comes next as the usual cause of childhood gut discomforts during the toddler and preschool years.

Then comes the worry stage of middle childhood and adolescence. This is the stage when the child's head brain starts to react to life's emotional quirks: social pressure, school pressures, and domestic issues. The emotions that the child feels in the head brain are reflected in the gut brain. *Emotional stresses* are the most common cause of recurrent abdominal pain at this stage. Now that you know the typical "growing pains" those guts go through, here's how you can help:

Causes

As you can see, these pains are *real* at all stages of childhood. They need real understanding and real help.

Constipation. This is by far the most common cause of chronic abdominal pain prior to puberty. Here are some clues to help you decide if constipation is the culprit:

- Your child may have symptoms of constipation such as straining hard to pass a bowel movement, pooping only once every few days, passing thick, hard stools or clumps of hard pellets, or spending more than five minutes passing a movement.

- As the colon contracts several times a day against the hard backed-up stool, your child will complain of cramping pain. Pain will subside after contraction stops, usually after ten to thirty minutes. The child "feels better" after eventually pooping. You note the child is free of gut pains for the next couple days, and then the cycle resumes.

If you think that constipation may be a cause of your child's abdominal pain, see page 240, Constipation.

Lactose intolerance or milk protein allergy. These two conditions are not the same thing. One is an inability to digest lactose sugar (intolerance), whereas the other is an allergic reaction to milk proteins. Symptoms for both include:

- stomach cramps after eating dairy

- gas pains and bloating

- intestinal cramps

- diarrhea

The pain subsides when dairy products are limited or eliminated from the diet entirely. See page 327 if you suspect a problem with milk.

Other food allergies. Besides milk, other allergic causes of abdominal pain include wheat (and other gluten grains), soy, corn, nuts, and shellfish. Gluten sensitivity (the protein that is in wheat, oats, rye, barley, and a few other grains) is the second most common trigger for intestinal pain after milk. See page 330 for more information on this often overlooked cause.

Heartburn, gastritis, and ulcers. *Gastritis* is the medical term for upset stomach; *gastroesophageal reflux* is the medical term for heartburn. Inflammation in the stomach is caused by overproduction of stomach acid. Ulcers occur when this acid erodes too far into the stomach lining. Older children will describe it as a burning or gnawing pain over the upper middle or left side of the abdomen, or even the middle of the chest. Younger children can't describe a pain as "burning." There are three main causes of this overproduction of acid:

- *Stress.* Emotional stress in children can cause increased stomach acid and stomach aches.

- *Infection.* The bacterium called *H. pylori* can infect the stomach and cause increased stomach acid and pain. This infection can run in families. It is diagnosed either by a simple blood test or with a biopsy taken during endoscopy of the stomach. The blood test is not very reliable for children younger than five years old.

- *Medications.* Some medications can cause stomach irritation. The most common culprits are aspirin and ibuprofen products.

Intestinal inflammation. If during middle childhood or adolescence your child has recurrent fevers, bloody diarrhea, joint pains, and bouts of "hurt bad" abdominal pains, you should suspect inflammatory bowel disease (see page 378).

Intestinal infections. There are a variety of bacteria and parasites that can infect the intestines. The pain can occur anywhere in the belly. The biggest clue that the abdominal pain may be due to an intestinal infection is the presence of *chronic diarrhea. Diarrhea* is the gut's way of quickly getting rid of anything (food or germs) that irritates. These infections are diagnosed by sending samples of the diarrhea to a lab for testing. See page 277 for more on diarrhea infections.

Behavioral causes. Children ages four to seven will sometimes experience belly pain based on a need for attention. The pain may or may not be "real"; however, if your child's need for attention is very strong, she may perceive the pain as real. This commonly occurs when a new baby arrives in the family: your older child may feel left out. It can also occur during a move, when starting a new school, when there's been a family tragedy or breakup, or at any other time when your child may feel left out, insecure, or worried about something. One way to approach this situation is to acknowledge your child's pain by saying something like "I know, dear, sometimes my tummy hurts too. But you will be okay." Do not give any special attention to it, and do not try to help your child find a remedy. For example, do not have her lie down while you rub her tummy to make it feel better. Make some effort to give her extra attention at times when she is *not* complaining. This will lessen her need to complain for attention. There is really no way to know for sure if the pain is due to behavior or illness. Use your instinct, and do not ignore the pain longer than you feel is appropriate.

Less common causes:

- *Tumors.* This is an extremely rare occurrence in children; do not jump to this as a probable diagnosis. An abdominal mass can often be felt by the doctor.

- *Organ problems.* Very rarely, one of the abdominal organs, such as the liver, gallbladder, pancreas, kidneys, or spleen, hurts, and this means your child needs medical attention.

- *Abdominal migraines.* This uncommon cause is related to migraine headaches. Just as enlargement of the blood vessels in the head causes pain, so can dilation of blood vessels in the gut. Blood vessel spasms in the belly cause episodes of unexplained pain, nausea, and vomiting. Sometimes migraine headaches occur simultaneously. There's no test to confirm this cause; the diagnosis is made based on the description of symptoms.

Diagnosis

Finding the cause of chronic abdominal pain is no easy task. Begin by considering all the above possibilities, treating constipation or gastritis if suspected, eliminating common food allergies, and creatively dealing with possible behavioral causes. If the pain is mild and not interfering with your child's life or sleep, then it is okay to spend several weeks doing this. If the mystery persists after these measures, or if the pain is moderate to severe, then it's time to make a pain diary and visit your doctor.

Create a pain diary. Your doctor will need to know many details regarding the pain in order to evaluate its cause. If you and your child are vague about the pain and unable to give many details, the doctor will have to rely more on invasive and expensive testing. Keep a diary for several weeks. Write down every day when the pain occurs, and state the following with each episode:

- time of day

- proximity to mealtimes

- severity on a scale of 1 to 10 (Does your child simply tell you her tummy hurts but shows no outward signs? Or does she double over in pain, holding her stomach and rolling on the floor?)

- length of each episode

- location of pain in the belly

- remedies that have succeeded or failed

- what your child was doing right before the pain occurred

- whether the pain awakens her at night

- whether it occurs only at school, or only at home, or both

DR. SEARS PAIN CLUE #1
Night-Waking Pain?
See a Doctor

As a general guide, any pain that awakens a child is more concerning and less likely to have a psychological cause than one that occurs only during the day.

- whether it also occurs on the weekends or only on school days (your child may be worried about school)

This information will be very valuable to your doctor, so come to your appointment well prepared.

DR. SEARS PAIN CLUE #2
Does Your Child
Circle or Point?

Those little hands are clues to when and when not to worry about abdominal pains. Tell your child, "Show me where it hurts." If he *circles* the belly button area and gives a *vague* and *inconsistent* description of the pain, this is less of a worry. If, however, he *points* to a specific location, is more specific about the pain, and always tells the same story, see the doctor.

Medical tests to find the cause. If tests are necessary to determine the cause, here is a typical protocol that your doctor might follow.

- *X-ray.* This may sound like an extreme first step, but one simple X-ray can be very helpful, and is easy to do and fairly inexpensive. It can diagnose such things as constipation,

swallowed objects, gallstones, tumors, and kidney stones.

- *Stool tests* for bacterial infections, parasites, and bleeding.
- *Blood tests* for food allergies, *H. pylori* infections, and organ dysfunction.
- *Abdominal ultrasound.* This is a non-invasive test (just like a prenatal ultrasound) that examines each specific organ in the abdomen for particular problems as well as for abdominal tumors.

DR. SEARS TIP
Try This Triple Treatment for
Any Intestinal Ailment

Before you undertake expensive and invasive testing to diagnose the cause of chronic abdominal pain, try taking these three steps first for a few weeks. They cover the most common causes of pain and are harmless to try, even if the problem ends up being something else:

- **Stop all dairy products.** This can help with constipation, milk allergy, and lactose intolerance.
- **Take probiotics.** These healthy germs can improve a variety of intestinal problems, including inflammatory bowel disease (IBD), constipation, and infections.
- **Drink aloe juice.** Available at most healthy grocery stores, aloe juice looks and tastes (almost) like water. Give about half a cup daily to relieve constipation and inflammation.

Seeing a specialist. If all the above measures don't yield a diagnosis and effective treatment plan, it's time to consult a pediatric gastroenterologist, who can take the diagnostic tests to a deeper level. Oftentimes, a "look see," such as an upper endoscopy or lower colonoscopy, is needed.

What to Do

Read about being good to the gut, page 25, for step-by-step home remedies for nearly every pain in the gut.

ACNE

Remember going through the pimple stage of adolescence? It's a topic of worry, especially among self-conscious teens. Acne is the most common skin condition for which teens seek medical attention. It's also a stage of parenting where you can shine. The more you understand about what causes acne, the more you can do to help your child get through this stage. Long after the pimples have gone away, your child's belief that she can trust you as a valuable resource will last forever. This is why we are going to give you a thorough course in the causes of acne and how to help your teen through it. Let's get started.

Causes

Let's go through the life span of a zit so you and your teen (read this together) can understand how these pimples begin.

Skin becomes more oily. Sebaceous glands are tiny oil-secreting glands located at the base of the hair shaft and most concentrated on the face, chest, and back, which explains why these are the three most frequent sites of acne. These glands secrete an oil that is important in maintaining healthy skin. In childhood, they are somewhat quiet, which is why childhood skin is not that oily. When puberty begins the hormones (androgens) trigger these glands to grow and secrete more oil, called sebum. In some preteens and teens, these glands are especially hyper-responsive to the hormones of puberty and secrete excess oil from the glands, which explains why acne can be more severe in some teens than others. This hormone sensitivity also explains why the severity of acne tends to be genetic. Your teen's zits are likely to be as severe as Mom's and Dad's were. Sebum secretion peaks during adolescence and gradually declines after age twenty.

Glands become plugged. All that excess oil is trying to get out of the glands up into the skin through tiny pathways called *ducts*. In the next stage of acne formation, these ducts become plugged with the thick oil and the accumulation of skin cells that are normally shed.

Blackheads and whiteheads form. A plugged duct is called a *comedo,* also known as a blackhead or whitehead. Contrary to what you may think, the black color of blackheads is not caused by dirt but rather by the oxidation of melanin, the normal dark pigment that is present in the skin.

Blackheads and whiteheads become infected. As a general principle, any bodily secretion, whether oil or water, that gets plugged up gets infected. This is when a blackhead or whitehead grows into a pimple. Nearby bacteria called *P. acnes*, which normally live on the skin, become trapped in the plugged pores, and this triggers an inflammatory reaction so that the skin gets red and swollen around the heads and keeps growing into the pimple.

DR. SEARS TIP
Don't Squeeze the Zits!

Oh, it's so tempting to pop those nasty, ripe mini-boils with your dirty fingernails. Don't! Usually this just increases the inflammation by driving the germs into the surrounding tissue, worsening the infection and leading to permanent scarring. Let your doctor or dermatologist pop the boil-like zits using the proper technique. Learn from your doctor how to use a sterilized needle and when and how to pop the zits when they are ripe.

What to Do

Now that you understand the stages of how acne develops, it's easy to understand what your teen and your doctor can do to treat it. You can't do much about increased oil production except wait it out; like most adolescent nuisances, this stage does pass. But you can do something about the formation of blackheads and whiteheads and whether or not these heads get infected. Your teen's personal acne-action plan is aimed at:

- keeping whiteheads and blackheads from forming

- unplugging the heads

- preventing these heads from becoming infected

Step 1: Talk with Your Teen

Most teens do not want a course in Dermatology or Acne 101. They just want to get rid of the zits. But it's worth giving some explanation of general skin care:

- The blackheads are not caused by dirt.

- Some teens get more acne than others not because of their personal habits but because of their genes. Some teens produce more oil in their skin.

- For girls, expect acne to flare up when the hormones do, during menstrual periods. These nuisances are called premenstrual breakouts.

- Don't pick the zits. That will make them worse and possibly lead to permanent scarring.

- Greasy cosmetics or hair grease can worsen acne.

- Junk food can cause junk skin (see why, page 30).

- Tight helmets, chin straps, or shoulder pads worn during sports may make acne worse. The rubbing of helmets and pads against the skin often produces "football player's acne."

- If your daughter must wear makeup when going out, be sure it's oil-free. There are special cosmetics that are more acne-friendly than others. She should always remove makeup at night.

- Acne medication should be applied before makeup.

- Be sure to use the treatment exactly as the doctor prescribes. It's normal for skin to "feel worse" before it feels better, especially during the first few weeks as the medication peels the skin and unplugs the pores. The itching and burning should subside after that. Be sure your teen uses the skin regimen long enough; otherwise the acne will come back and he'll have to start all over again.

- Humidify the bedroom air. Skin at any age does not like the dry air of central heating, which is why acne flare-ups are worse in the wintertime. (Dry air and lack of sunshine both contribute to wintertime acne. See Humidify Your Child's Air, page 24.)

- Harsh scrubbing can irritate the skin and sometimes make acne worse rather than better.

- Your teen shouldn't use anyone else's acne medication (especially prescription medicines).

- Applying too much medication too harshly can actually worsen the skin, causing it to be more red and irritated.

- Read more about general skin health, page 29.

Step 2: Learn Topical Tricks

Effective treatment of acne includes what you put *onto* the skin and *into* the skin. Let's begin with what to put onto the skin. Your doctor may suggest beginning with a topical benzoyl peroxide (BP). (Medications come in creams, gels, or lotions.) This formulation helps unplug the heads and oil ducts, thins the oil, and can kill some of the acne-causing bacteria. BP is the first step and mainstay of acne treatment. Begin with an over-the-counter 2.5 percent solution. Stronger concentrations may require a prescription. Try the mildest strength first, as the stronger the medication is, the more irritating it can be, leading to burning, redness, and drying of the skin. Here are instructions your teen can follow to apply the medication properly:

- Wash the skin with a *cleanser* (rather than soap) and one that says "noncomedogenic."

This means it cleans out the pores instead of plugging them. After applying the cleanser, rinse with warm water and pat (not rub) dry. Vigorous scrubbing can make acne worse.

- After normal washing, use an over-the-counter oatmeal-based scrub. Massage gently (not abrasively) in circular motions around the acne areas. The combination of a cleanser and a mild scrub removes the excess oil and some of the weaker heads.

- Apply a thin coat of the BP before bedtime to all the acne-prone areas rather than just dabbing it on the zits. Put a pea-sized dab on your fingertip and then spread it in an area a couple inches wide. Keep going around the face until you've covered it. For areas that you can't reach, such as the back, you may need parents to help. Do not "spot treat" your acne. Apply the gel over the *entire* face or affected skin. Oftentimes, this regimen is enough to control mild acne. Note that BP may bleach bedding and clothing. It's best to remove clothing or not lie down on bedsheets for around fifteen minutes after application to let the medication sink in.

- If the acne continues, you might be able to repeat the same regimen every morning depending on the strength of BP you are using and whether or not it's irritating your skin. If your skin is overly sensitive to topical solutions (too red, too itchy, or peeling too much), try using them every other night instead of nightly, to give your skin a rest.

Start off with a peel: One of the newer forms of treatment that dermatologists use is a *liquid nitrogen roll-on.* The doctor or nurse uses a cotton-tip applicator and rolls liquid nitrogen over the skin of the face to start the peeling process so that the prescription medications can begin to take effect sooner. This is the same medication that doctors use to freeze off warts. Some dermatologists will use other types of gentle chemicals to gradually peel off inflamed or scarred layers of skin.

DR. SEARS TIP
Find the Right Products
for Your Child

One of the teens in our family had some significant challenges with acne. He spent about three years using all available treatments (short of Accutane) and routinely went to a dermatologist for facial peels. Although there was some improvement, the problem remained what we would consider to be moderately severe. We heard about a new treatment option that uses more natural products along with ongoing facial treatments that were less irritating. We saw significant results right away, and after about three months the improvement was very dramatic. We now consider his acne to be mild, and the old scars are virtually gone. With acne treatment, it's important to consistently give a particular treatment several months to see if it's going to work. But if you aren't happy with your child's progress, make a change. For information on this revolutionary treatment, visit www.Dadashie.com.

Apply a topical retinoid: A derivative of vitamin A, this topical cream or ointment may be used instead of or in combination with some of the above treatments if the acne is getting worse. Topical retinoids keep the skin

from getting excessively oily but can also cause the skin to be excessively dry and irritated. Usually the doctor or dermatologist will try different types and strengths of these topical medications. Depending on the severity of the acne, your doctor may recommend a BP and/or a retinoid topical preparation: one applied before bedtime, the other applied in the morning.

It may take four to six weeks to notice significant improvement, yet the above regimen is effective 90 percent of the time. Although the dictum "no pain, no gain" is a bit of an overstatement, expect some unpleasant sensations at first. Although itching and peeling are listed as "side effects" on these medications, they are really the normal, expected effects. After all, these medications are really a skin peel. The medicines have to unclog the pores before they can work, so it's bound to be a bit uncomfortable. In fact, we tell our

DR. SEARS TIP
Let the Sun Shine In

Acne is usually worse in the sunless, winter months (and the dry air of central heating certainly doesn't help). When possible, expose the face to fifteen minutes of sunshine daily. But by all means avoid *sunburning* the face, which will increase scarring. Don't use prescription topical gels if your face accidentally gets sunburned, as the skin could peel and be very painful. Since many prescription acne medications increase the sensitivity of the skin to sunlight, be sure to remove them, or do not apply them, on the day you're going to let your face enjoy some sunshine. Instead, apply a light noncomedogenic sunscreen.

patients to expect a bit of redness, dryness, itchiness, and stinging for at least the first few weeks.

Step 3: Antibiotic Treatment May Be Needed

If the inflammation and the infection is getting worse, your doctor may prescribe a benzoyl peroxide/antibiotic combination gel instead of straight BP. The usual combinations are BP with clindamycin or erythromycin.

Oral antibiotic treatment. If the acne does not respond to topical antibiotics (the zits are getting bigger, redder, and more numerous), the doctor might prescribe an oral antibiotic. This will treat the skin from the inside and get rid of the offending bacteria. The two antibiotics that are often used are forms of tetracycline and erythromycin. It's important to know that it may take six to eight weeks of oral antibiotic therapy before the teen notices a significant improvement.

Mix and match. Depending on the severity of the acne, the doctor may use a variety of all these steps and medications to help your teen work out her own personal acne-action plan.

The Last Resort—Accutane (Isotretinoin)

Your teen may ask, "Why can't I take the miracle pill Accutane, like my friend does?" Because of the possible serious side effects listed below, doctors reserve Accutane for only the most severe acne that has not responded to the above steps. It's used for "cystic acne," in which the sores have gotten so numerous and are so large that the teen feels like he has hundreds of red, lumpy cysts

on his face and back. The reason Accutane is used in this most severe form of acne is that it is the most likely to lead to permanent scarring and "pock marks." The Food and Drug Administration (FDA) takes the prescribing of Accutane so seriously that dermatologists must obtain a special license in order to prescribe it. Because this drug can cause birth defects, don't be surprised if the prescribing doctor requires the teen to sign consent that she will not have unprotected sexual intercourse while taking Accutane. Routine blood work is required every few months while on Accutane. Be sure your teen's doctor is licensed to prescribe Accutane.

 DR. SEARS TIP Untreated Zits Can Become the Pits

Treatment of moderate to severe acne is very important, not only for the social effects it can have, but also for the long-term cosmetic effects. Untreated or undertreated acne can lead to lifelong scarring and pits. There are new dermatological procedures, such as laser treatments, that can help diminish some of these effects. However, the best treatment is prevention.

Don't Forget to Feed Your Teen's Skin

The pills-skills model of medicine as described on page 13 really shines for acne control. Treat skin from the *inside* by making sure your teen gets enough omega 3s, phytonutrients, anti-inflammatories, and hydration, all of which are outlined in the skin health section, page 29.

DR. SEARS TIP
Don't Feed the Acne

Although there are a lot of food myths surrounding the cause of acne, it's important that your teen learns that junk food can cause junk skin. It stands to reason that if severe acne is an inflammation of plugged oil glands, the better you can build the body's immune system and control inflammation, the better the skin. Be sure your teen follows the anti-inflammatory dietary suggestions listed on page 35. Teen diets tend to be deficient in the omega 3s that contribute to healthy skin. Though it may not be true that eating greasy foods causes oily skin, eating the right kinds of fats can contribute to healthier skin.

ALLERGIC REACTIONS (ANAPHYLAXIS)

Allergic reactions come in all shapes and sizes and vary from mild to severe. This section deals with the most severe form of allergic reaction, which is called *anaphylaxis:* swelling of the hands, feet, or face; difficulty breathing or swallowing; wheezing; feeling faint or dizzy; breaking out in hives; and drooling or vomiting excessively. If your child is having a less serious allergic reaction, see Hives (skin welts) without other signs, page 370; antibiotic rash or other antibiotic reaction, page 551; unknown rash, page 443; nasal allergies, page 131.

A severe allergic reaction (anaphylaxis) can produce shock and life-threatening respiratory distress. In severely allergic people, anaphylaxis can occur within minutes or up to several hours after exposure to a specific allergy-causing substance, such as bee stings and peanuts, although almost any allergy-causing substance — including pollen, latex, certain foods and drugs — can cause anaphylaxis. Sometimes the cause of anaphylactic reactions is unknown.

Symptoms of Severe Allergic Reaction

• Your child might break out in hives, and the eyes or lips might swell.

• Hives and/or swelling will become more severe, and the inside of the throat might swell as well, even to the point of causing difficulty breathing and shock.

• Dizziness, confusion, abdominal cramping, nausea, vomiting, or diarrhea might also occur.

How to Be Prepared

If your child has had an anaphylactic reaction in the past, carry rescue medications with you.

• Epinephrine is the most commonly used drug for severe allergic reactions. It is an injection that must be prescribed by your doctor (EpiPen or EpiPen Jr). Seek emergency medical attention immediately after injecting epinephrine.

• An antihistamine, such as diphenhydramine (Benadryl), should also be kept on hand. This long-acting medication is usually taken along with epinephrine, which is short-acting.

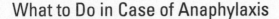

What to Do in Case of Anaphylaxis

- Call 911 or your local medical emergency number.

- Administer epinephrine as directed — usually by pressing the auto-injector against your child's thigh and holding it in place for several seconds.

- Have your child take an antihistamine pill or liquid if he is able to swallow without difficulty.

- Have your child lie still on his back with his feet higher than his head.

- Loosen tight clothing and don't give anything to drink.

- If there are no signs of circulation (no breathing, coughing, or movement), begin cardiopulmonary resuscitation (CPR).

 DR. SEARS TIP
Be Prepared

If your pediatrician prescribes an auto-injector of epinephrine, read the instructions before a problem occurs, and have your household members read them, too.

ALLERGIES

Allergies are a common occurrence among children. Because nasal allergies (also known as hay fever) are the most common symptom of allergies, we will focus on the diagnosis, treatment, and prevention of nasal allergies. This information may also help with other allergic conditions, such as asthma and eczema. Food allergies may also contribute to nasal symptoms. Please see our related sections on Asthma (page 151), Eczema (page 297), and Food Allergies (page 327) if your child's allergic problems include those areas.

Symptoms

Here are the main signs of nasal allergies to watch for:

- nasal congestion

- runny nose with clear mucus

- itchy nose

- crease across the top of the nose from constant wiping

- excessive sneezing

- itchy, watery, red eyes

- chronic cough

- wheezing

- snoring

All of these symptoms can also be part of a common cold. So how do parents decide whether their child has a cold or allergies? The best indicators are the duration and the repetitive nature of the symptoms. A common cold will only last one to three weeks, then fade away. Sinus infections can last longer, but those will progress to green nasal drainage, fever, and headache, obvious symptoms of infection.

Allergies, on the other hand, show several different patterns:

Symptoms for three weeks or longer. If symptoms last for more than three weeks and haven't worsened into a sinus infection or begun to subside, then it's probably allergies.

Recurrent symptoms. Allergies can occur for a day or two at a time, or can hit for a week or more, then fade away, only to recur again a week or two later.

Sudden resolution of symptoms. Colds will gradually linger and fade away over several days. Allergies, on the other hand, can be full-blown one day, then completely gone the next.

Predictable seasonal pattern. Some allergies will occur for a month or more during a particular season, usually spring or fall. It takes a year or two of observation to detect this pattern.

Recurrent infections. Children who repeatedly get sick with coughs, colds, sinus infections, or ear infections may have an underlying allergic trigger. Chronic allergic nasal congestion can be a breeding ground for bacteria and viruses.

 DR. SEARS TIP
Quick Diagnosis for Allergies

One easy way to determine if your child's symptoms are from allergies and not a cold is to give him an antihistamine medication (see treatment options below). If the symptoms improve for several hours, you know it's allergies. If they don't, it's probably a cold. This doesn't tell you what is *causing* the allergies. That takes a lot more work. Read on.

Here are four common situations that may seem like allergies, but are probably not:

- A child who clearly goes through a fever, cold, and cough illness for a week or two,

then has residual nasal symptoms for several weeks more. Colds can sometimes linger for up to six weeks.

- Dark circles under the eyes without nasal symptoms probably are not a sign of allergies. Some kids simply have that type of complexion.

- Chronic or recurrent cold and cough symptoms throughout the winter are usually just recurrent infections, as this is the season for it.

- Recurrent ear infections *without* chronic nasal symptoms are probably not due to allergies.

Causes

A foreign substance, called an *allergen,* enters the body through eyes, nose, lungs, stomach, or skin. If you are allergic to this allergen, your immune system's cells in the area will react by releasing a chemical called *histamine.* This chemical irritates the body tissues in the area. This irritation is designed to flush out or neutralize the allergen, but unfortunately it also results in the allergic symptoms we experience.

Family history plays a very big role as well. If one parent suffers from nasal or skin allergies, your child has a 25 percent chance of having allergies as well; if both parents have allergies, your child may have up to a 75 percent chance.

Over-the-Counter (OTC) Treatments

Before consulting your doctor, you can try several treatment options that should help relieve your child's symptoms:

Hose the nose. You can limit allergen exposure and decrease congestion simply by flushing out the nose twice a day with saline, followed by nose blowing. Saline nasal sprays for younger kids and nasal irrigation bottles for older kids and adults are available at any drugstore. Doing this before using any nasal spray medications helps the meds work better. See page 20 for more nose-hosing tips.

Short-acting oral antihistamines. These are the most effective OTC meds for decreasing symptoms, but they do cause drowsiness. Diphenhydramine (Benadryl) and chlorpheniramine (Chlor-Trimeton) are the two most commonly used. They last around six hours, but some formulations act up to twelve hours.

Long-acting, non-drowsy oral antihistamines. Loratadine (Claritin, Alavert) and cetirizine (Zyrtec) are twelve- to twenty-four-hour medications that work fairly well. Fexofenadine (Allegra) is due to change from prescription to OTC this year. They come in pill or liquid form, as well as soft tablets that melt in the mouth.

Combination oral antihistamine/decongestants. To help with severe nasal congestion and headache in addition to the allergic symptoms, try a combination. Various brands are available at a drugstore.

Proper dosing for children. Follow the directions on the bottle. Most come with dosing for kids four years and older. If the medication doesn't provide dosing for your child's age range, consult with your doctor's office.

Prescription Medications

If the OTC treatments don't bring sufficient relief, make an appointment with your doctor. Here are the treatment options at his disposal:

Long-acting, non-drowsy oral antihistamines. There are three main prescription brands: Clarinex (desloratadine), Xyzal (levocetirizine), and Allegra (fexofenadine, due to become OTC this year). Their effectiveness varies between people; one may not work well for one person, but another one will. Not all are approved for children younger than twelve years of age. One drawback in finding which one works best for your child is that most medical insurances will cover only one particular brand. You can save time with your doctor by finding out which brand your plan covers *before* your appointment.

Combination oral antihistamine/decongestants. Most of the prescription brands also come with a combination option.

Steroid nasal sprays. These are a very effective way to suppress allergies and, unlike the steroids used by bodybuilders, are very safe. They mostly act right in the nasal passage; very little to none is absorbed into the body. Nasal sprays don't work quickly, so they are not designed for occasional use. They work better when you stay on them for a while.

Antihistamine nasal sprays. A great alternative to the steroids, these can work just as well in some kids.

Combining prescriptions. For severe symptoms, a combination of oral antihistamines and steroid nasal sprays can be used.

Deciding Which Medications to Use

Here are some guidelines to follow when deciding which type of medication to use:

Occasional symptoms. If your child seems to have random allergic days here and there, an OTC oral long-acting non-drowsy antihistamine is best. If this doesn't work well, ask your doctor for a prescription one to use as needed.

Occasional nighttime symptoms. If random allergies mainly bother your child at night, first try an OTC short-acting medication, as these are very effective, and any drowsy effect will be gone by morning. Your second and third choices would be OTC long-acting antihistamines and then a prescription medication.

Seasonal prolonged symptoms. If you know the allergies are going to continue daily through spring or fall, first try an OTC long-acting, non-drowsy oral antihistamine. If that's not enough, try a prescription oral antihistamine or a nasal spray. Continue with whichever one works better. If neither works well alone, try using both simultaneously for a week. When the season is over, stop the medications.

Flare-up of severe congestion and headache. If your child's sinus complaints escalate while she is on allergy medications, add an OTC decongestant to relieve the headache and congestion until symptoms subside. In order to prevent these symptoms from worsening into a sinus infection, begin the nose-hosing and steam-cleaning techniques on page 20. An effective natural supplement for kids and adults that can also help support the sinuses (according to our experience in the office and our review of the research) is Sinupret, a blend of five herbs that help with sinus drainage and improve airflow through the nasal passages. Check out www.Sinupret ForKids.com.

Year-round allergies. If your child is going to need treatment every day of the year, an antihistamine nasal spray may be the best choice. A steroid nasal spray may be a good second choice. Add a prescription oral antihistamine if needed during flare-ups. Of course, if the allergies are this bad, you will want to focus more on investigating and preventing the allergies. Read on.

Tracking Down the Causes of Allergies

Although many parents would naturally want to find out what's causing the allergies in the first place, allow us to give you a little piece of advice. Doing so is time-consuming and complicated. Before you embark on such a journey, it's best just to wait and see if the symptoms go away over a few weeks. If the allergies continue beyond that time, or resolve but then recur, and are interfering with your child's day-to-day life, then it's worthwhile to launch an investigation.

Determining when and where the allergies occur will help you figure out the most likely causes.

Nighttime and upon waking. If your child seems to be fine during the day, but has allergy symptoms during the night and wakes up with severe symptoms in the morning, your child may be allergic to something in the bedroom. The most common bedroom allergens are dust, mold, and bedding. See page 135, Preventing Specific Allergens.

Seasonal allergies. If your child seems well all year, but suddenly develops allergy symptoms during a particular season (usually spring), or seems to have symptoms only on windy days, then she probably has allergies to particular pollens or plants that are prevalent during that season. These can cause symptoms during the day or night. See below, Preventing Specific Allergens.

School allergies. If your child only experiences symptoms at school or daycare, but is generally well at home and during the night and weekend, then the allergen is probably something at school. See below, Preventing Specific Allergens.

Friends' or relatives' houses. If you notice that your child only has symptoms at another person's house but not at school or your house, then he may be allergic to something unique to that house, such as smoking, pets, plants, or grass. The simple solution is to either not go there or give an antihistamine before going over.

Year-round allergies. If your child has allergies all year long, then the culprits could be any of the above as well as a possible food allergy. Secondhand smoke will also cause year-round symptoms.

If these distinctions allow you to narrow down the allergens to one or two possibilities that are easily prevented, then your job is fairly easy. The next section will guide your prevention efforts. However, if it's not yet obvious where to start, or if your child has year-round allergies, it may be best to skip right ahead to allergy testing. Finding out what your child is allergic to through testing will help you focus your efforts where they are most likely to help.

Preventing Specific Allergens

Food Allergies

Don't overlook these as a possible cause. See page 327 for a thorough discussion of food allergies. The most common foods that would cause nasal allergies or asthma are cow's-milk, wheat, and soy products.

Seasonal Allergies and Pollens

Pollens are tiny, dustlike, yellow microspores that are found in the middle of flowers. Wind picks up pollen, and it floats around in the air, sticking to anything it touches, such as hair and clothes, and ends up inside your child's nose and lungs. If you suspect that your child has seasonal allergies due to pollens, here are the steps you can take to minimize exposure:

* Stay indoors on windy days during pollen season and when the pollen counts are high, which you can track online.

* Don't allow your child to play in fields with flowers and tall grass.

* Keep all the windows and doors closed during your child's specific allergy season.

* Wash hats and jackets more frequently during pollen season.

* Give your child a bath and wash hair before bedtime to get the pollen out.

* Don't hang-dry your child's laundry outside, as it can pick up pollen.

* Install a special filter into your central heating and cooling system that cleans the air as it comes in from outside. You can buy these from a hardware store.

* Buy a portable HEPA filter to remove pollens, molds, spores, dust mite droppings, animal dander, and many other irritants. They cost $100 to $200 and will usually clean only one room. Or try an ionic filter. This type of filter costs about $400 to $600, but one unit will clean the entire house.

- Pollen counts are usually highest during late morning and early afternoon. Limit outside playtime to early morning, late afternoon, and evenings during allergy season.

- Put window air-conditioning units on recirculate to keep out the outside air.

- Keep trees and bushes near the house well pruned to avoid heavy vegetation.

- Keep your child from playing around freshly mowed grass.

- Put your child's clothes (which will harbor pollens) straight into the laundry room.

HEPA VS. IONIC AIR FILTERS: WHICH ONE TO BUY?

HEPA filters draw the air through the unit, filter it directly, then expel the clean air back into the room. They are fairly inexpensive, but one unit is usually needed for each room (unless a very expensive unit is installed into the central air-conditioning and heating system). Ionic air cleaners, on the other hand, disperse ions (charged particles) in all directions from one unit placed in the center of the house. These particles stick to most allergens in the air, causing them to fall to the ground. They are more expensive than one-room HEPA filters, but one unit will service the entire house. Either choice should help most allergies. If you try one type and don't experience much relief, try the other. Some air filters also utilize ozone to clean the air. This can irritate the lungs of asthmatics, so we don't recommend using the ozone feature if anyone in the family has asthma.

Dust Mites

Dust itself does not cause allergies. It is actually dust mites, microscopic organisms that live in dust, and the particles of feces that the mites excrete, that cause the allergies. Dust mites thrive in warm, humid environments. Here are some steps you can take to remove sources of dust from your house and limit the dust mite allergens in the air. Take all of the following dust-attracting items out of the bedroom: stuffed animals, books on bookshelves, piles of clothes, down comforters or feather pillows, upholstered furniture, stacks of boxes, items stored under the bed, wool blankets, heavy drapes and horizontal blinds, electric fans, and large houseplants. Take the following precautions with common bedroom items:

- Wash blankets, sheets, and pillowcases in hot water once a week to kill the mites.

- Use synthetic pillows that can be washed monthly and replaced yearly.

- Place cheesecloth over vents in the bedroom to catch dust. Change the cloth every few months when using the central air or heating.

- Keep the bedroom closet doors closed, and avoid storing toys, boxes, luggage, or heavy coats in bedroom closets.

- Dust with a damp cloth when cleaning.

- Vacuum the mattress every two weeks.

- Use an air filter as discussed above.

- Encase mattresses, box springs, and pillows with dust mite–proof zippered covers.

- Use a vacuum cleaner with a HEPA or other specialized filtering system that will prevent dust and other particles from spreading around the room.

Severe allergies. Here are some more expensive and less convenient measures that may prove necessary:

- Remove carpeting from the bedroom and possibly the rest of the house. Hardwood, tile, and linoleum can be kept virtually dust-free. Use throw rugs that can be washed frequently.

- Lower-pile commercial carpeting can be used if needed. It is less likely to trap dust mites.

- Control humidity. Place a humidity gauge in the bedroom and in other rooms as needed. Molds and dust mites thrive in high humidity. A humidity level of 25 to 40 percent is ideal. Run a dehumidifier when necessary.

- Clean out the central air ducts. This costs several hundred to over a thousand dollars to have done professionally. Do it at least every few years if not sooner.

Mold

This is another source of allergies that can be found throughout the house. Molds thrive in dark, cool, damp places. They release spores into the air that are then inhaled. An environmental testing company can test your house to see if mold is a problem. In some cases, the mold is too extensive to clean up, and you may need to move. Generally, however, the company can assist you in cleaning up the mold enough to decrease your family's exposure. Here is how you can limit mold in your house:

Throughout the house

- Clean mold-susceptible areas routinely with a mold-killing disinfectant such as a 10 percent bleach solution.

- Humidity control — follow the same precautions as for dust above.

- Mold-killing sprays can be sprayed into air-conditioning intake vents if you detect a musty odor.

- Ventilate the house by opening all the windows several times a week.

- Install filters in the central air and over vents in the house as discussed under dust control.

- Use HEPA or ionic air-filter units in the house.

In the bedroom

- Keep a nightlight on in closets. This can decrease mold growth.

- Regularly clean window frames with mold-killing solution.

- Wash wallpaper frequently with mold-killing solution if using a humidifier or vaporizer during dry weather (too much humidity can increase mold).

- Replace carpeting that has had repeated water damage.

In the kitchen

- Regularly clean the bottom of the refrigerator as well as around the rubber door gaskets.

- Wash garbage cans frequently with bleach.

- Run the exhaust fan when boiling water.

In the bathroom

- Run the vent fan in the bathroom during showers to prevent mold growth from the humidity.

- Clean shower, bathroom tiles, and toilets regularly with mold-killing solution.

- Clean the shower curtain regularly and replace it periodically.

- Regularly wash wallpaper and replace it if water-damaged.

Outside the house

- Remove damp piles of debris from the yard.

- Keep windows that are near moldy shrubbery closed.

- Prune shrubbery and trees regularly to avoid shading the house too much. Sunlight helps kill mold.

- Correct drainage problems. Pools of stagnant water or grass grow mold.

Pets

It's not actually the pet hair that causes allergies but the pet dander, tiny flakes of skin mixed with saliva that shed off animals and float around in the air. Cats, dogs, and birds all shed dander, even short-haired pets. The urine of rodents can also be allergenic. The easiest way to confirm a pet allergy is to have your child tested. If your child is allergic, but you feel that you can't give away the pets, these precautions may help:

- Give the house a frequent thorough cleaning to remove existing pet dander.

- Keep the pet out of your child's bedroom at all times.

- Keep the pet in one room as much as possible, and keep this room well ventilated to the outside.

- Keep the house well ventilated. Open the windows as much as possible to recirculate the air.

- Use a HEPA or ionic air filter as described in the seasonal allergies and pollen section.

- Wash your pet frequently to minimize dander shedding.

- Use a vacuum with a special filter to trap allergens.

- Try allergy-control solutions, which can be sprayed onto the carpet to deactivate accumulated dander.

Allergies at School

If your child seems to have symptoms only at school, here are several possible sources to consider:

- Pets in the classroom — often there is a class gerbil, rabbit, or other rodent. You can test this by asking the teacher to let someone take the pet home for two weeks and see if your child improves.

- Dust mites and mold — the classroom can contain all the same sources of dust and mold as your house. Talk to the school principal about a possible course of action.

- Portable trailers may harbor more mold than regular building classrooms. If your child's symptoms are worse in a trailer, have your doctor give you a medical excuse to change classrooms if practical.

- Plants and grass — there may be specific grass or pollens present only at school. It would be difficult to prevent exposure to these.

- Cockroaches in lockers or other areas — children can be allergic to the feces of these insects.

If you can't eliminate these sources, you may need to treat your child with medication.

Cigarette Smoke

Exposure to secondhand smoke is one of the most ignored and preventable causes of allergy symptoms and asthma. The best way to prevent this allergy is to stop smoking altogether. When this is not an option for the smoking family member, here are some precautions you can take:

- Never smoke around the child. This includes inside the house, in the car, and outside near the child.

- Never smoke in the house or car, even when the child isn't home. The smoke can linger for hours to days, and the child will constantly be inhaling the residual smoke. Smokers can't smell the residual smoke because they are used to it, but just ask any of your non-smoking friends; they will usually tell you your house has a very strong odor of smoke.

- Smoke outside away from any open windows so the smoke doesn't blow in.

- When smoking relatives come to visit, remember, this is your house. You make the rules. Tell them to smoke outside. See page 484 for more information.

Consulting Your Pediatrician

All of this information can be overwhelming. Don't despair! Try some of the more simple suggestions and observe your child for improvement. If you don't see any significant improvement, then it's probably time to discuss the allergies with your pediatrician.

What your pediatrician can offer you. Although your child's doctor may not be able to offer any additional advice on allergy prevention and control, she may be able to help you narrow down the cause of the allergies. She can also make recommendations on treating the allergies with medication and discuss the various forms of over-the-counter and prescription allergy medication. Finally, she can offer blood allergy testing to help you find the causes.

Consulting an Allergist

There are several services that an allergist can offer you that your pediatrician probably cannot:

Time. An allergist often has more time to sit down with you and discuss your child's allergies. The allergist may be able to pinpoint the most likely allergens affecting your child so that you can focus your prevention more precisely. The doctor can also spend more time educating you on allergy prevention.

Skin testing. An allergist's office can perform skin testing on your child to help identify specific allergens. A tiny needle is used to introduce potential allergens, such as dairy protein or pet dander, into the skin. The allergist can do either a small number of these at a time to test suspected allergens or thirty to forty different allergens (and skin pricks) at one visit to get a more complete allergy profile. A bump will form in the skin for each test that is positive.

Up-to-date treatments. An allergist is often more up to date than a general practitioner about the latest medications to alleviate allergy symptoms. He may also be more adept at using combinations of medications when needed.

Allergy shots. Allergy shots are long-term, time-consuming, and expensive treatment that involves several shots each week for the first few weeks, followed by one shot a week for a few months, and then one or two a month for a year or more. The shots slowly make your child less sensitive to his specific allergens. This is a very aggressive — but sometimes necessary — treatment.

ANEMIA

Anemia means "low blood hemoglobin." *Hemoglobin* is the substance that makes red blood cells red and carries oxygen to the blood to be delivered to the tissues. Children who don't have enough hemoglobin don't get enough oxygen to their tissues, which affects the whole body.

Symptoms

- Your child's skin appears pale, primarily on the face and earlobes.

- You may notice a more rapid heartbeat.

- The child may be excessively tired.

- Because anemia affects the neurochemicals in the brain, an anemic child may be irritable and have otherwise unexplained behavioral problems.

- Your baby or toddler may show slower than optimal growth.

Causes

- The child's body does not produce enough red blood cells, usually due to iron deficiency.

- Excess red blood cells are lost from the body, the most common cause being slight but chronic intestinal bleeding.

- An increased rate of breakdown of red blood cells, usually a hereditary quirk, causes the red blood cells to be broken down faster than the body can reproduce them.

Diagnosis

During their first few months babies have an excess of red blood cells and hemoglobin, but by around two to three months, this excess begins to dissipate, and babies begin making more of their own red blood cells. The most common cause of anemia in infants and toddlers is iron deficiency. Hemoglobin requires adequate iron to allow red blood cells to do their job. If infants don't get enough iron in their diet or lose too much iron through the red blood cells from minute intestinal bleeding, they will develop *iron-deficiency anemia*. This is why your health-care provider will routinely check Baby's hemoglobin (usually by obtaining one drop of blood by a simple finger stick) sometime between six and twelve months, and often up to age two if your infant shows any signs of anemia.

**DR. SEARS TIP
Take Iron-Deficiency
Anemia Seriously**

Children with iron-deficiency anemia not only have a tired body — they have a tired brain. New insights show that infants who have iron-deficiency anemia that has gone untreated for a long time are at increased risk for delayed physical and mental development. Sometimes a skin-prick test of hemoglobin in the pediatrician's office may be "low normal" (normal for an infant is between 11 and 13) but not optimal. It doesn't hurt to treat with iron or push iron-fortified foods in this situation to boost the levels up to high normal. If deemed necessary, a more accurate test will be taken to measure your infant's serum ferritin level, the actual blood level of iron. This test requires going to a laboratory and having your child's blood drawn. If your child's exam or dietary history suggests low iron even though the hemoglobin is in the normal range, your doctor may order a serum ferritin level before recommending supplements just to be sure.

What to Do

Pediatricians are very conscious about watching for signs of anemia and testing for it, including pinpointing infants who are at risk for developing anemia, such as premature babies who are born with low iron stores. If your doctor says your infant is anemic, here's what to do:

Give your infant more iron. If Baby's anemia is worrisome, your doctor may prescribe some daily iron drops in addition to increased iron in the diet. Be sure to give this iron-rich medication as prescribed, usually for a month or two after the hemoglobin returns to normal, in order to replenish your child's iron stores.

Use iron-fortified formula. A few infant formulas are labeled as having low iron. Switch to one with more iron if your doctor agrees.

Delay cow's milk for infants; limit it for toddlers. The Committee on Nutrition for the American Academy of Pediatrics recommends that parents delay using cow's milk as Baby's main source of nutrition until around one year of age for two reasons: cow's milk is low in iron (infant formulas are iron-fortified), and cow's milk can irritate Baby's intestinal lining, causing tiny amounts of bleeding and loss of iron. If intestinal blood loss is suspected, the doctor may check your child's bowel movements for traces of blood and have you decrease or stop your baby's milk intake. Because yogurt is less allergenic and more intestine-friendly than cow's milk, we recommend yogurt as the main dairy product starting from nine months of age.

**DR. SEARS TIP
Milk Limit**

Limit your toddler's cow's milk intake to no more than sixteen ounces a day.

Feed your toddler iron-rich foods. Top toddler iron-rich foods include the following:

- beef
- lamb
- dark-meat poultry
- fish (tuna and wild salmon)

- blackstrap molasses

- prune juice

- tomato paste

- potatoes with the skin (leave the iron-rich skin on homemade French fries)

- sweet potatoes

- beans and lentils

- raisins

- dried fruit (apricots, figs, peaches)

- iron-fortified cereals

 DR. SEARS TIP
Add Vitamin C to
Iron-Rich Foods

Vitamin C increases the amount of iron that is absorbed from the above foods, so encourage your child to drink a glass of orange juice with a meal, eat tomato-rich spaghetti sauce with homemade meatballs, and eat vitamin C–rich fruits and veggies with a meal. This is why Grandmother's advice to "eat your meat and veggies" is nutritionally correct for preventing anemia. Combining iron-rich foods with vitamin C–rich foods can double the amount of iron absorbed from the foods.

(See related topic, Blood in Bowel Movements, page 196.)

ANOREXIA

Much has been learned about anorexia over the past twenty years. In a society that seems to increasingly value the "supermodel" look perpetuated in the media, television, and movies, more and more individuals are at risk for this devastating illness. Adolescents and teenagers, especially young women, experience a great deal of peer pressure to maintain a certain lean "look."

The highest-risk group for anorexia is teenage girls. However, it is being diagnosed at younger and younger ages today, as girls are exposed to various media sources that pressure them to feel like they must lose weight. Anorexia is being diagnosed more and more among teenage boys as well.

Signs and Symptoms

Potential warning signs that may indicate your child is at risk for anorexia include the following:

- a generalized disinterest in foods

- a sudden unexplainable drop in weight or a drastic drop-off on the growth chart percentiles for weight

- weight below the fifth percentile

- a generalized malnourished appearance — looks like "skin and bones"

- fine, brittle hair

- dry skin

- the development of fine, soft, whitish hair, especially on the cheeks, known as *lanugo* hair

- obsessing about weight and appearance

- "overdoing it" when it comes to exercise, constantly feeling the need to be in the gym or involved in other high-intensity activities, such as running, in excess of what would be considered healthy

- irregular periods or cessation of periods, or failure to begin menstruating by an age when normal menstrual activity occurs

- ongoing dizzy spells or periods of passing out

- repeated, unexplainable episodes of nausea

- new onset of seizure activity

- symptoms of depression and/or anxiety

If your child or young adult is experiencing any or all of these features, consult your pediatrician.

What to Do

Consult your pediatrician. If your pediatrician suspects your child is exhibiting possible signs of anorexia, blood work must be performed to rule out serious illness. Anorexics can have severe and dangerous deficiencies of certain nutrients and electrolytes, especially sodium and potassium, which can lead to seizures and even death. Treatment of anorexia requires a multidisciplinary approach involving various health professionals. The pediatrician should closely monitor the patient's progress with frequent office visits to follow weight and height as well as with various blood tests to follow important electrolyte levels.

Consult a nutritionist. A nutritionist should closely monitor the patient's daily caloric intake, as well as make suggestions on healthy eating habits. It is especially important to find someone who has experience working with anorexic patients.

 DR. SEARS TIP
Model Healthy Weight

The seeds of anorexia may be planted early in life. It is very important for parents to send a healthy message to their children about their body types that says, "I like the way you are." Often, obsessive behavior regarding appearance and weight is learned by the children through the example set by their parents and friends. Teach your children what a healthy weight is. Encourage proper eating and exercise habits, and mirror that yourself. Take note of your adolescent's peer groups. Encourage friendships with individuals who are not overly obsessive about their appearance and their weight.

Consult a therapist. A psychologist and/or psychiatrist must also be involved in the patient's care. Anorexia is always accompanied by symptoms of depression and/or anxiety, which must be managed and treated. People suffering from anorexia carry with them a higher suicide risk, and this risk must be assessed. Certain behavioral therapies have also been shown to be effective in the treatment of anorexia.

Sadly, even with the best of treatment, anorexia is difficult to control and manage. It is often a lifetime affliction, with individuals fighting a constant battle to see themselves in a new light and live a healthy existence. Thankfully, over the past twenty years we have become much more effective at diagnosing and treating this debilitating disease.

DR. SEARS TIP
Food Fat and Body Fat Are Good!

Teen girls are bombarded with the scientifically incorrect message that "fats in food are bad." Wrong! They are also given the message that "fat on the body is bad." Wrong again! Teach your teen about *good* food fats (e.g., seafood, olive oil, flax oil, nut butters, and avocados). Healthy food fats help every organ of the body, especially the brain, grow properly. Although the term *lean* is important, you should show and tell your teen that *lean* means having just the right amount of body fat for her body type — not too much, not too little: "If you don't have enough body fat, you won't develop as well into a woman. The right amount of body fat makes the female hormone estrogen, which helps your breasts grow, causes menstruation to begin, and gives you those attractive girly curves. After all, if Mom didn't have enough body fat you wouldn't be here — she couldn't have conceived you or nursed you."

For more about healthy nutritional fats, see the Dr. Sears L.E.A.N. Kids Program, page 417, or see *The Family Nutrition Book*.

APPENDICITIS

Your previously healthy child starts feeling nauseated and her appetite is diminished, so you think she's coming down with the flu. Within hours or a day, she starts complaining of vague pain around her belly button. Within the same day that pain moves over to the lower right side just above the right hip bone or around into the back. You see your child grabbing the area. She says, "Mommy, it hurts me to walk." You feel her forehead and find that she has a low-grade fever. You call the doctor immediately. "I think my child has appendicitis."

Symptoms

Although there are many causes of lower abdominal pain (constipation, which tops the list; urinary tract infections, especially in girls; intestinal infections; flu; and food poisoning), if your child develops the following collection of clues, seek medical attention immediately:

• decreased appetite and nausea

• abdominal pain that begins with the "circle sign" (the child circles the belly button with the whole hand), which is followed within a few hours or a day by the "point sign," with the child pointing to the right lower quadrant of the abdomen in the area between the right lower ribcage and the pelvic bone, or around to the right back

• limping or holding the lower right side when trying to walk

• low-grade fever

• pain with jumping. Have your child sit on a table so his feet dangle about a foot from the floor. Ask him to jump to the floor. Alternatively, ask him to jump up and down in place. If he refuses to jump because "it will hurt" or if as soon as the child jumps he immediately grabs his lower right abdomen, you should suspect appendicitis, especially if some of the other signs above are present.

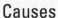

Causes

The appendix is a seemingly useless finger-sized "appendage" that hangs down from the beginning of the large intestine. This little wormy structure opens to the large intestine. If the opening gets blocked, such as with undigested food or a hard piece of stool, the appendix becomes inflamed and gets infected by the bacteria that live there. If the inflamed appendix, or appendicitis, is not diagnosed and removed, usually within twenty-four hours, it can "rupture," spreading bacteria and infection throughout the abdominal cavity and resulting in a serious total-body infection. The earlier the diagnosis is made and treatment begun, the less dangerous it is. Removing the inflamed appendix before it ruptures is the goal. The child is often well enough to leave the hospital the following day and bounces back quickly with full appetite and activity within a few days, with only a little tender area where the wound is healing and an inch-long scar to remind her of a "bad day."

 DR. SEARS TIP
Hold the Food!

If, based on the clues above, you believe your child might have appendicitis, don't let him eat (but he may drink clear liquids) before the doctor has an opportunity to evaluate him. Food in the stomach or intestine will only delay the anesthesia and surgery. The sooner the inflamed appendix is "in a pickle jar," the better.

What the Doctor Will Do

The doctor will see your child immediately and go through the following steps:

- He will listen to your history of the evolution of the signs and symptoms.

- He will say to the child, "Tell me where it hurts." The doctor is also looking for the point sign.

- He will examine your child's abdomen. You'll notice your doctor gently pressing in on the area of pain and then quickly removing his hand. If the child winces with this test, this is highly indicative of appendicitis. This test is called "rebound tenderness," meaning that when the doctor quickly removes his hand the inflamed appendix bounces up against the abdominal wall and causes pain.

- Your pediatrician may also do some other office tests, such as urinalysis to exclude a urinary tract infection, especially in girls, and a white blood count. Because the white blood cells are increasing to fight the infection, children with appendicitis nearly always have an elevated white blood count.

- The doctor will also examine your child's right hip, especially if the child is limping, because sometimes right hip problems, such as dislocation or infection, can radiate pain to the abdomen.

Sometimes the diagnosis is clear-cut, and your doctor will immediately call the surgeon and send your child to the hospital. In this case we tell parents, "That little appendix belongs in a pickle jar as soon as possible." If the diagnosis is still "uncertain" or "a possible appendicitis," the doctor may send your child for an X-ray, an ultrasound, or a CT scan of the area, which often can show an inflamed appendix.

You may have heard about children (and adults) having an appendectomy only to find the appendix was "normal." Even with modern diagnostic techniques, occasionally the diagnosis is questionable. Yet, the age-old appendicitis wisdom still holds: "When in doubt, take it out." This is because a ruptured appendix can lead to a serious abdominal infection.

 DR. SEARS TIP
Check the Throat

Sometimes children with strep throat first present with abdominal pain resembling appendicitis. This is because there are tonsil-like glands in the abdomen around the area of the appendix. When the tonsils swell in the throat, so do the lymph nodes in the abdomen; as a result, a sore throat can also lead to a sore abdomen. Once the strep throat is treated, the appendicitis-like symptoms magically go away.

ARTHRITIS

The general term *arthritis* means "pain and swelling of a joint." The most common form of arthritis, also known as *osteoarthritis,* occurs most often in older adults. It is the result of general wear and tear of the joint along with a slowly diminishing amount of cartilage that keeps the joints mobile. This type of arthritis is seldom seen in young people.

A second, less common form of arthritis is known as *rheumatoid arthritis*. Although this form of arthritis is still more common in adults, Juvenile Rheumatoid Arthritis can be seen in children from the ages of one to sixteen. Rheumatoid arthritis in children is quite distinct from its adult counterpart.

Juvenile Rheumatoid Arthritis (JRA)

Juvenile Rheumatoid Arthritis (JRA) tends to affect girls more often than boys. It is the result of an inflammatory reaction in certain joint spaces in the body. For unknown reasons, special cells in the body that are normally designed to attack only foreign substances as part of our normal immune system begin attacking cells within the joints. This causes an inflammatory reaction, and can lead to damage and possible destruction of areas in the joints, which is called an *autoimmune reaction.* JRA occurs in approximately 50 to 100 per 100,000 children in the United States, usually before the age of sixteen.

Symptoms

The most common symptoms are pain, redness, tenderness, and/or swelling at a specific joint. Knees, ankles, fingers, and wrists can all be affected.

 DR. SEARS TIP
FUO May Signal JRA

Preschool-age children may initially present with a *fever of unknown origin* (FUO, or as doctors muse, "*F*ailure to *U*ncover the *O*bvious"). The child may have periodic bouts of spiking fevers with no other signs or symptoms. Although this scenario usually means a viral illness, occasionally these bouts of fevers may be early signs of JRA, and the joint signs appear later.

Older children will be able to verbalize the discomfort of a certain joint. Children younger than three may find it difficult to communicate their symptoms to parents. Symptoms in toddlers may include lethargy, irritability, or reluctance to play. Over time, the course of this disease varies greatly from person to person. Symptoms might be present in one joint only or may slowly progress to multiple sites mentioned above. The pain and inflammation may be present on one side or both — for example, in one knee or both knees. Specific joint symptoms of JRA include the following:

- joint stiffness, especially when waking up in the morning

- limited range of motion of the joint

- hot, swollen, painful joints

- back pain

- unwillingness to use a certain joint

- slowed growth rate or uneven growth of arms or legs

Occasionally, children may experience system-wide symptoms along with the arthritis, including fever that fluctuates throughout the day, possibly along with a rash. Certain patients may also experience swollen lymph nodes or glands.

Diagnosis and Treatment

This diagnosis can be difficult to make, especially in young children. Often the diagnosis is made after an extended period of time, due to the progressive nature of this illness, and after putting all the above clues together. Your pediatrician may begin to suspect JRA if your child begins to experience symptoms spreading to various joints in the body. A full examination should be performed, giving special attention to the joints affected, the amount of pain on movement, and the range of motion of the joint. X-rays may be performed in order to look for any evidence of inflammation and

damage to the joints. When rheumatoid arthritis is suspected in adults, blood tests can be useful in diagnosis. However, in children, these types of blood tests are usually negative, even when the child has rheumatoid arthritis.

Treatment of JRA is based upon severity of symptoms. Early on, and in mild cases, anti-inflammatories are often used. In more advanced cases, or when there is evidence the disease is progressing, other prescription medications similar to those used in treating adult rheumatoid arthritis are given. These cases are usually treated by a pediatric rheumatologist.

What You Can Do

To soothe your child's inflamed joint or joints:

Strengthen the muscles. In addition to medical treatment, physical therapy and special exercise programs may be helpful. A useful medical teaching is that the joints are only as strong as the muscles supporting them. In consultation with your physical therapist, encourage a strength-building program that keeps the muscles strong around the most affected joints.

Keep your child lean. Being overfat and overweight harms the already inflamed joints in three ways:

1. Excess abdominal fat spews out inflammatory chemicals into your child's bloodstream, which increases the inflammation and wear and tear on the already inflamed joints, worsening the arthritis. (See iBods, page 35.)

2. Being overweight contributes to excess pressure on the inflamed joints, further aggravating the wear and tear on the hip, knee, and ankle joints.

3. Being overweight throws a child's walking off balance. An overfat child can have a waddle walk, which puts excess strain not only on the knees, but also on the lower back and hip joints, further aggravating arthritis in these joints.

Move the joints. JRA goes through "remissions" and "exacerbations," meaning it goes away for a time during which the child seems completely normal, and then it periodically reappears. During the remissions, capitalize on the principle of muscle, bone, and joint health: Use it or lose it. In consultation with your child's doctor and physical therapist, get your child into sports and exercise programs that move the affected joints.

**DR. SEARS TIP
Swimming Is Swell
for Swollen Joints!**

One of the safest and most effective exercises for arthritis is swimming, which is often possible during those flare-ups or exacerbations of JRA. Swimming moves the joints, yet the buoyancy prevents excessive weight-bearing and consequent wear and tear on inflamed joints. Your child's rheumatologist and physical therapist will explain to you when to rest the joints and when to move them.

Pump the joints. Surrounding all the joints in your child's body is a natural lubricant, called *synovial fluid,* which acts like oil to the moving cylinders of an engine. Besides being a lubricant, it also acts like a cushion and as a delivery vehicle for maintenance and healing nutrients to the joint. One of the most effective exercises, especially for the knees, is lifting one foot off the floor and moving the

lifted foot back and forth, or sitting and pumping both legs. This "pump it up" technique can be done with all the joints. The flexion and extension of the pumping motion sloshes the synovial fluid around the joints to bathe the inflamed structures with lubrication, nourishment, and repair substances.

Feed the joints. Read how food affects inflammation, and see the list of anti-inflammatory foods, especially the natural anti-inflammatory properties of omega 3s, on page 33. Be sure your child gets enough calcium for growing bones (see Nutrition, page 93). Long-term studies have shown that bone strength is mostly set in the early years of life. Children and adolescents who grow up with strong bones are much less likely to suffer arthritis in their aging years. These studies suggest that calcium

**DR. SEARS TIP
Keep an Eye on It!**

It is important that every child diagnosed with JRA gets regular eye exams from an ophthalmologist. For unknown reasons, children with this condition are at higher risk for certain potentially serious eye conditions, and they should get eye exams every three to six months, depending on the pediatrician's recommendation. If your child is diagnosed with JRA and experiences the following symptoms, see your doctor immediately:

- red eyes

- eye pain

- visual changes

- increasing pain when looking into lights

supplementation is more effective in building stronger bones at younger ages.

Long-Term Prognosis

The good news is that approximately 75 percent of children with JRA eventually end up in full remission with little loss of joint mobility and minimal deformity. Some children, however, will experience periodic flare-ups. Children and adolescents with the more severe form of JRA are at risk for progressing to the adult form of rheumatoid arthritis.

Are They Growing Pains or Something Worse?

We often see children in our office complaining of pain in their joints. Usually, there is nothing to worry about, and we can reassure parents that this is a normal part of a child's growth. Growing pains are a real thing and affect many children. They are caused when growth plates in the joints (especially the knees, ankles, and hips) go through rapid periods of growth spurts. Usually, children experiencing growing pains do not have the same severity of symptoms as children with JRA. We tell patients to look for warning signs such as pain and morning stiffness, swelling or deformities of the joints, or diminished growth. Additionally, children with growing pains are usually not slowed down much by this condition. Children with true JRA are often extremely affected by this condition, and it can interfere greatly with their activities. Of course, you should always have your pediatrician examine your child if she is experiencing pain in one or more joints. (For more information, see Growing Pains, page 346.)

Septic Arthritis

This is rare in children, but when it does occur, it is considered a medical emergency. It is essentially an infection of a joint space and can occur in almost any joint in the body. Most commonly affected are the hips and knees. This usually leads to the formation of an abscess and can lead to the eventual destruction of the joint itself. Septic arthritis can arise from the following causes:

Penetrating trauma. Although rare, this can lead to septic arthritis when a puncture or traumatic injury occurs in the area of a certain joint.

Body-wide infection. Bacteria can spread through the blood into the joint space, eventually leading to septic arthritis. The child will usually show signs of infection, such as high fever and lethargy, and will appear very ill. He may complain of extreme pain at a specific joint site.

Sexually transmitted disease. Although very rare, an infection from gonorrhea, which is a certain type of bacteria, can spread through the rest of the body and invade joint spaces, especially the knee.

Treatment

This serious infection usually requires hospitalization, intravenous antibiotics, and often surgical drainage of the abscess.

Psoriatic Arthritis

Psoriasis is a relatively common skin disorder among children and adults. The underlying cause is unknown, but it is believed to be an autoimmune disease in which the body's immune system attacks its own cells in the skin. This often causes very uncomfortable and painful outbreaks of scaly rashes on the skin. It is uncommon in young children, but up to one-third of patients with this disorder show symptoms before fifteen years of age. Some people with psoriasis will also develop underlying arthritis. This leads to the diagnosis of *psoriatic arthritis*. It is unknown why some people with psoriasis also develop symptoms of arthritis.

Inflammatory Bowel Disease (IBD)

Individuals who suffer from certain inflammatory bowel diseases (IBD), such as Crohn's disease or ulcerative colitis, can also begin to have symptoms of arthritis (see Inflammatory Bowel Disease, page 378).

ASPERGER'S SYNDROME

The Austrian physician Dr. Hans Asperger described this syndrome in 1944. Asperger's syndrome (AS) is part of the autism spectrum, but many Asperger's specialists prefer to separate this syndrome from autism because many of these children are very verbal and social and act quite differently from those with autism. We believe AS belongs in the overall spectrum of what we call "quirky kids." The most common characteristics of children with AS include the following:

- Their behavior is socially inappropriate. Some children are socially aloof; others are just socially awkward. Most of these children have trouble picking up on the usual social cues and responding appropriately. They may blurt out an opinion that is off the topic of discussion during a social conversation or right in the middle of class.

- They have difficulty with back-and-forth listening and speaking during normal conversation.

- They seem uncomfortable with appropriate eye-to-eye contact. They may be uncomfortable engaging in prolonged conversation and social interactions.

- They have difficulty forming close friendships.

- They may show quirky mannerisms, such as hand flapping.

- They may appear clumsy and inappropriate in their use of body language.

There is wide variability in the number and severity of these quirks.

Many children diagnosed with AS are bright and creative. These kids often think outside the box and, if given proper parental and professional help, they will often grow up to build better boxes.

What to Do

The brains of children with AS work differently, and oftentimes these differences can be channeled to work to the child's advantage.

Be your child's social chairman. Social quirks are usually what get these children into trouble. Notice which peers your child relates to appropriately and encourage those relationships. It's important that these children learn to form a few deep friendships with compatible peers. Although some do better with one-on-one relationships, others shine in group play. Invite temperament-compatible friends to your home for playdates and overnights.

Set your child up to succeed. You may discover that your child relates best to children who are equally bright and interesting, but he gets easily bored around children he perceives as boring. If you see him engaging in socially inappropriate behavior, help him work through it. Your child may need you to be his social counselor, such as when another child approaches him to play. He just may not get it, and you may need to tell him, "Johnny wants you to play with him."

Model socially appropriate behavior. Help your child become comfortable engaging in normal conversation. Encourage listening and eye contact; for example, say: "Jimmy, I need your eyes; I need your ears." Be animated with your facial gestures so that he becomes comfortable and enjoys looking at someone's face.

Encourage his special talent. Every child has a special talent. Discover it, run with it, and encourage its development. It may be a sport, art, music, or academics. If he succeeds in one endeavor and feels good about it, the "carryover effect" is likely to help him develop appropriate behavior in other situations.

Model empathy. These children often have trouble with empathy, the ability to get into the mind and behind the eyes of another person and imagine the effects of their own behavior on their friends. For example, they may laugh when a friend is sad. When your child shows emotions, such as being sad or happy, respond with empathetic responses, such as "I'm sorry" or "I'm happy too." If you see your child responding inappropriately to social cues, such as laughing at a sad person, remind him, "That's inappropriate!"

Consult an expert. There are specialists in AS in most major cities. Interview several to find the right match for your child.

LEARN MORE ABOUT IT

Visit www.Aspergers.com or see *The Autism Book* by Robert W. Sears, MD.

(See related sections, Autism, page 167, and Growing a Healthy Brain, page 14.)

ASTHMA

The term *asthma* simply means "wheezing." The wheezing noise is caused by air passing through narrowed airways in the lungs. With asthma, the airways are narrowed by two mechanisms:

- Constriction (also called bronchospasm). The muscles around the airways squeeze the tubes and make them narrower.

- Inflammation. The lining of the airways gets swollen and secretes extra mucus.

Treatment of asthma is aimed at relaxing the constriction to widen the airways and relieving the inflammation so that the lining doesn't swell and secrete so much mucus. The pills-skills model of medical care on page 13 really shines in the treatment of asthma. In addition to pills, such as medicines to relax the airways and suppress the inflammation, we will show you how to teach your child self-help skills to relax the bronchospasm and suppress the inflammation.

Symptoms

A child who wheezes once or twice doesn't necessarily have asthma. Asthma is a *chronic* condition in which a child suffers *repeated episodes* of wheezing or tight-chested breathing. These symptoms may occur on a daily basis or more sporadically. A child is not given the diagnosis of asthma until he has suffered several episodes or has recurrent bouts of wheezing.

Here are the four main signs to watch for in determining if your child has asthma:

- *Wheezing.* This is the hallmark symptom of asthma. Wheezing is a squeaky rattling sound during exhalation. When severe, wheezing may also occur during inhalation.

- *Tight-chested breathing.* Some sufferers will feel like their lungs are too tight to breathe in easily. They will raise their shoulders up and down to assist in breathing.

- *Retractions.* During an asthma attack, the skin in the neck area just above the sternum or in the upper abdomen just below the ribcage will "suck in," or retract, when the child inhales.

- *Chronic cough.* Some children will display a chronic cough day and/or night. This cough will generally be a shallow forced single cough (as opposed to the deep junky coughing fits of a chest cold). An asthmatic forces air into the lungs through back pressure (even though the cough is mainly going *out*).

Types of Asthma

In order to understand the cause, treatment, and prevention of asthma, it's critical to understand which type of asthma your child has. A child can have one, two, or all three types together.

Exercise-Induced Bronchospasm (EIB)

In this form of asthma, a child only experiences symptoms with exercise. The child fortunately does not have any wheezing or tight-chested breathing at night or during the course of normal daily activities. This is often referred to as "exercise asthma."

Reactive Airway Disease (RAD)

In this condition, a child only has wheezing or tight-chested breathing during a cold and cough illness. When the child is otherwise well, he has no trouble breathing, even during exercise. So this isn't really considered an actual type of asthma if there are no exercise or allergy-induced problems. Most children outgrow RAD as their immune systems mature and they get fewer colds.

Allergic Asthma

In this most troublesome type of asthma, a child has breathing difficulty whenever he is exposed to something he is allergic to. The severity and frequency of symptoms depends on what a child is allergic to, and how easy these things are to avoid. A person may only have symptoms once a year during an allergy season, or he may struggle almost every day or

 DR. SEARS TIP
Don't Forget GERD

One of the most common hidden causes of wheezing is gastroesophageal reflux. Regurgitated stomach acids trigger spasm and constriction of the airways. Treat the reflux (see GERD treatment, page 341) and the "asthma" goes away.

night if he has multiple food and environmental allergies. In general, if your child doesn't just have EIB- or RAD-related episodes, he probably has allergic triggers for his asthma.

Diagnosis

The first or second time a child wheezes it's usually assumed to be temporary wheezing situations triggered by a cold, an infection like pneumonia, or an allergy exposure. It won't be until such events repeat themselves a few more times, or persist for more than a few weeks at a time, that asthma will be suspected.

You and your pediatrician will then determine the type of asthma your child has based on the types of asthma described above. It helps if the doctor can examine your child while he is experiencing symptoms to confirm that he is indeed wheezing. If you suspect your child may have asthma but on examination the doctor has been unable to find any abnormal breathing signs, an allergist or pulmonary specialist can do pulmonary function testing (a simple test in which your child blows into a tube) to determine if your child's breathing is impaired.

Treatments for Different Types of Asthma

Treating asthma is definitely a team effort, and you, the parent, are the most critical part of that team. Treatment begins with a proper understanding of how each type of asthma is treated.

Treating exercise-induced bronchospasm (EIB). Your child may outgrow exercise asthma over the years. Be sure to encourage him to stay active in sports. Twenty to thirty minutes before beginning exertion, your child will use a bronchodilator inhaler like albuterol or an anti-inflammatory inhaler like cromolyn (see Medications, page 155). This will work to keep the airways from constricting during exercise. He can also repeat the inhaler during sports as needed. You may find certain sports (especially those with frequent bursts of sudden exertion, such as sprinting or tennis) cause more breathing difficulty than sports with continuous low-to-moderate exertion, such as long-distance running.

Treating reactive airway disease (RAD). Fortunately, children usually outgrow this tendency to wheeze during cold and flu infections. The main treatment is to use a bronchodilator inhaler or nebulizer (see Medications, page 155) such as albuterol at the first sign of a cold or cough coming on and throughout the duration of the cold. This helps your child stay ahead of the wheezing so the breathing doesn't become too labored. You should also follow our chest-clearing advice under Colds and Coughs, page 222. Boosting your child's immune system (see page 33) so he doesn't catch so many colds in the first place is helpful too.

Treating allergic asthma. Successfully treating this type of asthma depends on the degree of allergies. Children with a few identifiable allergies that can be easily prevented can overcome their asthma without too much effort. Those with multiple allergies will have to work harder to avoid exposure and may experience asthma for many years, or throughout life. The rest of our discussion will focus on preventing and treating allergic asthma.

Taking Control of Your Child's Asthma

Now that you have determined which type of asthma your child has, we will lay out the steps you and your child should take to take control of the asthma so it doesn't control you.

1. Maintain lung health. Read our section on general lung health (page 24).

2. Boost your child's immune system. Read our section on boosting your child's immune system (page 33).

3. Allergy-proof your home. The degree of allergy-proofing you need to do depends upon the severity of your child's allergies. Focus on allergy-proofing your child's bedroom first, since this is where he spends the most time. Dust-proof the bedroom as much as possible: Remove feathered pillows, stuffed animals, and fuzzy toys that collect dust; ban pets from the bedroom; run a HEPA or ionic air purifier to remove the allergens. During the winter months, turn down the central heat and use a vaporizer instead. Try to keep the humidity around 50 percent. If the air is too humid, it can trigger the growth of mold. If there is not enough humidity, it can thicken the secretions in the respiratory passages. There are many more allergy-proofing steps you can follow throughout the house. See our section on Allergies, page 131, for a more detailed list.

4. Keep an asthma diary. Write down each time your child wheezes. Here are the five most important things to track:

- How frequently the wheezing episodes occur.

- How severe they are. For example, does your child miss school, miss sleep, or need a trip to the emergency room, or is it just occasional episodes of noisy breathing that slow your child down a bit but don't really interfere with his life?

- What triggers the wheezing. As often as possible, try to identify the triggers. Become a parent detective. Did it occur when your child was playing outside, in the bedroom, around a smoker, when he was anxious or upset, or when a new pet came into the family?

- How often your child uses medication, which ones work, which ones don't.

- How many doctor's visits or visits to the emergency room your child has had in the past year. This entry is a very important part of your diary because, as you will learn below, it will help the doctor make an important decision: Whether your child needs medications only when the wheezing episodes occur or needs to be on daily preventive medicines to keep the wheezing from occurring. It also helps the doctor determine whether your child's asthma can be controlled with bronchodilator medications alone or if your child also needs anti-inflammatory medicines — and which ones. Be a keen observer and an accurate reporter of your child's asthma. This helps your doctor treat your child *appropriately* — neither too little medicine nor too much.

5. Monitor asthma with a peak flow meter. Your pediatrician can provide you with this tool to help you gauge your child's degree of wheezing. Your child blows hard into this simple handheld tube, which measures how much air he can rapidly exhale. You should determine what this reading is as a baseline when he is well (your doctor can tell you what it should be for your child's age and height). When your child begins wheezing, you can compare that peak flow reading to the normal reading.

DR. SEARS SUGGESTS: COLOR-CODE THE WHEEZING	
Green light: Don't worry.	Mild asthma attack — peak flow reading is 80% to 100% what it normally is.
Yellow light: Worry, start medicines.	Moderate attack — reading is 50% to 80% of normal.
Red light: Seek medical help now!	Severe attack — reading is less than 50% of normal.

6. Help your child learn to relax. Relaxing your child's brain relaxes the airways. Stress causes the muscles around the airways to constrict, which is why asthma is also called *bronchospasm*. This becomes a vicious cycle. When your child feels like he can't get enough air, he gets panicky and anxious, which constricts the airways even more and worsens the asthma. Teach your child relaxation techniques; for example: "As soon as you feel yourself beginning to wheeze, relax, sit still, think happy thoughts, and imagine yourself getting lots of air flowing through your lungs . . ." Read him a relaxing story or sing a soothing lullaby. Try to instill in your child's mind a confidence that he can control his wheezing. The loss of control is what causes children with asthma to panic, which makes the asthma even worse.

7. Consult your doctor. Bring your child — and your diary — to the doctor. Here's how a typical asthma evaluation will occur: After concluding that your child does indeed have asthma, the doctor will try to appropriately match the treatment for the severity of the illness. Based upon your history and your child's diary, the doctor will decide whether your child needs occasional medicine when the wheezing occurs or whether he should be treated with daily preventive medicines.

Medications

Occasional Asthma

This asthma is seasonal and non-serious. Your child might wheeze several times a year but does not miss much school, play, or sleep. If this is the case, the doctor will prescribe what are called *rescue medications*. These are used on an *as-needed* basis, when your child experiences asthma symptoms. The primary rescue med is albuterol. This non-steroid inhaler relaxes the muscles surrounding the airways so they stop squeezing the airways. It provides relief within five to fifteen minutes. During severe asthma attacks, a doctor may also prescribe a swallowed steroid for three to five days. Although it takes about eight hours to work, it is the most

 DR. SEARS TIP
Steroids Are Safe for Asthma

Using steroids and anti-inflammatory treatments in children concerns many parents, but extensive research has shown these to be safe and effective. We know that chronic, uncontrolled wheezing and asthma can cause growth problems and heart problems, so the remote possibility of medication side effects poses little risk compared to uncontrolled asthma.

effective way to rescue the sufferer from the inflammation within the airways that blocks breathing.

Your pediatrician will advise you to continue keeping your diary and using the peak flow meter. If your child's asthma is getting worse, he is missing more school days, has more trips to the emergency room, has more doctor's visits, and is using the rescue medications (an inhaler and possibly steroids) more, the doctor will then move to the next step.

More Severe Asthma

Some medications are designed to be used *daily* to prevent constriction and inflammation in the airways. This way, your child experiences few or no asthma symptoms at all. Of course, you would only begin one of these medications, called *controller medications,* if your child has frequent symptoms without the medications. If your child has symptoms for more than three days each month or has severe asthma attacks requiring doctor or emergency room visits more than three times each year, then a controller medication may be warranted. These medications fall into three categories:

- Inhaled controller medications. These include steroids and cromolyn, which suppress the allergic inflammation in the airways, and long-acting bronchodilators, which reduce constriction of the airways. They come as pump inhalers or disk inhalers.

- Swallowed controller medications. These include steroid pills and leukotriene inhibitors, which suppress the allergic inflammation in the airways. There are also

swallowed bronchodilators, but these are rarely used in children.

- Allergy medications. Using allergy pills or nasal sprays (see Allergies, page 131) may help prevent asthma symptoms during allergic seasons.

The doctor will help you decide if your child's symptoms are frequent enough to warrant use of a controller medication. They are often used more during allergic seasons or during cold and flu seasons to keep your child breathing better.

Possible side effects of asthma medications. The main side effect of bronchodilators (like albuterol) is that they may speed up your child's heart rate, which may make her feel jittery or hyper. This harmless, but still rare, effect is acceptable because wheezing must be treated. Steroid and other anti-inflammatory treatments have very few side effects.

How to administer inhaled medications. There are various techniques used to effectively give inhaled medications depending on a child's age:

- Infants will usually be prescribed a nebulizer machine. This small air pump turns the liquid medication into a mist that is inhaled over several minutes.

- Young children will be given an inhaler with a *spacer,* a tube that attaches to the inhaler. A parent pumps the inhaler into the tube space, then the child takes several breaths out of the tube.

- Older children can usually be taught to use a plain inhaler effectively by the doctor, pharmacist, or asthma educator.

DR. SEARS TIP
How to Properly Use a Standard Pump Inhaler

Proper use is key for inhaler effectiveness. Follow these simple steps:

1. Hold the inhaler about two inches away from the mouth (do not put it in the mouth).

2. Tell your child to exhale comfortably, then inhale deeply.

3. Spray the inhaler just after your child's inhalation begins.

4. Tell your child to hold the breath for a comfortable five to ten seconds, but no more.

5. Wait two minutes and repeat the dose (if you are prescribed two puffs). Disk inhalers work differently and instructions will vary between brands.

If your child's asthma seems to be controlled on the daily medicines for several months or longer, at some point your doctor may suggest coming off the daily medications and going back to just using rescue medicines when the attacks occur. Your doctor will constantly fine-tune your child's treatment to keep her wheezing-free enough to help her lead a happy and healthful life but not overmedicated to the extent that she experiences too many side effects. Again, being a keen observer and accurate reporter of your child's asthma symptoms helps the doctor treat your child appropriately.

Asthma Emergencies

Your child is likely to have an asthma attack from time to time. These can vary from mild to severe, and it's important that you know what to do ahead of time so that you can act without waiting to hear from the doctor. A peak flow reading (page 155) can be helpful in these situations if you have one. Following are some guidelines:

First asthma attack. If this is your child's first episode of wheezing, and you don't have any asthma medications, your pediatrician probably won't be able to prescribe you any over the phone without examining your child. You can start by trying the chest-clearing techniques on page 203. If this doesn't help, you should go to your pediatrician if the office is open or an urgent care or emergency room if it's after hours.

Mild asthma attack (in a known asthmatic). During a mild asthma attack, you will hear some wheezing sounds but your child shouldn't feel short of breath or bad enough to restrict his normal daily activities. You should see no *retractions* during breaths, your child shouldn't be raising his shoulders up and down to breathe, and his rate of breathing shouldn't be more than forty breaths per minute.

Administer your rescue inhaled medication (probably albuterol) and watch for improvement. As long as your child improves for several hours with each treatment, you can probably wait until the doctor's office opens. Continue your rescue medication as prescribed (generally every four hours) to keep your child stable.

Moderate asthma attack. You will notice retractions, your child's activity level will be decreased, and you may see him working harder with his shoulders to breathe. His breathing rate may be forty to sixty breaths per minute. Initial treatment is the same as for a mild attack, but you should keep a closer eye and ear on your child. If your child doesn't improve with treatment, call the doctor to discuss the situation.

Severe asthma attack. Your child will be working very hard with his shoulders to breathe, breathing rate will be over sixty breaths per minute, he may appear pale or have blue lips, and you will see marked retractions and very loud wheezing (or you may not hear wheezing because very little air is going in and out). If your child is having a severe attack, you should administer rescue medications as you go directly to the emergency room or the doctor's office. Call the doctor en route to discuss the situation. If you believe your child's breathing is severely impaired, call 911.

 DR. SEARS TIP
Develop a Written Asthma Action Plan (AAP)

Write a plan in consultation with your pediatrician that tells you exactly what medications to use and what action to take during any mild, moderate, or severe asthma attack.

What You Can Do

If your child has asthma and needs ongoing medications, don't just accept his fate and let the meds handle everything. Here are some important ways you should be involved:

Allergy prevention. We've already mentioned this. Do everything you can to get to the bottom of your child's allergies. See page 131. Get allergy tested if necessary.

Communication and observation. It's important to talk to your child about how his breathing feels. On a calendar, write down the days he uses an inhaler or other medication. Keep a log of his asthma attacks, even if mild, to show the doctor. Attend asthma education seminars at your local hospital. For older children, use a peak flow meter to keep track of your child's status.

Proper use of medication. Use controller medications as directed by your pediatrician. Failure to use these can lead to overuse of rescue medications, which can make them lose their effectiveness over time. Using controller

ASTHMA PREVENTION CHECKLIST	Yes	No
Did you work out an AAP with your doctor?		
Do you keep an asthma diary?		
Do you try to keep your child's bedroom allergen-free?		
Do you ban smoking around your child?		
Do you use a peak flow meter to grade severity?		
Do you understand when and how to use *rescue* meds?		
Do you understand when and how to use *controller* meds?		
Do you have a *nebulizer* for home use?		
Do you feed your child an immune-boosting diet?		
Do you teach your child relaxation techniques?		

medications on a daily basis is much safer than using rescue medications every day.

ATHLETE'S FOOT

If your child has itchy feet, then he most likely has athlete's foot. Don't worry, you didn't do anything wrong, it is just a very common fact of life. If your child has warm, damp feet (i.e., if he wears socks), then he'll probably get athlete's foot at some point in his life.

Athlete's foot is a red, scaly, cracked rash on the foot and between the toes that itches and burns. If scratched too much, the rash becomes raw and weepy. Shoes and feet might have an unpleasant odor. It is very common in adolescents and adults. In fact, about 75 percent of people have athlete's foot at some time. The medical term is *tinea pedis*.

Athlete's foot is caused by a fungus that likes to grow on warm, damp skin. This is a greater problem during the summer and in people who tend to sweat a lot. Contrary to popular opinion, athlete's foot is *not* very contagious. Your child can continue with gym, sports, and swimming activities. Normal laundry procedures are adequate, and no special precautions are needed in showers. With treatment, athlete's foot will clear up in a few weeks. However, it is very common to have recurrences, so you may need to follow our prevention tips below.

What to Do

Use antifungal cream. Most over-the-counter creams, like Tinactin, Lotrimin, and Micatin, work well. Apply to the rash and between the toes twice a day for one to two weeks (for at least seven days after the rash clears up).

Relieve itching. Itching is the most annoying symptom of athlete's foot and is usually worse at bedtime! Applying 1 percent hydrocortisone cream to the itchy areas should provide quick relief from the itching. Don't apply this very often as it doesn't help with the healing, only the itch. Frequent scratching will delay healing.

Keep feet dry. Because fungus loves warm, damp skin, it's important to keep things dry. Before applying the antifungal cream, rinse the feet in plain water and then thoroughly dry the feet. Avoid sweaty feet by using cotton socks, and change socks frequently or wear sandals or flip-flops as much as possible. Canvas shoes also breathe well, but tight-fitting shoes should be avoided.

 **DR. SEARS TIP
A Natural Treatment for Athlete's Foot**

For parents who prefer a more natural treatment, try a cream or powder with tea tree oil. This natural oil has antifungal properties and can be a great alternative for many fungal skin infections. Or try a solution of one ounce of white vinegar in eight ounces of water, applied twice daily.

Prevention

Simply keeping the feet dry as described above will usually prevent recurrences. Weekly soaks in a half water, half white vinegar solution will also work well. Soak the feet for about ten minutes, and then be sure to dry thoroughly, especially between the toes.

When to Worry

- the rash looks infected (yellow pus, spreading redness, or red streaks)

- the rash isn't improving after one week of treatment

- the rash isn't completely cured after two weeks of treatment

- the feet are very painful

What Your Doctor Might Do

For athlete's foot that is not responding to the above home remedies, your doctor will probably prescribe a stronger antifungal cream, and maybe some cortisone cream if the itching is severe. Even though these creams are generally safe, their use should be supervised by a physician.

ATTACHMENT PARENTING (AP)

You may hear the term *attachment parenting*, a style of baby care that is most likely to bring out the best in your baby and in your parenting intuition. Dr. Bill and Martha coined this term in 1980. We also reviewed the scientific literature on outcome studies in which researchers followed children who were the products of various styles of parenting to see how they turn out. After forty years of practicing pediatrics and witnessing the adult people these attachment-parented children turn out to be, we are convinced that this is the style of parenting that brings out the best in families.

The easiest way to understand attachment parenting is to imagine that you are expecting a baby. You and your husband live on a remote island. You will not have access to baby books, psychologists, pediatricians, and mothers-in-law. When your baby is born, you must rely only on your basic instincts to care for your baby. Attachment parenting is what you would instinctively do. Try to practice as many of the following Seven Baby B's as you can. You may not be able to practice all of them all the time. Do the best you can with the resources you have and your baby will someday thank you.

A grandmother who had attachment-parented her son recently shared with us: "The other day my daughter-in-law came up and hugged me and said, 'Thank you for raising such a sensitive and caring man.'"

The Seven Baby B's

1. Birth bonding. How you and your baby get started with one another during the sensitive period of the early weeks sets the stage for your relationship. Spend as much time in skin-to-skin and eye-to-eye contact as possible, even if medical complications disrupt this attachment time. Remember, you are the most valuable part of your baby's medical team. In fact, as former director of a university hospital newborn nursery, I (Dr. Bill) taught that attachment parenting was even more important for mothers of premature infants or those in the ICU. I called it *therapeutic touch* and *therapeutic milk*.

2. Breastfeeding. Besides giving your baby nature's perfect milk, breastfeeding is an exercise in baby reading. The skin-to-skin and eye-to-eye contact promotes bonding. You learn your baby's facial expressions and body language of hunger, and you nurse even before Baby has to cry to get fed. Your breast milk is the best "grow milk" for Baby, and the very act of nursing sets the stage for a lifelong relationship — Mom as comforter and a trusted resource. Try to breastfeed as often and as long as possible. In fact, long-term studies have shown that babies who are breastfed tend to be healthier, happier, and smarter. Yet, if a medical or lifestyle complication prevents you from breastfeeding, make bottlefeeding a time of high touch and high communication, always keeping in mind there is a person at each end of the bottle. Think of feeding time as a time of bonding and communication in addition to delivering nourishment.

3. Baby wearing. Carried babies cry less. Happy babies make for happy mothers. It's as simple as that. When new parents come into our office for their baby's first newborn checkup, we give them a crash course in baby wearing. We insist, if possible, fathers also attend the first visit. New moms enjoy watching me drape the baby sling over Dad, position Baby comfortably in the carrier, and watch Daddy and Baby stroll around the office. We've observed that carried babies spend more time in the state of *quiet alertness,* the behavioral state in which babies learn most about their environment and are most receptive to your interaction. Teaching dads how to wear their babies promotes father-infant attachment or "father nursing" — "nursing" implies comforting, not just breastfeeding. Yes, fathers can "nurse."

4. Bedding close to Baby. The American Academy of Pediatrics (AAP) recommends that babies sleep in the same room as mothers for nighttime attachment. Try the Arm's Reach Co-Sleeper, a bedside bassinet that attaches safely next to your bed for easier nighttime attachment parenting. See page 482.

5. Belief in Baby's cries. A baby's cry is a baby's language. Listen to it. Babies cry to communicate, not to manipulate. Early on as we were studying the effects of attachment parenting we noticed that attachment-parented babies cry less, and when they do fuss their cries are not as ear-piercing and disturbing. One reason is that an attachment-parenting mother is able to read her baby's pre-cry signals — a change in body language or facial expression — and then comfort Baby before he needs to cry. This is one of the reasons that attachment-parented babies *thrive* — that loaded medical word that means not only getting taller and heavier but growing optimally physically, emotionally, and intellectually. If babies don't waste a lot of energy crying, they can divert that energy into growing and developing.

6. Beware of baby trainers. Recently there has been a flurry of books that remind us of control methods used to train pets, a sort of rerun of the old "spoiling theory" that research disproved decades ago. I'm sure you've had well-meaning friends and relatives deluge you with their personal how-to's of baby training: "Get her on a schedule…" "Let him cry it out so he learns not to manipulate you…" and "You're spoiling her by carrying her so much…" While certainly some modification of attachment parenting may be necessary to help your baby fit into your lifestyle, if you are not cautious, baby training is a lose-lose situation. You lose trust in your ability to read and respond to your baby's cues and instead follow somebody else's printed formula dictating how you should respond to your baby: "Let her cry twenty minutes the first night, eighteen minutes the second night, and so on." The only person in the whole wide world who even has a clue how to respond to a baby is the very person who shared an umbilical cord with that baby — Mom. Also, Baby loses trust in the signal value of his cues. Baby cries and no one listens.

7. Balance and boundaries. "My baby needs me so much that I don't even have time to take a shower," lamented my tired wife, Martha, during one of baby Matthew's high-need stages. Later that day I posted a sign on the bathroom mirror: "Please remember what our baby needs most is a happy, rested mother." Just like the right dose of the right medicine is healing, an overdose of attachment parenting can sometimes hurt. In your zeal to give so much to your baby it's easy to neglect your own needs and those of your marriage. That's why early on when quizzing new mothers and fathers about their chosen style of parenting we ask, "Is it working for you? Is your baby thriving: physically, emotionally, and developmentally? Are you thriving? Do you feel happy about these Baby B's? If not, we may need to modify them a bit."

For more information, see *The Attachment Parenting Book* in the Sears Parenting Library.

ATTENTION DEFICIT DISORDER (ADD)

ADD and ADHD (attention deficit hyperactivity disorder) are definitely on the rise. Nearly 10 percent of schoolchildren are tagged with these labels, yet they are two of the most misunderstood, misdiagnosed, and mistreated problems in childhood. Think of the "D" in ADD as *difference* instead of *deficit* or *disorder*. In fact, a more accurate "D" word is *description*. ADD describes a child's way of thinking, learning, and acting. Some children are wired differently. They think differently, learn differently, and act differently. Consequently, they need a different style of parenting and teaching. However, ADD *can* become

a deficit disorder, and even a disability, if the child is not appropriately identified and managed.

Understanding ADD

There are four main features of ADD/ADHD:

1. Selective attention. Most children with ADD have problems paying attention to subjects that don't seem particularly relevant to them, yet they are actually able to pay deeper attention to things that the children perceive as important and particularly relevant to them. For example, a goalie on a hockey team goes into a state of hyperfocus when the guy with the puck is coming toward him. Yet he can zone into a state of inattention when the puck is at the other end of the rink. In school, the child with selective attention zones out, focusing on the bird in the tree outside the classroom window, and seems inattentive to the teacher describing the features of some irrelevant war that happened a thousand years ago. Yet if you give that same child a lead part in a play that reenacts the history lesson, he shines.

2. Distractibility. The child with ADD has difficulty filtering out clutter and distracting images and thoughts, so much so that his mind wanders off of the main subject and into seemingly irrelevant and distracting scenes. For example, during class while the teacher is outlining a math problem, the child sees a moth land on his desk. He focuses more on the moth and less on the math and oftentimes can't seem to get his mind off the moth. When given gobs of homework, he is so overwhelmed with all the stuff he has to read and learn that he has difficulty getting started.

3. Impulsivity. The child with ADHD leaps before he looks and acts before he thinks. This trait makes him more accident-prone and gets him into trouble with teachers and peers. The term *inappropriate* often characterizes his actions. He may shout out what he thinks is the right answer in class without waiting his turn. He may have trouble with empathy — the ability to get behind the eyes of another person and imagine the effects of his behavior on that other person. The impulse to push or shove a classmate clicks in quickly and strongly before the child even has the chance to think about the trouble he may get into or how the pushed classmate might feel.

4. Hyperactivity. While some children have what's called "silent ADD" (more common in girls), others get an "H" added for *hyperactivity*. It's not only that they are very active but that they are also "hyper" at inappropriate times, such as in the classroom or at the dinner table.

How to Tell If Your Child Has ADD

Here is a step-by-step approach:

1. Keep a diary. In your diary, list the behaviors that concern you, your child's teacher, and other persons of significance (e.g., scoutmasters, coaches). Try to put these under the three categories of "attention span," "inappropriate behaviors," and "learning difficulties."

2. Note the severity and progression of the concerns on your list. Are they getting better, worse, or not changing? How much are these behaviors interfering with your child's educational and social development and his level of happiness? Are they just quirky nui-

sances that don't seem to interfere much with learning and socialization, or are they progressing in severity so that they are interfering with your child's overall development and with your relationship with your child?

What to Do

If you decide that your child is happy, you've found an appropriate match between child, teacher, and classroom that works with your child's quirks, and he seems to be progressing, then perhaps you can afford to take the wait-and-see approach. With time and maturity your child might grow out of the tag of "ADD" and become, rather, a child with learning and behavioral differences. If, in consultation with your child's teacher and health-care provider, and in accord with your own parental intuition, you decide that ADD is interfering with your child's life and that he needs professional, educational, and parental help, go to the next steps described below:

1. Keep an ongoing diary. Keep your diary up to date. Professional counselors are likely to ask you, "What are your child's major quirks?," "Are they getting better, worse, or not changing?," and "How much are they bothering your child?" Your ongoing diary is important to providing this accurate assessment.

2. Read the pills-skills approach to management as described on page 13. It's important for you to insist that the health-care providers and other professionals helping you with your child's overall ADD management understand this pills-skills model. Pills-only will not work. All too often, a child with ADD or ADHD is hastily given prescription medications while the equally if not more important *skills* part of the overall treatment plan is ignored. With the pills-skills management approach, you first see if your child can be managed by skills-only. If not, then ADD medications may need to be added. In our experience, most children with ADD can be managed with the skills-only approach and some need the pills and skills, but the pills-only approach should never be used.

3. Interview significant others. Children with ADD have what are called *cross-situational* problems, meaning the main concerns listed in your diary occur at school, at home, with peers, and in other social settings. Interviewing other people is important because if these quirky behaviors occur only at school, then you would be less likely to tag your child "ADD"; instead, it could be that your child and school are mismatched. If, on the other hand, all or most of the people in your child's life have similar concerns, your child may indeed have ADD.

4. Make a classroom visit. Volunteer to "help" for a few days in your child's classroom. Observe the problem behaviors and note them in your diary. The goal is to structure the classroom to fit your child. Ask to have your child seated in the least distracting area, such as away from the windows, close to the teacher, and definitely away from other children with ADD.

5. Be sure your child, teacher, and classroom match. Some children are labeled ADD unfairly. Because these children think and learn differently, they often need a different style of teaching. Try to make sure your child's needs are met in school.

6. Begin the day with a brainy breakfast. The brain is affected — for better or worse —

by nutrition. If a child begins the day with a junky breakfast, expect junky behavior. It's as simple as that. For a list of suggested healthy, high-protein carbs and friendly fat-filled brainy breakfasts, check out *The Healthiest Kid in the Neighborhood* or *The N.D.D. Book* in the Sears Parenting Library.

7. Exercise your child. Recent studies have shown that many children tagged with ADD markedly improve and can often either come off their medication or lower the dose just by getting at least an hour of vigorous physical exercise a day. This is especially true of children with ADHD. Exercise seems to induce relaxing and focus-enhancing neuro-chemicals that promote better focus and reduce hyperactivity. We have helped several children in our practice by having them take periodic homework breaks and jump for five minutes on a mini trampoline, take a brief run, or have a mini workout with exercise bands. This physical activity can enhance mental activity.

8. Be sure your child sleeps well. Recent studies have uncovered that one of the most common causes of ADD and other learning and behavior problems at school is *lack of optimal sleep.* Many doctors believe that before treating a child with ADD medication, the child should have his sleep habits fully evaluated and be referred to a pediatric sleep specialist, if necessary. Medical and psychological problems that lead to poor sleep and consequently learning and behavior problems are obesity, anxiety, depression, allergies, and joint pains. One often-overlooked contributor to ADD is obstructive sleep apnea. The oxygen deprivation during sleep can affect brain function. See page 474.

9. Foster your child's special talent. Every child has a special gift or talent, such as a sport, art, or music. Discover this "special something" in your child's life and run with it. Children who have learning or attention differences often feel different, and to a child, feeling different often equates with feeling less. Self-esteem takes a nosedive, which further aggravates quirky behavior. When a child puts her special talent to work and succeeds at it, it raises her self-esteem. We call this the *carryover effect,* meaning success in one endeavor carries over to academic and behavioral success.

DR. SEARS TIP
Ten Things I Like About Me

Have your child make a list of the ten things that he likes most about himself and frame it on his wall. This becomes a constant reminder of all the qualities he appreciates in himself and takes the constant pressure off his ADD.

10. Frame your child positively. The concept of framing is an important skill for parents and teachers to learn in helping the child with ADD. This is especially true if a child has to stand in line to get his "focus pill" from the school nurse every day, has special tutoring, or is in some way singled out as having a problem. For example, you're attending a parent-teacher conference, and your child's disruptive behavior and inattentiveness comes up. When you hear from the teacher, "He sure is disruptive," counter with, "He does have an active personality." If the child is tagged as "stubborn," counter with, "He is very persistent." If someone says, "My, he's hyperactive,"

counter with, "He sure is enthusiastic and energetic." When the teacher, you, and your child repeatedly hear your child being framed positively, it changes the way everyone views him and helps them see the bright side of ADD. Most of these children are bright, funny, creative, and energetic. In fact, many creative people who have made this world a better place to live in, such as Wolfgang Amadeus Mozart and Thomas Edison, might today have been tagged ADHD. Your child's perception of himself depends upon how he perceives others perceive him. If he always hears negative tags like "lazy," "dumb," or "bad," sooner or later he's likely to live up to them.

You see where we're going with this management plan? You are now equipped with the management skills to help your child learn the way he is designed to learn and to help his attention skills. It's important that parents and other significant people in your child's life focus on all these skills before even thinking about going to behavior- and attention-modifying pills.

11. Seek the right professional help. Managing a child's ADD successfully requires a team effort of teachers, learning specialists, behavior therapists, psychologists, and sometimes a series of medical doctors, such as a child's primary-care physician or a neurologist. Hearing and vision tests should be done to be sure these are normal. And parents must be the team quarterback, coordinating all the input from the team members for the best interest of their child.

12. Try neurofeedback training. Neurofeedback for brain training is actually one of the oldest treatments around. It was developed in the sixties and used to help Top Gun fighter pilots focus better. Think of neurofeedback for the brain like weight training for the muscles. The child sits in front of a computer screen and tiny wires are pasted on his scalp to record brain waves. The child then essentially plays a video game, and his level of attention controls what happens on the video screen. If he loses focus or "spaces out," the images on the video screen change and give him instant feedback that he's not paying attention. As the child exercises the neuropathways to pay better attention, over time these pathways become stronger and more appropriate for the child's age. There are neurofeedback centers in nearly every major city. Visit the International Society for Neurofeedback and Research at www .ISNR.org.

13. Consider medication. Here are guidelines on when to consider medication:

- Consider medication when, despite trying all the skills in the pills-skills model, your child is still having learning or behavioral problems to the extent that his inattentiveness and inappropriate behavior are interfering with not only his learning but his overall self-esteem, development, and family communication.

- Use pills only in addition to, not instead of, the self-help skills mentioned above.

- In our opinion, mood-altering medications and "focus pills" should be prescribed only by medical professionals who specialize in the medical management of ADD. When using medication that messes with the brain, your child deserves a specialist. There is no one-pill-fits-all approach to ADD. Different medications in different dosages work for different kids.

- Market the pill as a "focus pill." Tell your child that the pill will only help all the other skills work better. You want to be sure that your child attributes his success mainly to his own efforts and not to the pills. In addition, some children feel that when they need to take a pill something is wrong with them and they perceive themselves as "sick" or "different" (which equates with being less), and this can sabotage your whole management plan. When your child is succeeding, be sure that you reinforce that *he* did it, and that the pill only helped.

- Keep a medication log in your diary. In order to arrive at the right medication, the right timing, and the right dose for your child, your doctor will need your feedback. Your diary may look something like this:

MEDICATION	DATE STARTED	DOSE	CHANGES NOTICED	SIDE EFFECTS

List the main concerns, such as impulsive behavior, inability to focus, and so on, and then grade the changes after each one of these concerns, such as "better," "worse," or "no change." List the name of the medication, the dose, and the times of the day you give it. When you see the doctor for "medication adjustment," bring in your diary. The observations you record (along with those of the teacher and other persons of significance) are absolutely necessary for the doctor to make the right medication adjustment. If your child really needs medication, it should work, and the effect should be obvious. Vague entries in your diary like "I think he's a bit better" don't count, as nearly all medications have a placebo effect, meaning that when we take a pill to feel better, we imagine that we are feeling better. That's why you need to be as objective as possible and pinpoint specific changes, such as "It takes half as long to complete his homework."

Be sure you also record possible undesirable side effects of a medication, such as insomnia, diminished appetite, medication roller-coaster effect (the child's behavior deteriorates at the end of the day when the effect of the medication wears off), unusual mannerisms such as facial twitches, or other unpleasant behaviors when on the medication. Mention these to your pediatrician.

AUTISM

Autism is a neurological and medical disorder in which the parts of the brain that control communication, behavior, social interaction, learning, and coordination aren't functioning

---

LEARN MORE ABOUT IT

The above step-by-step approach is simply meant to give you some guidelines to get you started. For an in-depth discussion of ADD:

- Read *The A.D.D. Book* by William Sears and Lynda Thompson. Dr. Thompson is director of the ADD Centre in Toronto, Canada; www.ADDcentre.com.
- Read *The N.D.D. Book: How Nutrition Deficit Disorder Affects Your Child's Learning, Behavior, and Health and What You Can Do About It — Without Drugs,* by William Sears.
- Go to CHADD — Children and Adults with Attention Deficit Disorder; www.CHADD.org.

---

properly. A child with autism doesn't process sensory input correctly and often can't turn it around as typical and understandable output. Each person is affected in different ways and to varying degrees. Some will show only a few autistic characteristics; others will display many or all.

Autism is perhaps the most frustrating disease that is affecting children today. Rates have risen dramatically in the past decade to the point that about 1 in 100 children is found to be on the autism spectrum (at the time of this writing). What makes it so difficult for parents is that autism seems to strike unexpectedly out of nowhere; a healthy and neurologically normal infant can suddenly regress into autism between ages one and two. Some infants don't regress backward, but simply stop progressing forward through normal social and language milestones. A few infants will show some autistic characteristics right from birth.

Equally devastating is the fact that when a child is diagnosed, the doctor can't explain why. There is no specific physical or medical abnormality that anyone can point to as the cause. Although little is known about the cause of autism, much is known about early detection and early intervention. Here is our guide to autism symptoms, screening for early detection, initial steps parents can take if a diagnosis of autism is suspected, and common treatment approaches that are currently being used or investigated.

For a more comprehensive discussion on autism diagnosis, treatment, and prevention, see *The Autism Book* by Robert W. Sears or visit www.TheAutismBook.com.

Signs and Symptoms

Your child may have autism if he

- uses little or no language, or uses language inappropriately or repetitively

- displays self-stimulating behaviors like hand flapping or repetitive movements

- doesn't understand typical social boundaries or how to behave and interact in normal social situations

- is obsessed with routines and "sameness"

- only eats certain foods and refuses to try unfamiliar ones

- engages in less imaginary and pretend play than do other children

- is noticeably hyperactive or underactive and sedentary

- has tantrums that are more extreme than expected

- plays alone in own world

- is obsessed with spinning objects, such as wheels or fans

- doesn't play with toys in the manner the toy is intended

- is overly aggressive or self-injurious

- has unusually high or low pain tolerance

- makes poor eye contact or may peer at objects sideways

- is bothered by large crowds, noises, and chaos

- may not want and may even be adverse to hugging and close contact

- studies interesting objects or events alone without inviting others to join in the fun (termed a lack of "joint attention")

- is bothered by sensations like clothing tags, shoes that don't feel right, smells, or the feel of grass or sand on the feet

Types of Onset

Autism comes in all shapes and sizes. It is a "spectrum" disorder, meaning it can range from extremely mild and barely detectable (as in Asperger's syndrome) to very severe. There are two very distinct patterns of onset that parents should be aware of:

Early-onset autism. Some babies show a lack of eye contact, interaction, interest in affection, and animated facial expression within the first few months of life. These babies are typically thought of as "easy babies," but they are essentially too easy. As they grow through the first year, they don't begin babbling at a normal age and their vocalization stays immature. After age one, they haven't developed words, and it becomes more apparent that they aren't interacting socially. By age two, more autistic signs appear and a diagnosis can be made. Such children are essentially thought to be born with autism.

Regressive autism. In this more common type, babies seem completely healthy, develop normally in every way, and may even begin to say several words. Then, between ages one and two, they either stop progressing in their development or actually regress and lose many of their age-appropriate skills, including language. Those who regress typically develop other signs of autism by age two, and the devastated and frustrated parents wonder where their child went. Those who don't regress but simply stop progressing often aren't diagnosed with autism until around age three.

Early Detection and Screening

The sooner autism is detected and appropriate developmental intervention is begun, the better the eventual outcome. Children who are diagnosed early (eighteen months to three years) and begin speech and language therapy, behavioral therapy, physical or occupational therapy, social development guidance, and medical therapy do better than those diagnosed and treated late (four years or older). Children who are treated at a younger age progress faster through developmental milestones, achieve a higher level of social function and interaction, learn better, and are more likely to grow up as "typical" children (or nearly so).

Screening tools used by the pediatrician. Doctors used to not take language delay or quirky behaviors very seriously, hoping, along with the parents, that the child would just grow out of it. Parents often used to hear, "Oh, he's just a boy. Boys talk late." No longer is this the case. With autism on the rise, doctors are more vigilant than ever, or they should be. Your doctor will likely ask you to fill out a standard social development screening questionnaire at your eighteen-month and two-year checkups. Following is a list of questions adapted from the CHAT, or Checklist for Autism in Toddlers:

- Does your child enjoy swinging or being bounced on your knee?
- Does your child enjoy physical affection and crave your attention?
- Does your child show interest in other kids?
- Does your child enjoy peek-a-boo, hide-and-seek, and other social games?
- Does your child play pretend games, such as a tea party, feeding a doll, or cooking?
- Does your child use the index finger to point to an object or to ask for something?
- Does your child play with toys the way they are intended (cars, blocks, dolls) instead of simply mouthing, fiddling with, or throwing them?
- Does your child bring you objects to show you?
- Does your child display any of the symptoms listed on page 168?
- Can your child say several easily understandable words at eighteen months and use two- or three-word sentences by age two?

It's important for parents to realize that almost every child will have one or two "no"s on this checklist, and that's not a cause for concern. This is a screening tool, not a diagnostic one, which means it is designed to find toddlers who *may have* a delay in development. It is not used to diagnose or label a child with autism based on just one or two criteria.

Your pediatrician will also observe how your toddler interacts during the appointment. Again, adapted from CHAT, he might observe the following:

- Does the child make sustained eye contact?

- Does the child show interest in something when the doctor points to it and says, "Look at that ___!"

- Does the child play with a toy appropriately? For example, if given cup and doll, does she give the doll a drink? Or when given a toy car does he push a car around making car noises?

- When the doctor says, "Where's the light?," does the child make eye contact with the doctor, then point at the light with the index finger?

- Can the child stack some blocks?

 **DR. SEARS TIP
Late Talking Only—
Probably Not Autism**

Like normal late walkers, many children, especially boys, are normal late talkers (see page 488). If this is the only developmental delay, without some of the other signs on the symptom list, then it is probably not autism. However, such a child should be carefully screened for autism.

Diagnosis

Screening tools don't make a diagnosis of autism. They simply help the doctor and parent decide if there may be a developmental problem and if further evaluation is warranted. If your child doesn't pass a screening test, or if some problems are suspected even without a formal screening test, it's time for a more thorough evaluation. Here are your choices:

State-funded regional developmental therapy center. These county centers provide developmental evaluations and a full spectrum of therapies for all types of developmental problems for children three years and younger. Your child can be evaluated by a doctor or other medical professionals through these centers free of charge (in most states).

Public school system. Once a child turns three, diagnostic and therapeutic services are usually managed by the local public school special education department.

Pediatric neurologist. This specialist can evaluate and diagnose your child. It is better to see one who takes a particular interest in or is part of a center that specifically treats autism.

Developmental pediatrician. This pediatric subspecialist will give a thorough developmental evaluation to determine if autism is likely.

Psychologist. Many pediatric psychologists are well trained in diagnosing autism.

Speech and language therapist. Often the first sign of autism is speech delay. A speech therapist can help you determine if your child's lack of speech is only a simple isolated delay or part of a larger developmental problem.

Other therapists. You can also take your child to a specific therapist that helps treat autism, such as an occupational therapist, a sensory integration therapist, or an Applied Behavioral Analysis therapist (see below) to get an opinion on these specific areas of development.

DR. SEARS TIP
Don't Take a Wait-and-See Approach

If there is a problem, the sooner your child receives therapy the better. If you decide to just wait and see, or if your doctor advises you to wait six months and come back for another look, you could be doing your child a disservice. If you seek further help, and it turns out your child is fine, all you've wasted is some time and money. But if you wait until the problems are bad enough that the diagnosis is completely certain, then you've missed several potential months or even years of early intervention.

Criteria for the Diagnosis

Specific and detailed criteria, called the DSM-IV criteria, have been established to make a diagnosis. A specialist will observe your child to see if he fits these criteria. Here is a brief summary:

- social impairment in non-verbal language (eye contact, facial expressions, posture, and gestures), peer relationships, interaction with others, and reciprocating emotions

- communication impairment in speech, or in the case of those who do speak, a failure to initiate or sustain conversations; the use of repetitive or out-of-context phrases; or a lack of pretend and imaginative play

- repetitive, obsessive, compulsive, or stereotyped behaviors such as fixations on patterns or routines, abnormal body movements, or intense preoccupation with a narrow range of interests

Other Forms of Autism-Like Disorders

There are other terms used to describe a child who is "autistic-like" but who doesn't meet all the criteria for a diagnosis of autism:

Pervasive Developmental Disorder Not Otherwise Specified (PDD-NOS)

This describes an infant or toddler who has delays in most areas of development, yet lacks enough of the typical signs of autism to be given that diagnosis. A toddler who is being evaluated by a specialist for developmental delays will often be diagnosed with PDD at first and then with actual autism six to twelve months later if autistic-like problems begin to show up. PDD is often autism waiting to happen. Treatment should be initiated right away, without waiting for a full diagnosis of autism.

Asperger's Syndrome (AS)

This disorder, also known as *high-functioning autism*, has one distinct difference from other kinds of autism: the child has normal language development. The AS toddler will often begin speaking at the same age as a typical child, and as he gets older, he can carry on a somewhat normal conversation. Yet, as he grows, he begins to display some autistic behaviors, mannerisms, and unusual social interaction. The diagnosis is generally made much later than it is for those kids with standard autism because of the normal speech development. Treatment is much the same as for autism. See page 150 for a more detailed discussion on AS.

Non-Verbal Learning Disabilities (NVLDs)

This diagnosis describes a child who doesn't understand many aspects of non-verbal language and social cues, yet does not have typical behavioral and neurologic features of autism. He will also suffer from some fine and gross motor incoordination because the brain has difficulty integrating spatial awareness. It differs from Asperger's syndrome (AS) in that a child with an NVLD knows and cares that he doesn't pick up on non-verbal cues. He knows he's different, and it bothers him. Kids with autism don't know they are different (unless they recover), and children with AS know but may not care (unless they recover). This is a diagnosis that is not yet well understood. Its underlying causes may be similar to autism, and it may be that it should be included within the Autism Spectrum Disorders.

Sensory Processing Disorder (or Sensory Integration Disorder)

This disorder occurs when a child's brain does not know how to correctly process sensory input. The brain receives signals from all five senses but doesn't know how to properly turn this information around into normal motor and behavioral responses. This not only results in difficulty handling many of the normal sensations of childhood (such as messy hands, tags on clothing, loud and chaotic play settings, various food textures, and walking barefoot in sand or grass), but also creates an overall disorganization within the brain that can manifest as attention problems, difficulty following instructions, challenges with balance and coordination, fidgeting and inability to sit still, and some social awkwardness. Language development is usually normal. Many children with autism have sensory integration problems, but the disorder can also exist by itself in an otherwise neurotypical child.

Treatment

There are many aspects of treatment for a child who has autism, both medical and behavioral. All are important and complement one another.

Behavioral therapy. The behavioral aspects of therapy focus on stimulating, teaching, and enhancing the parts of the brain that aren't functioning well. Most or all of the following approaches should be incorporated into a coordinated treatment plan:

- One-on-one programs with a therapist, like Applied Behavioral Analysis, Discrete Trial Training, and Floortime, teach specific and correct behaviors one at a time.

- School-based group programs, either with other children with autism and a high teacher/student ratio or in a classroom with typical kids, use a variety of techniques to teach kids various skills to help them learn how to function.

- Social skills training with one-on-one programs like Relationship Developmental Intervention or group social skills classes teach kids how to socialize with other children and overcome many autistic behaviors.

- Speech and language therapy helps bring out verbal communication, and non-verbal kids can learn to communicate using picture systems (like the Picture Exchange Communication System, or PECS).

- Occupational therapy (OT) helps with muscle coordination and strength.

- Sensory Integration OT helps children learn how to properly process touch, sound, taste, and smell sensations.

Medical therapy. The medical side addresses any health problems or conditions that may be common to autism. There are two basic approaches:

- Medications to treat seizures (if present) and to help regulate aggression, hyperactivity, and other challenging aspects of autism are usually managed by a pediatric neurologist or psychiatrist.

- Treating related medical conditions, such as chronic diarrhea or constipation, food allergies, intestinal infections, viral infections, vitamin and mineral deficiencies, metabolic problems, and heavy metal overload, all of which may play a role in exacerbating autistic symptoms, is an emerging field that is currently thought of as alternative medicine. As more research and experience comes to light, these approaches may become more and more popular. Dr. Bob covers these emerging therapies in more detail in *The Autism Book*.

For more information on autism, check out *The Autism Book* in the Sears Parenting Library, or visit www.TheAutismBook.com.

BACK PROBLEMS

There are a number of back problems that can develop during childhood. Some cause pain, and some don't. Some are minor and temporary, and others may be more serious and require prompt attention from a doctor. In this section we will discuss various back problems and show you how to approach your pediatrician for help. Here are signs to watch for that warrant a visit to your doctor:

Signs and Symptoms

These signs and symptoms accompanying back pain prompt a more urgent medical evaluation with further testing:

- accompanying muscle weakness, especially in the arms or legs

- abnormality seen in walking, or difficulty walking

- numbness or tingling traveling from the spine to the arms or legs

- inability to hold in urine, or inability to pass urine

- inability to hold or pass bowel movements

- back pain that wakes a child up at night

- other body-wide symptoms that accompany back pain, such as fever, weight loss, or ill-feeling

See your pediatrician immediately if any of these symptoms develop. Write a detailed history of the pain to share with the doctor, including where the pain occurs, when and how it began, how often it occurs, what makes it better or worse, and any recent changes in activities or sports that could have caused or aggravated the pain.

Your pediatrician will do a complete musculoskeletal and neurological examination of your child. Based on the result of the exam and your child's history, the doctor may advise just a brief period of observation, or he will obtain some imaging studies, such as X-rays, MRIs, or CT scans, in order to more fully evaluate the cause of the back pain and prescribe appropriate treatment.

DR. SEARS TIP
Should You See Your Pediatrician or a Chiropractor?

We believe it is useful to first see your pediatrician to make sure there is no urgent medical problem that requires immediate testing or treatment. If your pediatrician determines there is nothing medically wrong and that no testing is necessary, and diagnoses your child with simple back pain with no serious cause, then it's time to go see a chiropractor. Chiropractors are skilled in correcting the alignment of the muscles, ligaments, and bones of the spine. Such adjustments usually bring relief to general back pain. They can also be a great help in healing various neck and back injuries, such as muscle or ligament strain and whiplash, as well as more chronic conditions, such as scoliosis and other spinal deformities (discussed below).

Causes

The following are various causes of back pain, but it is important to note that diagnosis and treatment of back problems in pediatrics are extremely complex and beyond the scope of this writing. Talk with your pediatrician or orthopedic specialist for more information.

Back Muscle Strain

This is a common injury among active teenagers. The back consists of many large muscle groups that support the spine and are important for proper movement. Certain injuries and activities can lead to muscle strain:

- sports-related injuries

- improper lifting techniques

- lifting objects that are too heavy

- activities that place repetitive stress on the back

- sudden or abnormal twisting motions of the back

- trauma to the back

Such injuries occur when there is damage to one of the many muscles of the back. Patients will often complain of pain in a specific area of the back. This pain is usually not located directly over the spine itself but rather to one side or the other. Often certain movements, such as twisting or bending over, worsen the pain. Your pediatrician will perform a physical examination of the back in order to make this diagnosis.

Treatment. Treatment of back muscle strain can be difficult because it can take a long time for a muscle strain to heal. It is important not to make the strain worse. Activities that caused the strain in the first place should be avoided. Ice the sore area for twenty minutes several times each day for three days. A period of rest is sometimes needed to speed up the healing process. Occasional use of anti-inflammatory medications, such as ibuprofen, may help ease the pain. Even with the best of treatments, these injuries can take several weeks to heal. The take-home message in treatment for muscle strain is to avoid back movements or exercises that make the pain worse.

Backpack Pain

Backpack pain is an increasingly common problem now that children are carrying more books and heavier objects at a younger age. Growing backs and heavy packs are a recipe for sore back muscles, especially in young children. Carrying backpacks that are too heavy or worn improperly is one of the most common, and most preventable, causes of childhood back pain. A study of 1,700 children showed the heavier the backpack, the greater the incidence of back pain. A study of 345 children in grades five through eight showed that over half the children carried loads heavier than 15 percent of their body weight, and one-third of the children who carried these heavier weights had back pain severe enough to cause them to visit a doctor or miss school. Here's how to prevent backpack pain:

Pick the right backpack. Avoid backpacks with only one strap, as these models have been shown to cause the most pain. Buy a backpack that has two straps. Be sure the shoulder straps are wide and padded, and choose a model that has a waist belt. A hiking type of backpack with a metal frame distributes the weight more evenly across the back of the hips.

Lighten the load. Orthopedists recommend that a backpack and its contents should weigh no more than 10 percent of the child's weight. So, an eighty-pound child should limit the load to eight pounds. Put your child's backpack load on the bathroom scale, and you may be amazed at how heavy it is.

Wheel it instead of wearing it. Try a "wheelie," a backpack on wheels. This is the best way to get the load off your child's back.

Wear it wisely. The heaviest part of the pack should sit on the lower back, just at the top of the hip bones. Pack heavier items first so they rest lower on the back. Avoid placing a lot of weight on the upper back, as this causes the greatest amount of strain.

Pick up the pack properly. Show and tell your child to bend at the knees when picking up the heavy pack or other heavy objects instead of bending over stiff-legged, which puts excess strain on the back muscles.

Get a second set of books. Although this is the most expensive remedy, it works. Rather than have the child lug heavy homework books back and forth, buy or rent an extra set of the heaviest books to keep at home.

Lightening the backpack load is especially important for children who already show some curvature of the spine or asymmetry in the development of their back muscles. Often during an examination the doctor will notice that the muscles on one side of the back are more developed than the other side, causing the shoulder blades to be somewhat uneven. Wearing heavy backpacks could aggravate this asymmetry. Finally, if your child has to wear a backpack, in addition to following the above precautions, teach her how to strengthen her back muscles by swimming the breaststroke or through supervised strength training.

Lower Back Pain

If unexplainable and/or serious causes of back pain have been ruled out by your pediatrician, then your child will probably be given the diagnosis of generic low-back pain. This chronic condition is seen more commonly in obese, less-active children and adolescents. Of utmost importance in treatment of low-back pain is to *stay mobile and active!* We always tell our patients that a strong back is very important for healthy growth and performance.

Specific back exercises can be done to help strengthen the spinal column and the muscles supporting it. Becoming less active and less mobile only makes the problem worse! We tell patients to limit the use of anti-inflammatories as much as possible, as these only mask the symptoms. A heating pad applied to the area can provide relief at the end of a long, active day. Other potential complementary treatment options include chiropractic spinal manipulation and back massage.

Scoliosis

Scoliosis is defined as an abnormal curvature of the spine, usually present in the middle and/or lower portions of the back. Scoliosis usually has an unknown cause. Very rarely, scoliosis may be due to abnormal formation of the spine, or it may be secondary to other muscular or neurologic disorders, such as cerebral palsy or muscular dystrophy.

Symptoms of scoliosis often begin in early adolescence. Sometimes there is a little pain associated with scoliosis in the teenage years, but more commonly pain arises later in life. Often scoliosis is first noticed by parents who observe differences in shoulder height or clothes not fitting right.

Examining the spine. Your pediatrician will do a specific examination to screen for scoliosis. If suspected, the doctor may decide to do special X-rays to determine the degree of scoliosis. This is important because treatment is based upon the level of severity of the problem.

Treating scoliosis. Most cases of mild scoliosis do not require treatment at all. Often observation is all that is needed. Occasionally, special braces are needed if the scoliosis is severe or worsening. Rarely, surgery of the involved vertebrae is needed.

For a more detailed discussion of scoliosis, see page 455.

Spondylolisthesis

The spine is made up of many vertebrae that are normally stacked like blocks in line with each other. *Spondylolisthesis* (meaning "slippage of the spine bones") is usually caused by a defect in one of the small bones making up part of the vertebrae, so that one of the vertebrae slips out of position relative to the rest of the vertebrae. This can happen if a small fracture in a bone has failed to heal properly and the vertebrae slip as a consequence of this weakening. Spondylolisthesis usually occurs in the lower portion of the back, and it may gradually worsen over time. Children at risk are those involved in activities that place a great deal of stress on the lower back, such as gymnastics, football, cheerleading, and dancing.

Symptoms. There could be no symptoms at all or lower back pain that often travels down the leg and may be made worse by standing. Patients may also experience occasional muscle spasms of their hamstrings. Your pediatrician will perform a complete back and neurological exam when your child presents with these symptoms. If such an injury is suspected, your doctor will order X-rays or CT scans to get an in-depth look at the vertebrae.

Treatment. Spondylolisthesis is often treated with specific strengthening exercises. Activities that may worsen the condition, such as continuing involvement in football or gymnastics, should be avoided completely. Occasionally, a custom-made orthotic device similar to a back brace may help control the pain symptoms. Normally, as the child matures, the defect heals over time, and most children achieve full recovery with little or no back problems in the future. Very rarely, the slippage worsens. Further consultation is needed in these rare cases, which may require spinal surgery.

Kyphosis (Humpback)

This is defined as excessive curvature of the thoracic or mid-portion of the spine. Kyphosis occurs most commonly in boys in early-to-mid adolescence. Most of the patients we see with this condition are brought in by concerned parents or grandparents who have noticed a worsening change in posture over time.

Symptoms. Usually the child reports no symptoms at all, but has a clear slumped-over appearance, especially when sitting. However, patients with severe kyphosis may certainly report pain. Your pediatrician will have your child perform a series of flexion and extension maneuvers of the back to assess the degree of curvature. X-rays are often done to evaluate for any spinal deformities.

Treatment. Occasionally, this curvature will progress as the child grows and may affect his ability to perform heavy lifting or certain exercises in the future. The good news is that generally this does not occur. Most cases of humpback are simply caused by poor posture and can be corrected with routine back exercises, as well as by practicing good posture techniques. Only when there is a specific spinal deformity are other treatments needed, such as bracing or, in extremely rare cases, surgery.

 **DR. SEARS TIP
Stand Up Straight!**

Mom was right! It's important to encourage your children to practice good posture while sitting and standing. Don't nag them, but gently remind them from time to time to stand up straight if they are slouching.

Traumatic Injuries to the Spine and Neck

Blunt trauma to the back or being involved in an accident, particularly in an automobile, can cause injuries to the back and neck. Following a severe injury or accident, complete spinal X-rays are often taken to rule out serious injury to the spinal column.

Whiplash injuries. These are common in auto accidents, and usually involve strain of the upper portion of the spine, also known as the *cervical vertebrae*. If whiplash is diagnosed, a neck brace is occasionally worn for a short amount of time. This injury can take quite a long time to heal.

Fractures of the spine. These are rare in children and adolescents, but in severe accidents this can occur. If a fracture is diagnosed, immediate consultation with a back specialist is required.

Back sprain. This is often the result of a sports-related or automobile-related injury. X-rays should be performed to rule out anything more serious. See treatment options, page 174.

Other Very Rare Causes

The following are extremely rare causes of back pain in children and adolescents and can usually be ruled out with a detailed history and X-rays, CT scans, or MRIs:

Juvenile osteoporosis. This can cause a thinning and weakening of the spinal bones. It is very rare and usually only results from severe nutritional deficiency of calcium and/ or vitamin D. Signs of osteoporosis can be seen on a basic X-ray.

Benign and malignant tumors. These are exceedingly rare in young people and can usually be ruled out with a good history and physical exam, and an X-ray if needed.

Infections of spine. Also known as osteomyelitis, this is very rare in youngsters. It may result from surgical procedures of the back or lumbar punctures (also known as spinal taps), or it may be secondary to body-wide infection. This is almost never seen in healthy children.

 DR. SEARS TIP
Physical Therapy

For most types of chronic back pain or deformity, learning proper back exercises is very important. We recommend you have several visits with a physical therapist to educate yourself and your child on what types of stretching and posture exercises he should be doing for his specific back problem. A reevaluation every year may also be useful.

BAD BREATH (HALITOSIS)

Although bad breath is usually more of an annoyance than a medical problem, it may have an easily remedied underlying cause.

Causes

These are the seven most common causes of stinky breath in order of frequency:

- postnasal drip from a cold or sinus infection: In our experience, one of the most common hidden causes of persistent bad breath is a chronic sinus infection. Like water in a stagnant pond, fluid collects in the sinuses and provides a culture medium for bacteria. As bacteria collect in the retained mucus, the resulting decaying material gives off an offensive odor. Persistent bad breath is often a clue to an underlying sinus or tonsil infection. Chronic nasal allergies may also cause halitosis.

- deep pits in large tonsils that collect oral and nasal secretions and decomposing food (called tonsilloliths — see page 525)

- decaying teeth

- dry mouth: when the natural rinsing action of saliva lessens, bacteria grow in the mouth and release smelly gases. Encourage your child to drink at least three or four glasses of water per day.

- gastroesophageal reflux disease (see GERD, page 338)

- a stinky tongue: bacteria and secretions that have collected on the back of the tongue

- foreign body stuck in nose (see page 416)

What to Do

Bad breath is usually a sign that you should see your pediatrician to make sure your child doesn't have an underlying sinus or throat infection. Before the doctor's appointment, keep a home diary noting what the child's breath smells like, how often you notice it, and if there are any other clues that you have noticed, such as a runny nose, cough, tiredness, and hoarseness. The odor from regurgitated stomach contents in children with GERD smells more sour, and is most often noticeable after "wet burps." Do a home throat exam, checking for food residue stuck between teeth or even in the crevices of tonsils. Such *tonsilloliths* will look like white or yellow dried pus (see page 525). You should also check the tongue. Using a plastic spoon or toothbrush, scrape the back of your child's tongue. If the scrapings smell like your child's breath, it's probably due to the residue of postnasal drip or food accumulating on the back of the tongue.

Take your child to the dentist if neither you nor your pediatrician finds the cause of your child's halitosis. Dental plaque and impacted food or rotting teeth can give off an odor.

Home Remedies

In addition to diagnosing and treating the cause, try the following remedies:

• Dr. Sears's favorite remedies: The "nose hose" and "steam clean." (See page 20.)

• Although it's unlikely that a child can be taught to gargle, she can be taught to swish. Children over four should swish their mouths with a warm saltwater solution (one quarter teaspoon of salt to an eight-ounce glass of water). A children's

mouth-rinse solution from a drugstore can also help. We don't recommend children use an adult mouthwash, as it may contain alcohol that children could swallow.

• Brush the tongue with a toothbrush every night, reaching as far back as your child will allow.

• Teach proper tooth brushing. Teach your child to brush her teeth to get all the "sugar bugs" off.

BEDWETTING

Bedwetting, medically known as *enuresis,* is a common developmental nuisance. Around 15 percent of five-year-olds wet the bed, with boys outnumbering girls by four to one. Nearly all children eventually outgrow their bedwetting, yet up to 5 percent of children do experience an occasional wet night even during the teenage years.

Causes

In the first couple of years, the bladder-emptying reflex is automatic, and the child wets his diapers. Sometime around two years of age, a child becomes aware of bladder fullness and can consciously hold on to his urine and inhibit the automatic bladder-emptying reflex. Urine-holding stretches the bladder muscles and increases its capacity. Nearly all children can consciously inhibit the bladder-emptying reflex during the day. Nighttime control, the ability to unconsciously inhibit the bladder-emptying reflex, usually occurs sometime between three and six years of age, often later in boys.

Some children simply have anatomically

small bladders that are more easily overfilled. Also, studies suggest some children don't produce enough antidiuretic hormone (ADH), which is released by the pituitary gland during sleep and causes the kidneys to make less urine so that the bladder doesn't fill beyond capacity. Bedwetting continues if there is a developmental delay in the brain-bladder communication at night or if the bladder remains small and cannot hold urine all night. Time and maturity usually heal both of these conditions.

Sleep studies on bedwetters show that bedwetting is most likely to occur during the delta stage, or deep stage, of sleep. And, in bedwetters, this stage may be deeper and last longer.

The age of bladder maturity varies greatly from child to child, with boys being later than girls. Think of bedwetting as another developmental milestone. Just as there are late walkers and late talkers, there are late dry-nighters. Nighttime bladder control occurs when the child can unconsciously inhibit the bladder-emptying reflex.

Four Insights

1. Bedwetting is a sleep problem. Think of bedwetting as a communication problem between bladder and brain. The child sleeps so deeply that he sleeps right through his bladder signals. He is not aware of his full bladder at night nor has he achieved the developmental capability of keeping his bladder from automatically emptying. In fact, it would be more correct to use the term *sleep-wetting* rather than *bedwetting*.

2. Bedwetting is rarely a psychological problem. Now that you understand that there are anatomical and neurodevelopmental reasons why children wet their beds, you can lose the thought that your child is "just being lazy at night." Be sympathetic to your child, as you would if he had any other medical problem.

3. Bedwetting is treatable. Once upon a time, parents and doctors took the "he'll grow out of it" approach. Though this is true, and most do, with modern insights and management techniques, it is no longer necessary for a child to wake up in a wet bed and for you to have your laundry room full of urine-filled sheets.

4. Bedwetting may have a genetic component. If both parents were bedwetters after the age of six, the child has about an 80 percent chance of being a bedwetter. If only one parent was wet at night, the child has about a 40 percent chance of having accidents.

 **DR. SEARS TIP
He Wets It, He Washes It**

It's your child's bladder, and as he's learning how to control it, he should also be learning to take responsibility for where he wets. Cheerfully encourage him and help him do the laundry according to his age and level of maturity. Be sure his laundry chore is not perceived as punitive but rather as a natural consequence of wetting his bed. Besides, it's likely to motivate him to do more of the self-help bladder-training skills.

Nine Steps to Dry Nights

We have practiced this step-by-step method in our office for nearly thirty years. It's a time-tested approach that we estimate works in at least 70 percent of our patients. Although it may take all nine steps, the problem is usually solved sooner, and most children begin to experience dry nights within a few months.

1. Keep a diary. For thirty days, write on a calendar how often your child wets his bed. Put "W" for wet nights and "D" for dry. On the nights that show "W," record what's different about that day and evening, such as different diet, different activity, different stress level, or emotional upsets at school or home. Try to identify the trigger or persistent pattern. For example, does your child wet the bed less on weekends, when he's been more active and has less stress than during school days?

2. Consult your doctor. Although most of the time bedwetting is a developmental quirk, occasionally there are anatomical abnormalities or medical illnesses that interfere with bladder control. Your child's doctor will do a complete physical examination first to be sure there are no neurological quirks that could interfere with nerve supply to the bladder. Your pediatrician may watch your child urinate to be sure he has a strong, steady stream and that the opening where the urine comes out (the *urethra*) is not too small.

If a child's bladder is smaller than normal, the doctor may ask you to measure your child's urine volume. Here's how to do it: Have your child drink lots of water and hold his urine as long as possible. Then have him empty his bladder into a cup. Be sure to have him empty it completely ("grunt three times"). A child's usual bladder capacity is his age plus two ounces. A five-year-old should be able to hold seven ounces of urine. If your doctor suspects that your child has an anatomically small bladder, here is an exercise

that your doctor may recommend to stretch his bladder and help it hold more:

"Hold on as long as you can…" This is called *progressive urine withholding*: once a day encourage your child to drink lots of fluids then "hold it" as long as he can. Tell your child he is stretching his bladder capacity like a balloon so it can eventually hold more so he doesn't have to go so often. After a few weeks of these bladder-stretching exercises, do the measuring-cup method again to see if he has increased his bladder-holding volume. Don't bother doing these bladder-stretching exercises unless your child is willing and able to cooperate, which would usually be by eight or nine years of age.

 DR. SEARS TIP Don't Hold It!

Don't try urine-withholding techniques without the advice of your child's doctor. Generally, we want a child to purposely listen to his bladder signals and not ignore them. Progressive urine withholding is only a temporary technique to help increase bladder capacity. Also, we tend to use these willful urine-withholding techniques less in girls because their anatomy makes them more prone to urinary tract infections, and one of the best ways to lessen UTIs is to go frequently and keep the bladder empty. Boys with urinary tract abnormalities, such as reflux, should not try urine-withholding techniques.

If your doctor suspects a plumbing problem or a structural or functional abnormality of the urinary tract, he may refer your child to a urologist for an ultrasound or X-ray study to outline your child's kidneys, his bladder, and his whole plumbing tract. With the help of your diary, your child's doctor may look for some hidden causes of bedwetting that are outside his plumbing but can affect it, such as the following:

- *Large tonsils/adenoids.* In our experience, this is one of the most overlooked causes of bedwetting. Large tonsils and/or adenoids partially obstruct the breathing at night, causing obstructive sleep apnea, which interferes with normal sleep cycles. This, in turn, interferes with brain-bladder communication during sleep, resulting in wet sheets.

- *Constipation.* Full bowels can "crowd out" a full bladder. (See treatment of constipation, page 241.)

- *Food sensitivities.* Junk food in general can cause junk sleep, and bedwetting is part of it. Food sensitivities that have been implicated as contributing to bedwetting are artificial colorings and caffeinated beverages.

- *Stress.* A stressful day often leads to a wet night. See if you can remove some of the stress triggers in your child's life.

- *Attention deficit disorder (ADD).* Children with ADD are more likely to wet the bed, presumably because they don't have the attention span to sit or stand still long enough to completely empty their bladders during the day. For this reason, their bladder capacity may be smaller. Additionally, children with ADD often have poor-quality sleep, which can increase bedwetting at night (see ADD, page 162).

Only around 5 percent of children have a hidden medical cause for bedwetting. The rest of the time, it's simply a developmental quirk.

READ MORE ABOUT IT

Using a picture book such as *Dry All Night* by Alison Mack will help you explain to your child how his kidneys make urine and fill the bladder.

---

3. Play show-and-tell. With the help of drawings, talk about the brain-bladder connection with your child. Here's an example of how we explain bladder training to five- to seven-year-old children in our office: Draw a picture of the brain with "wires" connected to the bladder. Explain the brain-bladder communication to your child in terms that go something like this: "Your bladder is like a balloon the size of a baseball, and inside the balloon are tiny nerves, like feelers, that tell you when your bladder is full. When your bladder is full, it sends messages to your brain and the brain tells you to go pee. At night the brain is sleeping. When your bladder is full, it tells the brain, but the brain sort of says, 'Don't bother me. I'm sleeping.' The bladder becomes so full it's got to go, so you pee in your bed. We're going to do some fun things to help your brain listen to your bladder at night."

4. Go to bed with an empty bladder. Many children who are tired or in a hurry only dribble a bit when they go to the bathroom before going to bed. They go to sleep with a half-full bladder. Teach your child triple-voiding. Here's how you can explain this bladder-emptying technique to your child: "Grunt, grunt, grunt three times to squeeze your bladder so you push the pee out and go to bed with an empty bladder."

5. Have the brain-bladder before-bed talk. Just before bedtime remind your child how his brain and bladder talk to each other at night. As he dozes off, he's then programmed to get up when his bladder is too full. Just before he drifts off to sleep, have him repeat phrases that imprint on his brain, like a conditioned reflex, what he will do when his bladder feels full: "I will get up and go to the bathroom when I feel my bladder get big...I will splash water on my face to wake up and grunt three times." One of the last scenes that your child rehearses before drifting off to sleep is how he and his bladder are expected to behave at night. If you don't want to get up with him at night, put an alarm clock in your child's bedroom and set it to go off within two to three hours after he retires, or set it to go off before your diary tells you he usually wets his bed. Right before he goes to sleep, tell him what to do when the alarm goes off: "When the alarm clock goes off and you feel your bladder is full, walk to the bathroom and grunt three times to get it all out." Be sure to leave a series of nightlights on in the path from bedroom to bathroom. The older your child gets, the more responsibility he needs to take for his bedwetting. You should not have to get up in the middle of the night. It's his bladder. But be a supportive coach.

6. Do the shake-and-wake. Most children wet the sheets within a couple hours after going to bed. Some will wet later in the night. Regardless of your child's pattern, try the following drill just before you retire:

- Fully awaken your child and help him walk to the bathroom.

- Have him splash water in his face to completely awaken.

- Have him "go three times" to completely empty his bladder.

- Walk with him back to his bed.

When you wake him, remind your child to repeat the conditioned-reflex phrases he used before going to bed in step 5.

7. Reward dry nights. Just as you would motivate and reward a child for mastering a skill, such as improving his musical skills, reward him for mastering his bodily skills. Try a sticker chart. Make a calendar and put "W" for wet nights and "D" for dry nights. Let him place a sticker on the dry nights. After five straight stickers, he gets a privilege. For the child who requires a few months of nighttime bladder training, perhaps reward him if the next calendar month shows more dry-night stickers than the previous one. Oftentimes, a reward, such as an overnight at the home of a friend, will be enough motivation.

DR. SEARS TIP
Encourage Sleepovers

Although you may initially feel that a sleepover could be embarrassing to your bedwetting child, it can also be motivating. Besides, chances are that he has at least one other friend who is a bedwetter too. Start by encouraging sleepovers with your child's best friends, as they are unlikely to tease him. Present sleepovers to your child with a "no big deal" attitude. If your child feels that you're not "embarrassed" by his problem, he's less likely to be fearful. Notify the friend's parents of your child's bedwetting. They are likely to be understanding and may come up with ideas to make your child feel more comfortable. You could have your child take over a plastic sheet or safety-pin a garbage bag inside his sleeping bag. Also, encourage a week or two away at camp if your child wants to go. The more you can help him not feel embarrassed about the bedwetting, the less of a problem it's likely to be.

8. Go high-tech. If your child is still wet most nights, even after trying the above steps, and he is getting increasingly bothered by this nighttime nuisance, try a bladder-conditioning device. These devices, available from your pediatrician or online, consist of a moisture-sensitive pad the child wears inside his under-wear or that is built into a sheet. When a drop or two of urine strikes the pad it sets off a buzzer that is attached to the child's pajama top. The principle behind this technique is conditioned response. Every time a child's bladder gets full, the alarm goes off so that the child gets conditioned to the feeling of a full bladder and awakening. The aim of the game is to "beat the buzzer" and for the child to get up and go to the bathroom *before* the alarm goes off. We have used these devices in our pediatric practice for over twenty years and have found around a 90 percent success rate. We do a trial run in one of the exam rooms in our office by teaching the child and the parent how to use the device. We pretend that our exam room is the child's bedroom, and then we rehearse the drills that they will go through at night. Here's the rehearsal that we do in our office and one you can do at home:

- Go to the bathroom and "grunt three times" to get all the pee out.

- Hook the device up to your child according to the manufacturer's instructions.

- Explain to your child what's going to happen: "The buzzer will help your bladder and brain listen to each other at night while you're sleeping. Pretend your bladder is full and starting to stretch and it's time to get up. Imagine waking up and taking a trip to the toilet."

- Do a practice run. As your child is lying in bed, set off the alarm manually and have your child hop out of bed as soon as he hears it. Then walk him to the bathroom and remind him how to wake himself up by splashing water in his face. Have him "grunt three times" to get the pee out. Rehearse this drill three times.

The rest is up to the child. Above all, don't use the device without first going through the drills. You want your child to get used to the sound or vibration of the alarm so that it doesn't frighten him.

9. Drugs for dry nights? We strongly discourage using some of the older medications, such as antidepressants, for bedwetting. In our experience, the side effects, such as sleep disorders and anxiety, are worse than the nuisance of the bedwetting itself. A safe and effective medication is DDAVP (desmopressin acetate), which works by mimicking the natural action of ADH, the antidiuretic hormone, and lessens the production of urine at night. It's available in a nasal spray or tablet and is taken before bedtime for two or three months and then tapered off. Remember to use the pills-skills model for bedwetting. Pills alone won't do it, but usually pills in addition to the skills mentioned above will work. Most of the time skills instead of pills can cure bedwetting.

RESOURCES

The two bladder-conditioning devices we use in our practice are Nite-Train-R, available at www.nitetrain-r.com, and Potty Pager, available at www.pottypager .com.

BIRTHMARKS

Nearly all infants are born with or later develop pink, blue, or red patches on their skin. These are caused by extra blood vessels beneath the skin. Growing children have rapidly growing skin, which contains a vast highway of rapidly growing blood vessels. Areas that contain extra blood vessels show through the skin as birthmarks. Here are the two most common kinds you're likely to see:

Stork Bites

"Stork bites" are red patches most commonly noticed at the nape of the neck, the forehead, or on the eyelids. Medically speaking, these are known as *nevi*, but they have humorously been dubbed "stork bites." They are caused by extra blood vessels showing through areas of thin skin. As your baby grows and the skin in these areas thickens, these blotches will fade over time. Because forehead spots are often more prominent when baby cries, mothers dub them "forehead lights." These marks usually fade between one and two years of age.

Strawberries

"Strawberries" are another common birthmark. Medically speaking, these are called *hemangiomas* and occur because the blood vessels under the skin keep growing and growing until they push through the skin. Some get so large they resemble a strawberry. They usually appear in the first year, reach their peak size by a year or two, and begin to shrink between the ages of three and five, and nearly all of them are completely gone by teen time. The rate of growth and shrinkage varies a lot from child to child; when the center of the strawberry starts turning gray, the blood vessels have stopped growing and the strawberry is beginning to shrink and fade. These are harmless, not precancerous, and rarely need any treatment. Occasionally, these strawberries need shrinking by laser surgery or other treatments, especially if they appear in areas that interfere with organ function, such as on the eyelids. Although most toddlers don't even notice these "special spots," discourage the habit of picking on these curious red bumps, which may cause them to bleed or become infected.

Blue Spots on Back

These common bruise-like bluish marks on the lower back and buttocks are called "Mongolian spots" because this genetic quirk was first identified among Mongolians; such marks are also common among children of Asian, Latino, African, and Native American descent. These spots are caused by excess concentration of pigment-containing cells called *melanocytes*.

What to do. These common spots are harmless, are not precancerous, and usually partially fade by the school-age years. Occasionally, they may persist to a slight degree throughout adulthood.

Although these spots are harmless, they sometimes get parents into trouble. We have seen cases in which parents have been falsely accused of abusing their children because these birthmarks were mistaken for "spank marks." We advise parents to take pictures of the spots and file them to protect themselves against these accusations. It is our practice to note these spots in the child's chart and mention this possibility to the parents. When enrolling your child in daycare, mention these "special spots" to the daycare providers so they won't misidentify them as spank marks.

Explaining these spots to your child.
Around three years of age, when children are old enough to understand these marks, play show-and-tell. Tell your child that he was born with these "special spots" and show him pictures. Reassure him that many children have these "special spots" and that they usually fade over time.

BITES: HUMAN, ANIMAL, AND INSECT

Human Bites

It's inevitable. Put two toddlers together to play for an hour, and someone's likely to get bitten. Although most such bites aren't serious, here are some steps you should follow to clean the wound and decide if a doctor's visit is warranted.

Treatment

If the skin isn't broken, then you don't have to do anything. But children's teeth are sharp, so if blood was drawn, follow these steps to flush out as many germs as you can:

- Irrigate the wound. You can rinse the wound with a strong stream of water from a kitchen sink or shower; however, such water isn't sterile. If possible, it's better to go to a drugstore and buy a bottle of sterile saline and an irrigating syringe (no needle). Flush the wound with eight to sixteen ounces of saline. A bottle of sterile water can also be used.

- Use an antiseptic solution. Diluted hydrogen peroxide (half water, half peroxide) or very diluted Betadine (one part Betadine to ten parts water) can also be swabbed onto the wound to kill any germs. Follow this with another saline rinse so that the irritating antiseptic doesn't remain in the wound.

- Apply an antibiotic ointment and a bandage.

When to Worry

Most wounds don't need a doctor's visit, but here are a few situations that do require a trip:

- Stitches. See page 259 to help you determine if stitches are needed.

- Bites to the face, hands, fingers, feet, or toes that break the skin. These have a high infection rate from mouth bacteria and may need antibiotics. Don't worry if it's just a minor puncture from the tips of the teeth.

- If you notice the wound becoming infected (red, draining pus, swollen and painful around the wound), see a doctor.

Animal Bites

Domestic pets cause most animal bites. Dogs are more likely to bite than cats, but cat bites are more likely to cause infection. Bites from non-immunized domestic animals and wild animals carry the risk of rabies. Rabies is far more common in raccoons, skunks, bats, and foxes than in cats and dogs. Rabbits, squirrels, mice, and other rodents rarely carry rabies. If an animal bites your child, follow these guidelines:

Treatment

Treatment depends on the severity of the wound.

Minor wounds. If the bite barely breaks the skin (draws little to no blood), and the animal is not likely to carry rabies, treat it as a minor wound. Wash it thoroughly with soap and water, apply an antibiotic cream to prevent infection, and cover the bite with a clean bandage.

Deep wounds. If the animal bite deeply punctures the skin or the skin is badly torn and bleeding, apply pressure with a clean, dry cloth to stop the bleeding and see your pediatrician (or go to an emergency room if after hours).

When to Worry

Infection. If you notice signs of infection such as swelling, redness, increased pain, or oozing, see your pediatrician immediately. Depending on the severity, source, and location of the bite, the doctor will probably prescribe an oral antibiotic to prevent infection. Bites to the face, hands, and feet are more likely to become infected. Bites to more central parts of the body are unlikely to become infected.

For suspected rabies. If you suspect the bite was caused by an animal that might carry rabies (see above), see your pediatrician immediately or go to an emergency room. The medical staff will help decide if you need a rabies vaccine. If the bite was caused by a domestic pet, try to obtain immunization information from the owner to confirm that the pet had a rabies shot. If the animal is wild, or seems domesticated but the owner cannot be found, do not try to catch the animal. Contact animal control (you can dial 911 if unable to find the number) for assistance. The animal can be quarantined and tested or observed for rabies.

DR. SEARS TIP
Get a Tetanus Booster

If your child's last tetanus shot was more than five years ago and the wound is deep or dirty, your child should get a booster within forty-eight hours of the injury.

Snake Bites

Most people don't encounter snakes in daily life. But children who live in rural areas likely will, and it's useful to know what to do in the event of a snake bite. If you are able to identify the snake without risking further bites or injury, do so. Knowing whether or not the snake is poisonous is important.

What to Do

Cleanse the wound. Wash the wound thoroughly with soap and water. Look for, and remove, any pieces of dirt or snake fang that might have broken off.

Immobilize the limb. Continued use of the limb can help the venom spread more quickly. Using a sling for the arm, or limiting the amount of walking if bitten in the leg, is helpful. Use a splint if available, but be careful not to wrap the limb so tightly that you cut off blood flow. Don't allow this to significantly delay your access to emergency care.

Seek emergency care. If you are very certain that the snake is non-poisonous, it is okay to not go to the emergency room and simply care for the wound at home as you would any other cut. If you aren't sure, or if you know that the snake is poisonous, go to the nearest emergency room without delay.

Remove any jewelry. If the limb swells, jewelry may need to be cut off.

Get a tetanus shot. The same guidelines apply as with animal bites.

Consider anti-venom. If the snake is positively identified as poisonous, the doctor will decide with you whether or not to administer anti-venom. Symptoms of venom exposure include shock, muscle weakness, fainting, difficulty breathing, and nerve dysfunction. These may occur within hours or may be delayed. The doctor will help you decide the appropriate time of observation in the hospital.

What Not to Do

Do not ice the wound. This may decrease blood flow to the wound and increase the risk of tissue damage.

Do not try to cut or suck out venom. Cutting increases the risk of infection and tissue damage, and sucking has not been shown to effectively remove venom.

Do not use a tourniquet. Reducing blood flow to the arm may increase the risk of tissue damage.

Bee Stings

Bee stings are very painful and usually obvious when they occur, if the bee is noticed. Some stings occur when a bee is stepped on with bare feet or while a child is sitting on the ground. If you don't see a bee, you will likely find the stinger still in the skin at the site of the sting.

What to Do

Remove the stinger. You can use tweezers or your fingernails.

Ice it. Apply a cold washcloth dipped in ice water or a baggie filled with ice water (ice applied directly to the skin is usually not tolerated by a child) as long as the child will allow it until the sting feels better. You may need to repeat this periodically over the next few hours.

Take an antihistamine. If the area begins to swell, apply some diphenhydramine (Benadryl) cream as directed on the tube. If the swelling persists or progresses quickly, give your child an oral dose of diphenhydramine (see page 549 for dosing). You can repeat this every six hours as needed.

When to Worry

The only worry with bee stings is a severe allergic reaction. Fortunately most children are not allergic. If your child has symptoms of a severe anaphylactic reaction (wheezing, difficulty breathing or swallowing, swelling of the hands or face — see page 130) call 911 or proceed to an emergency room right away. Once it is known that a child is allergic to bee stings, a prescription EpiPen adrenaline injection can be carried around with the child to prevent a severe reaction in the event he is stung again.

Spider Bites

The vast majority of spiders are harmless. There are only two types of spiders to worry about in North America: the black widow and the brown recluse.

Black Widow Spider Bites

The black widow is a shiny, black spider with long legs and a red (sometimes orange) hourglass marking on its torso. It is about one inch in length, including the legs. Black widow bites cause immediate pain and swelling near the bite. Painful muscle cramps may occur for six to twenty-four hours. These bites are rarely fatal except occasionally in younger children or if there are multiple bites.

What to do. Apply ice to the bite area (this will help reduce the spread of venom), then *immediately call your physician or go to the nearest emergency room.* Do not apply a tourniquet, but keep applying the ice for at least twenty minutes. When you arrive at the emergency room, your child's vital signs will be monitored and anti-venom administered if the bite is severe. Medications may also be given for the painful muscle cramps.

Brown Recluse Spider Bites

This spider is smaller than the black widow and harder to recognize. It is about ½ inch in length, including the legs. It is brown and has a dark, violin-shaped marking on its head. The brown recluse tends to hide in corners of the attic, so be careful when you're digging through boxes up there. These bites cause a delayed reaction of local pain and a blister that forms four to eight hours later. The center of the blister will turn dark (bluish-black) and an ulcer or crater will form. This crater is the serious part of a brown recluse bite and may require skin grafting if it becomes large enough. These bites are rarely fatal.

What to do. Wash the bite area thoroughly with soap and water, apply ice, then call your pediatrician. If possible, save the spider for identification. For severe bites, the area might need to be surgically drained and cleaned.

Other Spider Bites

Most spiders — including the tarantula — cause local reactions that are not dangerous.

Spider bites are usually painful and swollen for a day or two, like a bee sting.

Home remedies. First, wash the area with soap and water. Next, apply meat tenderizer to the bite. This is best done by rubbing the bite with a cotton ball soaked with a one-half meat tenderizer/one-half water solution. Continue applying this solution for about ten minutes. Use ice if you don't have any meat tenderizer. If pain and swelling persist, try oral or topical diphenhydramine (Benadryl).

When to Call the Doctor

- The bite becomes a blister.
- The bite turns dark (purple or bluish-black).
- Your child develops muscle cramps.
- The bite looks infected, with pus draining.

Prevention

- Have your child wear gloves when working around stacked wood, drainpipes, rock piles, window wells, or outdoor planters.
- If you find a black widow or brown recluse spider, spray the area with insecticide.
- When the weather turns cold, be prepared for spiders that try to move inside. Repair cracks in doors or windowsills and spray these areas with insecticide.

 DR. SEARS TIP
Nature Lesson

Instead of killing every harmless spider we see at home (such as daddy longlegs), we try to discuss with our kids how spiders help keep flies and mosquitoes at bay. We like to leave such spiders alone or safely take them outside.

Mosquitoes, Fleas, and Other Bug Bites

Most insect bites are harmless in the long run. There is usually no reason to see a doctor to identify what type of bites they may be, because the treatment is all the same: minimize itching and prevent infection. A doctor usually wouldn't be able to determine what type of creature had your child for lunch anyway.

What to Do

Follow these tips to ease the itch and prevent infection:

Cool it down. Dip a washcloth in ice water and apply it to the bite area. An ice cube rubbed around individual bites works too.

Medicate it. One of our favorite instant-relief treatments is a topical anesthetic gel (Itch-X) applied to the bites. This may sting if the bite has been scratched open, but it works very well otherwise.

Coat it. Soothing pink calamine lotion can ease itchy bites. Do not use calamine lotion on the face for open bites as the powder left over once the calamine dries may stay in the bite and cause a small scar.

Note: for tick bites, see page 517.

Scorpion Stings

Scorpion stings can be quite scary, as scorpions are classically thought of as being deadly. However, most scorpions in the United States are actually non-poisonous. The poisonous species live primarily in the desert regions of the southwestern United States. If you are able to catch the scorpion without risking another sting, do so. It will be useful to identify the species as poisonous or non-poisonous.

What to Do

- Wash the wound with soap and water.

- Cool the area with ice (do not put ice directly on the skin; use an ice pack or a bag of ice) for ten minutes on and ten minutes off to slow the spread of the venom.

- Remove any jewelry.

- Keep the area of the body that was stung as still as possible to slow the spread of venom.

- Do not cut into the wound or try to suck out the venom.

- If you are able to catch the scorpion, you can call the poison control hotline at 1-800-222-1222. They will be able to help you identify the scorpion.

Emergency Care

If the scorpion is identified as poisonous, or if you are uncertain, proceed directly to an emergency room while tending to the preceding steps. Symptoms of scorpion venom exposure are similar to those of other poisonous bites, and include shock, difficulty breathing, and neurological symptoms. These may begin within two hours of the sting. If you are certain it is non-poisonous, observe your child at home. A tetanus shot is generally not needed, as scorpion stings are not very deep.

BITING BEHAVIOR

Parents naturally worry about why their otherwise adorable little child bites the very hands that care for him, but try not to take this and other annoying behaviors, such as hitting and yelling, personally. The nips and slaps that most parents are exposed to are common behaviors of the child who doesn't yet have the verbal language to communicate his needs, so he uses his hands and mouth. Sometimes these little nips are playful communications; other times they reveal frustrations. Once a child has the verbal skills and language to communicate his needs, these annoying behaviors will cease.

What to Do

Track the trigger. What triggers the biting or hitting? Is your child tired, hungry, or bored, or are there too many kids in too small a space? Try to remove the triggers in order to squelch the behaviors.

Play show-and-tell. Show and tell your toddler that biting hurts. Gently and lovingly press his forearm against his upper teeth and show him the resulting marks on his arm. Use this self-biting demonstration immediately after your child bites so he makes the connection. Do this in an instructive way, not a punitive way. You want him to learn, "See, biting hurts!"

Don't bite him back. This often-given advice is unwise because it models to the child that biting is okay. After all, the child concludes, "Whatever Mommy and Daddy do is okay for me to do, too."

Remove him from other little biters. Your child may be learning these annoying behaviors at daycare or from other toddlers. If possible, limit exposure to these other children. If your child is exposed to too many biters, hitters, and screamers, he may pick up that these are "normal" behaviors and incorporate them into his own behavior.

Use alternative behaviors. Redirect those slapping little hands into more acceptable physical alternatives, such as "Give me five!"

Try a timeout. If the biting behaviors are not improving with the above strategies, have a timeout. Two-and-a-half-year-old toddlers can make the connection between annoying behaviors and their consequences.

 DR. SEARS TIP
Don't Ignore It!

Although sometimes the "ignore it and it will go away" response does work in suppressing annoying behaviors, we prefer that parents help the child work through these behaviors by teaching him more acceptable ones. This approach has a double benefit. It helps you develop creative parenting skills, and it teaches your child that you are a valuable resource, an impression you want to build into your children early on so they call upon you for help later when the stakes are much higher.

BLADDER INFECTIONS (URINARY TRACT INFECTIONS)

One of the kidney's main jobs is to filter the blood of waste products and produce urine. The urine then travels down a tube into the bladder. This tube is called the *ureter*. Urine then passes through the bladder into another tube called the urethra and into the diaper or toilet. Bacterial infections can occur at any point along this "plumbing" system, which is called the *urinary tract*. Doctors usually refer to bladder infections as UTIs for short, although most of these infections involve only the bladder or urethra.

Why Kids Get UTIs

Normally, urine is sterile, and as long as the plumbing system works like it should, urine keeps flowing and the child urinates easily. A principle of the human body is that fluid that gets stuck anywhere eventually gets infected. So any malformation, habit, or medical problem that slows the passage of urine sets the child up for a urinary tract infection. Because a girl has a shorter urethra that is connected to the vagina and because the vaginal bacteria can travel more easily through the urethra into the bladder, girls tend to have more UTIs than boys. Here are some reasons why children get UTIs:

Malformation of the kidney or bladder systems. Any developmental obstruction (an anatomical malformation of the kidneys or any obstruction of the tubing carrying the urine) that keeps the urine from flowing normally can lead to an infection. A common malformation is called *bladder reflux:* the valves where the ureters enter the bladder malfunction, allowing urine to reflux from the bladder back up into the ureters and kidneys so that the child never totally empties the bladder. This retained urine is prone to infection. The back pressure from the urine flowing the wrong way may also cause kidney damage if it persists for many years.

Constipation. Golf-ball-like stools in the lower intestines can press against the bladder, keeping it from completely emptying.

Urine-holding. Sometimes children "forget" to go. They don't want to lose their place in line, or they're too embarrassed to ask the teacher to go. Normally, when the bladder gets full, sensors will tell the brain, "Got to go!" Some children, especially boys, don't pay enough attention to their bladder signals. Remember, the bladder has to empty routinely to prevent infection. Children are especially prone to ignore their urge-to-go signs while playing video games.

Symptoms of UTIs in Babies

The younger the child, the more challenging the diagnosis. Because babies can't tell you if they hurt, and they urinate frequently anyway, the signs of UTIs are not as clear-cut, especially in the early months. Here are two potential signs:

 DR. SEARS TIP
When in Doubt, Check It Out

As you can see, signs and symptoms of UTIs in babies are vague, which is why when your baby is sick without an obvious cause a pediatrician will nearly always check your baby's urine, for two reasons. First, recurrent, undiagnosed UTIs can lead to kidney damage. Second, what may start as a mild UTI can, if left undetected and untreated, progress so that the bacteria get released into the bloodstream, making an infant extremely ill and even requiring hospitalization. The earlier the UTI is diagnosed and treated, the better the outcome.

Fever of unknown origin. If your baby has a fever, and neither you nor your doctor can tell where the fever is coming from, suspect the urinary tract.

Baby is sick, but with no obvious cause. The baby is lethargic, vomiting, feverish, and "just not herself."

Testing a Baby's Urine

Since you can't just tell a one-year-old to "go pee in a cup," the following describes what you and your doctor might do in order to diagnose your baby:

Bag Baby. The nurse in your doctor's office (or the parent) can put a special bag over the vagina or penis and then wrap the diaper over it. The nurse will clean out the area first with a wipe to get rid of the bacteria that normally reside in this area. Nurse or feed your baby. As soon as the baby urinates into the bag the nurse or doctor will do a urinalysis, which may reveal a UTI. Bag specimens are not usually sterile, but at least they are a convenient place to start. If the bag specimen does not show clues of a UTI (presence of blood, white blood cells, or nitrites — a substance produced by bacteria), a UTI is unlikely, though still possible. If, however, the specimen shows evidence of a UTI, a culture may be sent to the lab (see below).

Have a cup ready. Wash the penis or labia and feed your diaperless baby. Have a sterile cup ready to catch the urine, sort of a "midstream specimen." Although this method of urine collection is more challenging, it is more accurate than a bag specimen. The doctor will perform a urinalysis and send this specimen off to a laboratory for a culture to grow the bacteria. A urine culture will yield two pieces

of valuable information: (1) whether or not your baby has a UTI; (2) the offending bacteria if the culture is positive. The laboratory will then do an antibiotic sensitivity test to show what antibiotics are most effective against the offending bacteria.

Catheterized urine specimen. If Baby is very ill and a very accurate diagnosis is required, the doctor may do a *catheterized urine specimen* by inserting a tiny catheter tube through the urethra into Baby's bladder. Naturally, this is a more painful way of collecting the urine, but it is the most accurate way to identify the offending germ since no harmless germs that normally live around the penis and vagina can contaminate the collected urine sample.

Symptoms of UTIs in Children

The older the child, the more definite the symptoms. The most common ones include the following:

- frequent urination
- sudden urges to urinate, but only producing small amounts at a time
- abnormal smell or appearance of the urine
- pain or burning with urination
- fever: not present when only the bladder is infected, but will usually be part of a more serious kidney infection

Treatment

If, based upon the above symptoms, your doctor suspects a UTI, she will check your child's urine in the office to confirm. Your child will be asked to give a "midstream urine sample" or "pee in a cup" after cleaning her labia or washing his penis. Obviously, you will need to help your child do this. The doctor may then send the sterile specimen to a laboratory for a culture to identify the germ.

If the symptoms and the urinalysis are positive for a UTI, your pediatrician will prescribe the antibiotic most likely to be effective. If, on the other hand, the diagnosis is still questionable, the doctor may wait for the urine culture results before prescribing an antibiotic.

When to treat before getting the culture results and when to take a wait-and-see approach is a judgment call based upon how definite the symptoms and how bothered your child is.

If you and your doctor decide on a wait-and-see approach for mild bladder infection

DR. SEARS TIP
Collecting a Urine
Sample at Home

If you suspect your child has a UTI, you will want to properly collect a urine specimen to take into your pediatrician's office. Here's how:

- Do a "clean-catch midstream" sample. The best time is the first urination in the morning.

- Clean the penis or labia.

- Have the sterile cup (or a jar that you have previously sterilized with boiling water) ready. Be sure your child urinates a few seconds, then collect a sample. You'll only need about a half inch of urine in the cup.

- Take the sample to your doctor's office right away. If your appointment is later in the day, store the sample in the refrigerator.

symptoms without fever, you can start flushing out the infection by having your child drink three glasses of cranberry juice (or take a cranberry extract from any health-food store) and take vitamin C (250 mg for kids one to four; 500 mg for kids five and up) twice each day. By the time you get the urine culture results back, your child may be feeling better. You may not even need antibiotics at that point, even if the culture is positive for infection. You should discuss this option with the doctor.

Symptoms of a More Serious UTI or Kidney Infection

The goal of diagnosis and treatment of the UTI is to prevent the infection from spreading up into the kidneys. If it does, here are symptoms that suggest your child is developing a kidney infection:

- acting and appearing much more ill than with only a bladder infection

- high fever that can spike to 104 degrees

- pain in the side or lower back in the area of the kidneys

- lower abdominal pain

- chills and shaking

- vomiting

If the doctor suspects a kidney infection, the same urine tests will be done to confirm the UTI. Your pediatrician may also draw blood to see if the infection has gotten into the bloodstream, which is common with a kidney infection. Treatment of a kidney infection usually requires a stronger antibiotic given by intramuscular injection or intravenously. Depending on its severity, your child may need to be hospitalized for a few days while the antibiotics take effect.

Prevention

The two simple goals to prevent UTIs:

- keep germs out of the urine

- keep the urine flowing

Here's how you can help your child have fewer UTIs and help treat them when they occur:

Avoid local irritations. Strong soaps, bubble bath, and tight clothing can irritate the urethra in girls. You can lower your little girl's risk of getting a UTI by avoiding long periods of sitting in soapy or bubble baths. Let her play in the bath with just warm water and use soap only at the very end of the bath, right before she is ready to get out.

Teach proper wiping. Teach your little girl to wipe from front to back, not back to front, to prevent vaginal germs from entering the urethra.

Teach bladder signals. Encourage your child to "go" when his bladder tells him to (see the dialogue modeling how to teach your child to listen to his bladder signals under Bedwetting, page 179).

Treat constipation. Keep those little bowels moving (see Constipation, page 240).

Teach bladder-emptying techniques. Hurried children often don't empty their bladders. Teach your child to "grunt three times and squeeze all the pee out." (See further bladder-emptying techniques under Bedwetting, page 179.)

Give daily juice. Encourage your child to drink a glass of cranberry juice or take a cranberry extract supplement (from any health-food store) every day. Also, offer a daily serving of blueberries. The phytonutrients in these berries keep bacteria from adhering to the bladder wall and therefore lessen the chance of infection.

Recurrent UTIs: What Your Doctor Might Advise

If your child is getting recurrent UTIs, it's important to be sure there is no structural abnormality of the urinary tract. The goal is to minimize UTIs in order to protect the growing kidneys. This is why your doctor may suggest a thorough examination of your child's urinary tract to be sure it is structurally normal, including these tests:

- An ultrasound may disclose major structural abnormalities.

- A VCUG — *voiding cysto-urethrogram*. With this test, the radiologist inserts a catheter through the urethra and injects dye into the bladder. While the child is emptying her bladder, X-ray pictures are taken. This test is very useful because it detects the most common abnormality causing recurrent UTIs — *vesico-ureteral reflux* (VUR), or bladder reflux. It is the most common test performed for a child with recurrent UTIs.

If your child has a mild degree of reflux, the doctor may take a wait-and-see approach in the hope that the valves will mature and correct themselves. Or, while they're growing, the child may be treated with daily antibiotics to keep the urine sterile while you and your child conscientiously practice the bladder-training techniques mentioned above (see page 195). If the reflux is severe or not correcting itself, the doctor may recommend surgical correction of the valves. Sometimes this can be done as an outpatient endoscopic procedure. There is a new procedure called *deflux,* where your doctor injects a healing gel into the area of the defective valve; it is a much less invasive procedure than surgical correction. It is estimated that around 1 percent of all children have some degree of VUR.

BLISTERS

Blisters are usually caused by friction or burns (see page 205 for burn care). It is usually best to leave the blister intact. Unbroken skin over a blister provides a natural barrier to bacteria and decreases the risk of infection. Protect a small blister with an adhesive bandage, and cover a large one with a porous, plastic-coated gauze pad that absorbs moisture and allows the wound to breathe.

If a blister is large, under a lot of pressure, or in an area that has a lot of friction, you can drain it to relieve some of the pain. Here's how:

- Wash your hands and the blister area with soap and water.

- Swab the blister with antiseptic or rubbing alcohol.

- Sterilize a clean, sharp needle by wiping it with rubbing alcohol.

- Use the needle to puncture the blister at several spots near the edge. Let the fluid drain, but leave the overlying skin in place. Note: You can reassure your child that he will not feel any pain when you prick the blister.

- Apply an antibiotic ointment to the blister and cover with a bandage.

After several days, cut away any dead skin with scissors sterilized with rubbing alcohol. Keep the open blister covered with antibiotic ointment and a bandage.

Signs of infection. Call your doctor if you notice:

- pus

- redness

- increasing pain

- warm skin

Prevention. It's important to recognize where a potential blister might develop before it does. You can often anticipate "hot spots" when wearing a new pair of shoes. Also, keep in mind that long walks or hiking trips are common times for blisters to erupt on the feet. Biking or waterskiing can lead to blisters on the hands. Check for areas of chafing or redness and use gloves, socks, a bandage, or similar protective covering over the area being rubbed. Special athletic socks are available that have extra padding in critical areas. Moleskin can be attached to hot spots on the inside of the shoe to prevent or reduce rubbing.

BLOOD IN BOWEL MOVEMENTS

The two most common causes of specks of blood in Baby's bowel movements are rectal fissures and food allergies.

Rectal fissure. This is a tiny tear in the lining of the rectum. A clue that a rectal fissure is the cause is only a few specks of *bright red* blood. Oftentimes, the doctor may be able to see the tear when examining your baby's rectum. The most common cause of rectal fissures is constipation. (See page 240.)

Food allergies. The second most common cause of blood in bowel movements — and one that is more concerning and possibly harmful — is blood loss from irritation of the intestinal lining due to a food allergy. The two most common offenders are milk and wheat. A clue that the blood in the bowel movements is due to food allergies and not a rectal fissure is that food allergies usually produce darker red or even black specks of blood because bleeding occurs higher up in the intestines. Also, the stools tend to be more watery, looser, mucousy, and greenish. Bowel movements with a rectal fissure tend to be firmer, not mucousy or greenish.

DR. SEARS TIP
The "Target Sign"

Because food allergies produce acidic bowel movements, a clue that your child may have them is a red, burn-like rash around the anus, which results from the acid irritation from frequent stools. If you see this "target sign" and your child has other signs and symptoms of food intolerances (abdominal pain, bloating, skin rash, and stool with the characteristics described above), be sure to alert your baby's doctor.

When to Worry; What to Do

Babies seldom lose enough blood from a rectal fissure to become anemic. Besides stool-loosening strategies, apply a dab of glycerin or other emollient around Baby's rectum to ease the passage of the stool across the fissure. Glycerin suppositories can also help.

Take blood loss from food allergies more seriously, as food-allergic infants can lose enough blood to become anemic. See your doctor within the next few days. (See related sections: Anemia, page 140, and Food Allergies, page 327.)

BODY ODOR IN YOUNG CHILDREN

For most pre-pubertal children who develop underarm odor, it's nothing more than an offensive quirk. Contrary to popular belief, sweat doesn't stink. It's what happens to the sweat once it gets on the skin that gives it the odor. Some children sweat excessively, a quirk called *hyperhidrosis.* And some children start the increased sweating of puberty earlier than others, even as early as six to eight years of age. Although how much your child sweats is genetic and individual, the good news is that you can do a lot to help how much that sweat smells.

DR. SEARS TIP
Use the Term *Quirk* a Lot

In discussing a lot of unusual behaviors, physical findings, and bodily nuisances, use the term *quirk* rather than *illness, disease,* and so on. A *quirk* simply means a harmless difference and does not leave the child feeling self-conscious or unnecessarily worried. Explain to your child, "We all have quirks, and this is yours, but here's how we can deal with it." By using the term *quirk* you help your child create a "no problem . . . no worry" attitude. In our pediatric practice we use the term *quirk* a lot and find it is a less judgmental and worrisome term.

Causes

First, let's understand how your child sweats and how to keep it from stinking. Some children have more active sweat glands and harbor more bacteria on their skin. There are several million sweat glands throughout your child's body. In early childhood these are undeveloped, so your child sweats less. Around middle childhood, the sweat glands are better developed. At puberty, they've reached full development and begin to really take off. Your child's body produces two types of sweat. Sweat glands that are located over the smooth surfaces of the body secrete a sweat that is mainly water and nearly odorless. Sweat glands near hairy areas, such as the groin and under the arms, secrete sweat that contains some proteins and fatty substances. The bacteria that normally live on the skin feast on the fatty substances, thus releasing the odor. That's an important point to remember: bacteria feasting on sweat produces the odor. Naturally, then, the way to stop the odor is to control the bacteria.

Excessive underarm odor can be a sign of early or precocious puberty. Be sure to mention this quirk to your child's doctor on her next regular checkup. Your doctor will then check your child for other signs of precocious puberty such as underarm or facial hair, breast enlargement, or pubic hair. If there are no signs of precocious puberty, consider this problem harmless and not a clue of a possible medical problem.

Six Ways You Can Help Your Child Lessen Body Odor

1. Help your child understand her sweating quirks. Excessive sweating is an inherited tendency, especially increased sweating on the palms of the hands and soles of the feet. If your child inherits this tendency, present it as just a quirk. It doesn't mean anything is wrong with her, it's just that some people sweat more than others. Explain that part of body hygiene is to learn how to manage your quirks. Some people sweat more when eating spicy foods. Emotions can cause you to sweat, particularly on the palms of the hands and around the upper lip. This does not mean anything is wrong.

2. Keep the skin clean. As you learned above, it's the bacteria feasting on the fatty chemicals in the sweat that causes the odor. So the less bacteria on the skin, the less the odor. Play show-and-tell. Teach your child that the odor of sweat is caused by these bacterial feasts. She'll understand how using soap and water to wash off the "bugs" will keep her sweat from smelling. When a child understands why she needs to wash, she will be more likely to do it. Be sure your child rinses well. Teach your excessive sweater to take frequent *mini baths* by washing under her arms several times a day, especially after play. Instruct your child to dry very thoroughly. Leaving moisture on certain areas of the skin, such as in the skin folds under the arms, in the groin, and between toes, can further increase bacterial growth. Again, remind her that the less time the bacteria has a chance to feast on sweat, the better.

3. Air the sweat. The sweat that stinks the most is located in the areas of the body that are covered, such as under the arms and the groin. Wearing loose-fitting, cotton clothing that allows the skin to breathe and air to circulate in these areas should delay the bacterial feast and the consequent odor.

4. Feed the skin pure food. What your child eats can affect how the sweat smells. It stands to reason that if sweat is part of your body's garbage-disposal system, the less garbage you put into the body, the less there is for the body to process. In our pediatric practice, we have many such testimonies. Mothers who fed their children "pure" diets (going organic and eating real, unprocessed foods) notice diminished odor in their children's sweat. Your child needs to learn that junk food produces junk sweat.

5. Use deodorants if necessary; do not use antiperspirants. As the name implies, deodorants are scents that mask the smell of sweat. Antiperspirants, on the other hand, are chemicals that actually plug the sweat pores and diminish sweating. We discourage the use of antiperspirants prior to puberty because many contain irritating chemicals. Also, plugging pores sets the stage for inflammation. Use the mildest deodorant that does the job. Underarm rashes are especially common in children who use deodorants. It's okay for your child to use deodorant, but in addition to, not instead of, all the other sweat-control tricks mentioned above. Once excessive sweat becomes more noticeable (during puberty), an antiperspirant/deodorant is appropriate.

6. Don't act offended. It's better not to make a big deal of your child's body odor. Young children are sensitive and often conclude "if my sweat smells, I smell." That's why if your child does ask, you should explain that some people have this quirk and that it's one of life's little nuisances that you will help her deal with. The less your child perceives it bothers you, the less it will bother her.

BOILS

A boil is a tender, red lump on the skin similar to a large pimple. Boils can occur anywhere on the body, but are most common on the armpits, buttocks, shoulders, neck, and face.

Causes

A boil is the result of a bacterial infection of a hair follicle or sweat pore on the skin. *Staphylococcus aureus* (commonly known as "staph") bacteria are normally present on our skin and usually do not cause problems; however, these bacteria can get into and infect the sweat pores or hair follicles, resulting in inflammatory substances (increased blood flow, white blood cells, and other immune-fighting chemicals) all coming to the site to fight the infection. This causes a pus-filled boil to develop. Boils can also develop when surface bacteria penetrate through areas of broken skin, such as a scrape or cut. Children with diabetes, eczema, a weakened immune system, or anemia are more prone to getting boils, so let your doctor know if your child has had more than three bouts with boils.

What to Do

Your child's immune system will usually fight the infection on its own over a couple of days, and the boil should slowly improve. You can aid in the healing process by doing the following:

Wash the boil. Wash the boil gently several times a day with soap and warm water.

Soak the boil. Take a clean cloth, soak it with hot water, and apply it as a hot compress to the area of the boil for fifteen minutes three or four times a day. This will help kill the bacteria in the skin and bring the boil to a head so that it is ripe for draining. (Be sure not to use water that is so hot that it will burn.)

Let the boil pop on its own. *Do not* attempt to burst or pop the boil. This can cause the infection to get into the lower tissue layers of the skin. You may notice a white or yellow head developing in the middle of the boil. This may or may not burst. If the boil bursts, continue warm-water soaks to help remove all the pus. Wash the area with soap and water. Apply a topical antibiotic ointment to help speed the healing.

Cover the boil. When the head of the boil opens, cover it with a sterile dressing to prevent the infection from spreading.

When to Worry

See the doctor if any of the following symptoms develop:

- The boil is not improving.

- The boil is getting larger rather than smaller.

- The boil does not come to a head.

- Your child begins complaining of increasing pain.

- Reddish streaks spread out from the boil.

- Your child develops a fever.

- Several boils develop on the skin.

- Your child has underlying medical problems, such as diabetes or immune deficiency.

- The boil is near your child's eyes.

Your doctor may prescribe an oral antibiotic and provide further wound-care instruction if the above symptoms occur. A boil that continues to get worse can form an *abscess*. In this case, the boil needs to be surgically drained to completely clear the infection. This can usually be done as a brief, outpatient procedure. Some large abscesses may require brief hospitalization along with further treatment with intravenous antibiotics to completely clear up the abscess.

Prevention

Children can keep getting boils or can even spread them to other family members. This can be minimized by taking the following steps:

- Read Boosting Your Child's Immune System, page 33.

- Once a boil is draining, keep the area clean and covered with sterile wound dressing.

- Use special antiseptic soaps for one to two weeks following a boil.

- Wash all your child's bedding, washcloths, and towels in hot water following a boil.

- The bacteria that lead to boils often come from the nasal passages. Applying a prescription antibiotic ointment inside the nostrils for several weeks can eradicate the bacteria. If your doctor suspects your child or another family member is a carrier of staph, the doctor may culture the nasal passages.

- Your doctor may take a sample of the drainage of the boil or perform other blood tests to rule out any underlying medical conditions.

- See related section: MRSA, page 406.

BREATHING DIFFICULTY

Infants and children may experience breathing difficulty for a variety of reasons. This situation usually requires an evaluation by a doctor. Here is our guide to help you understand the best course of action to take:

Symptoms

It's important to distinguish what type of breathing trouble your child is having. This will help you narrow down what is causing it and what you can do to help.

Wheezing. This is a high-pitched, whistling, crackly sound. If your child has asthma or has wheezed before, then you are probably already familiar with this. If you only hear wheezing during exhalation, this is a good sign that the situation isn't too serious. If your child is wheezing while breathing both in and out, this is more serious. Wheezing sounds usually don't clear up after a cough. Harmless chest congestion, which can sound like wheezing to a novice parent, does clear up after a nice strong cough.

Stridor. This term describes a hoarse, raspy sound while your child breathes in. You may also notice your child has lost his voice and may have a funny-sounding cough, like a seal barking.

Retractions. This term refers to skin drawing inward while a child breathes in. You can see retractions in the abdomen (below the ribcage) or in the neck area just above the ribcage. Retractions are a sign that your child is having trouble drawing air into the lungs.

Rapid breathing. If a child is breathing more rapidly than normal (more than thirty to forty breaths per minute), this is a sign that the lungs are having to work harder to bring in oxygen.

 DR. SEARS TIP
Fever and Rapid Breathing

If your child's breathing is rapid during a high fever, don't worry just yet. Rapid breathing is a normal response to fever as a way to breathe off some of the excess heat. Before you worry that something might be wrong with the lungs, bring the fever down first. If the rapid breathing persists once the temperature is lowered, see or call your pediatrician. See Fever, page 317.

Labored breathing. Labored breathing refers to when a child has to use his shoulder muscles to help draw air into the lungs. Your child will raise his shoulders up with every breath. He may also lean forward and brace his arms against something.

Non-Serious Symptoms

Some parents see or hear some abnormal breathing sounds and patterns and worry that something serious may be going on, when in reality it's nothing to worry about. Here are some harmless signs to recognize:

Chest congestion. If you hear loose rattling sounds in the lungs that clear easily after your child has a good cough, this is probably just harmless mucus in the upper airway. Such harmless sounds are also normal while an infant feeds.

Nasal congestion. An infant with a severe stuffy nose can appear to be struggling for every breath, and a parent may worry that something is wrong with the lungs. If your infant is snorting his way through every breath, try our nose-clearing techniques described on page 20. You will probably see any difficulty temporarily relieved.

Gasping or straining during coughing. Children can make all kinds of funny sounds while coughing. Don't worry about anything you see or hear during this time. What's important is how your child is breathing when not coughing.

Causes

There can be many causes of difficult breathing. Review these possible causes and decide which description fits your child best:

Asthma attack. If your child is wheezing for the first time, it may be an asthma attack. You may also notice labored breathing and retractions. You can read more about how to tell and what to do in our asthma section, page 151.

Respiratory syncytial virus (RSV). RSV is a common cold virus that infects the lungs of infants and causes runny nose, cough, and wheezing. You may also notice retractions. See page 451 if your infant has these symptoms.

Allergic reaction. If your child just ate something suspicious or was just stung by an insect and is wheezing, this may indicate a

troublesome allergic reaction. See Allergic Reactions, page 130.

Reactive airway disease (RAD). RAD occurs when a normal cold virus causes some minor lung irritation and triggers wheezing. It is a mild form of asthma, but only occurs during cold viruses. See page 151 if your child has a cold and wheezing.

Croup. This viral illness usually causes stridor along with a raspy voice and unusual cough that sounds like a seal barking. See page 250 if this describes your child.

Pneumonia. This infection often causes rapid and labored breathing, even when the fever is down. See page 434 for more details.

Inhaled foreign body. If your child may have choked and inhaled an object, you may hear stridor or wheezing and perhaps labored breathing. See page 218.

When to Worry

Besides the information for each specific situation above that you will find elsewhere in this book, here are some guidelines to follow to help you decide if your child's situation is urgent:

- Mild wheezing or chest congestion without rapid, labored breathing or retractions — this means your situation can probably wait until the office next opens. Try the chest-clearing techniques we suggest on page 203.

- Mild stridor without rapid, labored breathing or retractions — in this case, you should give your doctor's office a call to let them know so that they can help you decide if you should be seen.

- Any situation with rapid, labored breathing and retractions should be evaluated by your doctor right away, or in an emergency room if it happens after hours.

BRONCHITIS

Bronchitis is an infection of the upper airways in the lungs. A common misconception is that bronchitis is always bacterial and requires antibiotic treatment. This is not the case. Bronchitis can often be viral, especially in infants and children. However, a viral cold and cough can turn into a secondary bacterial infection as bacteria grow in all that mucus that sits in the upper lungs during a cold. Here is our guide to understanding, diagnosing, and treating bronchitis:

Symptoms

The inflamed upper airways (whether from a virus or a bacteria) will generate more mucus and thicker mucus in bronchitis compared to a common cold and cough. You will notice these symptoms:

- junky-sounding cough
- congested breathing and rattling in the chest
- chest or throat pain while coughing

What to Do

Treatment is similar to our suggestions for a regular cough and cold, with an emphasis on clearing out the chest congestion:

Steam cleaning. Take the time to allow your child to breathe deeply through the mouth in a steamy bathroom or try the other methods we describe on page 20 at least three times each day.

Chest clearing. We suggest you don't use a cough suppressant during the day (unless the cough is really bothering your child). Encourage your child to cough periodically to clear out the chest. An expectorant cough syrup (see page 222) can help loosen up the thick mucus and make it easier to cough out. Natural herbal supplements (like Bronchipret; see page 224) can also help.

Chest percussion. After your child steams or takes an expectorant, spend a couple minutes gently clapping on the front, sides, and back of the ribcage. This helps shake the mucus loose and will facilitate coughing it up.

DR. SEARS TIP
Is Swallowing Mucus Okay?

Many parents express to us their worry over the fact that their child won't spit out the mucus they cough up. They worry that swallowing it prolongs the illness. This isn't true. As long as a child is coughing the mucus out of the lungs, it doesn't matter where it goes (into the trash can, sink, or into the tummy and eventually the toilet).

When to Worry

There's no need to rush into the doctor's office during the first several days of a junky cough to rule out bronchitis, as most bronchitis in children is viral. Here are some signs to watch for that may indicate a bacterial infection bad enough to need antibiotics:

- Moderate to severe chest or throat pain while coughing. Viral bronchitis doesn't cause much painful irritation to the airways. Bacteria, on the other hand, can really make things sore and create significant pain during coughing attacks.

- Fever more than five days or high fever more than three days. These warrant a trip to the doctor.

- Rapid, labored, or wheezy breathing. If your child's breathing is steadily worsening, see a doctor right away. This may indicate pneumonia (see page 434) or an asthma attack (see page 151).

BULIMIA

Also known as *bulimia nervosa,* this condition consists of bingeing and purging activities, usually secondary to a distorted body image. This illness is much more common in women than men, and adolescent girls show the highest rates. The bulimic usually goes through episodes of extreme overeating, accompanied later by self-induced vomiting and/or laxative use to purge her body of the excess food she consumed. Diuretics, laxatives, and enemas may also be used. The bulimic usually experiences a sense of loss of control in her eating habits. She tries to correct this with purging behavior. This illness can have a long course, often over several years and even decades, and if not properly treated it can lead to severe long-term health problems.

Signs and Symptoms

Binge eating and purging. Binge eating and purging behaviors are usually done very secretively. If your child's weight seems to be much lower than you would expect for how much food she eats, she may be purging.

Self-induced vomiting. This is a typical clue to the illness of bulimia.

Scars on knuckles. The hands are often used to induce vomiting, and the teeth can cause wounds to appear on the knuckles.

Inappropriate use of laxatives or diuretics. Your child may appear to be overly reliant on these medications.

Cavities and eroded enamel of teeth. The constant exposure to stomach acids in the mouth can erode teeth and enamel, causing severe cavities.

Electrolyte imbalance. Repeated episodes of vomiting can lead to low levels of electrolytes in the body, especially potassium. This can cause severe health problems and even death.

Severe dehydration. The overuse of laxatives, diuretics, and repeated vomiting can cause children to lose too much body fluid volume.

Overly obsessed with weight. Your child may constantly check her weight and express her dissatisfaction with her overall body weight.

Overachieving personality. Your child may appear overanxious about perfection and achievements.

Signs of depression or other mood disorders. High rates of depression are seen among bulimics.

Long-Term Complications

- severe dental cavities from the constant exposure to stomach acids

- tears in the esophagus from repeated vomiting and consequently severe gastrointestinal bleeding and possibly death

- chronic constipation from long-term laxative abuse as the body builds up a tolerance to laxatives

- dehydration from excessive loss of body fluids

- pancreatitis — the pancreas over-secretes digestive enzymes because of the bingeing and purging, possibly causing inflammation of the pancreas that can be fatal

- electrolyte abnormalities, especially low potassium, which can lead to heart arrhythmias and sudden death

- severe mental problems, especially major depression, because of the sense of guilt and lack of control

- risk of suicide (Suicide rates are higher among bulimic individuals.)

Note that signs of both bulimia and anorexia (see page 142) may be seen in the same individual at the same time. People suffering from both these illnesses have a worrisome long-term prognosis. Although the cause of bulimia is unknown, it is thought to be linked to several social and possibly genetic causes. There are often major family problems present. People who are considered perfectionists or who place an overemphasis on physical appearance are at higher risk for this disease.

Treatment

Those suffering severe medical complications as described above may require hospitalization for treatment. Once life-threatening complications have been resolved, long-term treatment is necessary. Consultation with a nutritionist is important in order to lay out a healthy eating plan. Behavior-modification techniques have been shown to be very beneficial and should be performed by a specialist experienced in treating bulimics. Psychiatric consultation may be required. Antidepressant drugs are sometimes used in addition to other mood-altering techniques. An evaluation of suicide risk is also vital.

Many great support groups to help sufferers, such as Overeaters Anonymous and the American Anorexia/Bulimia Association (www.AABAinc.org), exist and can provide great resources to help guide one's recovery.

 DR. SEARS TIP
Counsel the Whole Family

Bulimia must be seen as a group or family problem, not just a problem with the child. It is necessary to include group or family counseling along with the above-mentioned treatment methods. Getting help for the family can often help the individual.

BURNS

We often get calls in our office from a frantic parent whose child was just burned. We highly recommend that parents read this section *before* a burn happens and pay special attention to the suggestions for prevention. Most burns are caused by hot water or drinks. Other causes are fires, hot ovens, stoves, grease, curling irons, hair dryers, space heaters, steam vaporizers, and irons. The severity of a burn and treatment is determined by its size as well as how deep the burn is. They are rated as first-, second-, or third-degree burns.

DR. SEARS TIP
Don't Break the Blister!

It's usually best to leave the blister intact. Unbroken skin over a blister provides a natural barrier to bacteria, decreases risk of infection, and speeds healing.

First-degree burns. Only the outer layer of skin is burned. The skin will be red, swollen, and painful, without any blistering. First-degree burns can usually be treated at home unless they affect large areas of the hands, feet, face, or groin.

Second-degree burns. These involve both the outer and inner layers of skin. The burn will be much more painful, the skin will be very red, and blisters will develop. Home treatment is usually okay if it is a small second-degree burn (smaller than two inches in diameter). Seek medical attention for larger second-degree burns or any burns on the hands, feet, face, groin, or buttocks, or over a major joint.

Third-degree burns. These burns are usually *painless* (because the pain nerves were destroyed) but are the most serious. Third-degree burns involve all layers of the skin; even fat, muscle, and bone may be affected. The burn areas may be charred black or appear dry and white. Call your physician for small third-degree burns (smaller than a quarter). Go straight to the emergency room for larger third-degree burns.

What to Do

Cool the burn as soon as possible. Immediately get the burned area under some cold water. Running cold tap water over the burn will suffice for the first few minutes. If possible, add some ice cubes to a tub of water and immerse the burned area. Continue cooling the burn for fifteen minutes. Don't submerge severe large burns in ice-cold water — this can cause shock.

Do not apply butter or ointments.

Cover a large burn. Use a clean, wet cloth or plastic wrap to cover the burn loosely. This will lessen the pain and keep the burn clean while you head to the emergency room.

Call your physician about the following:

- A third-degree burn.

- A second-degree burn that is *larger than two inches* across. This may require a prescription burn cream called Silvadene.

- Any burns *on the hands, feet, face, groin or buttocks, or over a major joint.*

CALL 911 if there is any difficulty breathing or if injuries are severe.

Home Care

After you follow the first-aid directions above, minor burns can usually be cared for at home.

Pain relievers. Use ibuprofen to ease the pain. Mild first-degree burns can be sprayed with sunburn sprays.

Leave blisters intact. The outer covering of a blister is the best protection from infection.

Wash the burn area with warm water once a day. Don't use any soap unless the area is dirty (soaps can slow the healing process).

Keep it moist with antibiotic ointment. You should put an antibiotic ointment on the burned areas and cover with a loose bandage. Once a day, wash the area with warm water, apply antibiotic ointment, and cover with a clean bandage.

Use non-stick gauze. When the blisters open to expose the raw, red skin beneath, start placing a protective, sterile non-stick gauze over the ointment so the bandage doesn't stick to the burn. Change the bandage daily. Continue this for a week or two until the red, raw skin looks more like normal skin (pink and dry).

Remove dead skin. Use sterile scissors to cut away the dead skin (a day or two after a blister opens); wiping with a wet washcloth will also remove any loose skin. This is important for preventing infection.

When to Call the Doctor

Call your pediatrician if any of the following occur:

- The burn starts to look infected (increased redness or oozing pus).

- Pain or redness increases after the second day.

- Fever occurs.

- The burn is not mostly healed by day ten.

**DR. SEARS TIP
Keep an Aloe Plant**

One of the best treatments for first-degree burns (like sunburns) is the juice from an aloe plant. Tear off a leaf, squeeze some juice onto your hands, and gently apply to the burn.

Long-Term Care

Sun protection. This is one of the most important factors in scar prevention. For up to a year after a burn, the skin will continue to look a little pinker than the surrounding skin. This fresh skin is much more susceptible to sun damage, which can lead to permanent scarring. Always use an effective sunblock, hat, or sun-protective clothing.

Scar creams. There are some commercially available creams designed to be used long-term after a burn or cut. These are applied every day and are often recommended by plastic surgeons to reduce scarring. The most popular cream currently available is called Mederma, which is offered over the counter at most pharmacies.

Chemical Burns

If a chemical burns the skin, follow these steps:

1. Remove clothing that has been contaminated by the chemical. Do so carefully, without rubbing any chemicals onto other parts of the body. Cut clothing away with scissors if necessary.

2. Flush the skin with cool, running water for fifteen minutes. This will remove the cause of the burn.

BURN PREVENTION

All parents will think about these things *after* a burn has happened. Our goal is that you think about them *before* an accident happens:

- Never drink anything hot while holding a baby. It is very easy to spill hot coffee, tea, or cocoa if Baby grabs for the cup. Never step over a child while carrying a hot beverage.
- Use the back burners on a stove, and keep pan handles turned in.
- Keep hot items away from the edge of a table.
- Don't leave an iron, curling iron, or hair dryer unattended. Curious fingers will get burned as they grab for the interesting object.
- Be sure the hot-water heater is set no hotter than 125 degrees or at the low-medium setting. If set any hotter, your child could be scalded in just a few seconds if he accidentally turns on the hot faucet. Use a cooking thermometer to test the temperature of the hot water from your faucets.
- Be careful with hot-steam vaporizers if you have young children. Severe burns can occur if they get too close. It's safer to use a cool-mist humidifier instead.
- Teach your child about "hot" things. Toddlers will usually recognize a fire in the fireplace as "hot." When you're using items without the telltale flame (such as an electric stove, an iron, or a hot-steam vaporizer), tell your child, *"Hot — ouchy!"*

3. Wrap the burned area loosely. Use a dry, sterile dressing or a clean cloth.

Minor chemical burns usually heal without further treatment. Give ibuprofen for pain (see page 553 for dosage). Sunburn spray or aloe can also help with discomfort.

Seek Emergency Medical Assistance If:

- Your child shows signs of shock, such as fainting, looking pale, or having difficulty breathing.
- The chemical burn penetrated through the first layer of skin, and the resulting second- or third-degree burn covers an area more than two to three inches in diameter.
- The chemical burn occurred on the eye, hands, feet, face, groin, or buttocks, or over a major joint.

Not sure whether a substance is toxic? Call the poison control center at 1-800-222-1222. If you go to the emergency room, bring the chemical container or a complete description of the substance with you for identification.

 DR. SEARS TIP Lock It!

Be sure to store unsafe chemicals in a place where kids cannot get to them. Child locks on cabinets are not secure enough for something as important as your child's safety. Use locked cabinets that are up high and out of your child's reach.

Electrical Burns

An electrical burn may appear minor or not show on the skin at all, but the damage can extend deep into the tissues beneath the skin. If a strong electrical current passes through your child's body, internal damage, such as a heart rhythm disturbance or cardiac arrest, can occur. Sometimes the jolt associated with the electrical burn can cause your child to be thrown or to fall, resulting in fractures or other associated injuries.

Dial 911 or call for emergency medical assistance if your child has been burned and is in pain, confused, or experiencing changes in his breathing, heartbeat, or consciousness.

While waiting for medical help, follow these steps:

1. Look first. Don't touch. The person may still be in contact with the electrical source. Touching the person may pass the current through you.

2. Turn off the source of electricity if possible. If not, move the source away from both you and your child by using a non-conducting object made of cardboard, plastic, or wood.

3. Check for signs of circulation (breathing, coughing, or movement). If absent, begin cardiopulmonary resuscitation (CPR) immediately.

4. Prevent shock. Lay your child down with the head slightly lower than the trunk and the legs elevated.

5. Cover the affected areas. Cover any burned areas with a sterile gauze bandage, if available, or a clean cloth. Don't use a blanket or towel. Loose fibers can stick to the burns.

CANCER SYMPTOMS

A detailed discussion regarding cancer diagnosis and treatment is beyond the scope of this book. We do, however, want you to be aware of the primary symptoms of cancer in children so you can bring any concerns to your doctor. Symptoms will vary depending on the body system that is affected. Here are the most common cancer types in children and the accompanying symptoms:

Leukemia and Other Blood Cancers

These are the most common types of cancer in children. The signs can be subtle early on but will eventually become very noticeable. Children may experience one of these symptoms for a variety of harmless reasons, but two or more of the following may be a concern:

- Fatigue. Gradually worsening fatigue and low energy levels can be a sign of the anemia associated with blood cancers.

- Easy bruising. Bruises that routinely occur unexpectedly after minor trauma, seem larger than normal, or persist longer than expected can be a concern.

- Easy bleeding. Frequent bloody noses that are difficult to stop, bleeding gums, or blood in the stools or urine is a worry.

- Frequent and prolonged illnesses. A child who becomes unusually ill on an ever increasing basis is a red flag.

- Aching bones. Although this is a subtle sign, it can be a worry when combined with other symptoms.

- Swollen lymph glands. It is normal to feel some small lymph nodes around the neck and in the groin. Increasingly swollen glands in these areas or in the armpits may be a worry.

Blood cancers can be easily screened for with a simple blood test. Speak with your pediatrician if your child has two or more of the above symptoms or if one sign worries you.

Bone Cancer

Here are signs to watch for that may indicate that a tumor is growing within a bone:

- Lump or swelling. Any hard mass or increasingly swollen firm area over a bone is a concern.

- Gradually worsening local pain. Any pain that occurs in one consistent area of a bone and gradually worsens is a worry.

- Limping. Bone cancer in the legs will create a gradually worsening limp that doesn't resolve within a couple weeks.

- Fracture after minor trauma. A bone with cancer will break very easily.

Bone cancers can be detected with an X-ray. Ask your doctor about any of the above concerns.

Tissue Tumors

Some tumors can grow within muscle or fat tissue or right under the skin. Here are some signs:

- Mass or lump. Any unusual lump that you didn't feel before should be brought to the attention of your child's doctor.

- Pain. Worsening pain in a specific body part or abdominal organ may be a worry.

Abdominal Tumors

Belly aches are the most common pain complaint among children, but abdominal tumors are the least common cause of such pain. Here are some concerning signs to watch for:

- chronic abdominal pain that is not relieved by addressing the common causes discussed on page 117

- swelling or bloating that persists after addressing common causes

- hard mass felt anywhere in the abdomen

- blood in the stools that persists after addressing constipation and food allergies

Skin Cancer

Every child begins to develop moles within the first few years of life, and these may gradually grow larger in the coming years. Skin cancer is extremely rare in children, but it is important to know how to recognize when a mole might be a problem. See Moles, page 399.

Brain Tumors

Parents tend to think the worst when a child complains of recurrent headaches, but brain tumors are extremely rare. See Headaches, page 349, for symptoms of brain tumor.

CANKER SORES

These are large white and red sores in the mouth that result from trauma such as biting the tongue or bumping the lip. They usually occur just one or two at a time. They are generally caused by a herpes virus that has been living within the nerve tissue for years and flares up during trauma or illness. They last for about a week and can become quite painful. Large sores can cause pain over an entire cheek or chin area. There is no useful treatment to help them go away more quickly. Over-the-counter numbing gel can be applied to provide short periods of relief during mealtimes. If your child has multiple mouth sores at once, see page 404 for information on mouth sore illnesses.

CARSICKNESS

Tiny tummies are especially prone to motion sickness during car travel. Motion sickness occurs when the brain receives confusing messages from the stomach and eyes. When your child is buried in the backseat, her eyes see only the stationary back of the seat, but the motion sensors of the inner ear tell the brain the body is moving. Some children have more sensitive equilibrium centers than others. Unsettled equilibrium centers unsettle the brain, which upsets the tummy. Try these ways to settle little traveling tummies:

Plan ahead. Try to time your travel for naptime. Sleep can settle queasy insides. And, as an added bonus, you arrive at your destination with a happy and well-rested child.

Tank up your child. Eating stimulates a part of the nervous system that can help calm down a queasy stomach. Give your child a light meal of non-fatty foods — such as cereal, pasta, and fruit — before traveling. Take along some stomach-friendly snacks, such as home-made cookies and a cool drink in a carton with a straw, to satisfy the hungry traveler.

Tank up the car. Because children are sensitive to exhaust and fumes at gas stations, try to fill up the gas tank when your child is not in the car.

Plan a straighter route. When possible, use straight roads and freeways. Winding roads and frequent stops and starts upset tiny tummies.

Make frequent pit stops. Treat travel like infant feedings: short, frequent trips rather than lengthy ones. When driving long distances, prepare to make frequent rest stops.

Provide a seat with a view. Children get carsick if they can't see out the window, but don't compromise safety for a view. For kids over twelve, sitting in the front seat and looking forward triggers less motion sickness. For young kids, use a government-approved booster or car seat, preferably one that's high enough for your child to see out the window.

Natural remedies. Ginger and peppermint are old-fashioned but possibly effective remedies. Acupressure applied to the inside of the wrist, one to two inches above where the wrist bends, may help some people.

Provide fresh air. Fresh air is a tummy rumble's best friend. Open a window on each side of the car for cross ventilation. Avoid substances that pollute the air inside the car, such as perfumes and cigarette smoke.

Take along tunes. Keep favorite music just for travel and add an occasional surprise. Keeping little ears focused on catchy tunes will keep their minds off their tummies.

Keep up the chatter. If you can keep your eyes and mind on the road while at the same time engaging your child verbally, the trip will be more pleasant for both of you. Keep chatting with your child in a way that invites her responses (unless it's naptime, of course). If your child is bored, she has more time to think about her queasy tummy. A happy, occupied child means fewer whiny demands for stops.

Play games. Playing a mind-engaging game that requires concentration also keeps a child's mind off her tummy. Try games like "I Spy" that keep your child focused on objects far away, such as billboards, buildings, and mountains. Focusing on attractions farther away is usually more tummy-friendly than focusing on close-up coloring books. Watching DVDs or playing handheld video games may contribute to nausea in some kids.

CAT SCRATCH DISEASE

Cat scratch disease, also known as "cat scratch fever," is a bacterial infection that is spread from cats to humans. Approximately twenty thousand cases of cat scratch disease occur each year in the United States.

Symptoms

Clues that your child has developed cat scratch disease include:

- recent history of cat scratch or bite

- a blister or small, painless bump that develops several days after a scratch or bite

- nearby lymph nodes that become tender and swollen a couple of weeks following a scratch or bite (The most likely lymph nodes to be involved are at the elbow, armpit, neck, or groin; swelling can last up to four months.)

- fever, usually low-grade

- fatigue

- headache

- loss of appetite

- in rare cases, other organs, such as the liver, spleen, or lungs, become infected

- very rarely, inflammation of the brain, resulting in seizures

Causes

Cat scratch disease is caused by bacteria called *Bartonella henselae* that is spread between cats via fleas. Cats with this bacteria do not get sick and have no symptoms from the bacterial infection. The bacteria lives in the cat's or kitten's saliva and can live there for months at a time. Humans are infected with cat scratch disease when they are bitten or scratched by the cat. It is not contagious, but multiple family members can become infected from the same cat.

Treatment

Your pediatrician will begin by taking a history and doing a thorough examination. If cat scratch disease is suspected, he may prescribe a course of antibiotics to treat the disease. This will usually lessen the duration of infection and the severity of the symptoms. Rarely, lymph nodes become so inflamed and painful that they need to be drained. To confirm cat scratch disease or to rule out any other causes of swollen lymph nodes, the doctor may perform blood tests and/or lymph node biopsies. Warm compresses over the areas of lymph node swelling can ease discomfort, along with anti-inflammatories, such as ibuprofen.

If your child develops a high fever while on antibiotics, the lymph nodes become increasingly large and painful, or the child seems very sick or develops any other symptoms, seek medical treatment again.

CELLULITIS

Cellulitis is a bacterial infection within the skin and usually requires prompt antibiotic treatment. Here is what you need to know:

Symptoms

Cellulitis can be distinguished from other non-infectious rashes by the following five signs:

Redness. The infected skin will turn from pink to red over the course of twelve to twenty-four hours and spread outward in an ever-widening pattern.

Heat. The area will feel significantly warmer to the touch compared to surrounding skin. Place the back of your fingers or hand on one area and compare the temperature to an adjacent area.

Swelling. The infected area will appear slightly swollen. Cellulitis around the eyes (called *periorbital cellulitis*) will cause redness and moderate to severe swelling of the eyelids.

Pain. The affected area will be painful to touch.

Fever. Cellulitis may not cause fever in the early stages, but a fever will likely begin after one or two days of infection.

Many non-infectious or non-serious skin conditions may have one or two of these signs. But if three or more of these are present, cellulitis is likely.

Causes

Cellulitis is always caused by bacteria, most commonly *strep* or *staph*. The bacteria often get introduced into the deep skin layers through a cut or insect bite. Rarely, a sinus, ear, or eye infection may spread to the skin, causing cellulitis in the surrounding area.

Treatment

Oral antibiotics may effectively treat cellulitis if started early. Some cases, however, will require intravenous antibiotics for one or two days in a hospital to halt the progression of the infection. Soaking the infected area with a washcloth dipped in warm water for fifteen minutes every few hours can also help.

When to Worry

If you suspect that your child has a cellulitis infection developing, see a doctor that same day (even if this means going to an urgent care center or emergency room). Do not wait until the next day. If oral antibiotics don't halt the spread of the redness within twelve hours, call your pediatrician right away.

CHEST PAIN

Heart problems and heart attacks are almost unheard of in children, so if your child is complaining of chest pain, don't rush off to the emergency room just yet. Virtually all types of chest pain in children and adolescents are caused by something other than heart problems. Here is our guide to helping you figure out what's causing the pain and when to seek medical attention.

Causes

Here are the various causes of chest pain in children. Even though heart problems are the least likely, we'll start with that first just to put your mind at ease.

Heart attack. This causes sudden, severe, squeezing pain right where the heart is. Other symptoms include shortness of breath, a feeling of not getting enough oxygen, rapid breathing, sweating, rapid pulse, and pain shooting down the left arm. If this describes your child, hopefully you have already put the book down and are calling 911. Realize, however, that heart attacks are virtually unheard of in children.

Heartburn. Stomach acid can move up into the throat and be perceived by a child as chest pain. Upon questioning, your child may describe it as a "burning" pain and may report a sour taste in the mouth or some minor regurgitation. See Abdominal Pain, page 117.

Costochondritis. This term describes inflammation of the cartilage where the ribs join the sternum. Some cold and cough viruses will irritate this cartilage (for reasons unknown) and create some significant pain.

You can test this by pushing on each rib right next to the sternum. Your child will let you know (quite loudly) if you come to one that is inflamed.

Rib injury. A bruised or cracked rib, or a pulled rib muscle, is very painful, and a deep breath, a cough or sneeze, or swinging the arms will make the pain worse. Pain when pushing on the injured area is also a clue to rib injury.

Bronchitis. Junky cough and chest or throat pain indicate bronchitis. This cause can be distinguished from costochondritis by the fact that bronchitis ribs aren't painful when pushed on. See page 203 for details.

Pneumonia. Bad cough, fever, and rapid or labored breathing with pain may indicate pneumonia. See page 434.

Sore muscles. This is often an overlooked cause. Ask your child if he has recently done some exercises he isn't used to (such as pull-ups or push-ups). Sore muscles may be indicated if pressing on the pectoral (chest) muscles and swinging the arms cause pain.

Asthma. Children with asthma tend to get muscle spasms in the chest because they have to work harder to breathe from time to time. These sharp pains only last a few seconds.

Anxiety. This cause shouldn't be overlooked in a teenager. Anxiety can cause real chest pain (from stress hormones and adrenaline). Anxiety may be the cause of chest pain if symptoms seem to occur around the same time, or in relation to a certain emotionally stressful activity, every day.

Treatment

It's not always easy to determine the exact cause of a child's chest pain. One easy way is to try various treatments, from most convenient to least, and see which one works. Here are some ideas:

Antacids. Let your child eat a Tums or drink some Mylanta or Maalox. If the pain goes away quickly, then it was heartburn. See page 122 for more details.

Ibuprofen. This treats inflammation (as in costochondritis) and pain (as in bruised or cracked ribs or sore muscles).

Antibiotics. This would be a treatment for bacterial bronchitis or pneumonia.

Menthol rubs. Rubbing this into sore chest muscles should ease the pain if muscles are the problem.

Counseling. If you suspect anxiety, a few sessions talking with a professional or a known mentor may yield some improvement in your child.

CHICKEN POX

What used to be a routine childhood illness is now becoming a thing of the past. However, it still occurs often enough that your kid may still be one of the "lucky" ones to catch it. It is very contagious and is transmitted like a common cold. Here is our guide to recognizing and getting through chicken pox.

Symptoms

Chicken pox virus causes fever and a characteristic, itchy rash. The problem is, you can't really tell that the rash is chicken pox until a day or two have gone by. When you see any sudden unusual red bumps on your child's skin, you may need to quarantine her for a day until you know for sure. Here is how you can tell:

Red bumps (day 1). On the first day you will see between five and twenty red bumps on your child's trunk that look like insect bites. They will probably itch, and your child will have a fever and not feel very well. You may or may not realize this may be chicken pox, and there's no way to know until day 2.

Blisters (day 2). By the second day you will notice that the red bumps from the first day have now turned into small, clear fluid-filled blisters. You will also see more red bumps appearing and spreading out around most of the trunk and starting on the upper arms and legs. By now your child will be very itchy as well as feverish.

Crusts (day 3). The original red bumps from day 1 that turned into blisters on day 2 will now have opened up to form crusts. The day 2 red bumps will now be blisters, and you will see new red bumps forming all over the body as well as the face (possibly a few hundred).

What makes chicken pox recognizable is this three-day pattern of red bumps turning into blisters then into crusts, with new batches of red bumps appearing every day for three or four days.

 DR. SEARS TIP
Don't Rush to the Doctor on Day 1

Your pediatrician won't really be able to determine if your child has chicken pox until the red bumps turn into blisters. The best time to see the doctor is the day after the rash begins.

Treatment

The goals of treatment are to minimize the itching, limit the scratching (which can create skin infections and increase scarring), and generally try to keep your child comfortable:

Cut the fingernails. This decreases the trauma to the spots when your child can't resist that urge to scratch. Wearing long sleeves and pants also makes the spots less accessible.

Relieve itching. There are many ways to reduce itching during chicken pox:

- Oral diphenhydramine (Benadryl). This is the most effective way to treat itching. See page 549 for dosing.

- Oatmeal baths. You can buy products at a drugstore.

- Cool washcloths held on any particularly itchy spots may help.

- Anti-itch creams, such as calamine or diphenhydramine, can also help. Do not use pink calamine lotion on open pox; this may increase scarring.

Don't treat fever. Interestingly, studies have shown that allowing a child to have a fever of 101 degrees or lower shortens the duration of the illness. So don't be too quick with the medications. It is okay to treat a fever with acetaminophen or ibuprofen if it goes above 101.

Warning: Don't use aspirin. Giving aspirin during chicken pox (or the flu) creates an unusual life-threatening immune reaction called Reye's syndrome.

Antiviral medications. Acyclovir (available in liquid or pill as a prescription) is a very effective treatment that, if started within seventy-two hours (forty-eight hours is even better) of the first signs of rash, can decrease the itching, fevers, overall sick feeling, and size and number of spots. However, it is quite expensive, and has a higher rate of side effects than basic antibiotics. For those reasons, it isn't really recommended for healthy children under twelve years of age (although it can be used at the parent's and doctor's discretion). Any older teen, adult, or person with a compromised immune system who would be expected to suffer a more difficult course of the disease should take acyclovir. See your doctor on the second day of illness if you want to consider this treatment. This way, enough time has passed to confirm the diagnosis and the treatment window for starting acyclovir is still open.

Contagious period. A child can return to normal life as soon as there is no fever for twenty-four hours *and* all the blisters have opened up into dried crusts (usually at least one week). It may be best to wait one more day after you feel your child has met these criteria.

What to Do If Your Child Is Exposed

The incubation period for chicken pox is between ten and twenty-one days. This means that anyone exposed to the disease who isn't vaccinated will probably get sick between ten and twenty-one days later. Begin checking your exposed child carefully every day at that point before letting him out of the house, and isolate him at the first sign of fever or not feeling well. Here are some other steps you can take:

Get your child vaccinated. If your child has already had the shot, you don't need to worry. Sometimes, however, the vaccine doesn't work perfectly, and your child may still get a mild case. That's actually an advantage though, because then he'll probably have better immunity for the future.

If your child hasn't been immunized previously, you can get him the vaccine within seventy-two hours of exposure, and he will likely not get sick (or only have a mild case).

Get an acyclovir prescription. Make an appointment with your pediatrician and discuss whether or not you want your children to take this medication. Any adult or teen in the house may also want to be armed with a prescription. Having this on hand allows you to start the treatment during the first forty-eight hours of illness. Don't be too quick to jump on the medication though. You want to wait until there are at least several dozen spots and some have turned into blisters so that you are sure of the diagnosis.

When to Worry

Although most children sail through without any trouble (the fatality rate is only 1 in 65,000 cases), there are some rare complications to watch out for:

Bacterial skin infection. If you notice any spots turning particularly red, or any crusts continuing to ooze after a day of opening, this may indicate a bacterial infection. Fever lasting more than five days is one sign that a bacterial infection may be setting in. Your pediatrician may want to treat this with topical or oral antibiotics.

Pneumonia. Bacterial pneumonia is known to happen toward the end of chicken pox (the reasons for this are unknown). See page 434 to review pneumonia symptoms. See your pediatrician if this occurs.

Brain infection. A rare complication of chicken pox is the spread of the virus into the brain. This causes severe headaches, dizziness, stiff neck, difficulty walking, and other neurologic signs. Go to an emergency room if your child has these symptoms.

Pregnancy and newborn babies. Women who are immune to chicken pox don't need to worry if they are exposed during pregnancy. However, if a susceptible woman is exposed to chicken pox during the first half of pregnancy, problems can occur with the fetus. Contact your obstetrician right away. Another serious situation is when a pregnant woman breaks out with chicken pox right at the end of her pregnancy (between five days before delivery and two days after the baby is born). The newborn baby will suffer a very serious, and potentially fatal, case.

Shingles (Reactivated Chicken Pox)

Shingles, also known as *herpes zoster,* is a common outbreak of painful sores on the skin, seen often in adults and the elderly. Shingles is a reactivation of the virus that causes chicken pox. Following recovery from chicken pox, usually in childhood, the chicken pox virus remains dormant inside some nerve cells, usually around the chest. Periods of illness, stress, or anxiety will lower the immune system and allow the virus to wake up and cause an outbreak of sores where the nerves end in one area of the skin. Although seen most commonly in adults, approximately 5 percent of cases of shingles happen in children younger than fifteen years old.

Symptoms of shingles. Prior to the rash, several days of vague symptoms such as these may occur:

- pain in different areas of the body

- itchy skin

- low-grade fever

- fatigue

- headache

Parents will notice a rash resembling early chicken pox (or even like flea bites) on their child's skin, usually on the chest and back. The child may complain of a burning, painful sensation on that area, sometimes even before the sores are noticeable. The virus is contagious only by direct contact with secretions from the spots.

Diagnosis and treatment. Shingles has a very characteristic appearance and distribution on the body. Most cases are diagnosed without any testing needed. Antiviral medication may lessen the duration of the rash and intensity of the symptoms, but there is no cure. The rash usually lasts for two to three weeks, with the area slowly crusting over and disappearing over that period of time. Antiviral medications are most effective when used within the first three days of the rash appearing on your child's body. Unfortunately, shingles often recurs throughout one's lifetime. With prompt diagnosis and treatment, the symptoms can at least be lessened.

CHOKING

Many children choke on food or liquid when it accidentally "goes down the wrong way,"
into the windpipe. Soft food or liquids will usually get coughed back up after a few moments of gagging and hacking. Solid food like grapes or hot dogs can get stuck in the airway, which is a much more serious problem. With a complete blockage of the windpipe, your child will panic, unable to cry, speak, cough, or breathe. Within one to two minutes, your child could be unconscious, so you must act fast. We hope that you are reading this ahead of time for your own education and to be more prepared. If your child is currently choking, you should be on a speaker phone with 911 and allow them to direct you. For information on cardiopulmonary resuscitation (CPR), including rescue breathing and chest compressions, see page 244.

If your child can make crying or coughing noises, then he is not seriously choking. Encourage him to keep coughing. He should clear his airway within a minute or so. Don't give anything to drink unless he is choking on something dry and flaky (such as crackers); extra fluids can make the problem worse. If your child turns blue or becomes unconscious, call 911.

If your child stops breathing, can't cough, or can't make any noise then you need to try to dislodge the object.

What to Do

Dislodging an Object

For children OLDER THAN one year old, perform the Heimlich maneuver:

- Yell for help and ask someone to call 911.

- Hold your child from behind (like a "bear-hug") with your hands below his lower ribs, but above his belly button. Make a fist

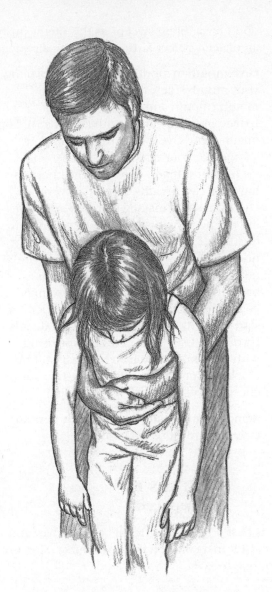

- Repeat this thrust ten times rapidly until the object is dislodged.

- If the child is too heavy to hold with your arms or has become unconscious and is too limp for you to hold up, lay him down on his back. With both hands on his belly, just below the ribs, give upward thrusts to dislodge the object.

For children YOUNGER THAN one year old, use back blows and chest thrusts:

- Call 911 BEFORE beginning the Heimlich or back blows for infants under one year. The sooner help arrives, the better.

- While sitting down, place your infant facedown at a slight downward angle on your forearm. (See illustrations on page 220.)

- Give five quick back blows with your hand between the shoulder blades. This forces air out of the lungs in an effort to dislodge the object.

- If your infant is still not breathing, flip your infant over and perform five rapid chest thrusts using two fingers placed on the lower third of the breastbone.

- Alternate between five back blows and five chest thrusts until the object is dislodged.

- Avoid abdominal thrusts (the Heimlich maneuver) with infants under one year because you can damage the liver or spleen.

If the Object Is Dislodged, but Your Child Becomes Unconscious and Stops Breathing

Begin mouth-to-mouth breaths:

- Open the mouth and look for any obstructing objects. If you can see an object, try to remove it with a sweep of your finger, but

with one hand and wrap the other hand around it.

- With a sudden thrust, pull your hands upward and backward (as if trying to lift the person up) to squeeze the air out of the lungs and pop the object out.

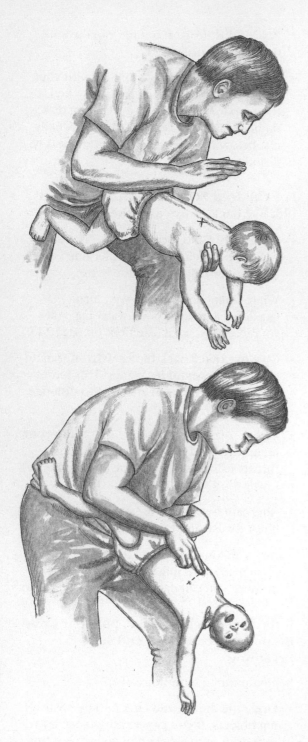

don't try a "blind sweep" as this might push an unseen object farther down the airway.

- Give mouth-to-mouth breathing by placing your mouth sideways over your child's mouth (mouth and nose for infants). Exhale into the mouth with a tight seal. For infants, only give a brief puff of air. You should see your child's chest rising with each breath. If you don't see the chest rising after two breaths, reposition your child's head by making sure you aren't flexing the neck up or down and try two more breaths. If the chest rises this time, continue giving one breath every five seconds until help arrives or your child begins breathing on his own. You will also need to begin checking the pulse and consider starting CPR. See page 244 for CPR details. If you don't see your child's chest rising with your breaths, the airway may still be blocked. Repeat the Heimlich maneuver or chest thrusts and back blows again.

- Remember to recheck the mouth periodically for any loosened objects.

 DR. SEARS TIP
Be Prepared

It is best to learn the Heimlich maneuver and full CPR in a certified training course. Sign up for one today!

Strategies to Help Prevent Choking

Children can choke on foods and other objects. Here are some simple tips to help avoid a potentially life-threatening situation:

Foods

- Avoid giving young children hard foods: Nuts, popcorn, gum, hard candy, sunflower seeds, orange seeds, cherry pits, watermelon seeds, raw carrots, raw peas, raw celery, and hard fruits like raw apples are all choking hazards. Most children under four years old will not understand the need to chew thoroughly or to spit the item out.

- Chop soft foods into small pieces: hot dogs, sausage, large pieces of meat, grapes, gummy candy, caramels, and so on are choking hazards.

- Be sure that babysitters and older siblings know not to give these foods to younger children.

- Teach children to chew food adequately before swallowing.

- Don't let your children fill their cheeks like a chipmunk.

- Crying or laughing with a full mouth should be discouraged.

- Don't let children chew gum while playing sports.

Toys

- Don't let infants play with toys that have small removable parts — they are easily swallowed or choked on.

- Be sure older siblings keep their small toys (Legos, doll accessories, and so on) put away in a safe place.

- Keep rubber balloons out of reach of small children; they are a serious choking hazard, both inflated and deflated.

Household Objects

- Be sure to dispose of small button batteries properly.

- Be sure to clean up completely after a party; there may be many potential choking hazards on the floor within the reach of your child.

- Perform a brief visual sweep of the floor around your baby any time you set him down.

CIRCUMCISION DECISION

Whether to leave your infant's foreskin intact or to have it removed is a question that parents-to-be often have. Circumcision is the surgical removal of the sleeve of skin, called the *foreskin,* that covers the head of the penis, called the *glans.* Once upon a time, circumcision was considered routine for most American newborns, and it still is in a few religious cultures. As with so many "routine procedures," many parents are now making more informed choices. The American Academy of Pediatrics (AAP) now advises that circumcision no longer be considered a routine procedure. Instead, it should only be done based on a strong preference on the part of the parents. Here are some considerations that may help parents make an informed choice:

Is the foreskin necessary? The foreskin protects the sensitive glans of the penis. The foreskin also secretes a protective coating and lubricant called *smegma*. Removal of the foreskin removes this protective tissue.

What happens if the foreskin is left intact? Although the foreskin appears tight in the first year, there is certainly enough of an opening through which Baby can urinate normally. In the first year or two, the foreskin requires little or no attention. The secretions (smegma) are simply washed off as part of the normal bath routine. Every time Baby gets a normal erection (which happens many times each day), the foreskin stretches itself and retracts gradually over the next few years. The more it naturally retracts, the easier it is to keep clean. As part of his normal bath routine, the older child should be taught to gently retract the foreskin and clean out remaining secretions. This becomes a natural part of his hygiene, in the same category as washing his hair.

Should I retract the foreskin? No, never forcibly retract the foreskin. Here's why: The foreskin naturally adheres to the glans, especially in the first year or two. If you forcibly retract the foreskin, you unnaturally break down the tissue adhesions between the foreskin and the glans. Traumatized tissue overreacts by rapidly growing back, causing even more adhesions, which become painful when the foreskin does naturally retract. Bottom line: Don't interfere with nature! Let the foreskin naturally retract.

Are there any medical reasons that favor circumcision? Over the last few decades there has been a lively debate on whether there is any medical justification for routine circumcision. The general conclusion at this writing is that there is not enough medical benefit to justify routine circumcision, provided foreskin hygiene is practiced diligently. The question of whether urinary tract infections (UTIs) are more common in uncircumcised males is still unanswered, as UTIs are rare in males anyway. The AAP has called into question the validity of the studies suggesting an increased incidence of UTIs among

uncircumcised males. A study in the *New England Journal of Medicine* did show that circumcised men are less likely to be infected with the human papillomavirus (HPV), a sexually transmitted disease. The conclusion was that female partners of circumcised men may be less likely to develop cervical cancer caused by HPV. This is still open to debate. It was once thought that cancer of the penis was more common in uncircumcised males, yet after thoroughly reviewing all of the studies, the AAP concluded that there is no medical reason to recommend routine circumcision for male infants.

Can something be done to ease the pain? Yes. It is now standard procedure to use a local anesthetic, which is injected around the base of the penis to numb the foreskin.

COLDS AND COUGHS

This is a very broad topic, but most colds start off the same. Your child catches a minor cold or cough. It either stays mild and goes away after a week or two, or it worsens into a more bothersome infection. Here is everything you need to know to work through your child's illness:

Symptoms of a Routine Cold

- duration between a few days and three weeks

- several days of green mucus

- up to five days of fever

- some chest congestion and junky-sounding cough

- some mild ear pain

- some headache and sinus pressure

- some sore throat

- some coughing spells that trigger gagging and vomiting

- some fussiness and night waking

- some loss of appetite

Causes

Cold viruses. Most colds are caused by the common cold virus. These normally last for a week or two and usually include some fever and a "green mucus" phase. Fortunately, cold viruses usually clear up without any antibiotic treatment.

Bacteria. There are several bacteria that cause cough and cold symptoms. You can expect a few days of fever and some green mucus. Even bacterial colds and coughs often go away without antibiotics. The body's immune system can usually do the job.

Flu virus. Cough and runny nose can also be part of the more troublesome flu. This usually includes high fever, body aches, nausea/vomiting, and other flu symptoms. See page 325 if you think your child may have the flu.

 DR. SEARS TIP
Is It a Regular Cold
or the Flu?

During flu season, every person who catches a cold wonders if it's the dreaded flu. The best way to tell is that the flu generally causes a lot more aches and fever right at the beginning, along with the variety of respiratory and intestinal symptoms. A common cold usually starts out with minor sore throat and runny nose, then becomes a full-blown cold.

When Not to Worry

Knowing when to worry and not to worry starts with a good understanding of what a normal cold virus acts like. There are two general courses you can expect from a normal cough and cold illness; gradual onset and sudden onset. As long as your child's condition follows these descriptions, you can rest assured that it's probably not bacterial.

Gradual onset. Some colds start off with clear runny nose and mild dry cough, but the child generally feels well. Over several days the mucus gets thicker and turns yellow or green. The cough worsens and sounds junky. After several days, fever sets in (usually not above 102 degrees) and may last anywhere from one to five days. Just when you are thinking of going to the doctor, things begin to improve again. The nose clears up a bit, fever breaks, appetite comes back, and your child is left with a lingering junky cough and mild nasal congestion that doesn't seem to bother him too much. After about two to three weeks total, your child is as good as new.

Sudden onset. Other colds and coughs will come out of nowhere with severe symptoms right away, including fever, aches, and decreased appetite and activity level. Cough and nasal congestion are thick and bothersome. After just a couple days of this, things begin to improve. Your child's fever breaks, and he seems to feel like his normal self again. The thick nasal congestion and junky cough continue, but it doesn't slow your child down. Minor symptoms linger for a week or two and eventually clear up.

As long as your child's illness fits within this general description and you are able to keep her comfortable enough with the various treatment approaches described below, you can rest assured that your child should get through the illness without needing medical care.

Treatment

Here are some ways you can keep your child's nose and chest clear and help him get over the illness more quickly:

Hose the nose. Keeping the nose clear of thick mucus is one of the best ways to prevent bacterial infection. See details on page 21.

Boost the immune system. Echinacea, vitamin C, and zinc are useful supplements that might help the immune system fight off illness. See page 33 for more information and dosing.

Sleep upright. Place a pillow under your infant's mattress, or prop your child's head up on several pillows, while sleeping. This will help him breathe easier.

Steam cleaning. Run a hot-steam vaporizer in the bedroom over night. (Warning: these can be a burn hazard to curious hands. Teach your child about the danger of hot steam before using.) If your child wakens during the night with severe congestion, sit in a small bathroom with the hot shower running for several minutes for some quick relief. Older children can sit with their face over a pot of hot water (not at the stove, please). Add a few drops of eucalyptus and/or lavender oil to a warm bath, hot shower steam, facial steamer, pot of hot water, or vaporizer. These natural vapors can help congested chests and noses.

Clap on the chest and back. With an open palm, firmly clap on your child's chest, sides, and back while steaming to help loosen up chest congestion.

Natural sinus and respiratory remedies. Numerous herbal supplements are available at pharmacies and health-food stores. We have tried many of them ourselves and with our patients over the years, and two that we feel work well and have clinical research demonstrating their safety and effectiveness are Sinupret and Bronchipret (available in drugstores and health-food stores). These herbal blends work by loosening up mucus, helping with mucus drainage, opening up breathing passages, and supporting the immune system. For more information visit www.SinupretForKids.com.

Over-the-counter (OTC) cold and cough medications. Although these don't help the infection go away faster, they can make it more tolerable while it runs its course. But these medications can be confusing to new parents. Many parents have stood in the medicine aisle at the local drugstore staring at the many different options. Choosing between cough suppressants, expectorants, antihistamincs, and dccongestants or any possible combination of these can literally give parents a headache. As of this writing, OTC cough and cold medicines should not be given to children under four years of age. Here is a guide to help you sort through the various options:

- Treat your child's specific symptoms. If, for example, your child simply has a bad cough, but no nasal congestion, then you probably don't need a multi-symptom cough and cold medication. You only need a cough suppressant.

- Only treat if needed. If your child's cold symptoms are not interfering with his sleep or daily activity, then you probably don't need to use medication. Often the most effective treatments for colds are "non-medical" such as nasal saline spray, hot steam, and simply drinking plenty of fluids.

- Understand the four major cold medication ingredients:

Nasal decongestant —This helps mostly with stuffy noses by slightly decreasing mucus production and shrinking the swelling in the nose, thus allowing air to flow through the nose. Side effects may include excitability and possible interference with sleep.

Antihistamine —This helps mostly with drying up a very runny nose by decreasing mucus production in the nose. The most likely side effect is drowsiness, which is fine at night, but could interfere with daytime activities.

Cough suppressant —This helps with a persistent annoying cough by suppressing the cough reflex in the throat and lungs so that the mucus or irritation there won't trigger coughing. There are no likely side effects.

Expectorant —This helps when your child has thick chest congestion by loosening thick mucus, making it easier to cough up. There are no likely side effects.

DR. SEARS TIP
Choosing the Right Medicine

The brand name of the medication is not important, and you shouldn't get confused by the long scientific names of the ingredients. Decide which symptoms require treatment. Under the brand name on the front label will be listed the types of medication (e.g., decongestant, cough suppressant, etc.) that are in the bottle. This should make your buying decision easier. It is okay to use more than one medicine at a time, as long as you are not overlapping any of the above four types of medications. For example: you could use an antihistamine/decongestant combination along with a cough suppressant/expectorant combination.

MATCH THE SYMPTOMS WITH THE RIGHT MEDICATIONS

Symptoms	Recommended medication	Explanation
dry cough	cough suppressant	If your child has an annoying cough, especially from a dry, itchy throat, but not a lot of runny nose or congestion, use a cough suppressant alone.
mild productive cough	expectorant	If your child's cough is very mild — only a few coughs per hour — and it is not interfering with sleep, or if he has chest congestion with mucus that is difficult to cough up, use an expectorant.
cough, chest congestion	cough suppressant, expectorant	If your child has a wet, productive cough that is interfering with sleep or daily activity but does not have a bothersome runny nose or sinus congestion, use a cough suppressant and expectorant combination. It is okay to use a cough suppressant alone if that is all you have.
nasal congestion	decongestant, expectorant	If your child has nasal congestion without severe itchy, runny nose, a decongestant should help. An expectorant can help if the mucus is really thick, but it is not necessary. Decongestants can interfere with sleep (unless they are combined with an antihistamine) so this medication is best for daytime use.
cough, chest congestion, nasal congestion	cough suppressant, expectorant, decongestant	If your child has a wet, productive cough with chest congestion and nasal or sinus congestion but not itchy, runny nose, use a cough suppressant/decongestant combination. An expectorant can help if the mucus is really thick, but is not necessary. Decongestants can interfere with sleep (unless they are combined with an antihistamine) so this combination is best for daytime use. Some preparations will also contain acetaminophen (fever reducer), which will help relieve any aches or fever that your child may have.
nighttime cough, nasal congestion, runny nose, chest congestion	antihistamine, decongestant, cough suppressant, expectorant	This combination is great for an itchy, runny nose, nasal congestion, and frequent cough that interfere with sleep. This is good for nighttime use because the antihistamine will make your child drowsy. Some preparations will also contain acetaminophen (fever reducer), which will help relieve any aches or fever that your child may have.
runny nose, nasal congestion	antihistamine, decongestant	Like above, but without the annoying cough. This combination is great for an itchy, runny nose, and nasal congestion that is interfering with sleep. This is good for nighttime use because the antihistamine will make your child drowsy. Some preparations will also have acetaminophen (fever reducer), which will help relieve any aches or fever that your child may have.

When to Worry

The mucus that collects in the ears, nose, throat, and lungs during a common cold is a breeding ground for bacteria. If these germs multiply enough to take hold, a secondary bacterial infection sets in. Here's how to tell:

Ear infection. The most obvious sign that an ear infection has set in is ear pain. Fever is usually present. Infants who are too young to communicate ear pain specifically may be fussy and pull on their ears. But not all ear infections require urgent medical care or antibiotics. See page 285 for more details on how to tell if your child's ear symptoms warrant a doctor's visit.

Sinus infection. Nasal congestion, thick yellow or green mucus, sinus headache or pain around the nose, eyes, forehead, and/or cheeks, and fever usually indicate a sinus infection. Sinus infections don't necessarily need antibiotics during the first few days of infection. Your child's immune system may be able to fight it off. If troublesome sinus pain and fever persist for more than a few days, give your pediatrician a call. See page 472 for more details.

Bronchitis. Bronchitis is an infection of the upper airways and causes a mucousy productive cough and possibly throat and chest pain with cough. Most cases of bronchitis in children are actually viral and don't need antibiotics. However, if the pain is severe and fever persists for more than a few days, bacterial infection is likely. See page 203 for more information.

Pneumonia. Symptoms of pneumonia include shortness of breath, rapid breathing, chest pains, severe cough, fever, lethargy, wheezing, and sometimes vomiting. Usually a doctor can diagnose pneumonia by assessing the symptoms and listening to the lungs. Occasionally an X-ray of the chest may be done if a definite diagnosis is needed. See page 434 to read more.

Coughs That Require Specific Treatment

There are three types of coughs that need a different approach from the common cough and cold:

Croup. This describes an infection of the vocal cords and upper lungs. A unique feature of croup that sets it apart from common coughs is that the cough sounds like a seal barking. The child may also have a raspy voice while talking, breathing, or crying. If this sounds like your child, see Croup on page 250 for details.

Whooping cough. This type of cough is caused by one specific bacteria called *pertussis*. After about one or two weeks of normal cough and cold symptoms, the child begins to have more severe coughing fits lasting for thirty seconds to one minute. The spells are so severe that the child can barely breathe until the fit is over. He will then take a deep recovery breath that has a "whooping" sound. If this describes your child, see page 540 for more details.

Infant wheezing. Some infants will experience tight coughs, labored breathing, and wheezing during normal chest colds. Although this isn't asthma, it is usually treated in a similar way during infancy. See respiratory syncytial virus (RSV), page 451, if your infant has these symptoms.

DR. SEARS TIP
Is It a Cold or Is It Allergies?

Many parents come into our office at the start of cold symptoms because they want to know whether their child has a cold or allergies. The truth is, the doctor probably won't be able to tell for sure until the symptoms have persisted for a couple weeks. And there's really no good reason that you have to distinguish between these two conditions right away because the initial treatment is the same: nose hosing, steam cleaning, and OTC decongestants or natural treatments. You can make a logical guess on your own using the following chart:

Cold virus:	Allergies:
Deeper, more productive cough	Clear runny nose
Fever, not feeling well	Dry cough, throat clearing
Nasal congestion	Known to have allergies before
No prior history of allergies	Nasal itching, sneezing
Thicker nasal discharge	Not feeling sick

See page 131 for a more detailed discussion on how to determine if your child has allergies.

When to See a Doctor

One of the most common dilemmas for any parent is deciding when to take your child to the doctor when she has a cold, cough, and fever. You don't want to make an unnecessary, and costly, trip if you don't really need to. But you don't want to wait too long and delay treatment for a serious infection. If you are ever in doubt, err on the side of caution. Here are general signs to watch for that mean it's time to give your pediatrician a call during normal business hours for an appointment:

- Fever over 103 degrees for more than forty-eight hours. This doesn't necessarily mean your child needs antibiotics, but it is worth checking out just to make sure no special treatment is needed.

- Any fever for five days or more. Most viral infections don't have fever for more than five days, so a visit to your doctor is warranted.

- Symptoms of a bacterial infection as described on page 227.

- Rapid, labored breathing. If your child is working harder than normal to breathe, using her shoulders to inhale, acting short of breath, or breathing faster than sixty breaths per minute for infants under one year, fifty for kids age one through four, and forty for kids over four years, these may be signs of severe pneumonia or an asthma attack. Your child should be seen by your doctor right away, or go to an emergency room.

Deciding When Antibiotics Are Needed

Your doctor will generally prescribe antibiotics for most moderate to severe bacterial complications of a cold. However, not all bacterial infections require antibiotics; a healthy immune system can fight these off. Because of antibiotic overuse and emerging bacterial resistance, doctors are now more careful with these prescriptions. Mild ear and sinus infections usually don't need antibiotics. Bronchitis without fever generally doesn't either. If your child does need antibiotics, see page 549 for tips on how to take them properly and how to prevent side effects.

Returning to School or Daycare

Most colds and coughs will remain contagious for the duration of the illness, which can be weeks. It's unreasonable to keep a child out of school or child care for that long. But sending him back early will expose other kids. One thing to keep in mind is that kids are most contagious during the first few days of illness, so it's likely that the other kids were already exposed to the germs before your child was sick enough to stay home. When you do send your child back, she'll probably still be contagious, but that's life. Be sure to instruct her to wash her hands frequently, not share food or drinks, and not kiss anyone until she's better. Here are some ways you can decide when your child should return:

Fever. Once your child is fever-free without any fever-reducing medications for twenty-four hours, she may return.

Constant cough and runny nose. Give your child a natural or medicated cough and cold remedy when she wakes up. If the cough remains frequent, and the nose doesn't slow down, keep her home.

Green nose. This too may slow down or dry up with cold medication, but if not, keep her home. This is where it's tempting to go on antibiotics so the green will go away sooner. But if your child isn't ill enough, it's better to stay off the antibiotics. A good steam cleaning and cold medication in the morning should be enough to minimize the green so that she can go to school.

DR. SEARS TIP
Green Isn't Necessarily Mean

There is a common misconception that a green nose is more contagious. That's not true. The initial clear and runny phase of a cold is more easily passed on to others through coughing and sneezing. But it's the *virus* that is contagious at that point. Once the nose turns green, any *bacteria* that are growing can be contagious if another child comes into close contact with the snot. If a child keeps her hands to herself and washes them frequently, a thick green nose won't be passed around as easily.

COLD SORES

Cold sores, otherwise known as *fever blisters*, occur outside the mouth around the lips. They are caused by the herpes virus. They may begin as very tiny dots that are unusually painful. Over several days, they will grow into blisters that last for about a week. Several may appear at the same time. Various over-the-counter (OTC) cold sore remedies are available to help the sores go away more quickly. If recurrent episodes tend to flare up into painful and unsightly sores, a topical prescription ointment, called *acyclovir*, can be used to minimize the sores.

COLIC

Colic is one of the most misunderstood terms in pediatric care. Recently, new insights have demystified colic and revealed not only what it is but also how to treat babies who are truly in pain. The term *colic* comes from the Greek word *kolikos,* meaning "suffering in the colon." In simple jargon, colic is a pain in the gut. *Colic* is the term used to describe frequent, inconsolable outbursts of painful crying that come and go throughout the day in an otherwise happy baby. Pediatricians often tag an apparently healthy, thriving infant with colic if Baby's crying jags follow what is called the *rule of threes:*

- begin within the first three weeks of life

- last at least three hours a day

- occur at least three days a week

- continue for at least three weeks

- seldom last longer than three months

Three things parents should remember about the term *colic*:

- Colic is a description, not a diagnosis.

- Colic often has a cause.

- Replace the term *colic* with *hurting baby.*

In tracking down the cause and formulating treatment for the colicky baby, the first thing we did in our pediatric practice was to drop the term *colic* from our diagnosis list and instead use the term *hurting baby.* Besides being more accurate, use of this term motivates doctor and parents to keep searching for a cause and keep working at ways of helping their baby feel better. This label was also therapeutic for parents. By viewing your baby as "hurting" instead of "crying," you are more likely to show the same empathy that you would for a baby who was hurting because of an identifiable medical cause, such as an ear infection. Instead of regarding crying as an annoying tool babies use to "manipulate" their parents into holding them a lot, which tops the list of colic myths, using the term *hurting baby* brings out the best in the parents and the doctor. The parents feel more empathetic for the baby and don't blame themselves when their baby cries so much (while their friends have such "good babies"). In addition, the doctor can click more into the medical mind-set of a "healer" in order to heal the hurt instead of glossing over it.

What to Do

Now that you and your doctor have canned the term *colic* and approach your child as a hurting baby, here is a step-by-step approach to tracking down why your baby hurts and what to do about it:

Step 1: Keep a colic diary. Recording your baby's outbursts is helpful for two reasons: you may uncover clues that help your baby's doctor diagnose a hidden medical cause of why your baby hurts, and, by trial and error, you will develop your own home remedies and comforting tools. Record the following in your diary:

- What triggers the outbursts of crying? What turns them off?

- How frequently do they occur and how long do they last?

- Does Baby awaken in pain at night, or are the crying jags mainly a daytime occurrence? Night waking in pain usually means a medical cause of Baby hurting.

- Are these episodes getting better, worse, or staying about the same over time?

- Do the episodes consistently seem to be related to feeding: method of breastfeeding, type of formula, type of bottle? What changes in feeding techniques or formulas have you tried?

- Does your baby spit up frequently? How often? With how much force? How soon after feeding?

- If breastfeeding, do you notice any correlation between what you eat and how much your baby fusses?

- Does your baby seem to have "gut problems"? Is she bloated? An air swallower? Gassy?

- Record your baby's bowel movements. How frequent are they? Are they easy to pass? Are they soft or hard? Do you notice any changes in the frequency or characteristics of the stools in response to a change of feeding?

- What changes or comforting techniques have you tried?

- What consistently works? What doesn't?

Step 2: Video record your baby's episodes. To help your doctor appreciate how devastating these painful episodes are, videotape a few of your baby's crying jags and bring it with you as part of your baby's medical evaluation. We have found that watching the distress tape helps us appreciate whether Baby is just crying or really hurting, and the type of cry often gives a clue to the diagnosis.

Step 3: Schedule a medical evaluation. Don't settle for just a five-minute squeeze-in appointment. To thoroughly evaluate a hurting baby, your pediatrician needs time. Request an extended office visit, preferably the last one of the morning or when the doctor usually schedules consultations. To get the most out of your "hurting baby medical evaluation," do the following:

- Bring along your diary and your videotape.

- Don't hold back how much your baby's crying bothers you. As one exhausted mother told us, "I'm camping out in your office until you find out why my baby is crying."

- If possible, both mother and father should attend the doctor's visit. Mothers downplay how much Baby is crying and the impact on the family because of the myth that Baby must be crying because of "something Mother is doing or is not doing." Fathers will often tell it like it is: "My wife is burning out, and our baby's crying is taking a toll on our nerves."

Step 4: Suspect an underlying medical cause in these cases:

- The baby frequently awakens in pain (hypersensitive babies who cry a lot for no obvious medical reason often sleep well at night).

- The "colic" is not going away.

- The baby's cry is so intense that your intuition tells you, "My baby hurts somewhere."

- The baby is not thriving; for example, his weight gain is poor, and he has frequent respiratory and intestinal illnesses.

Causes

The five usual medical causes of the "hurting baby" are:

1. Gastroesophageal reflux disease (GERD). In our experience, this is the most common cause of "colic." The regurgitated stomach acid causes "heartburn." Clues from GERD are:

- Baby frequently spits up soon after feeding, or some reflux comes halfway up.

- Baby is in more pain when lying flat.

- Baby seems more comfortable when being held in the upright position.

- Baby is restless and suffers frequent, painful night waking.

- Baby shrieks in pain after a feeding.

If you suspect GERD as the cause of your baby's "colic," see a complete discussion on diagnosis and treatment of GERD, page 338.

2. Overactive let-down of breast milk.
Some breasts respond "too well" to Baby and release a rush of milk during the first few minutes of a feed. Baby gulps his way through, swallows too much air, and gets gas pains. This "fore" milk is also higher in lactose sugar than the high-fat "hind" milk, which also creates more gas during digestion. Talk to a lactation consultant, or call La Leche League (1-800-LA-LECHE) for tips on how to slow your let-down and increase hind milk.

3. Food sensitivities to a breastfeeding mother's diet. Sensitivities to foods in a breastfeeding mother's diet is next on the list of hidden causes of "colic." Although there may be others, in our experience the following are the most common fuss foods that breastfeeding mothers report:

- dairy products

- egg whites

- cruciferous vegetables (cabbage, broccoli, onions)

- spices and foods with strong flavor (such as garlic)

- caffeine-containing foods (soft drinks, coffee, chocolate, cold remedies)

- soy products

Here are some clues that your baby may be sensitive to a food in Mother's diet:

- Baby keeps pulling off the breast during feeding and crying as if in pain. Feeding time can be difficult for the allergic baby and frustrating for the breastfeeding mother.

- Baby seems gassy or bloated after a feeding.

- Baby's painful episodes occur within a few minutes after feeding.

- Baby's bowel movements are watery, mucousy, and sometimes "explosive."

- The "target sign," a circular, red rash, is visible around Baby's anus. (Food sensitivities cause the stools to be more acidic, thus causing a burn-like rash.)

- Baby's behavior significantly improves during Mother's elimination diet.

Starting an Elimination Diet

- List the fuss foods that are most suspect, particularly those Mother enjoys or tends to "overdose" on. Food sensitivities are often dose-related, meaning Baby is not bothered if Mother drinks one glass of milk but gets fussy if Mother downs three glasses. Mother should eliminate the most suspicious fuss foods from her diet for at least two weeks, and, if Baby improves, Mother can add them back into her diet one by one.

- If you're uncertain which foods may be the culprits, start with the most common — dairy products. The proteins in dairy products have been scientifically shown to produce colicky symptoms in allergic babies. If there is no obvious improvement after a week or ten days, eliminate wheat. There is minor evidence that the gluten in wheat can also cause Baby to react. The other foods on the "fuss food" list are more anecdotal. In our experience, most babies whose colic is due to food sensitivities do better when a breastfeeding mother either eliminates or reduces the amount of dairy products and/or wheat in her diet.

If Baby is still severely colicky even after eliminating the most suspect fuss foods from Mother's diet, try the following more drastic elimination diet. Most mothers should not go to this extreme unless they have to. They may become undernourished themselves. Mothers of colicky babies need extra energy, not less.

- For a period of one to two weeks, Mother should eat only turkey, lamb, potatoes (baked or boiled), sweet potatoes, squash, pears, and rice and millet for grains. She should drink an unsweetened calcium-supplemented rice beverage in place of milk. During this time, Mother may need to take a calcium and multivitamin supplement and an omega-3 supplement. Above all, Mother should not undernourish herself.

- Be sure to keep a diary and write down three or four of Baby's most common fussing patterns (e.g., night-waking frequency and severity). Be as objective as possible. In attempting to find the cause and help Baby feel more comfortable, it's easy to lose objectivity. Usually if Baby's fussiness is due to some food in Mother's diet, there will be no doubt. Most fussy babies will respond to a change in Mother's diet dramatically within a few days.

- If Baby's fussy episodes are objectively and dramatically relieved according to Mother's diary, she should gradually add other foods into her diet, starting with the least allergenic foods, such as salmon, avocado, sunflower seeds, and more fruits and vegetables. The last foods to add would be those on the "fuss food" list.

"When can I eat a regular diet again?" Mother may wonder. Most breastfeeding babies will outgrow their food sensitivities by eight months of age, when the intestinal lining is more mature and able to screen out offending allergens. But the timing and response to food allergens varies widely from baby to baby.

4. Formula allergies. Babies may have intestinal sensitivities and show colicky behavior after ingesting two ingredients in some infant formulas: cow's milk proteins and lactose sugar. If a formula allergy is suspected based on the breastfeeding sensitivity behavioral clues listed on page 232, try the following steps in consultation with your baby's doctor:

- Switch to a pre-digested formula, such as Alimentum or Nutramigen, in which the cow's milk protein has already been broken down and is less allergenic. Formulas labeled as "sensitive" or "gentle" that are partially pre-digested (not to the extent that Alimentum or Nutramigen are, but possibly enough to help) can also be used and are less expensive.

- If lactose intolerance is suspected (Baby only has gastrointestinal symptoms such as bloating, gas, and diarrhea), try a lactose-free formula.

- The American Academy of Pediatrics (AAP) Committee on Nutrition recommends that soy formula *not* be used routinely in colicky infants because one-third of infants who are allergic to cow's milk protein are also allergic to soy.

- In the case of formula sensitivities, especially lactose sensitivity, the amount the baby is fed is often the problem. So, remember the Dr. Sears rule of twos: Feed Baby *twice* as often, *half* as much. When Baby gets less formula at a time, the proteins and lactose don't overwhelm the immature intestines. Sometimes just changing the volume and frequency of the feedings will be more comfortable for Baby.

See page 331 for more details on formula allergies.

5. Sensory processing disorder (SPD). Although most babies with colic probably don't have sensory processing disorder (SPD), this newly recognized developmental disorder (also known as *sensory integration disorder*) may play a role in causing colicky symptoms in some infants. In SPD, an infant's brain can't correctly process certain types of sensations, so many of the normal sensations of daily life can be irritating rather than comforting to a baby's brain. Instead of being soothed by swaddling or snuggling, for example, a baby with SPD may be overstimulated and irritated by feelings of confinement and want to be able to move more freely. He may prefer to be held upright instead of in a cradle position. The feeling of clothing against a baby's skin may be irritating and cause a baby to feel restless, especially at night. Sounds may startle a baby with SPD, and a loud, chaotic environment can cause nervous and insecure feelings. The constant irritation and overstimulation that the brain of a baby with SPD has to deal with can result in colicky symptoms throughout the day. Fortunately, SPD is treatable with sensory integration occupational therapy. See page 463 for more details.

**DR. SEARS TIP
Some Colic Doesn't Have a Correctable Cause Other Than Tincture of Time**

In our practice we find that the above steps help most cases of colic improve or resolve. But some babies won't show much improvement, despite all efforts. Some colic may not be caused by food, formula, or reflux problems at all. Fortunately, most babies get much better by four months of age as the intestines mature, so if you can't seem to figure out why your baby is fussy, you can be reassured that things should get better soon.

Ten Tips for Comforting Colic

Traditionally, colic has been "treated" by laying a reassuring hand on the tummy of the baby and the shoulders of the parents and temporizing, "Oh, he'll grow out of it!" Most approaches to colic are aimed more at helping parents cope than at relieving Baby's hurt. By maintaining the mind-set "the hurting baby" rather than "the colicky baby," you and your pediatrician form a partnership to persevere in finding the cause and the remedy for your baby's pain.

Although parents need to keep experimenting with comforting measures that work, most of them come down to motion, untensing tiny tummies, and administering the right touch at the right time. The following ten tips should help:

1. Slower, more frequent feedings. Overfeeding can increase intestinal gas from the breakdown of excessive lactose, either in Mother's milk or formula. As a rule of thumb, feed Baby twice as often and half as much. A baby's tummy is around the size of her fist. To appreciate the discrepancy between usual feeding volume and tummy size, place Baby's fist next to a bottle filled with four to six ounces of formula. It's no wonder tiny tummies get tense.

2. Colic carries. Here are some time-tested colic carries that work particularly well for fathers. We call them "favorite fuss-busters."

- *Football hold.* Drape Baby stomach-down along your forearm. Place Baby's head near the crook of your elbow and his legs straddling your hand. Grasp the diaper area firmly and press your forearm into Baby's tense abdomen. Or you can try reversing this position so that his cheek lies in the palm of your hand, his abdomen along your forearm, and his crotch area snuggled into the crook of your elbow.

- *The neck nestle.* Snuggle Baby's head into the groove between your chin and chest. While swaying back and forth, croon a low, slow, repetitive tune, such as "Old Man River."

3. Colic dances. The choreography that works best to contain colic is movement in all three planes: up and down, side to side, and forward and backward — essentially the movement that baby was used to while in the womb. Common dance positions are the neck nestle, the football hold, and the colic curl (described below). Our favorite colic-soothing dance is one we call "the elevator step." Bounce up and down, heel to toe, stepping at a rate of sixty to seventy beats per minute (count "one–and–a–two–and–a . . ."). This rhythm corresponds to the uterine blood flow pulse rate that Baby was used to. A comforting ritual that works for many is one we call the "dinner dance." Some babies love to breastfeed in the sling while you dance. Your movement, plus Baby's sucking, is a winning combination for settling even the most upset baby. Babies usually prefer dancing with Mother. After all, she is the dance partner Baby came to know even before birth. This explains why some fathers get frustrated when they try to cut in, offering some relief to worn-out dancing moms. Nevertheless, many fussy babies like a change in routine and welcome Dad's different holds and steps. And don't forget to invite Grandmother to the dance. She has patient and experienced arms and probably some pretty fancy footwork from her days as a baby-dancer.

4. Baby bends. When Baby is at the peak of an attack, here are two time-tested favorites:

- *The gas pump.* Lay Baby on her back on your lap with her legs toward you and her head resting on your knees. Pump her legs up and down in a bicycling motion while adding a few attention-getting facial antics.

- *The colic curl.* This is a favorite of babies who tense their tummies and arch their backs. Hold Baby in a sitting position facing forward in front of you and fold your arms under his bottom. Lay Baby back so his head and upper back are against your chest with his lower body curled slightly upward in front of you. Or, try reversing this forward-facing position: Baby's feet up against your chest as you hold him. In this position, you can maintain eye contact and play facial-gesture games with your baby.

5. Baby bounces. While laying a securing hand on Baby's back, drape him tummy-down over a large beach ball and roll him back and forth in a circular motion. If you have a large beach ball (or purchase a "physio ball" from an infant product catalog), use it for the baby bounce. Hold Baby securely and close enough to engage in an eye-to-eye gaze and slowly bounce up and down while sitting on the ball. We (Dr. Bill and Martha) still have "the big red ball" rolling around our house as a memento of our bouncing past. We used to call it "kangaroo time." A father in our practice scheduled his daily exercise routine during Baby's evening fussy times. While holding Baby in the neck nestle position, he bounced gently and rhythmically on a small trampoline. This took the tension out of Baby and pounds off Daddy. Parents would need to take special care to keep their balance and make sure Baby isn't bouncing too hard.

DR. SEARS TIP
Get Relief—for Mom!

If your baby's fussiness is getting to you to the extent that you are losing your mercy, it's time to get some relief. One time a mother who was burning out from comforting her fussy baby came into our office with her fussy baby and her two-year-old, who was sporting a T-shirt that said, "Mom is having a bad day. Call 1-800-GRANDMA."

6. Tummy tucks. Place a rolled-up cloth diaper or a warm-water bottle (not hot!) enclosed in a cloth diaper under Baby's tummy during gas pain. To further relax a tense tiny tummy, lay Baby stomach-down on a cushion with her legs dangling over the edge while rubbing her back.

7. Tummy touches. Place the palm of your hand over Baby's navel and let your fingers and thumb encircle Baby's abdomen. Let Baby lean her tense abdomen against your warm hand. Dad's bigger hands provide an added touch. Practice the "I love U" touch. This is a time-tested infant-massage technique. Picture an upside-down "U" over the surface of your baby's abdomen. Underneath are your baby's tense intestines, which need relaxing, out of which you are trying to massage the gas. Rub some warm massage oil on your hands and knead Baby's tense abdomen with your flattened fingers in a circular motion. Start with a downward stroke for the "I" on Baby's left side, then massage along the upside-down "L" along the top of your baby's abdomen, and then massage along the upside-down "U," stroking upward along the right, across, and down the left side. Try this abdominal massage with Baby on your lap and his feet facing you.

8. Warm touches. Try the warm-fuzzy (another favorite for dads). While lying on a bed or floor, drape Baby tummy-to-tummy, skin-to-skin with her ear over your heartbeat. The warmth of your body plus the rise and fall of your chest is a proven fussbuster. Taking a warm bath together in this position can be extra soothing.

9. Babywearing. The most time-tested method for calming colic is wearing Baby in a sling during fussy periods or, preferably, as a preventive measure before the evening outburst. Anthropologists who have studied infant care practices throughout the world have noted the correlation that carried babies fuss less. We use the term *babywearing* because *wearing* means more than just picking up Baby and putting her in a carrier when she fusses. It means carrying Baby several hours a day before Baby needs to fuss. Mothers who do this tell us, "My baby seems to forget to fuss." One mother in our practice had a colicky baby who was content as long as she was in a sling. But she had to return to work when her baby was six weeks of age. I wrote the following "prescription" to give to her daycare provider: "To keep Baby content, wear her in a sling at least three hours a day."

One theory about colic is that it is a symptom of disorganized biorhythms. During the nine prenatal months, the womb environment regulates Baby's systems automatically. Birth temporarily disrupts this organization. The more quickly Baby gets outside help with organizing these systems, the more easily she adapts to the puzzle of life outside the womb. By extending the womb experience, the babywearing mother and father provide an external regulating system that balances the irregular and disorganized tendencies of a baby. It helps to think of the womb experience lasting eighteen months — nine months inside the mother and nine months outside.

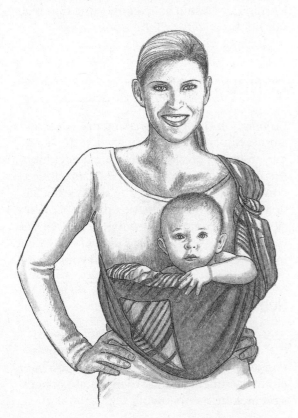

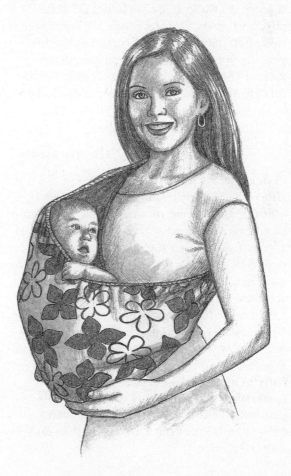

An experienced babywearing mother in our practice believes that wearing her baby after a feeding promotes "digestive organization."

10. Magic mirror. This trick has pulled many of the babies in our practice out of crying jags. Hold the colicky baby in front of a mirror and let him witness his own drama. Place his hand or bare foot against his image on the mirror surface and watch the intrigued baby grow silent.

When Will It Stop?

Seldom do the colicky outbursts continue past four to six months of age, although some fussy behavior may last throughout the first year. By six months of age, exciting developmental changes occur that lead babies to the promised land of colic-free living. They can see clearly across the room; babies are so delighted by the visual attractions that they forget to fuss. They can play with their hands and engage in self-soothing finger-sucking. Babies can enjoy more freedom to wave their limbs freestyle and blow off steam. Also, during the second half of the first year, Baby's intestine is more mature, and food allergies and reflux subside. If you are right in the middle of the colicky months, it's hard to imagine that the crying will ever end. But it will. Hang in there. Rely on some help from others to get you through. In just a short time, your baby will be consistently happy again, and you can move on and enjoy parenthood.

To read a more in-depth discussion of the causes and treatment of colic as well as to learn parent-tested colic-comforting tips, read our book *The Fussy Baby Book*.

DR. SEARS TIP
Plan Ahead for "Happy Hour"

Colicky babies seem to go to pieces in the late afternoon or early evening and, by a quirk of injustice, at the very moment when your parental reserves are already drained. If your baby is a "p.m. fusser," plan ahead for "happy hour" before Baby's colic occurs. Prepare the evening meal in advance. Frozen, precooked casseroles are ideal meals during the colicky stage. Treat Baby and yourself to a late-afternoon nap. Upon awakening, go immediately into a relaxing ritual, such as a twenty-minute baby massage, followed by a forty-minute walk with Baby in a sling (a good time for your exercise). With this before-colic ritual, Baby is conditioned at the same time each day to expect an hour of pleasure rather than an hour of pain.

CONCUSSION

Concussion (meaning "shaking up") describes a brain injury that can result when the head hits an object or when a moving object hits the head. A child or young adult can suffer a concussion during a sporting event, car accident, fall, or other traumatic episode. Concussions are uncommon in younger children. See Head Injuries, page 351, for tips on evaluating minor head trauma in infants and young kids.

Symptoms

Any child who suffers a significant blow to the head should be evaluated for a possible concussion. Symptoms that may suggest your child has suffered a mild-to-moderate concussion include the following:

- brief loss of consciousness (lasting less than one minute)

- headache

- short-term memory loss of events occurring close to the time of injury

The above symptoms are signs of a mild concussion. If your child exhibits any of the following symptoms, take him to an emergency medical facility immediately:

- continued loss of consciousness

- diminished level of consciousness

- drowsiness or difficult to arouse

- vomiting

- continuing confusion

- signs of convulsions or seizure

- pupils that are unequal in size

- pupils that react slowly to light

- difficulty walking

- muscle weakness

What Your Pediatrician Will Do

If your pediatrician suspects concussion, he will perform an initial neurological examination. He might ask your child questions such as what month or day it is, what city you live in, or the score of the game your child was playing when the injury occurred to test his level of confusion and consciousness. The doctor will look for physical signs such as difficulty walking, weakness, or eye abnormalities. Depending on the child's symptoms, the doctor might perform a CT scan or an MRI of the head to evaluate the extent of the injury and rule out bleeding inside the head.

Your pediatrician may use various scoring systems in order to classify concussions as mild, moderate, or severe (also known as grade 1, grade 2, and grade 3). He will consider the following:

- whether or not the child lost consciousness, and for how long

- the length of time the child experienced confusion or disorientation

- the presence or absence of other symptoms of more serious concussion

Treatment

In most cases, a child with a concussion is simply watched for resolution of symptoms. In the very rare case that a severe concussion results in brain injury or bleeding, hospitalization and possible surgery may be required.

Returning to Sports

Determining when a young athlete can get back on the field depends entirely on how severe the concussion is and for how long the child has been symptom-free. Only a doctor can clear your child to return to sports activities. Another factor in the doctor's decision is whether or not your child has suffered his first concussion or has suffered multiple concussions in the past. Even professional athletic teams are taking concussions more seriously now because of the possible consequences of repeated concussions.

Potential Long-Term Complications

In most cases, suffering one concussion — especially if it is mild — will result in no long-term complications. Problems may arise down the road in cases in which a child suffers two or more concussions or the concussion was severe. After each concussion, a medical assessment should be done in order to determine an athlete's risk for more severe brain injury if another concussion is suffered. Some people who have suffered multiple or severe concussions complain of long-term problems with headache, blurred vision, and occasional confusion. Remember, brain injuries are highly individualized and vary from person to person. Evaluation and treatment for concussion must take many factors into account, and treatment for one person may not be the same for another.

 DR. SEARS TIP
Second-Impact Syndrome

Second-impact syndrome can result if a second concussion is suffered before the first heals. Second-impact syndrome can lead to severe brain damage. This is why it is of utmost importance that an athlete not participate in any athletic activities until symptoms from the first concussion have completely disappeared for at least one week. If your child has suffered a concussion, *do not* let him participate in athletic activities until he is cleared by a physician.

CONSTIPATION

Virtually every child experiences an episode of constipation at least once. Although it can be quite painful and scary for both the child and parents, with the proper treatment it should pass easily enough. Some children, however, will suffer chronic constipation.

Along with the proper diet and stool-softening supplements, our guide to childhood constipation should help you and your child overcome this problem.

Symptoms

Constipation can sometimes pass unnoticed by parents and cause recurrent abdominal pain. Here are some clues that your child might be constipated:

- straining hard to pass a bowel movement (but not complaining)

- large, loglike stools

- having a bowel movement only once every few days

- taking a long time to pass a stool (more than five minutes on the potty)

- passing large quantities of stool at once

- passing small pellets (or clumps of pellets)

- small stool marks in the underwear

If your child is pooping only once every few days, but she doesn't have belly aches and the stool looks soft and reasonably sized, this is not constipation. Most infants will stool several times daily in the early weeks. Some will begin to have less frequent stools and may even slow down to one poop every four to seven days. If your baby is pooping comfortably, and what comes out is soft, then you don't have to worry.

What Your Pediatrician Will Do

Your pediatrician can assist you in several ways. He can order a belly X-ray if the diagnosis of constipation needs to be verified (large logs of poop are easily seen on X-ray), can feel hard lumps of stool in your child's belly if the situation is severe, can help rule out other causes of abdominal pain, or can perform a rectal exam to help get out any impacted stool if needed.

What to Do

This section deals mostly with chronic or recurrent constipation. If this is your child's first episode, and she is simply having a hard time passing a stool, don't bother reading all these details. Here's a quick fix: Buy some pediatric glycerin suppositories and a fiber drink mix (such as Benefiber or Fibersure for kids one year and older). Insert a suppository once or twice a day (read the directions) and give her the fiber drink for a few days. This combination should get the stool out and help keep it soft. If this doesn't bring relief, you can buy a pediatric enema (you'll really need to read *those* directions). See your doctor if an enema doesn't help.

Besides our quick-fix solution, which can be used during the first episode and any flare-ups that occur, there are many things you can do to fix the underlying situation. The first step is to eliminate possible causes, and the second is to use natural supplements or medications to relieve the problem.

Eliminating Possible Causes

Constipation can be caused by any of the following:

Introduction of solids at six months. Back off on what you've started and give your baby some pureed prunes or peaches every day to get things moving again.

Constipating foods. If your child is overdosing on, or has just started eating, any of the foods on the chart below, take them out of your child's diet, even if he's been eating them for years:

Apples	Nuts
Bananas	Rice
Carrots	White bread
Corn	White potatoes
Dairy products	

Potty training. If your toddler has recently been feeling pressured to use the potty, back off on training and try again in several months.

Stress or worry in older kids. Address and openly talk about any family, school, or social issues that might be affecting your older child.

 **DR. SEARS TIP
Got Too Much Milk?**

A common, yet often overlooked, cause of constipation in a toddler is the introduction of milk. An older child who overdoses on milk can also get backed up. Try going milk-free for a month or two and see if things improve.

Natural Treatments for Constipation

Once you've dealt with the possible causes, here are some useful items to add to your child's daily diet to get him moving again. Start with the foods, then add the next thing on the list every few days until you get results:

Bowel-friendly foods. Feed more of the following foods:

Apricots	Plums
Citrus	Prunes
Flax oil	Raisins
Grapes	Salad
Green veggies	Whole-grain bran cereals
Peaches	Whole-grain breads

Probiotics. These healthy bacteria, available as a powder or liquid at any health-food store, can help regulate bowel function. Look for the ingredients lactobacillus and/or bifidus.

Fiber drink mixes. Benefiber, Fibersure, Citrucel, and others are an effective way to keep things moving, especially in finicky toddlers who won't eat enough natural fiber foods. Older school-age kids might be more compliant with a fiber-filled diet so you don't have to rely on fiber mixes.

Smoothies. Incorporate natural supplements and fiber foods into a smoothie.

Aloe juice. This healthy beverage, available from any health-food store, is a great stool softener. Give about a quarter cup daily for babies over six months and toddlers, half a cup for preschoolers through age nine, and one cup for older kids.

Healthy oils. Oils such as flaxseed oil or fish oils may help. Mineral oil (about one to four teaspoons daily — adjust as needed), used for several days, can really make the stools slide along, although it has no nutritional benefit.

Concentrated fruit spreads. Available at most health-food stores, these spreads contain several fruits that can stimulate the stools.

Magnesium supplements. About 100 to 200 milligrams daily (vary the dose to resolve the constipation without making the stools too loose), available from any vitamin store, can help in kids two years and older.

Follow the Dr. Sears rule of twos. Eat *twice* as often, *half* as much, and chew *twice* as long. This way of eating increases the digestion of foods at the top end to save overloading the bottom end.

DR. SEARS TIP
The Sipping Solution for Constipation

Making a fruit, yogurt, and ground flaxseed smoothie (see recipe, page 15) is one of the healthiest treatments for constipation, and one we use frequently in our medical practice. Since the blender does much of the digestion, the gut has to work less and there is less undigested food to reach the colon.

Medications for Constipation

When the above measures don't help, or your child needs faster relief, here are some over-the-counter (OTC) medications you can try for kids two years and older:

Colace. This stool softener helps things pass more easily.

Miralax. This agent helps draw more water into the colon to soften stools and move them along.

Senna. This herb is incorporated into some OTC medications and stimulates the colon to push the stools along. Although other medications can be used for weeks or months, the colon can become dependent on senna if it is used daily for more than a week.

Prescription medications. There are several that can be prescribed by your pediatrician. These aren't really any stronger or better than the OTC choices.

Reprogramming the Constipated Colon

A healthy colon likes to be empty. When stool begins to fill and stretch the lower colon, it naturally contracts and pushes out the poop (that's the natural feeling you notice when you have to go). A chronically constipated colon will have become so accustomed to being full of stool and overstretched that it will have lost its ability to push out the poop. You will need to continue your treatment measures for at least three months (remember, senna-based treatments are not recommended for this long-term use) to keep the colon empty so it can shrink back to normal size. After three months, you can wean off treatments to see if your child can go on his own again.

If your child is having trouble with soiling his pants, see page 485 for tips on how to help your child resolve this embarrassing problem.

CONTACT DERMATITIS

Contact dermatitis is characterized by a red, raised, and sometimes oozing irritated rash. The classic example of this is poison ivy, but many things can come into contact with the skin and trigger a reaction.

Types

There are two general types to watch for:

Isolated patches. This classic type generally occurs on a few isolated areas that are exposed to the environment, such as the ankles, legs, and arms. The trunk is also fairly common. Because this is particularly itchy, the red, raised bumps and patches tend to spread out in scratch lines.

Generalized rash. This type occurs over larger areas of the body, such as entire extremities, and appears as generally red skin with numerous small red bumps.

Causes

Occasionally the cause is obvious, such as when children come home from a camping trip with poison ivy. More often the trigger is unknown. Virtually all types of contact dermatitis look alike, so don't expect your doctor to be able to tell you the exact cause. Fortunately, most cases are one-time occurrences. The best course is to simply treat the dermatitis without an involved investigation. If the problem becomes recurrent, then it's worthwhile to track down the culprit. Here are the most common possibilities:

- Plants and bushes — Poison ivy and oak thrive during the warm half of the year. But many common plants can also trigger a reaction. If your child has recently crawled through some bushes or played in a tree, this is a likely cause.

- Household cleaning solutions or chemicals — These can be irritating to the skin.

- Personal care products — New soaps, shampoos, lotions, detergents, and other common daily items may trigger a generalized rash.

Treatment

Over-the-counter medications. Try these treatments before consulting your doctor:

- Hydrocortisone, extra strength — Apply this two to three times daily for several days.

- Anti-itch creams — Several different creams are available. Try alternating one with hydrocortisone.

- Pink calamine lotion — This helps dry out the rash and decrease itching. Apply after the other creams have soaked in.

- Oatmeal bath — A nice soak in one of these can help.

- Oral antihistamines — Diphenhydramine (Benadryl) is the most effective for itching but can cause drowsiness. See page 548 for dosing. Non-sedating ones are an option.

Prescription medications. If home treatments don't provide enough relief or the rash doesn't improve after a few days, your doctor might prescribe the following:

- Stronger hydrocortisone cream — This can be very effective but can take a day or two to start working.

- Stronger antihistamines — A very effective but sedating antihistamine, called hydroxyzine, is available for tough cases. Non-drowsy long-acting prescription antihistamines also work well.

- Oral steroids — This is the most effective treatment, but it is reserved for severe cases or prolonged moderate ones.

Prevention

If you or your children are planning an outdoor trip that will put you at risk of contact dermatitis, here are some precautions you can take to decrease the risk:

- Poison ivy and oak prevention lotion — This lotion neutralizes the irritating oils from the plants if they get on your skin. Apply to exposed areas of the skin each morning prior to venturing out. It is available at sporting goods stores.

- Poison ivy rinsing lotion or soap — Take a shower and use this to rinse any poison oils off the skin at the end of each afternoon.

- Clothing — Wear long pants tucked into socks and tuck in shirts. Avoid touching shoes and ankles with bare hands.

- Avoiding the culprits — Try to stay on paths when hiking to avoid poisonous plants.

If you know your child has sensitive skin and has reacted several times in the past, take these precautions:

- Use natural, organic household products as much as possible, as these may be less irritating to the skin.

- Once you find soaps, shampoos, and laundry detergents that don't cause any skin trouble for your child, try to stick to those and avoid buying different brands.

- Always wash new clothes before your child wears them to remove any irritating chemicals that may linger from manufacturing.

CPR (CARDIOPULMONARY RESUSCITATION)

CPR (cardiopulmonary resuscitation) is designed to support or revive any person who has stopped breathing or whose heart has stopped beating. The best way to learn CPR and be prepared for an emergency is to take a certified, hands-on course at your local hospital. You can find a course near you by visiting www.americanheart.org. Following is a brief discussion of the basics of CPR, but this is by no means a replacement for a full CPR course. If you are currently involved in a life-threatening emergency, call 911 and follow their instructions. See page 218 for information on what to do if a child is choking.

Initial Assessment of an Unconscious Child

When you find a child (or anyone else) unconscious, gently shake him and ask if he is okay in a very loud voice. If there is no response, the next step you take depends on the child's age:

Children Eight Years of Age and Younger

If you are alone, immediately assess if the child is breathing by placing your ear near his mouth to listen and feel for breaths while you look to see if his chest is rising and falling. If

he is not breathing, begin rescue breathing as described below for a period of one minute *before* you call 911. A child is most likely to have stopped breathing and lost consciousness due to choking, and it's more of a priority to first try to clear the airway and provide breaths during this first minute than to call 911. If someone is with you, direct him or her to call 911 without delay and then return to help you.

Children Older Than Eight Years and Adults

If you are alone, call 911 before you begin rescue breathing. For older kids and adults, direct cardiac arrest is more likely than choking, and accessing emergency services as soon as possible is the top priority. If someone is with you, direct her to call 911 and then return to help you. Then begin rescue breathing.

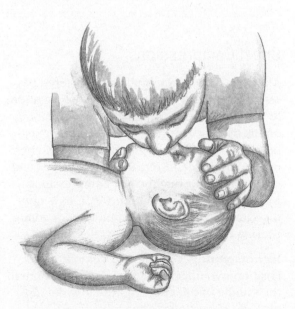

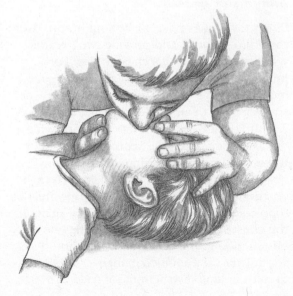

Rescue Breathing

The first step is to determine whether or not the child is breathing by positioning the child's airway and checking for breathing:

Position the Airway

It's important to make sure the child's head and mouth are in the proper position to allow for breathing. Gently lift the child's chin with one hand and push on the forehead with the other hand to tilt the head slightly back.

Look, Listen, and Feel for Breathing

Place your ear near the child's mouth to listen for breathing sounds. You can also feel his breath against your cheek and look for chest rise and fall. If the child is breathing, continue to observe him until emergency help arrives. If the child is not breathing, continue with CPR.

Administer Breaths

Pinch the child's nose, place your mouth over the child's mouth, and provide two breaths while watching for his chest to rise. For infants less than one year of age, place your mouth over his mouth *and* nose and provide smaller puffs of air while watching for chest rise. If you see the chest rise as you provide a breath, proceed to chest compressions below. If the child begins breathing on his own, observe him until emergency help arrives. If you don't see the chest rise with your breaths, reposition the head and chin and try again. If the chest still does not rise, there may be an obstruction in the airway and you should administer the Heimlich maneuver according to our choking instructions on page 218.

AEDS: AUTOMATED EXTERNAL DEFIBRILLATORS

These lifesaving devices assess the status of a victim's heart and can provide an electrical shock if needed during certain types of cardiac arrest. They are now commonly found in large businesses, airports, and other public places. An AED is unlikely to be available during the first few minutes of CPR, but if and when one does become available, stop chest compressions, turn on the unit, and follow the verbal instructions. You will be directed to attach wires to the victim's chest and, depending on the type of cardiac arrest, you may or may not be instructed to allow the unit to provide a shock that may restore the heart to normal rhythm and function. The AED may instruct you to continue chest compressions and rescue breathing once it has assessed the status of the heart.

Chest Compressions

After you have successfully administered two rescue breaths, it's time to turn your attention to the heart. If the child has begun breathing on his own again, this means the heart must be functioning and no compressions will be needed. If the child remains unconscious and is not breathing, begin chest compressions. Although the timing of compressions is now the same for all ages, the technique for administering chest compressions varies greatly:

Infants younger than one year of age. Position two fingers on the infant's sternum in the middle of the chest right below the nipples and press down one inch.

Children ages one through eight years. Place the heel of one hand on the sternum right between the nipples and press down approximately one and a half inches.

Older children and adults. Place the heel of one hand on the sternum between the nipples and place your other hand over it. Lean your body over the victim, lock your elbows, and use your body weight to press down two inches.

Administer thirty chest compressions at a rate of one hundred per minute. It should take you approximately twenty seconds to give thirty compressions, or a little faster than one per second. Then stop and provide two rescue breaths again. Continue on this cycle of thirty compressions, then two breaths, until an AED device arrives, emergency personnel arrive, or you notice the child begins moving or breathing on his own.

CRADLE CAP

Cradle cap is a crusty, plaque-like rash on a baby's scalp that results from the buildup of extra skin cells.

Causes

Infants grow very rapidly, and so does their skin. The skin cells of an infant regenerate very quickly. At the same time, special glands in the skin of the scalp, known as *sebaceous glands,* are secreting an oily substance called *sebum,* which helps keep the skin moist and healthy. However, an excess of this oily substance, probably due to the leftover maternal hormones that were transferred to the infant at birth, can lead to a buildup of dead skin cells that stick to the scalp, resulting in cradle cap. Medically known as *seborrheic dermatitis,* most infants have some degree of cradle cap. Occasionally, it can be seen around the ears, the neck, and the eyebrows. Cradle cap usually appears within the first three months of life and subsides by six months of age.

What to Do

Unlike eczema (which can be itchy and uncomfortable), cradle cap seldom bothers babies. The unsightly appearance of the rash, however, may bother parents. Most of the time little or no treatment is needed and cradle cap will often subside on its own. But if the scales build up into thick crusts, here is a tried-and-true regimen we use in our pediatric practice:

Oil your baby's scalp. Massage a vegetable oil (such as olive oil) into the crusty scales to soften them. Let the oil soak in for at least fifteen minutes and then remove the crusty scales with a soft hairbrush or comb.

Shampoo your baby's scalp. Use an over-the-counter tar-based shampoo once a week to prevent the recurrence of the scaly crust. A baby shampoo with tea tree oil is a good natural alternative. Take extra care to avoid getting the shampoo into Baby's eyes. Cradle cap is usually more crusty over the soft spot because parents are afraid to wash, or sometimes even touch, this area. Because the soft spot is really quite thick with fibrous tissue underneath, it's okay to shampoo and scrub that area as firmly as you do the rest of the scalp.

Humidify your baby's scalp. Dry, crusty skin usually worsens during the winter months of dry, central heating. Use a humidifier (see page 24) to humidify Baby's room.

Expose your baby's scalp to a bit of sun.
Be sure your baby gets enough fresh air and
enjoys the therapeutic rays of a few minutes
of sunshine on his scalp. If practical, try for
exposure to at least fifteen minutes of sunshine on Baby's skin and scalp each day during the cold winter months.

Go fish! Omega-3 supplements can help
soften dry, flaky, and inflamed skin. If breastfeeding, Mother should take an omega-3 supplement; if formula-feeding, parents should be
sure to use DHA-enriched infant formula. (See
more helpful hints under general skin care,
page 29.)

As the hormones and oil glands get their act
together during those early months, you will
find that the cradle cap gradually subsides,
and your baby will begin to sprout a "cap" of
soft, silky hair instead.

CRANIOSYNOSTOSIS

A newborn's skull is made up of many individual bones that lie close together and are inter-
connected by fibrous tissue. This allows the
newborn skull to be more flexible and accommodate the child's growing brain. There are
small spaces called *sutures* separating these
individual skull bones. The presence of these
sutures is important for normal skull and
brain growth and development. As a child
gets older, and once full brain growth has
been achieved, the bones of the skull eventually fuse together. *Craniosynostosis* (meaning
"fusing of skull bones") is a condition that
develops when the sutures (or the spaces
between the skull bones) fuse together too
early. This can interfere with normal brain and
skull growth and, if left untreated, can lead to

developmental and other medical problems
down the road.

It is unknown what actually causes craniosynostosis. It occurs in approximately 1 out of
every 2,000 births, affecting males twice as
often as females. Craniosynostosis does
appear to have a genetic component, as cases
can run in families. However, most children
with craniosynostosis have families without a
history of the condition. It is thought that perhaps the genetically inherited form of craniosynostosis may occur concurrently with other
genetic disorders.

The severity of craniosynostosis depends
upon how many of the skull sutures are
involved, which skull bones are involved,
and how early the sutures begin fusing
together.

A related condition is called *positional plagiocephaly*, in which the skull shape becomes
asymmetrical from an infant always sleeping
with the head in only one position (instead of
rotating the head to face various directions at
night). The pressure of the heavy head pushing against the mattress in only one area all
night for months will make that area of the
head flat. See Flat Head, page 324, for more
information.

Signs and Symptoms

Any or all of the following symptoms may suggest the presence of craniosynostosis:

- unusual or irregular head shape

- your baby's head growth slows over time,
  indicated by a drop in head size percentile
  over time

- hard, raised ridges along the lines of the
  sutures of the skull

- early disappearance of the "soft spot" on the top of your baby's skull

- developmental delays (if undetected and not treated early)

- poor feeding

- increased sleepiness and/or irritability

See your doctor if any of the above clues are present in your infant.

DR. SEARS TIP
Watch the "Soft Spot"

The "soft spot" on the top of your baby's head is the meeting point for four separate skull bones. Also known as the *anterior fontanel,* the "soft spot" usually slowly disappears over the first year of life. Inform your pediatrician at a checkup if you notice the "soft spot" has disappeared prior to your child's first year of life.

Diagnosis

Diagnosis begins with a complete history and physical examination of your child. After thoroughly examining your child's skull and facial structures and plotting the growth rates of your child's skull, your pediatrician may consider further testing. You should also inform the doctor if there is a family history of craniosynostosis or other head or face abnormalities, because this may indicate other genetic disorders.

If the overall percentiles of your child's head circumference are dropping lower and lower, there may be cause for concern. Your pediatrician can further discuss what this may mean.

Specific tests that may be run if your doctor suspects craniosynostosis include the following:

- X-rays of the skull and facial bones

- CT scans of the head and facial bones, which will produce an image of the bones, brain, and other structures of the head

Treatment

The treatment for craniosynostosis depends on the extent of the condition, the location and number of sutures and skull bones involved, and the presence of any worsening symptoms or developmental delays in your child.

In most cases, surgery is recommended. The goals of surgery are to insure there is enough room in the skull to allow for proper brain growth and development, to relieve any possible pressure on the brain due to early closing of the sutures, and to improve the overall appearance of the child's head and face. Surgery is usually done before the child is one year of age, as the bones at this age are much softer, more flexible, and often respond well to surgery. In severe cases, surgery may need to be performed at a very early age.

Long-Term Prognosis

How well a patient does with this condition depends entirely on how severe the deformity is and how early surgery is performed to correct the problem. If craniosynostosis is detected early and surgery is successful, this condition can usually be reversed, and in such cases children do well later in life. If not corrected, craniosynostosis can lead to increased pressure inside the skull, seizures, and developmental delays. Talk to your pediatrician if you have any concerns about the size or shape of your newborn's or infant's skull.

CROUP

Your child has had a mild cold for the past day or two; then around bedtime, you start to hear it: That barky, raspy cough that sounds like a sea lion asking for his next meal. If you have heard a "croupy" cough before, there's no mistaking it. If your child has never had croup, it can be a frightening experience.

Croup is a very common illness that most children will catch at some point, so it's best to be ready for it when it happens. It is a viral infection that affects mostly younger children (under five). It causes swelling in the child's vocal cords, and this causes the barky cough. The area of the vocal cords is the narrowest part of the air passages, and any swelling from infection may narrow the airway enough to obstruct breathing. Croup usually lasts five to six days and is worse at night. The symptoms tend to peak on the second and third night. Croup may hit without warning, or it may begin as a cold that gradually escalates into a croupy cough.

Is croup contagious? Yes, it is about as contagious as the common cold. Good hand washing is important to prevent spread.

Symptoms

Besides cough and cold symptoms, your child may show most of the following:

- Barky cough. A child will sometimes awaken from sleep with a croupy cough,

and it can be frightening for both the child and parent.

- Fever. There will often be a fever, but usually below 104.

- Hoarse voice. This is also from the swelling of the voice box.

- Stridor. This is the most concerning symptom of croup. Stridor is a harsh, raspy, whooping, gasping sound when your child breathes in. This can make breathing very difficult.

- Retractions. When you watch the little dent in the child's neck just above the breastbone, it caves in with each labored breath. This is a sign of serious croup and immediate treatment is needed.

- Symptoms you shouldn't see. If your child has some of the above symptoms of croup, but also has severe drooling, difficulty swallowing, and can barely get any air, this might be a sign of *epiglottitis*, a very rare but life-threatening throat infection that is more serious than croup. Call your doctor.

Signs of Non-Serious Croup

It's important to watch the behavior of your child and see how the croup is progressing. If your child is smiling, happy, playful, looking around, interested in the environment, and his breathing is not obviously bothered by the croup, *these are good signs.* He may have a barky cough but is *not* having stridor or retractions. As a final reassurance, if your barking child is able to lie down and sleep without too much interruption, then his breathing is probably not jeopardized.

Signs of Serious Croup

Here's when to be concerned: The child whose airway is significantly obstructed will have a worried look on his face and will not be interested in any play or interaction, as if he's concentrating his energy on getting air. The child won't lie down; he just sits up and barks, and he can't sleep. He will have retractions and stridor. The stridor will sound worse when your child is agitated or crying and seems to lessen when the child is resting peacefully.

Treatment

Keep your child calm. Croup can be frightening for your child, and crying will make the stridor worse. It is important to keep your child relaxed by cuddling and staying calm yourself. Sit your child upright in your lap, play soft music, sing lullabies, read a story. If breastfeeding, offer the great pacifier.

Steam things up. Humidity helps clear the child's breathing passages. Turn on the hot shower in your bathroom and close the door. While keeping your child calm, sit with him on your lap in the steamy bathroom. You should see some improvement in about ten minutes.

Cool mist. If you have a cool-mist humidifier or vaporizer, let your child breathe directly in front of the stream of mist. Once the child improves, keep the mist flowing near the bed for the rest of the night. If you only have a hot-mist vaporizer, you can still use it, but don't let anyone get too close, as you or your child can get burned.

Cool night air. Have your child sleep with the window open. The cool, humid night air is ideal for soothing croup. The combination of a hot-mist vaporizer running in the room all night and the night air coming in through the window is probably the most ideal humid and slightly cool environment for croup. If necessary, bundle up your child and take him outside into the cool night air for ten minutes or take a slow car ride with the windows open. The misty night air is why babies with croup often improve en route to the emergency room.

Treat the fever. Use acetaminophen or ibuprofen. See page 552 for dosing help.

DR. SEARS TIP
Be Cautious with Cold Medications

Important: For a child with croup, do not give antihistamines or decongestants without your doctor's advice. These may dry the narrowing air passages that the moisture is trying to open.

The above suggestions usually work well within about twenty minutes (an hour for the fever), and your child should be able to settle back down to sleep. Keep close watch over your child by sleeping in the same room for the rest of the night, as another croup attack is likely and the above treatments will need to be repeated.

Expect croup to worsen at night and improve during the day. A twenty-minute walk in the evening air can get ahead of the croupy throat swelling before bed. After three or four days, the croupy cough will change into a loose, mucousy cough, which will last a week or two.

When to Go to the Emergency Room (or Doctor's Office)

After trying the above treatments, assess how your child is doing. If he seems to be improving (retractions and stridor are lessening, color is returning to child's pale cheeks) then continue with the steam and a watchful eye and ear. If you feel your child is getting worse despite the above treatments, go straight to the emergency room. Your doctor won't be able to treat this over the phone, so it may be best to go to the emergency room instead of paging your doctor and waiting for a call back.

Watch for these emergency signs; if any of them arise, take Baby directly to the nearest emergency room:

- The retractions become more labored and your child's inhaling changes from a low-pitched stridor to a whistling sound.

- Your child becomes paler.

- The child can't speak or cry because of shortness of breath.

- The child is struggling more to get each breath.

- The child begins to drool excessively or has difficulty swallowing.

- The retractions are increasing, but the sound of breathing is decreasing.

Emergency Room Treatment for Croup

What will they do for you in the emergency room? As the staff evaluates your child, they should encourage you to hold him in your lap to help keep him calm. They might measure his blood oxygen level with an oximeter or "pulse ox," which uses a small light source that is wrapped around a finger or toe and helps determine if your child is getting enough air. They may have your child breathe some humidified air for twenty minutes or more. If your child's croup is severe enough, they might give him vaporized epinephrine to breathe with the humidified air, which works quickly to open the airways. The emergency room physician might recommend a short course of steroids, which will help keep the air passages open over the next few hours to days. Your child will only be on the steroids for a few days, and there are no side effects to worry about when steroids are used for a short time. The first dose often needs to be given as an injection, as the child with severe breathing difficulty will have trouble taking an oral medication or may throw it up.

CRYING IT OUT

"Our baby cries until I pick her up. My friends tell me to just let her cry it out, but that doesn't feel right to me. Should I let her cry it out?"

Your feeling is right and your friends' advice is wrong. "Let-your-baby-cry-it-out" is the worst advice you can get. It is *biologically incorrect*. Studies show that when a mother hears her baby cry, the blood flow to her breasts increases, and she has a hormonal urge to pick up and nurse her baby (*nurse* here meaning comfort, not just breastfeed).

Studies have shown that babies who receive an appropriate and nurturing response to their cries tend to cry and whine less as they get older, whereas babies who are parented in a more restrained way, left to cry themselves to sleep and rigidly scheduled instead of having their needs appropriately met, tend to either withdraw or cry and whine more. Let's go through the phrase "let your baby cry it out" to show you why it's unwise advice:

"Let your baby…" The best person who can tell if and how long to let Baby cry is the very person who shared an umbilical cord with that baby — Mom (or whoever is the primary caregiver). A person who has no biological connection to your baby, does not know your baby, is not invested in your baby, and isn't there at 3 a.m. when your baby cries should not pontificate on how you should respond to your baby's cries.

"cry…" A baby's cry is her language, designed for the survival of the baby and the development of her parents. Analysis of a baby's cry shows two distinct phases. The opening sounds of a baby's cry are called attachment-promoting sounds. They trigger a sensitive "need to respond" feeling in the mother. If these opening cues are not listened to, many babies go to the next phase of the cry, a more shrill and disturbing sound that can actually trigger feelings of annoyance instead of sensitive feelings in the mother. Responding earlier to a baby's cry is easier on both mother and baby.

"it…" The "it" is not an annoying habit. Babies cry to communicate, not manipulate. The "it" is an emotional and physical need. When your baby cries, he is telling you, "I need something" or "Something is not right. Please make it right."

"out." If you let your baby cry it out, something goes out of your relationship with your baby — trust. Letting your baby cry it out is a lose-lose situation: Baby loses trust in the signal value of his cries, and you lose trust in your ability to appropriately respond.

DR. SEARS TIP
Learn to Read Baby's
Pre-Cry Signals

As you and your baby grow together and naturally work out the cry-response communication, you'll begin to read your baby's pre-cry signals: a bit of body language, such as flailing arms or facial grimaces. By your responding to these cues, your baby learns that he doesn't have to escalate to crying to get his needs met. In effect, you are teaching your baby to communicate better.

Get into the mind of your baby and imagine what his cries mean to him. Baby's cry is his communication tool; if no one listens, Baby has two choices: Either he can cry louder and harder and produce a more disturbing signal, or he can clam up, withdraw, and become a "good baby" (not bother anyone). We have noticed that parents who fall victim to the cry-it-out method eventually become less sensitive to their babies. Because these parents desensitize themselves to the signal value of their baby's cry, the cry doesn't bother them. Insensitivity is what gets a new parent into trouble. Eventually, a distance develops between the insensitive parent and the less-trusting baby.

As your baby grows and learns other ways to communicate his needs, how quickly you respond to your baby's cries will become a cry-by-cry call. As you and your baby rehearse this cry-response communication hundreds of times in the early months, and as Baby learns self-soothing strategies, you'll eventually know when a cry is a "red alert" and needs immediate attention and when a cry does not need such an immediate response. Certainly, you

DR. SEARS TIP
Get Behind the Eyes
of Your Baby

The most practical parenting tip the Sears family would like to share with new parents is this: Whenever you wonder how to respond to your baby in any given situation, immediately ask yourself: "If I were my baby, how would I want my mother/father to respond?" Follow this instinctive guideline, and you'll nearly always get it right.

don't have to respond as quickly to the cries of an eight-month-old baby as you do to a one-week-old infant.

Two Cry-It-Out Stories from Our Practice

Some Babies Cry Because They Hurt

A mother brought her six-month-old infant into our office for consultation. He had suffered frequent crying jags since shortly after birth, some so severe that Mother had rushed him to the emergency room because she was so worried. Mother had been told by her friends that she was spoiling her baby, and she should just let him cry it out. She had also been told by several doctors that she was an overreactive mother. This mother was truly being a mother. She opened up the conversation with: "Dr. Bill, I know something is wrong with my baby. His cries tell me that." Mother was right! A thorough medical evaluation revealed that the baby suffered from severe gastroesophageal reflux disease (GERD). He cried because he hurt. By the time this diagnosis was made, the baby had already developed ulcers in his esophagus from the acid eating away at the lining. He required surgical correction of this problem. (See related sections: Colic, page 229; and GERD, page 338.)

Beware of Baby Trainers

A couple brought their three-month-old baby into our office for her routine checkup. I (Dr. Bill) had seen this baby since birth, and this family had been thriving. The first clue of a change: Although previously Mother had been wearing Baby in a sling, they were now carrying the baby in a plastic infant seat, and they plopped the baby down several feet away from them. Next, the father proudly said, "You know, Dr. Bill, she's such a good baby. She doesn't cry." The second clue! Father went on to boast, "And she sleeps through the night!" As I examined the baby, I noticed that she seemed distant. She avoided eye-to-eye contact and didn't seem connected. The third clue: Her weight and height had barely progressed from her previous checkup.

Because of these three clues, I asked the parents if they were doing anything differently. They mentioned they had gone to a baby-training class that taught them: "Don't let your baby control you," "If you let your baby cry it out, she'll learn to self-soothe," and "If you get her on a schedule life will be so much easier for you." These new and vulnerable parents had fallen prey to the let-him-cry-it-out crowd of baby trainers, and the whole family was paying the price. Baby was not thriving and the parents had desensitized themselves to the cues of their baby. I explained to the parents what was happening. Mother broke down and said instinctively, "My gut feeling told me this wasn't right." I advised that they simply go back to doing what was working for them before and not subject their baby to someone else's training methods. The attachment plug had been pulled and Baby had stopped thriving. She needed to reconnect with her parents.

At her checkup one month later, the baby was thriving. Her growth and development were back to the appropriate milestones. Father humorously quipped, "She's not such a 'good baby' anymore." We all knew what he meant: Baby cried to express her needs, and they were now appropriately met.

CURVATURES OF FOOT AND LEG

Growing feet and legs go through many changes in the early years. Most babies are born with curved legs and feet that turn inward. These gradually change as walking begins, and most children end up with straight legs and feet. Some, however, will retain abnormal curvatures, commonly known as *bowed legs* or *pigeon-toeing*. Here is our guide to understanding these lower extremity quirks and when to seek your doctor's advice. Some related foot problems you can find on other pages include Flat Feet, page 322, Toe Walking, page 520, and Feet, Smelly, page 317.

In-Curving of the Feet (Metatarsus Adductus)

Sometimes infants have straight legs, but their feet curve in. In fact, most newborns have in-curved feet, again because of their scrunched-up position in the womb. (Remember those adorable ultrasound pictures?)

Treatment. Special stretching exercises for feet that are more curved in may be beneficial. At least six times a day, or with every diaper change, hold the back of the foot firmly with one hand and the front of the foot with the other and gently and gradually straighten the foot. Hold the foot in the straight position for at least five seconds. Most cases of curved foot disappear by six months of age. In cases when the infant's feet are still curved inward by four to six months of age, special shoes may be used (fitted by an orthopedist) until the child begins to walk. Usually special shoes are all that is required to treat this condition. Sometimes short-term casting to keep the feet straight may be used. Only in very rare cases is surgical correction necessary.

When to worry; what to do. Here's how to tell whether or not your baby's feet are normally in-curved and will straighten with a tincture of time or if and when they need orthopedic treatment. Hold the back of your baby's foot around the ankle with one hand and the front of your baby's foot with the other. Hold the back of your baby's foot still and try to straighten out the front of the foot with the other. If you are able to straighten the foot with *gentle* pressure on the front of the foot, this is likely to be a normal newborn in-curved foot that requires no treatment and will self-correct with time. If, however, the curvature seems so rigid that you are unable to straighten it or you notice another clue — a deep crease on the bottom of the foot just in front of the heel where the foot curves in — this developmental quirk is called *clubfoot* and merits an evaluation by a pediatric orthopedist.

There are varying degrees of clubfoot. Some can be straightened successfully by a painless treatment called serial casting: plastic casts resembling little white boots are placed on Baby's feet and changed every few weeks. Each time the cast is changed, Baby's feet will become straighter. After the castings, Baby wears special shoes (they don't look obviously left or right but are rather straight or curve out the opposite direction) for several months to keep the growing feet straight. A clubfoot usually occurs in only one foot, yet normal *positional curvatures* usually occur in *both* feet or legs.

Bowed Legs

Bowed legs is the name given to the condition where a child's knees remain apart when the feet are placed together. All infants are born somewhat bowlegged due to the way the legs are folded inside the uterus. The infant's bowed legs usually begin to naturally straighten out between twelve and eighteen months as the child begins to walk and bear weight on the legs. In rare cases, bowed legs can be a sign of rickets, which is a vitamin D deficiency. Children with underlying rickets tend to have more severe cases of bowed legs. Your pediatrician can perform blood tests if rickets is suspected in your infant.

When to worry; what to do. Almost all cases of bowed legs are "treated" simply with observation of the child as she grows. Further treatment is needed only in very severe cases. In rare cases, X-rays and other treatments may

be necessary if your child shows the following symptoms:

- The bowlegged appearance is getting worse.
- Bowed legs persist past age three.
- Your child trips a lot.
- Your child is having problems walking or running.
- The bowlegged appearance is more severe on one side than the other.

Occasionally surgery is done to correct the deformity if it persists into adolescence. The long-term prognosis for bowed legs is usually very good, as this condition corrects itself over time in the vast majority of children.

Pigeon-Toed (In-Toeing Due to In-Curving of the Legs)

Pigeon-toed is the term used to describe infants and children who *toe-in* or walk like pigeons. All newborns come into the world pigeon-toed because their feet spent many months scrunched up in the womb. Dr. Robert Salter, who wrote the book on children's feet, says, "Infants are born pigeon-toed because there is no standing room in the womb!" This temporary developmental quirk usually straightens out by two or three years of age. Children can in-toe because of curvatures of two areas of the bones: inward curvature of the lower leg bones, called *tibial torsion,* or curving inward of the upper leg bones, called *femoral anteversion.* Because the feet follow the legs, if the bones curve in, so will the feet. These conditions have been found to have a genetic basis and may run in families.

Causes

Twisted shin (tibial torsion). Like curved foot, twisted shin is thought to arise while the child is still in the womb because the legs are rotated to fit in such a small space. Following birth, the leg bones begin to slowly straighten themselves out. Twisted shin occurs when the large bone in the lower leg (known as the tibia) is twisted inward just below the knee. This in turn will cause the foot to twist inward as well. The knee itself will be in a straight ahead position, with only the lower leg being curved inward. This is most commonly noticed by parents around the time the child begins to walk. They are often concerned that this will lead to long-term problems with walking or coordination.

To tell whether your child is toeing-in from a curved tibia or a curved femur (discussed below), observe your child standing. If the kneecaps turn inward toward each other, dubbed "kissing kneecaps," it's likely to be femoral anteversion. If the kneecaps keep facing forward, the toeing-in is likely to be due to tibial torsion.

Twisted thigh (femoral anteversion). Twisted thigh occurs when the child's thigh bone (known as the *femur*) turns inward. This condition may not become noticeable until the child is between two and six years of age. All infants are born with some degree of inward twisting of the thigh bone, which usually improves during the first few years of life. Twisted thigh bone can be distinguished from the above two causes of in-toeing by the fact that both the knees and the feet will turn inward. Again, this may not become apparent until the child has been walking for some time. Because this condition can take years to improve on its own, many parents worry when the condition is still present in their five- or six-year-old child.

Treatment

The good news is that almost all cases of in-toeing resolve on their own. This process can be slow, often not disappearing until the child is between six and eight years of age. Even in cases where this condition takes several years to improve, bracing, casting, and special shoes have not been shown to be very helpful. Usually the only treatment that is required is time. In very rare cases in which the curvature is severe enough to make walking difficult, surgery can be done to rotate the lower leg bones outward in order to cause the feet to point straight. Thankfully, surgery is almost never required.

When to Worry; What to Do

Although all beginning walkers trip a lot, in normal development toddlers trip less as they grow. If your in-toeing child is *tripping more,* be sure to mention this to your doctor. Another concern is limping. As we discuss on page 388, limping always warrants a thorough medical exam.

Although it's true that most children will outgrow their in-curved legs and feet, there are things parents can do to help those growing legs straighten out.

Discourage tummy sleeping. In the first nine months, back sleeping is the safest position for SIDS prevention (see why and how, page 505). Don't let your baby sleep on her tummy with her feet curved in underneath her — sleeping in this position is the most common cause of in-curved legs and persistent pigeon-toeing. In our practice we have had a few toddlers who were persistent tummy sleepers. All attempts to get them to sleep with their legs straight out failed. As a last resort, here's what worked: We encouraged the mothers to put their infants to sleep at night in pajamas where they had sewn the legs together so they couldn't roll over, at least until the children got into the habit of sleeping on their back or sides with their legs straight or only slightly curved. If your child is a confirmed tummy sleeper, before you go to bed yourself, pull his feet out from under him.

Sit pretty! Some toddlers and older children like to sit on their legs, with their feet curved underneath their bottoms. This causes the lower leg bones to curve inward. Instead, teach your child to sit cross-legged ("criss-cross applesauce"). Sitting in the "W" position with the upper legs curved inward and the lower legs flared outward can cause persistent curvature of the upper legs. Besides causing persistent in-curving of the upper leg bones, it's a no-no for the knee joints, as it stretches the knee ligaments and aggravates the knock-kneed appearance. Again, sitting with the feet straight out or Indian or tailor style is the preferred sitting position for treating knock-knees, pigeon toes, or any other leg-bone curvature quirk. Sitting and sleeping with the legs straight capitalizes on a developmental lesson from nature: As the twig is bent, so grows the tree. Because growth occurs mainly during sleep, if the child sleeps with the legs curved inward, those little "twigs" are likely to continue growing that way.

Lift flat feet. Children with flat and pronated feet soon learn that if they curve their feet inward, it makes an arch and it's sometimes easier to walk. (See page 322 to see which flat feet need treatment and why.)

It may be comforting to know that many successful athletes are pigeon-toed and run just fine. In fact, some coaches believe that being pigeon-toed can be an advantage for sports that require sharp running and turning, such as football, basketball, and tennis.

DR. SEARS TIP
No Tripping, No Worry

As a general guide, if your child does not trip a lot during normal walking and running, the in-toeing will not bother him and there is no need to worry.

Out-Toeing

As the name implies, out-toeing is the opposite of in-toeing and occurs when the toes and feet point outward instead of straight ahead or inward. Out-toeing is often first noticed by parents when their child begins to stand or walk.

Causes. Although not as common as in-toeing, out-toeing is seen quite often in our practice. Out-toeing is usually a result of excess outward rotation of the leg bones, which usually starts when the child is still in the womb, and it is related to being in the cramped spaces of the womb for nine months.

Treatment. In the vast majority of cases, out-toeing slowly corrects itself with time. Normally, as the child begins to walk, the feet begin to turn inward into more of a straight-ahead position. This may take a long time, however — up to six to eight years to fully correct. In only very rare cases is further treatment needed. Talk to your doctor if your child begins to exhibit any of the following conditions:

- The out-toeing affects how your child walks or runs.

- The out-toeing affects only one foot.

- The child complains of pain upon walking or running.

- The out-toeing seems to be getting worse.

- Your child is still showing signs of out-toeing by six years of age.

Very rarely, surgery is needed to correct the underlying structural problems.

CUTS, SCRAPES, AND STITCHES

We'll start with the first question parents have.

Does it need stitches?

- Any cut that is gaping open (regardless of size) and is longer than a half inch (one centimeter) probably needs stitches (or at least some type of closure, like skin glue or steri-strips).

- Cuts on the face that are longer than a quarter inch (half a centimeter) may need stitches.

The sooner a wound is closed, the lower the chance of infection. Try to see a doctor within four hours, although many wounds can still be stitched later than this (see below for full discussion on lacerations).

Home Care for Cuts and Scrapes

Minor cuts and scrapes usually don't require a trip to the emergency room but proper care is important to avoid infection. Here are some useful tips to help you care for simple wounds:

Stop the bleeding.

- Minor cuts and scrapes usually stop bleeding on their own. If they don't, simply apply gentle pressure with a clean cloth or bandage.

- Be sure to apply pressure continuously for five to ten minutes. Some wounds may require pressure for twenty minutes. If you keep checking to see if the bleeding has stopped, you might damage or dislodge the fresh clot that's forming and cause bleeding to resume.

- If the blood spurts with a pulsation or continues to flow after constant pressure, seek immediate medical assistance.

Clean the wound.

- Thorough cleaning is important because it reduces the risk of infection.

- Rinse out the wound with clean water using a large syringe, if available. "Ouchless" alcohol-free antiseptic rinses also work well. Rinse solutions out of the wound after a minute to avoid tissue irritation. Try to rinse out any visible dirt.

- Don't use hydrogen peroxide on an open wound because it can interfere with blood clotting, irritate open cuts or scrapes, and may delay healing.

- If dirt or debris remains in the wound, use tweezers cleaned with alcohol to remove the particles. If dirt is still embedded in the wound after cleaning, see your pediatrician.

- Clean the area around the wound with soap and a washcloth (but avoid getting soap in the wound — it can irritate it).

Apply an antibiotic. After cleaning the wound, apply a thin layer of an antibiotic ointment such as Neosporin, Polysporin, or other triple antibiotic to help keep the surface moist. These ointments discourage infection and allow the body's healing process to work more efficiently.

Keep things dry, yet moist. We recommend keeping the scab moist with ointment and a bandage, but you don't want the surrounding skin to remain so wet that it gets "pruney." Use a breathable bandage and let the wound "air out" several times a day. For large areas of raw skin, such as "road rash" from a bike accident, it is very important to prevent a dry scab from forming by keeping the entire wound moist with an antibiotic ointment or burn cream (Silvadene) for a week or two until new skin has formed. If a large scab dries out, it will shrink and crack, leading to infection, delayed healing, and scarring.

DR. SEARS TIP
Activ-Flex Band-Aids

Activ-Flex is one kind of Band-Aid we recommend. We have used them in our family for years for small burns, cuts, and abrasions. They are waterproof and provide a built-in lubricant, which speeds healing.

Cover the wound.

- A good bandage will help keep the wound clean and keep out harmful bacteria.

- Change the dressing at least daily, more often if it gets wet or dirty.

- After the wound has mostly healed (about three to five days), infection is less likely, and exposure to the air will speed healing.

Watch for signs of infection. Visit your doctor if you see any of these signs:

- pus draining from wound

- increased pain, redness, or swelling after forty-eight hours

- still not largely healed after a week

Stitches

How soon to see the doctor for stitches. Most cuts can generally be closed as long as twenty-four hours after the accident. Some cuts should be closed sooner, but it is generally safe to wait at least eight hours to have a cut closed. Therefore, if the cut occurs at night, it is usually okay to wait until the next morning, as long as you can get the bleeding to stop.

Very important: If you do decide to wait, rinse the cut with clean water or sterile saline from a drugstore to remove any dirt. Do not let the cut dry out. Wet some gauze and tape it over the cut. Change this every two hours to keep it moist. If you cannot do this, then put some antibiotic ointment on the cut and cover it with gauze or a Band-Aid. Repeat this every few hours until you see the doctor in the morning.

Four Options for Closing a Cut

There are four ways to close a cut. Your doctor will discuss these options with you.

1. Steri-strips. Also known as "butterfly" strips, these narrow strips are placed over the cut, and have a bit of tension to keep it closed. They are generally kept on for two to five days, and are used for cuts that are small, not gaping open, not very deep, and not over a joint or area of skin tension. If they stay in place for at least three days, the outcome can be just as good as stitches or even better because you avoid the "railroad track" appearance of some stitch lines. Although they are quick and painless to use, they will not stay in place as long as stitches. Benzoin adhesive liquid can be used to help them stick longer.

2. Stitches. There is little to no risk of stitches being pulled off too soon. An obvious disadvantage is the time and pain involved in suturing.

3. Skin superglue. This is a great invention! If it's applied by a skilled physician, wounds can be quickly and painlessly closed without any stitches. It is a good choice for clean, straight cuts that are not too gaping nor under tension. If you are hesitant to put your child through the trauma of stitches, but steri-strips are not enough, then this is a great option. If done well, the cosmetic outcome is the same as with stitches.

4. Staples. These are special medical staples that are often used in the scalp (within the hair). They are very fast to administer and close the cut almost as well as stitches.

Who Should Do the Stitches?

Should you go to a plastic surgeon, your family pediatrician, or an emergency room doctor? No matter who does the stitches, there will be at least a slight scar. Even the best plastic surgeon in the world will leave one. It is, however, important to minimize the scar. Parents naturally worry about this. Here are some suggestions to help you decide where to have the stitches done:

Plastic surgeon. For cuts on the face, we recommend a plastic surgeon, especially if the cut is large. An emergency room doctor or pediatrician could easily handle very small cuts on the face (especially if the cut is suitable for glue or steri-strips), but a plastic surgeon will be most able to minimize the scar. You can have the stitches done in the surgeon's office or in an emergency room by the surgeon.

Emergency room doctor. ER doctors have more experience with stitches than pediatricians, given that they perform the procedure several times a day.

Your pediatrician. For simple cuts anywhere besides the face, your pediatrician's office is probably the best place to go for the stitches, unless the office is very busy that day.

 DR. SEARS TIP
Tetanus Shot

If your teenager's last tetanus shot was more than five years ago, and the wound is deep or dirty, she should get a booster shot within forty-eight hours of the injury. Any child who is not vaccinated for tetanus should get a shot for any deep, dirty wound. A simple scrape or minor cut that doesn't warrant an emergency room visit probably has no risk of tetanus.

Wound Care After Closure

Ask your doctor for specific guidelines on proper wound care. Here are some general guidelines to follow:

• For the first forty-eight hours do not allow the wound to get wet in the bath or shower. Steri-strips are an exception. Keep them dry for at least five days. After that, you may get them wet to encourage them to come off. Do not pull them off unless they come off easily.

- Keep the wound covered for at least forty-eight hours. After two days, it is less important to keep covered, but it helps to protect the stitches from dirt and bumps.

- Avoid the buildup of a scab. A thick scab on the wound can increase scarring and prevent the skin from healing well. A crusty scab can also grow over stitches, making their removal difficult. Dab the scab with diluted hydrogen peroxide (half water/half peroxide) and then gently remove any loose scab. Do not pick away any scab that is still firmly stuck. Let the peroxide loosen it first. Do this twice a day.

- Apply antibiotic ointment twice a day.

When to Have Stitches Removed

Be sure to ask the doctor who puts in the stitches when they should be removed. Here are our general guidelines:

Face. Three to five days. Why so soon? By five days the stitch thread starts to react with the skin, and this can leave a mark for each stitch. If the skin is not turning red where the stitches enter, then it is best to wait the full five days. If a stitch reaction is occurring sooner, see your doctor to discuss having them removed sooner. Do not wait more than five days. When they are removed, the doctor may put steri-strips over the cut to provide a few more days of strength.

Body and scalp. Seven to ten days.

Extremities. Ten to fourteen days. If the stitches are over a joint area that bends and stretches, then you should wait fourteen days. If not, then ten days is enough.

How to Minimize a Long-Term Scar

Sun protection. Damaged skin is very susceptible to permanent discoloration from the sun for up to six months following an injury. It is very important to minimize sun exposure on the healing cut. Keep it covered with a hat or clothing as much as possible. When necessary (especially for long days at the park, beach, or swimming pool), apply a strong sunscreen or even a zinc oxide sunblock (the white stuff that doesn't soak in). Do not apply sunscreen until two weeks after the cut.

Fish oil supplement. You can buy these oils in a health-food store. They contain all the essential fats necessary for skin to grow and heal itself. Although it has not been proven to minimize scars, it theoretically should help. Give one teaspoon each day to infants and two teaspoons to children. Do not apply the oil to the cut.

Vitamin E oil. You can rub this oil onto the cut after the stitches are removed. There is not a definite proven benefit, but it may help the healing.

Scar-prevention creams. Available over the counter, creams such as Mederma may help reduce scarring.

CYSTIC FIBROSIS

Cystic fibrosis is a disease caused by a defect in one of the genes. Today there are approximately thirty thousand children and adults in the United States living with cystic fibrosis. About a thousand new cases are diagnosed in this country each year. Most children with cystic fibrosis are diagnosed by age two. A small number of people aren't diagnosed until their teenage years or later.

Symptoms

There are several common symptoms for cystic fibrosis, listed below, although type and severity of symptoms can vary greatly:

- newborns who have no bowel movements within the first one to two days of life

- infants who have stools that are light-clay-colored or very pale and often have an abnormally foul smell

- frequent respiratory infections, such as sinusitis, bronchitis, and pneumonia

- persistent and ongoing cough and/or wheezing

- failure to gain weight properly in infancy and childhood

- stunted growth

- fatigue

- persistent diarrhea

- salty taste on the skin

The Cause

Cystic fibrosis is caused by a defect in the gene known as the *CF gene*. The CF gene tells the body how to produce mucus in our systems. When the CF gene is defective, it instructs the body to produce mucus that is thicker and stickier than it should be. This causes an abnormal buildup of sticky mucus in the respiratory and digestive tracts and leads to serious and often life-threatening infections of the lung and gastrointestinal

tract problems. Cystic fibrosis is more common in people descended from northern or central Europeans.

Diagnosis

Cystic fibrosis may be suspected if an infant or toddler exhibits the above symptoms. Talk to your pediatrician if you are concerned that your child is exhibiting many of the above-mentioned symptoms. There are several types of tests that can indicate cystic fibrosis. The one most commonly done is known as a *sweat chloride test* and is considered the most accurate test in diagnosing cystic fibrosis. In some states, genetic testing for a defective CF gene is part of the normal newborn blood screening test done at birth. If cystic fibrosis is confirmed, further testing will be performed, such as testing of the gastrointestinal tract, a stool test, and an evaluation of pancreas and lung function (these are two of the most commonly affected organs in cystic fibrosis). All family members of a person diagnosed with cystic fibrosis should be tested to determine if they are carriers of the defective gene. A person needs two defective copies of the CF gene to have cystic fibrosis. People who are carriers have only one defective CF gene and one normal CF gene. These people will not have cystic fibrosis, but they can pass it on to their children if their partners also carry one defective copy of the CF gene.

Treatment

Early diagnosis can improve the length of survival and quality of life. Decades ago people with cystic fibrosis rarely lived into their twenties. Today, even with the best medical treatment, the average life span is thirty-seven years. However, some people will survive into their forties.

Treatment of cystic fibrosis requires a comprehensive approach involving several medical specialties. Many communities today have specialized cystic fibrosis clinics. There are many different treatment options, depending on a person's individual situation and severity. Following is a list of some of the potential treatments:

• Treating respiratory infections with antibiotics. Some people are placed on antibiotics long-term to reduce the number and complications of these repeat respiratory infections.

• Vitamin supplementation. People with cystic fibrosis often become deficient in several vitamins, especially vitamins A, D, E, and K.

• The pancreas, an organ that produces enzymes to help with digestion, is affected by cystic fibrosis. People with cystic fibrosis will need daily oral supplementation with prescription digestive enzymes.

• Inhaler medications to improve lung function.

• Daily prescription medication to help thin the mucus in an individual's airways and digestive tract.

• Special drainage techniques to help drain the airways of the thickened mucus.

• If available, and if a patient is a good candidate, a lung transplant may be performed.

Again, treatment for cystic fibrosis needs to be individualized. Talk with a cystic fibrosis specialist if your child is affected by this disease.

Long-Term Complications

Sadly, as mentioned above, the average life span of an individual with cystic fibrosis today is thirty-seven years. With early and aggressive treatment, the quality of life can be vastly improved. The most common complications of cystic fibrosis are repeated lung infections and lung damage, chronic respiratory failure, liver disease, heart failure, and diabetes.

DAYCARE DECISIONS

Once your child begins daycare, expect more frequent illnesses. Germs are one of the few things children share, and studies show that children get more respiratory and intestinal infections once they begin daycare. Two common decisions parents are faced with are:

• What can I do to keep my child from getting sick at daycare?

• When is my child too sick or contagious to go to daycare?

Play the numbers game. The fewer infants your baby is exposed to, the lower the chance of picking up infections. Too many babies in too small a room is a breeding ground for germs. Be sure the rooms are well ventilated with fresh air and that children are encouraged to play outside a lot. This lessens the chances of germ-sharing.

Review the daycare's hygiene policy. Licensed daycare centers should have policies for infection control. Ask to see them. Be sure they have thorough hand-washing policies before and after diaper changing, and that soiled diapers are carefully disposed of. Be sure they enforce thorough hand washing after children and daycare providers use the bathroom. Ask what their policies are for admitting potentially contagious children. Be sure they have a policy that requires parents to send a doctor's note stating whether or not a sick child is contagious.

Feed your child immune-boosting foods. The best foods to boost your child's immune system are:

- foods that contain omega-3 fats: fish (especially wild salmon), omega-3 fish oil supplements, and flax oil

- vitamin C–containing foods: citrus fruits, guava, kiwi, papaya, strawberries, and tomato paste

- vitamin E–containing foods: whole grains, peanut butter, green leafy vegetables, sweet potatoes, and nut oils

- immune-boosting spices: ginger, cinnamon, and turmeric

Encourage your daycare to serve children immune-boosting and not immune-depleting foods (added sugar or high-fructose corn syrup). A helpful immune-boosting resource to give your daycare provider is our book *The Healthiest Kid in the Neighborhood.* See Feed Your Child's Immune System, page 33.

Teach your child to cover his nose and mouth when coughing or sneezing. Show and tell your child how — and why — it's important to cover his mouth and nose when he sneezes or coughs: "When you sneeze or cough tiny droplets of mucus, like tiny balloons, carry germs from your nose and throat through the air and other children may breathe them in and get sick." Show your child how to sneeze or cough into his elbow or arm. This is better than the hand (which touches his surroundings and spreads the germs).

Keep immunizations and medical check-ups up-to-date. Be sure your child's immunizations are current. If in doubt, call your health-care provider to find out. During routine checkups ask your doctor if there are any seasonal illnesses going around and what extra precautions you can ask your caregiver to take to avoid these.

Should Your Child Stay Home?

How do you tell if your sick child should stay home or go to daycare? Here are the most frequent illnesses that are of concern:

Fever. Any fever 100 degrees or higher usually indicates some sort of contagious infection is going on. Plus, a febrile child will likely need extra tender-loving care that she can't get in a large daycare. The general rule on fevers is that they should be gone for at least twenty-four hours (without having needed any fever medication to hide it) before a child returns to daycare.

Colds. Colds are most contagious during the first few days when the mucus is clear and runny. They remain slightly contagious until the nose stops running. It just isn't practical to keep a child home for two weeks every time she catches a cold. It's a simple fact of child care that mild colds will be running around with the children. The decision to keep your child home or send her should be based on how sick your child feels. Here are some general guidelines: If your child is happy and playful, and the runny nose and cough are mild, it's appropriate to send her to daycare.

If, on the other hand, your child has a fever and is generally acting sick, she should stay home so you can provide the extra care she needs. Whether the nasal secretions are green or clear doesn't really matter; both are contagious. Some child-care centers, however, have a "no green" policy. But before you rebook your whole day based on what's coming out of your child's nose, here's our nasal drainage tip: The goop in the nose is always thicker upon awakening in the morning because the secretions have collected there during the night. Give your child a "nose hose" and a "steam clean" (see pages 20 and 21) and then reassess the nasal secretions. If the remaining secretions are clear and your child seems well, she does not need to stay home.

Coughs. Most coughs are not stay-home-from-daycare illnesses. Coughs usually bother children more during the night. Coughs are contagious, but that goes with the territory. Some viruses produce nuisance-type dry coughs that linger on for several weeks, but they are only minimally contagious once the nose has cleared up and your child may attend daycare. If the cough is accompanied by fever and green or snotty nasal discharge, and your

DR. SEARS TIP
Not All Coughs and
Sneezes Are Colds

Coughing and sneezing can be due to an allergy and not contagious. Here's how to tell an allergy from a contagious cold: The child with an allergy has wheezing, a clear runny nose, itchy eyes, and no fever, and is not that sick. The child with a cold has thick, snotty mucus, may have a low-grade fever, and has a generally unwell appearance.

child is acting generally ill, he should not attend daycare and needs medical attention. Once the fever breaks and the child seems better, he can attend daycare.

Ear infection. Unless accompanied by fever, cough, and a snotty nose, ear infections are generally not considered contagious, and you can send your child to daycare as soon as she feels better and is being treated appropriately. Ear infections usually follow a cold, and by the time the cold germs enter the middle ear, the cold is no longer very contagious.

Eye drainage. Sometimes a daycare will refuse admission to a child with eye drainage. Here's how to tell if your child is contagious. In the first six months of life, eye drainage is most likely due to a blocked tear duct (see page 303) and it is not contagious. Watery eye drainage during an allergy is not contagious. Goopy drainage from the eyes accompanying a cold (but without red eyes) usually means an underlying sinus infection. In this case, if the child feels well enough to attend daycare then he may do so, with a doctor's note. If the whites of the eyes are red and irritated, and there is eye drainage, this is probably conjunctivitis (see Pink Eye, page 307) and is contagious. The child should not attend daycare until he has received medical treatment. The American Academy of Pediatrics (AAP) recommends that a baby may attend daycare once appropriate treatment for the conjunctivitis has begun. You will probably need a doctor's note to this effect.

Sore throats. The two most contagious causes of sore throat are viral throat infections and *strep throat* (see page 500). As a general rule for both of these contagious illnesses, consider your child contagious until the fever has been gone for at least one day.

DR. SEARS TIP
The Face Tells It All

Mothers use the term *peaked* for the facial appearance of a sick-looking child. You won't find this term in any medical books, but it's a mother-approved description of a child who needs tender-loving care at home and should not attend school or daycare. A persistently peaked face usually means the cold has progressed to an underlying sinus infection and needs medical attention.

Diarrheal illnesses. Diarrhea-producing illnesses are the most contagious daycare germ. If your baby has frequent, watery, mucousy, or bloody diarrhea, this is a sure indication that she is probably contagious, especially if the diarrhea is accompanied by a fever and vomiting. Keep your child home from daycare until:

- there is no fever

- the child is adequately hydrated and no longer acting sick

- the stools are no longer watery, explosive, or bloody

During the recovery stage of gastroenteritis, be prepared for your child's stools to remain more frequent and looser for several weeks while the intestines are healing. This is called the *convalescent stage* of intestinal illness, during which your baby is no longer contagious and may attend daycare.

Head lice. Most school nurses and daycare providers are unnecessarily "nitpickers" and may ban your child from school or daycare until they no longer see the nits. The Committee on Infectious Diseases of the American Academy of Pediatrics (AAP) discourages "no nit" policies in schools and daycare because even though head lice are a nuisance and can be transmitted easily from child to child, they don't carry disease.

Impetigo. Impetigo is a skin infection common in preschool-age children. When the normal skin barrier to germs has been broken down (such as by irritation, a cut, scratch, or bite), bacteria such as staph or strep can infect the irritated skin, resulting in dime-sized blisters that may ooze a honey-colored pus. If the impetigo is mild, being treated with appropriate antibiotic ointment, and covered with a bandage, your child may attend daycare. Be sure to cut his fingernails short and show and tell him not to touch or rub the infected areas. If the impetigo is widespread to the extent that the infected areas cannot be covered, it is wise to keep your child home from daycare or school for at least forty-eight hours after the antibiotic treatment has begun. (For more information, see page 378.)

DEHYDRATION

Your child has been sick for three days, refuses to eat, may be vomiting and have diarrhea, will only take a few sips of juice, seems less active, and is urinating less often than usual. You begin to worry about dehydration. Here are some tips to help you determine how dehydrated your child might be and what steps you can take to evaluate and correct this.

Symptoms

Signs of adequate hydration. If your child has most or all of the following signs, then

you can be reasonably sure he is not significantly dehydrated:

- moist, shiny mouth from saliva, pools of
  saliva under tongue or lips

- moisture present in eyes, tears dripping out
  when crying

- urinating at least every four hours

- active, playful, running around, tearing up
  the toy room

Mild dehydration. Most children will
become mildly dehydrated during the course
of any illness simply because they won't drink
as much as usual. This is not dangerous. Common signs of mild dehydration include:

- less activity than usual, but still alert and
  playful

- lips slightly dry

- urinating slightly less frequently

Moderate dehydration. Many children will
progress to this stage during an illness. In general, this stage is not dangerous, but proper
hydrating measures are needed. Signs include:

- less active and playful, but still alert

- lips are dry and chapped, inside of mouth is
  slightly dry

- no tears when crying, but eyes still appear
  moist

- urinating about half as often as usual

- urine concentrated yellow

Severe dehydration. Children rarely reach
this stage. If they do, however, immediate
medical attention is required. Signs include:

- limp, inactive, makes minimal eye contact,
  and does not respond to your voice or
  touch — the definition of lethargic

- lips chapped, inside of mouth is dry and
  sticky with no saliva

- no tears, eyes are dry and sunken in

- no urination for twelve to eighteen hours,
  along with these other symptoms

- extremely unusual fussiness along with the
  other symptoms

 **DR. SEARS TIP
Not Enough Wet Diapers?**

Most parents worry about dehydration more
than necessary. We get many calls in the office
from worried parents saying, "My sick baby
hasn't peed all day." If the child's overall signs
and behavior fit in the mildly dry category,
that's okay. Many routine illnesses may cause
mild dehydration, which is harmless. In order
to progress to moderate or severe dehydration, a child really needs to be experiencing
vomiting and/or diarrhea. Most fevers, colds,
and sore throats don't make a child dry
enough to cause worry.

What to Do for Mild to Moderate Dehydration

First, read the relevant sections of this
book for specific treatment ideas on the
source of your child's dehydration (vomiting,
diarrhea, fever, cough, throat infection,
mouth sores).

Most children can stay adequately hydrated
or rehydrated by taking small, frequent sips of
clear liquids such as:

- breast milk
- white grape juice diluted by half with water
- Pedialyte or other oral electrolyte solutions
- frozen juice slushy

What to Do for Severe Dehydration

Go to the ER. If your child is severely dehydrated, go to the nearest emergency room for evaluation and intravenous fluids. This state is too serious to attempt home rehydration.

DENTAL PROBLEMS

Kids can experience a variety of dental illnesses and emergencies. Yet often a dentist isn't available after hours if something urgent arises. Here is our guide to several of the tooth-related problems you may encounter with your child and what you can do.

Tooth Trauma—Fracture, Chip, or Knocked Loose

No matter how watchful parents are, toddlers and young children are still bound to trip and fall, and those teeth are sometimes the first thing to hit the ground (or any other hard surface). It is not always clear what to do in an after-hours dental emergency. Try calling your own dentist for advice. Some pediatric dentists provide emergency care, and you may be able to find one in a phone book or get a referral from a friend or neighbor. Don't automatically just go to an emergency room. Call ahead and find out if they even provide emergency dental services with an on-call dentist. Most smaller emergency rooms probably don't.

Tooth knocked loose or pushed back. Mildly loosened teeth often heal well without any intervention. The main worry is that if the tooth is knocked too far out of place or pushed too far up into the gums, the root may be damaged and the tooth may eventually die. This isn't much of a concern for baby teeth. Adult teeth, on the other hand, can be expensive to replace. Deciding what should be done with the tooth is a case-by-case decision. If an adult tooth is extremely loose or pushed far out of place or up into the gums, it may be worth it to try to maneuver the tooth back into place in order to improve the chance that the root will survive. The sooner this is done, the better, even if it is after hours. If the tooth is barely loose or only slightly knocked out of place or barely pushed up into the gums, this can wait until the next morning to be seen by a dentist.

Tooth knocked out. When baby teeth are knocked completely out, it's often not worth the trauma of trying to re-implant them. There are, however, some advantages to maintaining proper spacing of the eventual adult teeth by re-implanting a baby tooth. For kids four and older, the adult teeth are just a couple years away; re-implanting a baby tooth is probably not necessary. For younger kids, it may be more worthwhile. It is useful to place the tooth into a glass of milk until you can get to a dentist.

Tooth fractures or chips. The first rule of a chipped or broken tooth is find the missing piece! It will make the dentist's job, and the cosmetic outcome, much better. If almost half of the tooth is broken off, this may involve the living center of the tooth (the pulp); the sooner this is reattached, the better. You can keep the broken piece in milk. If the chip is only a small corner or the tip of the tooth, this can wait until the next day.

Lacerations Within the Mouth from Dental Trauma

Large cuts or gashes on the inside of the mouth are common in face and dental injuries. If the teeth are intact, and the only problem is an internal cut, don't worry. This doesn't need to be stitched or seen in an urgent care center. We don't suture lacerations inside the mouth. If the cut went all the way through to the outside of the face, this is another story. The outside may need to be stitched if it is gaping. Such "through and through" cuts may also require antibiotics to prevent infection.

Dental Abscesses

A child can develop a deep infection within the gums around the root of a tooth. This will present as mild tooth pain that quickly increases over one or two days to a pretty tough toothache. You will notice a red, painful, swollen lump on the gums that is very tender to the touch. The nearby tooth will also be tender when you press firmly on it. This isn't really an emergency if you notice it after hours (unless there is fever). Ibuprofen can help with the pain. Call your dentist in the morning for an urgent appointment. It's better to have a dentist examine an abscess. If your dentist isn't available, see your regular doctor. An antibiotic will probably be prescribed, which will begin treating the infection until you can see the dentist.

It is important not to be fooled by a simple canker sore. This can act just like an abscess from a pain-and-tenderness standpoint. But when you look way up between the cheek and gums, you'll see an obvious canker sore and won't need to waste a trip to the doctor.

Cavities

No matter how well you brush your child's teeth, cavities can still happen. We won't take the time to explain all the ins and outs of how to find and fix cavities. We have witnessed a very wide range of opinions from various dentists on how aggressive to be with cavities, sedation, and choice of filling material to use. We don't believe there is a right or wrong approach to pediatric dentistry. But we do recommend you obtain more than one opinion if any dentist suggests an approach that feels too invasive to you. Here are some of our thoughts:

Should you get the cavity fixed? Some believe that every cavity should be fixed right away and others take a wait-and-see approach, observing minor cavities and only fixing those that worsen over time. Our experience with our own children has been a less aggressive approach. If a minor cavity is spotted, but hasn't gone too deep and is in a baby tooth that will fall out in a few years anyway, we believe you can wait and observe it, if your dentist agrees. On the other hand, some cavities, especially those on the molar, might go unnoticed until significant decay occurs. These may not be able to wait.

Should you use heavy sedation, full anesthesia, or try to get it done without? This really depends on the child and the location and number of cavities. One of our young kids had a cavity in a front tooth at an early age that wasn't too deep yet. One dentist suggested we do general anesthesia in her office to make the procedure as easy as possible. We didn't feel comfortable with that. We got a second opinion and elected to have it filled while it was still an easy job to do, instead of waiting. We decided to try to go without sedation. After some squirming and fussing by our child, we consented to some nitrous oxide (laughing gas) to take the edge off. And it did. The procedure went very easily, and our child was able to sit right on Mom's lap the whole time. Another one of our young kids used an oral sedative called Versed for a cavity repair, which also went well.

Our personal preference is to try fixing cavities with minimal sedation if possible. However, we do realize that kids with multiple cavities, especially in the back of the mouth, probably do need some extra sedation. Some will even need general anesthesia. You shouldn't proceed with any such procedure until you are comfortable with the dentist you've chosen and have gotten more than one opinion.

DEVELOPMENTAL DELAY

Every baby develops at his own unique pace. Some will walk by eight months, and others will take their own sweet time and take the first steps around fifteen months. Some will talk up a storm by fifteen months, and others will be just starting their first words. In this section we will give you some general guidelines on how to determine if your baby's development is delayed enough to worry. We will only be focusing on motor and social development in this section (movement skills). For speech delay, see page 488. For autism, see page 167.

Signs

Development varies greatly, so it's not always easy to determine when a baby is delayed enough to warrant therapy. In part II of this book, we show you the expected milestones for every age and checkup with your doctor. Any infant who is two to three months or more behind in any major milestone should be evaluated by the doctor. *The milestones and ages listed below are delayed ages, not the usual expected ages.*

Gross motor delay. These are the major body movement and strength skills. If your baby is missing any one of the following by the indicated age, let your doctor know:

- lifting head up off the floor during tummy time by four months

- rolling over both ways by seven months

- sitting up for at least a few seconds by nine months

- crawling or scooting along on bottom by twelve months

- pulling self up to standing while holding on to couch by fourteen months

- taking walking steps alone by seventeen months

Fine motor delay. These are the coordination and hand and eye movement skills. If your baby is missing any one of the following by the indicated age, let your doctor know:

- following you with eyes from side to side and grasping firmly on to your finger by four months

- reaching out purposefully and attempting to grab on to an object (such as a rattle) by six months

- accurately and playfully grabbing a toy quickly by nine months

- using pincer grasp (thumb and forefinger) or holding a cup to drink by twelve months

- pointing with index finger or stacking blocks during play by fifteen months

- attempting to feed self with spoon or mimicking actions like hair brushing or talking on the phone by eighteen months

Social delay. These are the interactive skills that a child develops. Let your doctor know if your baby is missing any one of the following:

- smiling responsively by four months

- laughing out loud; emitting various types of cries and waving hands or kicking legs to indicate wanting something by six months

- mimicking facial expressions and sounds and interacting with self in mirror by nine months

- responding to name, waving bye-bye, and lifting arms to be picked up by twelve months

- understanding *no* and other simple words and looking around to find something when you say "where is _____" by fifteen months

- recognizing facial parts, asking for something by pointing, and laughing at funny things by eighteen months

Just because your child isn't doing one of these items doesn't necessarily mean there is cause for concern. But your doctor should be made aware of it so he can do a thorough overall developmental assessment.

DR. SEARS TIP
Attachment Parenting –
the Best Rx for Development

Science is very clear on this point: attachment parenting (a continuous hands-on, face-to-face, interactive style of parenting) stimulates babies to develop faster in all areas. If your baby is beginning to show any delay, increase the Baby B's of attachment parenting. See page 160.

Risk Factors for Delay

Any baby can show some delay, but certain babies have a higher risk and should be watched more closely:

- premature babies

- babies with a difficult delivery

- babies with birth defects

- babies with a recognized neurological disorder such as seizures

- babies who needed to be hospitalized for illness in the early months

- babies exposed to illicit drugs or alcohol during pregnancy

- babies with older siblings with significant delays or autism

Treatment

A wait-and-see approach is definitely not the way to go if a significant delay has been identified. Here are some very important steps you need to take.

Become your baby's personal therapist.
No one can provide the daily stimulation a
baby needs like Mom and Dad. You have
probably already been doing this all along, but
you might need to step it up a bit. The more
you interact socially with your child with animated facial expressions, talking, singing, smiling, and laughing, the faster all areas of
development will progress. You should also
pay attention to the motor skills, but not at
the expense of social stimulation.

State-funded evaluations. Most counties in
the country have a state-funded program that
will do a thorough developmental evaluation
on your baby and provide the appropriate
stimulation services on a weekly basis. Take
advantage of this free service; it's your tax dollars at work.

Private therapy. Many insurances are beginning to pay for developmental therapy. Parents
who have the insurance can supplement their
baby's therapy with a private occupational or
language therapist. Social skills classes can
also be attended with other infants and
parents.

DIABETES IN CHILDREN

Diabetes is an illness that causes the body to
not make enough insulin (Type-1 diabetes) or
not utilize insulin efficiently (Type-2 diabetes).
Here are the most important points parents
should know about preventing the disease
and treating the child with diabetes:

Type-1 Diabetes

Type-1 diabetes (which used to be called juvenile or insulin-dependent diabetes) can start
anytime in infancy or childhood. Unlike in diabetes in adults and Type-2 diabetes, which can
come on very gradually, in Type-1 diabetes in
children the pancreas suddenly stops producing insulin, causing the child to get very sick
very fast (over just a few days).

Signs and Symptoms

Signs and symptoms of Type-1 diabetes
include the following:

Child urinates frequently. In order to flush
out the high blood sugar that's accumulating
in your child's bloodstream, the kidneys produce more urine. This is often one of the earliest signs of diabetes.

Child often complains of thirst. Because
the child is urinating so much and losing so
much fluid, she will often complain of being
very thirsty.

Dehydration and weight loss. Losing a lot
of fluid very fast causes the child to get tired,
lethargic, and dehydrated, with dry mouth, dry
eyes, and dry skin, and to quickly lose weight.

Rapid breathing. The high blood sugar
causes chemicals called *ketones* to build up in
the blood, which, in turn, cause the child to
breathe fast. You may even smell the ketones
on his "fruity" breath.

Treatment

Once your pediatrician examines your child
and puts all these clues together, your child
will be hospitalized immediately, rehydrated
with intravenous fluids, and given insulin to
bring down the high blood glucose. This biochemical state is called *diabetic ketoacidosis*,
and it is a medical emergency that doctors are
trained to recognize right away. In an otherwise well or slightly ill child, you wouldn't

need to wonder whether he had diabetes. Because these symptoms occur so quickly, over a matter of days, you are unlikely to miss it.

Type-2 Diabetes

Unlike Type-1 diabetes, which is a genetic or immunologic non-preventable disease, Type-2 diabetes is nearly always due to preventable unhealthy lifestyle and nutrition habits. With Type-2 diabetes the child's pancreas still produces insulin, but because of a metabolic quirk the cells become resistant to the effects of insulin, which is why this type of diabetes is called *insulin-resistant diabetes*. There are millions of microscopic "doors" on each cell of the body, and insulin acts like a "doorman" to usher just the right amount of sugar into the cells for energy. In this type of diabetes, these "doors" don't open efficiently, preventing insulin from doing its job. It could also be called an *insulin inefficiency*.

Signs and Symptoms

Unlike those with Type-1 diabetes, most children with Type-2 diabetes don't look or act very sick. Some may urinate a bit more frequently and be a bit more thirsty. (Drinking a lot of liquids in an otherwise well child is seldom a sign of diabetes, even though pediatricians frequently get the question "He drinks a lot. Could he have diabetes?")

The most common clue that your child may be pre-diabetic is a large waist size. Excess abdominal fat, also dubbed *pre-diabetic fat,* increases the risk of developing Type-2 diabetes because this excess fat churns out biochemicals that interfere with the action of insulin.

If your doctor suspects pre-diabetes, he may order blood tests, such as blood sugar, blood cholesterol, and a general lipid panel. Children, especially teens, with Type-2 diabetes are often more prone to develop the "highs"— high blood pressure, high blood sugar, high blood cholesterol — a cluster of biochemical problems known as the *metabolic syndrome*.

Causes

The two most common causes of Type-2 diabetes are eating junk food and sitting too much. In fact, the epidemic of junk-food eating and too much sitting has led the Centers for Disease Control (CDC) (the government think-tank that predicts health trends) to issue a shocking prediction that unless American families change their eating habits and lifestyle, one in three children is destined to later become diabetic. This dire prediction refers to Type-2 diabetes.

Risk Factors

Genetic risk. Some cultures have a higher risk of developing Type-2 diabetes, including African Americans, Native Americans, Hispanics, and Pacific Islanders.

Obesity. The good news is that obesity is preventable. Because the risk of obese children developing Type-2 diabetes is climbing higher and higher, most pediatricians now describe obese children as pre-diabetic.

Look for the following risk factors in your child:

- eats a lot of fast food and packaged foods
- drinks a lot of sweetened beverages
- has increasing waist size and extra abdominal fat
- has a large, stocky body type

- has a family history of diabetes, or one or both parents have a large body type

- craves sweets and other refined carbs

Prevention

- Reread the section on healthy eating and our L.E.A.N. Kids Program, page 417.

- Avoid sweetened beverages.

- Avoid foods with high-fructose corn syrup.

- Follow the rule of twos: eat *twice* as often, *half* as much, and chew *twice* as long. Grazers have steadier levels of blood sugar.

- Get lots of exercise. Children who move a lot tend to put on less excess abdominal fat. A lean waist is one of the top preventive medicines for Type-2 diabetes.

For more about the effects of diet and exercise on diabetes, see these two references by the Drs. Sears: *The Healthiest Kid in the Neighborhood* and *Dr. Sears L.E.A.N. Kids.*

DIAPER RASH

Diaper rash is something that every parent and infant will have to deal with at some point, especially in the baby's first year of life. The following section will give you some tips on how to minimize this problem.

Causes

Infants have extremely sensitive skin around the diaper area. The combination of a moist environment, exposure to urine and feces, and the rubbing of the diaper makes fertile ground for diaper rash. Baby's skin can become irritated and cracked, and may even bleed. To make matters worse, bacteria and/or yeast can take advantage of this situation and make diaper rash worse.

Prevention

Some babies won't get diaper rash. However, most babies do suffer flare-ups from time to time. Here's how to help prevent diaper rash:

Make frequent diaper changes. Stools are very irritating to young skin. Newborns should have their diapers changed at least every two hours. You can wait a little longer after the first few weeks. However, always change your newborn's diaper as soon as you notice it is wet and/or contains stool.

Try different brands. Baby may be sensitive to certain chemicals or fibers. Switch brands, try organic or even cloth diapers, until you find one that's friendly to Baby's bottom.

Clean the diaper area well. This helps keep Baby's skin rash-free.

Use unscented baby wipes. The chemicals in scented wipes can irritate the skin.

Use clear diaper ointment. Petrolatum or lanolin products are great for treating and preventing mild rashes.

Use white zinc oxide cream. Your baby may need this thicker cream. There are several brands containing zinc oxide, the best barrier to use for preventing and controlling diaper rash.

What to Do

Even the most diligent parent can't prevent the occasional diaper rash flare-up. Here are some ways to get these under control:

Rinse off Baby's bottom with water. Wiping the area of diaper rash with baby wipes can cause further irritation and worsen the flare-up. Instead, use a bulb syringe with water to gently wash away the stool and urine from the baby's diaper area. If some urine or feces remains, gently blot with a baby wipe.

Use more generous amounts of diaper cream during flare-ups. Zinc-oxide diaper cream is good for mild-to-moderate diaper rashes. We recommend Triple Paste or Butt Paste (available over the counter [OTC] at pharmacies or drugstores) for rashes that are more severe. Apply diaper cream with every change.

DR. SEARS TIP
Air It Out

Let Baby go without a diaper as much as possible — at least a half hour, several times a day a day, if not more. One good way to do this is to lay Baby down on a towel bottom-end-up without any diaper cream on. Air is great for soothing an irritated diaper area.

Different Types of Diaper Rash

There are several different culprits that may lead to diaper rash.

Contact diaper rash. This is the typical type of diaper rash discussed above, caused by Baby's sensitive bottom coming into contact with diapers and stools.

Yeast rash. This rash appears as a solid red, lightly raised area around the anus and/or genitalia with scattered red bumps spreading outward. It is treated with an OTC anti-fungal cream. See page 542 for details.

Seborrhea diaper rash. This is a skin condition that can affect the face, neck, scalp, and even the diaper area. It appears as a scaly, red, flaky rash that can be quite itchy and irritating. Your pediatrician can diagnose the diaper rash as a seborrhea diaper rash. Treatment usually involves using a steroid cream (such as 1 percent over-the-counter hydrocortisone) two to three times a day. Do *not* use steroid creams for more than a week unless instructed to do so by the doctor.

Impetigo. This bacterial infection of the skin can occur on any area of the body, including the diaper area. Impetigo appears as a red, blister-type rash with a honey-colored crust. Treatment involves a prescription antibiotic ointment as instructed by your physician. See page 378 for more on impetigo.

Bacterial pimples. Some babies (especially toddlers) will have numerous red pimples with small white heads that differ from the oozing, crusty patches of impetigo. These are caused by bacteria in the stool. Treatment involves washing the bottom more frequently with warm soapy water and applying OTC or prescription antibiotic ointment, if it persists.

Intertrigo. This rash can occur in skin folds on any area of the body. The skin creases in the groin area are especially susceptible to intertrigo. It is caused by the constant friction of skin on skin, and the skin inside the folds will have a red, burn-like appearance. Intertrigo is usually effectively treated with clear diaper ointments.

Allergy rashes. Rashes may also be a sign that your baby is allergic to some type of food. An allergy rash will usually appear as a reddish ring around the baby's anus. It can be caused by certain foods in a mother's diet that the infant gets through the breast milk. Common culprits are acidic foods (such as citrus and tomato-based foods), wheat products, and dairy products. There are many other potential causes of allergies that can lead to diaper rash. Breastfeeding moms may need to eliminate certain foods from their diet if they notice their babies have flare-ups when they eat these foods. See Food Allergies, page 327, for more information.

Chafing rash. Older toddlers experience a lot more diaper friction from running, climbing, and bending. It's typical to have some dry, red patches on the buttocks and legs from the waist and leg bands. A clear ointment (or potty training!) will help minimize this irritation.

See your pediatrician if your baby has a rash that does not improve after a week of treatment or is getting worse. Regular well visits are also a good time to discuss diaper rash with your pediatrician. If your baby has a rash at the doctor visit, show it to the doctor. Pediatricians have a lot of experience in distinguishing one type of diaper rash from another. The good news is that as children get older, particularly after the first year, diaper rash becomes much less of a problem.

DIARRHEA

Diarrhea is an unpleasant experience for everyone involved, from the child who suffers through the intestinal discomfort to the parent in charge of cleaning up the mess. Fortunately, most causes of diarrhea are not serious and will pass without any treatment. Here are some guidelines to help you and your child get through this messy experience without too much trouble.

Symptoms

Diarrhea is defined by:

Increased frequency. If your child begins having bowel movements more than twice as often as usual, this may indicate an intestinal condition.

Looser consistency. If the stools become more loose, watery, mucousy, green, or runny than usual, this is considered a significant change.

Rest assured that all infants and children will have brief changes in stool consistency as a normal part of life. If you see one or two stools that are suddenly different from normal, don't worry yet. Wait until your child has had several diarrhea stools before you begin to track down the cause.

Causes

Milk protein allergy. This is the most common non-infectious cause of diarrhea in infants and toddlers. Breastfed babies can be allergic to cow's-milk proteins in Mom's diet that pass through the breast milk. Formula-fed infants may be allergic to a milk-based formula. Toddlers tend to eat more dairy products and may begin to experience more discomfort.

Allergic diarrhea doesn't usually cause sudden symptoms, such as fevers and vomiting, as infectious illnesses do (see below). Instead, allergic diarrhea tends to be more chronic, without other signs of illness besides mild abdominal discomfort. Wheat and soy allergy are the next most common culprits in allergic diarrhea.

Infectious diarrhea. A variety of bacteria and viruses can cause diarrhea, usually accompanied by fever and vomiting. The presence of these infectious symptoms is a sure sign that your child's diarrhea is infectious instead of allergic.

- Viruses — Rotavirus and the flu are the two most commonly identified viral diarrhea illnesses. There are several others as well, but because none are treatable, it usually isn't necessary to determine which virus is the culprit.

- Bacteria — *E. coli* and salmonella are the most common bacterial causes and are often due to food poisoning. Several others are also possible. The most notable feature of bacterial diarrhea that sets it apart from all other causes is blood in the stool. Bloody diarrhea can indicate a severe bacterial infectious diarrhea that should be evaluated by a doctor.

- Parasites — A variety of intestinal parasites can be contracted during travel to third-world countries. A telltale sign of parasitic diarrhea is watery stools that last more than two weeks.

Diarrhea due to antibiotic use. Many children get one or two courses of antibiotics each year, and this is a fairly common cause of diarrhea. In most cases the diarrhea is tolerable and can be minimized with probiotics (see Treatment, below) while the antibiotic is continued. If the diarrhea is severe and/or bloody, stop the antibiotic and contact your doctor. See Treating Antibiotic Side Effects, page 551.

When Not to Worry

Most infectious cases of diarrhea, whether bacterial or viral, will resolve without any special treatment. As long as your child is adequately hydrated, is feeling generally well, and has no blood in the stools, you can rest assured she should get better within a week or two.

Fever, abdominal pain, and vomiting are often an expected part of the initial phase of diarrhea illnesses and are usually not an indication that anything more serious is going on. See the sections on these specific symptoms to determine when you should seek medical attention.

When to Worry

Here are some signs that indicate you should seek medical care from your doctor within one day:

- bloody diarrhea

- moderate dehydration — see page 267 for information on how to gauge your child's level of dehydration.

- accompanying fever for more than three days

- jaundice — yellow eyes or skin; this may indicate viral hepatitis, which should be evaluated by a doctor

- weight loss or lethargy

Treatment

Allergic diarrhea. If you suspect your infant or child has allergic diarrhea, the first step is to eliminate the most common cause — cow's-milk products. A breastfeeding mom should eliminate these from her diet for about three weeks to rule this out. If formula-feeding, change to a soy-based infant formula and let your doctor know at your next checkup. For toddlers and older, take cow's milk, yogurt, and cheese out of their diet for three weeks (see page 330 for more details).

Infectious diarrhea. There is no medical treatment for viral diarrhea. Even most bacterial causes aren't treated with antibiotics, which can make diarrhea worse. Some are, however, and your pediatrician can decide if treatment is needed if the diarrhea is bloody.

Home Treatment

Other than antibiotics, there are no prescription treatments for diarrhea. You can safely try the following treatment steps to improve your child's diarrhea no matter what the cause:

- Give probiotics — commonly known as acidophilus, these are the beneficial bacteria that normally live in our intestines and help keep our digestive system is healthy. Infections, allergies, and antibiotics can deplete these useful germs. See page 551 for details.

- Feed the BRAT diet — feeding your child bananas, rice or rice cereal, applesauce, and toast or bread for several days can minimize the diarrhea.

- Avoid certain foods — minimize cow's milk intake, avoid apple, pear, and cherry juice (the particular type of natural sugar in these can worsen diarrhea), and limit stool-softening fruits, such as plums and peaches, until your child's diarrhea improves.

- Keep your child hydrated — diluted white grape juice (half water) is one of the best hydrating drinks. Oral electrolyte solutions are okay but usually not necessary unless directed by a physician.

- Use soy formula — prolonged diarrhea can irritate the intestines to such a degree that they lose their ability to digest milk-based infant formula. Switch to soy formula until the diarrhea resolves.

- Use extra diaper rash cream — don't wait for a rash to appear. Liberally apply any zinc oxide white diaper cream with each diaper change to stay ahead of the irritation. See Diaper Rash, page 275, for more ideas if the rash worsens.

Over-the-counter anti-diarrhea medications should not be used in children twelve years and younger unless directed by a physician. By slowing down the stools, the toxins secreted by the infectious germs will cause more inflammation to the intestines and may worsen your child's condition. Older children can better tolerate these toxins and will greatly appreciate the relief such medications provide.

What Your Pediatrician Can Do

Infectious bacteria or parasite. If a bacterial infection is suspected, the doctor can send stool samples to a laboratory for testing. It usually takes two to three days to get results. Viral causes can also be tested for if you and the doctor wish to confirm that a severe case is just rotavirus. Your doctor can also assess the level of dehydration to determine if a trip to the emergency room for intravenous (IV) fluids is necessary.

Allergic diarrhea. If you suspect this cause, but a dairy-free diet doesn't give relief, the doctor can order blood tests for food allergies to look for other offending foods.

Antibiotic reaction. Rarely, a child will experience chronic loose stools for months or longer after antibiotic use. This can indicate persistent intestinal yeast overgrowth. Probiotics may be enough to fight off the yeast, but your doctor may prescribe an anti-yeast medication for a few weeks. Stool tests can be done to confirm yeast.

DIMPLE, SACRAL

If you notice a tiny "hole" near the base of your baby's spine, this is called a *sacral dimple*. As the two sides of your baby's spinal bones grow together in the womb, the skin covering the spinal bones is left with a crease marking where the bones have grown together. Sometimes an opening remains in the crease of skin, called a *dimple*. Your doctor may point this out to you during your baby's routine checkup.

What to Do

Most of these dimples are a harmless remnant of embryonic growth and need no treatment. Yet some of these openings may extend deeply into the skin and form a connection to the spinal cord. Medically this is known as a *tethered cord*, which means the spinal cord is connected to the skin below the birthmark. A tethered cord needs to be surgically relieved so it does not affect the growth of the spinal cord. Dimples that cause no harm and need no treatment have these characteristics:

• They are shallow. Often the doctor can see the bottom of the "hole" with a penlight.

• They are low down — they occur beneath the line where the buttock folds begin.

• They are tiny and do not contain any hair or extra tissue growth.

Sacral dimples that may need treatment or surgical removal have these signs:

• They tend to occur higher on the spine.

• They have hair growing in them.

• They have a skin tag or a mole growing out of them.

• They are deeper.

If you are uncertain how deep the dimple extends, your pediatrician may order an ultrasound or MRI of the lower spine to detect whether or not the dimple extends into the spinal cord and warrants treatment. A dimple that is higher on the spine and has a visible growth on it can be like the tip of the iceberg signifying various degrees of defects in the spinal cord, such as spina bifida. An MRI would reveal this.

DROOLING

Once teeth start pushing their way through the gums, the saliva faucet turns on. In fact, any irritation in the mouth (such as a toothache, a canker sore, or teething) increases saliva production. There is a normal balance between saliva production and saliva swallowing. But some babies produce saliva faster than they can swallow, leading to excess drooling.

Saliva sounds. When your child is going through what we dub "drool days" (usually just before new teeth are about to erupt), expect a whole symphony of throaty sounds. When saliva puddles in the back of the throat the air flowing through the saliva produces a variety of throaty noises which we dub:

• "gurgles" for noises in the back of the throat

- "snurgles" for sounds that are a combination of a snort and a gurgle that seem to be coming from the back of the nose

- "blurp" or "burble" for the burping sound passing through the saliva

While excess saliva can cause a few quirky sounds and rashes, saliva prepares the intestines to handle solid food and facilitate digestion. Here's how:

- Saliva contains a substance called *epidermal growth factor,* which helps mature the intestinal lining.

- Saliva neutralizes stomach acid and helps heal and lubricate the lining of the esophagus that may have been irritated by Baby's frequent spit-ups and regurgitation of stomach acids.

- Saliva contains enzymes to help pre-digest solid foods before they hit the intestines.

What to Do

While saliva is important for the body, here are some ways to handle some of the nuisances of excess drooling:

Prevent the drool rash. Drool rash is like a diaper rash on the cheeks and chin. When chubby cheeks rub against a drool-soaked bedsheet, a rash develops. Dab excess drool off the skin with lukewarm water and pat dry. Use a barrier ointment, such as Aquaphor or Soothe and Heal, just before naptime and bedtime. Lanolin ointment works too.

Prepare for drool stools. Another nuisance of this drippy stage is that just as the face end reacts to excess saliva, so does the bottom end. Saliva is a natural laxative, so expect looser stools and more diaper rash during

teething times. Apply barrier cream around Baby's anus just as you did on her face.

Once the teeth are in and Baby's swallowing mechanism matures enough to catch up with the saliva production, this drippy stage will pass.

 DR. SEARS TIP
The Saliva "Cold"

Excess saliva that puddles in the back of the throat can cause a cough, sort of like postnasal drip. In fact, when you place your hand on the back of your baby's chest, the rattle you feel and hear is not really coming from the chest but from the air passing through the puddles of saliva in the back of the throat. This is not really a cold (saliva rarely runs through the nose), but just the normal throaty noises of drool days. Whereas colds are noisier at night, saliva throaty noises subside because saliva production naturally lessens during sleep.

DYSLEXIA

The term *dyslexia* is the name given to a specific type of learning disability that usually presents in childhood. Approximately one in every five people in the United States has some type of learning and/or reading disability. The majority of reading and learning disabilities are attributed to dyslexia.

Symptoms

When most people think of dyslexia, they imagine individuals who mix up their letters or read words backward (for instance, the word *saw* appearing like the word *was*). The truth is that this is only part of the problem of dyslexia, and mixing letters or words up is quite common in young children. In fact, there are actually many different types and forms of dyslexia.

Signs of dyslexia can be difficult to distinguish from normal childhood reading and development. Before your child reaches school age, some early signs of dyslexia may include:

- beginning to talk late

- difficulty with short sentences

- difficulty rhyming words

- adding new words to vocabulary slowly

Possible signs of dyslexia in school-age children (children six years of age or older) may include:

- reading words more slowly than their peers

- difficulty recognizing different words and letters on a page

- reversing letters that appear similar (such as replacing "d" with "b")

- reversing words containing the same letters (the above-mentioned reversal of *was* for *saw*)

- trying to read words from right to left

- difficulty recognizing spacing patterns in a series of words

- difficulty with sounding out or pronouncing many types of words

- reading at a lower than expected level for their given age

It is important to know that before the age of six, many of the above-mentioned signs occur in children who do not have dyslexia. However, the problems stated above persist in children who have dyslexia. Some parent may fear that dyslexia is a sign of lower intelligence. In fact, most people who suffer from dyslexia have average or above-average intelligence.

Causes

Researchers are still trying to pinpoint a specific cause of dyslexia. It is believed that dyslexia is caused by problems in specific areas of the brain concerned with language and processing words. We do know, however, that dyslexia appears to run in families and therefore most likely has a genetic basis.

Diagnosis and Treatment

Most cases of dyslexia are not diagnosed until the child starts school and concerns arise among the teacher and/or parents that the child may not be reading as well as the other children. Treatment of dyslexia depends upon how severe the disability is. Most cases of dyslexia can be treated very successfully with the help of several specialists, including a speech or language therapist, an educational therapist,

 DR. SEARS TIP
Don't Delay an Evaluation

The earlier dyslexia is diagnosed, the better the long-term outcome. Parents, if you have any concerns that your child may not be "up to speed" in the classroom, talk immediately to your child's teachers and pediatrician about your concerns.

and occasionally child psychologists. Thankfully, most children with dyslexia are able to stay in a regular classroom and do not require long-term remedial education.

Long-Term Complications

Some children with dyslexia will suffer some type of emotional and psychological difficulties from the stigma of this type of learning disability. Sadly, those that suffer the most are those that don't get the help they need, especially if that help does not come at an early age. Children who struggle with dyslexia may withdraw from reading because they feel embarrassed or "stupid." This can turn into a vicious cycle that will only get worse unless the child gets some help. It can cause a further stunting of intellectual and emotional growth. Unfortunately, some people with dyslexia never get the help they need, and the problems continue into adolescence, young adulthood, and even later in life.

The good news is we are much better at recognizing dyslexia now than in years past. Today a child with dyslexia can be properly diagnosed and treated, whereas previously the child may have only been labeled "slow" or "of lower intelligence" and may have never had the chance to get that help.

EARACHES

Nearly every child experiences at least one earache, especially during infancy and the preschool years. Unfortunately, earaches usually come at the most inconvenient times, such as in the middle of the night or while traveling. Here are some causes of sore ears and methods to relieve the pain:

Causes

There are two areas of a child's ear that may get sore:

Middle ear pain. As fluid builds up in the middle ear cavity due to either infection or allergy, it causes pressure on the eardrum. Also, the same fluid that drips from a runny nose clogs the eustachian tube — the tiny tube that connects the middle ear to the throat and equalizes the air pressure on both sides of the eardrum. When the eustachian tube gets clogged either by fluid or due to air pressure changes on an airplane, pain in the middle ear results.

Ear canal pain. If the ear canal is inflamed or infected with swimmer's ear, it can also be painful (see page 507 to see how to distinguish between middle ear and ear canal pain).

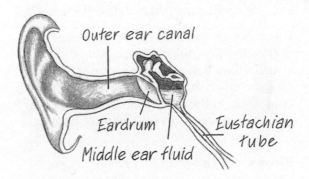

Outer ear canal

Eardrum

Middle ear fluid

Eustachian tube

Treating Generic Ear Pain

When you aren't sure what is causing the pain but need to provide relief until you can see a doctor, try these remedies:

Use gravity. Encourage your child to rest or sleep with the painful ear upward. This allows fluid in the middle ear to drain from the eardrum and reduce pressure.

Clear the nose. The eustachian tubes connect the back of the throat and nose with the ears, so if the nose is stuffy, the eustachian tube is likely to be also. To keep the ears clear of fluid and pain, it's important to clear the stuffy nose. (See nose-hose and steam-clean techniques, page 20.)

Wiggle away the pain. Popping open a plugged eustachian tube can often relieve ear pain. Grab the earlobe between your thumb and forefinger and pull down and out four times. This maneuver pulls on the ear canal structures next to the eustachian tube and may help to pop it open. If this maneuver causes more pain, your child probably has "swimmer's ear." See page 507.

DR. SEARS TIP
Diminished Hearing Is a Clue to Eustachian Tube Blockage

If you notice your child is saying "What?" or seems distant while you are talking to him, suspect fluid behind the eardrum and a plugged eustachian tube from an allergy or a cold. Fluid in the middle ear diminishes hearing, even though the child may not have pain.

Blow away the pain. If you suspect your child's ear pain is due to a clogged eustachian tube (such as during an allergy, cold, or during air travel), have him gently blow up a balloon. Balloon blowing will often pop open the eustachian tube and relieve the pain, just as yawning or squeezing the nose and blowing out pops open the eustachian tubes for adults.

Try eardrops for ear pain. Over the years we have heard many mom-approved natural ear-pain remedies, such as mullein garlic oil, olive oil, and aloe vera oil. While it's preferable to have a doctor examine your baby's ear

before using eardrops, during those middle-of-the-night earaches it's okay to use one of these warm oils, even though you don't know exactly why the ear hurts. Here's how to use them:

- Have your child lie down with the affected ear up.

- Drop four drops of warm (not hot!) oil into your child's ear canal. The oil should easily drip right off your fingertip. To get the oil to reach the painful area, gently pull on the earlobe to help the oil find its way down the canal and soothe the painful eardrum.

Your pediatrician may prescribe anesthetic eardrops and may recommend over-the-counter pain-relieving medications, such as acetaminophen or ibuprofen (see dosages, pages 552 and 553).

EAR, FOREIGN BODY IN

Clues that your child might have a foreign body, such as a toy part or an insect, stuck in the outer ear canal are:

- He admits to putting part of a toy into his ear.

- He complains of hearing a buzzing sound in his outer ear.

- There is a thick, smelly discharge from one ear that can't be attributed to swimmer's ear (see Swimmer's Ear, page 507).

What to Do

As Grandmother advised, "Don't put anything smaller than your elbow into your ear!" If you suspect that something is stuck in your child's ear canal, don't put anything into your child's ear to try to get it out yourself. Better to let the doctor do it by using a special light and forceps or a loop to grab the foreign body. Sometimes the doctor will use an irrigation technique similar to a dental water pick on a low setting to flush out the foreign body and the resultant drainage or wax that has accumulated.

After the foreign body is removed, the doctor will advise you to watch for signs of an external ear infection (see Swimmer's Ear, page 507). Sometimes the lining of the ear canal will be scratched from the foreign body or during removal, making the lining prone to infection.

EAR INFECTIONS (OTITIS MEDIA)

Your infant has a cold for a week, and suddenly one night she wakes up screaming. You take her to see the doctor the next morning and, sure enough, she has an ear infection. This scenario happens to nearly every child at least once. The medical term for ear infection is *otitis media*, which means "inflammation of the middle ear." Your child's hearing depends upon the eardrum and the structures in the middle ear working properly. Repeated infections can scar the eardrum, prevent it from vibrating properly, and interfere with hearing. For this reason, it's important to be vigilant about treating your child's ear infections properly, especially in the early years when your child is developing speech and language abilities.

Signs and Symptoms

With older children, it's easy to know when they have an ear infection because they'll complain of pain and notice they can't hear well out of the infected ear. But in infants and younger children, diagnosing an ear infection may not be so easy. Here are clues you can look for to help you decide when to see your pediatrician:

- Your child exhibits cold signs and symptoms, such as a runny nose, for a few days.

- He seems "sicker" than you would expect with a common cold.

- Eye drainage: "snotty eyes" accompanying a snotty nose may mean an ear infection.

- Your child is increasingly cranky and irritable following a cold.

- Your toddler's behavior deteriorates during a cold.

- He wakes at night in pain.

DR. SEARS TIP
Got an Ear Infection?

Increasingly snotty discharge (eyes and nose) plus increasingly irritable behavior — suspect an ear infection.

- Your child doesn't like to lie flat (the infected fluid presses on the eardrum).

- Fever may or may not be present with an ear infection.

Causes

When a child catches a cold, excess mucus becomes a breeding ground for bacteria, which spread through the nose, throat, and

DR. SEARS TIP
Beware of Drainage

If you see drainage coming out of your child's ear, do not put oil or prescription numbing drops in the ear without your pediatrician's advice. These haven't yet been determined safe to use with a ruptured eardrum, and the pain usually subsides once the fluid pressure has been relieved anyway.

sinuses. The bacteria and secretions migrate up the eustachian tube (the narrow tube that runs between the back of the nose and the ear) and into the middle ear space behind the eardrum, causing an infection. Mucus and pus from the infection collect, causing the eardrum to turn red, inflamed, and bulge outward. This is what the doctor sees when examining the ear. If the pressure from the trapped and infected fluid builds up too much, it can rupture the eardrum, which is when you may notice discharge, like snotty-nose fluid, in the ear canal.

Because a child's eustachian tube is short, wide, and straight, it is easy for germs to travel into the ear during a cold. As your child grows, the eustachian tube becomes longer, narrower, and slants at a more acute angle. This makes it more difficult for germs and fluid to collect in the middle ear. That's why most children outgrow their susceptibility to frequent ear infections.

Middle ear mucus or fluid doesn't always become infected. Chronic allergies or a mild cold may create some harmless fluid buildup, a situation called *serous otitis media*.

What You Can Do

While you're waiting to see the doctor, or in addition to what your pediatrician recommends, try these home remedies:

Give acetaminophen or ibuprofen. Try these over-the-counter pain relievers (see pages 552 and 553 for dosage).

Oil the ears. (See oiling techniques, page 284.) Administering warm mullein garlic oil eardrops (from a health-food store) is a tried-and-true natural pain reliever and antibiotic. Warm olive oil is another option for pain relief.

Have your child lie with the sore ear up. To let gravity keep the infected fluid from pressing on the eardrum, encourage your child to nap and sleep with the infected ear upward.

DR. SEARS TIP
Middle-of-the-Night Earaches

Although doctors and parents have professions that require giving up the right to a full night's sleep, it is seldom necessary to consult your doctor in the middle of the night if your child awakens with an earache unless he seems seriously ill. The only treatment the doctor might offer that you could not manage yourself would be an antibiotic, and this would not immediately relieve the pain or begin to take effect for at least twelve hours. The above treatment steps should be enough to get your child through the night.

What Your Doctor Might Do

Treating an ear infection is a partnership between parents and pediatrician: you comfort your child's pain, boost your child's immune system, and use preventive home remedies; the doctor treats the infection.

"Does my child always need antibiotics for an ear infection?" Not necessarily. New insights into the treatment of middle ear infections reveal that many mild ear infections will often resolve without antibiotics. For mild ear infections, the American Academy of Pediatrics (AAP) recommends the "wait-and-watch" approach. Based on the most recent studies, here is the approach that we use in our pediatric practice:

Watch and wait. If the child has a cold with fluid in the middle ear, but no fever and no bothersome ear pain, we generally do not treat with antibiotics. The fluid will usually drain out of the middle ear on its own (see self-help techniques for clearing plugged eustachian tubes, page 284) and antibiotics are at this stage unnecessary. "Watch" does not mean do nothing, but rather carefully observe your child for signs that she might be getting sicker. "Wait" simply means that the doctor might not immediately prescribe antibiotics, and you can focus on natural treatments instead.

If ears worsen. Remember, fluid trapped anywhere in the body, especially behind the middle ear, is like a culture medium for germs to grow in. If the infection worsens, the doctor may go to Plan B: prescribe antibiotics. *Call your doctor if:*

• Ear pain increases.

• The cold worsens, accompanied by increasing fever and overall discomfort.

Your pediatrician will prescribe the antibiotic according to the severity of your child's ear infection. If it's a mild ear infection, most doctors begin with the standard antibiotic amoxicillin (the pink stuff). If the infection is more severe and/or your child has a past history of not responding well to amoxicillin, your doctor may use Augmentin, which is a combination of amoxicillin and clavulanic acid, a preparation that is effective against many amoxicillin-resistant germs. If your child is allergic to penicillin-derived antibiotics or if these "first-line" antibiotics aren't effective, your doctor may use what are called "second-line" antibiotics, cephalosporins. The doctor's prescribed antibiotic course may vary from five to ten days, depending on the type of antibiotic prescribed, the severity of the infection, and whether or not your child also has an accompanying chest or sinus infection, which usually requires a longer course of antibiotic treatment. Remember, it may take twenty-four hours for the antibiotic to start working, so continue your pain-relieving and comforting home remedies. See page 549 for tips on taking antibiotics and preventing side effects.

Recheck ears. Be sure to complete the whole course of the doctor-prescribed treatment regimen, even if your child "feels better after twenty-four hours." Stopping the antibiotic too soon risks a recurrence. Be sure to have your pediatrician recheck your child's ears, usually a week or so after the treatment is finished. During the recheck, the doctor will examine the eardrum to be sure the infection is completely cleared. He will also check the middle ear to be sure all the fluid has completely drained out. Sometimes the doctor will use a special pneumatic otoscope to check the vibration of the eardrum. Even though it's common and usually harmless for fluid to take a few weeks to drain completely from the middle ear following an infection, if too much middle ear fluid remains for too long, it may restrict the vibration of the eardrum, which can diminish hearing. Also, if the fluid stays there more than a few months it may congeal into a sticky gel, a condition called *glue ear*, which may need to be removed by an ear, nose, and throat (ENT) specialist as an outpatient surgical procedure. This is why ear rechecks are necessary.

DR. SEARS TIP
Keep a Diary

As part of your parent-pediatrician partnership, it's important for you to keep an accurate diary of your child's ear infections: how often they occur, how severe they are, and the treatment that works best. This information is vitally important to a doctor to know if and when a child needs antibiotic treatment, which antibiotic to prescribe, and how long to use it. For example, if several entries in your diary reveal that the last two times he had a cold it progressed into an ear infection, the doctor may bypass the "watch and wait" stage and go directly to antibiotic treatment.

You may have several entries that reveal "that antibiotic didn't work" or "that antibiotic gave her horrible diarrhea." This information will be helpful to your pediatrician when prescribing an antibiotic.

Prevention

Infants and preschool children are more prone to ear infections for two reasons: their immune systems are still developing, and the short, wide, horizontal eustachian tube allows infected secretions to easily go from the nose and throat to the middle ear. As your child grows, the immune system strengthens and the eustachian tube becomes longer, narrower, and at more of an angle so that secretions do not accumulate within the middle ear as easily. Try these preventive measures:

Breastfeed as long as possible. Breastfed infants have fewer ear infections, which is thought to be primarily due to the increased natural immunity provided by mother's milk.

Bottlefeed upright. If your baby is prone to ear infections, feed your baby upright at least thirty degrees and keep him upright for at least thirty minutes after feeding. Upright feeding not only keeps the milk and formula out of the middle ear but also allows the stomach contents to empty. Babies who are prone to reflux (see Gastroesophageal Reflux Disease, page 338) are more prone to ear infections because some of the regurgitated stomach contents can get into the eustachian tube and trigger a middle ear infection. (Breastfeeding lying down seldom causes ear infections because the swallowing mechanism is different and breast milk is less irritating to the tissues. But if a breastfeeding infant has recurrent ear infections, it might be helpful to breastfeed Baby in a more upright position.)

Keep your child's environment as free of allergens as possible. Allergens such as house dust, mold, cigarette smoke, and animal dander cause fluid to build up in the nasal passages and the middle ear. Fuzz-proof your baby's sleeping environment by keeping stuffed animals, real animals, and other fuzzy things at a distance while Baby sleeps. Since animal dander is a common allergen, pet-purify Baby's bedroom. A HEPA or ionic air purifier may help. (See more tips for controlling allergies, page 131.) Food allergies, particularly dairy and wheat, can also contribute to middle ear fluid. (See more about food allergies, page 327.)

Don't smoke around Baby! The incidence of nearly every illness, especially allergies, asthma, and ear infections, goes up if Baby is exposed to cigarette smoke. (See Smoking, page 482.) Smoke irritates Baby's nasal passages and increases the accumulation of ear fluid in the eustachian tubes. This association is dubbed *smoker's ear*.

DR. SEARS TIP
Integrative Medical Professionals Can Help

Chronic ear infections may be improved with osteopathic care. Osteopathic physicians are actually the same as medical doctors, but they use more natural treatments. They are trained in certain touch and massage techniques that can improve the drainage of fluid out of the ears through the eustachian tubes.

Lessen pacifier use. A study published in the journal *Pediatrics* showed a correlation between the frequency of pacifier use and ear infections. Even though it is strictly a statistical correlation and the possible cause-and-effect relationship is unknown, it could be that persistent pacifier use interferes with normal eustachian tube function.

Use discretion with daycare. Although this isn't always possible, if you can make arrangements that avoid putting your child in a large-group daycare, you decrease the exposure to germs and also lessen the number of colds and ear infections. If you can't afford this move year-round, at least see if you can make a change for the winter months.

Boost your child's immune system. See page 33 on how you can boost your child's immune system.

Use the "nose-hose" and "steam-clean" methods. The more you can keep the nasal secretions thin and draining, the less likely the secretions are to get thick and goopy and plug the eustachian tubes. (See pages 20 and 21.)

Treat colds earlier and more aggressively. If your child has a history of ear infections resulting from colds, at the first sign of a cold begin the "nose hose" and "steam clean" regimen, as well as the other methods on page 20 for keeping nasal passages clear. Sinupret herbal nasal remedy (see page 224) can also help. If your child has a history of colds settling in the middle ear, your pediatrician may prescribe an antibiotic earlier. You could also begin garlic oil eardrops once a day as a preventative before your child even begins complaining of ear pain.

Complications

Although most ear infections clear completely with the above parental and physician management, here are some complications parents should be aware of:

Eardrum rupture. Occasionally, the pressure from the fluid buildup in the middle ear may cause the fluid to leak through the eardrum into the ear canal. You will see — and smell — snotty-nose, white fluid coming from your child's ear. Sometimes a bit of blood will also be present in the leaky fluid. Try not to let the term *ruptured eardrum* frighten you. Once the fluid pops through the membrane, the pressure and the pain are instantly relieved. In fact, in the pre-antibiotic era, doctors used to "lance" the eardrum to relieve the pain and drain the infection. If ear drainage occurs, your pediatrician may prescribe some antibiotic eardrops to supplement the oral antibiotics. In the follow-up appointment, the doctor will check to be sure the "hole" from the eardrum rupture has healed.

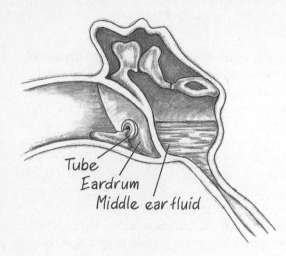

Tube
Eardrum
Middle ear fluid

Hearing loss and speech delay. Recurrent ear infections may diminish your child's hearing and cause speech delay, especially if they occur during infancy and toddlerhood, the stage of speech development. This is why ear infections need to be carefully treated: not too aggressively, with too many antibiotics, but aggressively enough to prevent hearing loss.

Mastoiditis. The ear infection may spread into the mastoid bones behind the ear. Signs of this rare complication are:

• The area of the protruding bone right behind the ear becomes red, swollen, and tender to touch.

• The earlobe may protrude more than normal.

If these signs of mastoiditis occur, seek medical attention immediately.

Ear personality. Chronic ear fluid makes a child chronically uncomfortable. When cou-

pled with diminished hearing, these can lead to what we call an "ear personality." Babies with recurrent ear infections show behavioral changes simply because they do not feel well or hear well, and therefore do not act well. Once constant ear infections are properly treated, parents notice "my baby acts so much better."

What About Ear Tubes?

If your child's ear infections are increasing in frequency and severity, your pediatrician or ENT specialist may recommend "ear tubes." Here's what you should know about this minor surgical procedure:

Who needs them? Although the decision varies from child to child, you and your pediatrician might consider ear tubes if your child:

• has more than four infections in a six-month period or five to six in one year

• has had persistent ear fluid for more than four months

• is developing speech delay and/or hearing loss

• is becoming resistant to the usual forms of treatment

How is ear tube surgery performed? An ENT specialist administers light anesthesia and pokes a tiny hole in the eardrum to drain the fluid. The doctor then inserts a plastic tube about the size of an eye-glass screw into this opening in each eardrum. This outpatient surgical procedure takes around twenty minutes. The tubes usually stay in place six to twelve months and fall out by themselves. After they fall out, the residual hole nearly always heals by itself.

When are tubes needed? Sometimes the fluid in the middle ear (medically called *middle ear effusion*) stays there so long it gets thick and glue-like (called *glue ear*), so that all the prescription medicines and home therapies in the world simply won't remove the fluid. Also, if the fluid stays in there too long, it can cause two problems: damage to the middle ear structures and diminished hearing with consequent speech delay. During the surgery the doctor removes all of the middle ear fluid. If the fluid builds up again, it can simply drain out the middle ear through the tubes. These tubes allow you to preserve the child's hearing while the eustachian tubes grow and begin to function normally. Parents often notice that their child's speech and hearing improve within a day or so after the surgery.

EAR PAIN ON AN AIRPLANE

The rapid change in cabin pressure can cause pressure to build up in the middle ear and cause pain. This is especially true if Baby has a cold or allergies that plug the eustachian tube, the natural pressure equalizer leading from the nose and throat to the middle ear. If your child is recovering from an ear infection, unless advised otherwise by your child's doctor, it's usually okay for the child to go on an airplane. Ear pain usually occurs on landing and is only sometimes a problem on takeoff. Try these ear-comforting tips when the plane ascends and descends:

• Let Baby breastfeed or bottlefeed, and encourage the older child to drink something. The swallowing mechanism can pop open the eustachian tubes.

• Humidify dry cabin air. Place a washcloth moistened with warm water in front of your baby's nose to humidify the little breathing passages. Place a drop of saline solution or breast milk into Baby's nose every hour.

• Awaken Baby. This is probably the only occasion you'll ever want to awaken a sleeping baby, since the eustachian tubes often don't work well to equalize pressure when Baby is asleep.

• Encourage the older child to talk, blow his nose, blow up a balloon, blow bubbles through a straw into a glass of water, yawn, or move his jaw to open his mouth widely. Although we don't normally recommend gum, chewing gum on takeoff and landing can help older kids.

• Have your child hold his nose while blowing with his lips closed to puff out his cheeks.

• Don't try to mute the crying child, since crying may pop open the eustachian tubes.

Preclean the nose. A few times a day for a few days and a few hours before the trip, do the "nose-hose" and "steam-clean" remedies described on page 20.

Don't bother with decongestants. Studies have shown that decongestants and antihistamines are of no use during plane rides.

 **DR. SEARS TIP
No New Medicines in Midair**

Never give a child a medicine (such as a sedative, decongestant, or antihistamine) that you haven't given the child several times before. The last place you want your child to have a hypersensitivity reaction to a medicine is 35,000 feet in the air.

EAR PIERCING

We generally discourage ear piercing for young children for many reasons:

- Poking metal earrings through skin creates an entryway for germs, potentially resulting in infected earlobes.

- Chronically irritated or infected skin, especially in children, tends to over-heal and grow over the backing of the earring. In our practice we have had to extract the back of a stud that has become embedded in the tender earlobe skin.

- The post from the earring can be jammed into the skin of the head during a fall or when playing sports.

- If the earlobes get infected and the earrings need to be removed, this painful procedure can result in scar tissue, leaving a tiny bump on the earlobe.

- Sizing is difficult for children's ears. If the posts are too short, the backs can easily become embedded in the child's earlobes and create infection. If the posts are too long, they can poke into the sides of the head or catch on hair or clothing.

It's best to wait until your child is at an age (at least eight years old) where she can responsibly care for her pierced ears.

 DR. SEARS TIP
Signs of an Infected Earlobe

The earlobe is tender, hot, red, and swollen around the piercing, and there may be pus.

If you do pierce.

- Remove the earrings at least once a week and soak them in alcohol.

- Clean the pierced area with a cotton-tipped applicator soaked in antiseptic solution (like peroxide), then rinse.

- If the earrings are in, pull the post forward to clean the area between the ring and the front of the earlobe. Then, pull the post from behind to clean the area between the back of the earlobe and the clamp of the post.

- Discourage your child from squeezing or tugging on her earrings.

As an alternative to ear piercing, try painting her toenails a pretty pink color. It's a much safer adornment.

EAR TAGS

Ear tags, also known as *preauricular tags,* are harmless physical quirks that babies may be born with. They appear as tiny flaps or bumps, usually around the size of a pencil tip or slightly larger. Treatment depends upon their size. If the tag hangs from the earlobe by a thread of skin or thin stalk, the doctor may tie a suture thread around the narrow piece of skin. This cuts off the blood supply and the tag eventually falls off, or the doctor can painlessly cut it off. If the tag is tiny but does not have a narrow base and is deeper in the ear canal, it's best to leave it alone. If the tag is large (larger than a pencil eraser), but does not have a narrow stalk, removal (if desired) will require a surgeon. This can be done at any age.

Although nearly all of these tags are harmless, statistically there is a tiny association between ear tags and an increased chance of having abnormalities of the kidney. This is why sometimes — in the case of very prominent tags — your doctor may advise an ultrasound of your child's kidneys to exclude this association.

EAR TUGGING

Most ear tugging is a harmless mannerism in the same category as hair pulling, thumb sucking, and nail biting. This quirk is especially common in toddlers who like to pull on all of their appendages as they're exploring and discovering their body parts. If your child is otherwise well and has no other clues to an underlying illness, then let it be. Other possibilities to consider:

Ear wax. This can plug the ear, and a child will tug on the ear to try to relieve the plugged feeling.

Ear infection. Ear tugging alone is seldom a sign of an ear infection. Usually an ear infection follows or accompanies a cold. If you are concerned about a possible ear infection, see page 285.

Fluid in the middle ear. Sometimes a cold or allergy can clog the eustachian tube, which equalizes pressure between the throat and middle ear. This can cause pain behind the eardrum. When an adult's eustachian tube is clogged, such as during air travel, he swallows, yawns, or does a lot of jaw contortions to pop the eustachian tube open. Children may tug at their ears to pop open the eustachian tube. Suspect middle ear fluid if your child has other signs of a cold or allergy, such as a runny nose. By examining your child's ears, your pediatrician can tell if there is fluid behind the ears or if the eustachian tube is blocked. (To pop open a clogged eustachian tube, see page 284.)

Teething pain. This is the most common cause of ear tugging in an infant. The pain in the gums can radiate up through the jaw to the ear, and pulling on the ears is how a baby tries to cope with this pain. See page 509 for tips on teething.

EAR WAX

Ear wax is formed by oil glands in the lining of the ear canal. The wax forms a protective coating against germs and irritation of the lining of the ear canal. It is part of the ear canal's self-cleaning mechanism, and it gradually works its way out, carrying with it germs, dust, and other debris. But some children make too much wax, which can plug the ear canals and diminish hearing. Some even produce so much wax you can see it sticking out of the ear canal.

What to Do

If the wax is not uncomfortable and is not interfering with hearing, leave it alone. If it is irritating or diminishes hearing, it can be safely removed in the following ways:

- Use a wax-dissolving solution containing hydrogen peroxide, available over the counter. Have your child lie down with the affected ear up and put four drops of the wax-dissolving solution into the ear canal.

Your child should lie still for ten minutes. This should soften the wax enough for you to then be able to gently flush it out with warm water, either with a bulb syringe or by allowing the shower stream to flow into the ear.

• If your child is still uncomfortable, your pediatrician can remove the wax with a special instrument. Just before your appointment, put the wax-softening drops into your child's ear to make it easier for the doctor to remove the wax more comfortably for your child.

Never try to stick anything into your child's ear canal to remove the wax, as this could damage the ear canal or eardrum. Let the doctor do it.

EATING PROBLEMS

The three main nutritional concerns parents share with us in our practice are:
"Our toddler is such a picky eater."
"Our child doesn't eat enough."
"Our child eats too much."
We're going to address the first two concerns together here, since the underlying worry seems to be that the child isn't getting adequate nutrition. Here are some tips from the Sears family kitchen on how to coax the most nutritious foods into those selective little mouths with minimal mealtime hassles:

Sixteen Tips to Feed the Picky Eater

"Doctor, my child is such a picky eater." We hear this complaint all the time in our practice. But once you understand the basic principles of toddler behavior, nutrition, and growth patterns, you'll understand why most two-year-olds pick and peck.

• During the first year, babies eat a lot because they grow a lot. The average infant triples her birth weight by one year. But the normal toddler may increase weight by only one-third or less between the first and second birthday.

• Many toddlers burn off excess body fat for energy, so they grow more proportionally in height than weight and go through a normal shedding-of-baby-fat stage.

• Tiny children have tiny tummies, about the size of their fist. Next time you put a heaping plateful of pasta in front of your picky eater, compare it with the size of his fist and you'll see why he doesn't "clean his plate."

• Changes in emotional and motor development also bring about changes in eating patterns. Toddlers do just that — toddle. They don't sit still to do anything, especially to eat. This is why grazing on small, frequent mini-meals is more compatible with a toddler's tiny tummy and busy schedule.

• Toddlers' eating habits are as erratic as their mood swings. Your child may eat well one day and seem to eat practically nothing the next. She may adore fresh vegetables one day and then refuse them the next. Toddlers like to binge on one food at a time. The only thing consistent about infant feeding is inconsistency.

This patternless eating might be worrisome, but it is completely normal. If you added up the nutritional value of everything your child ate for a week, you'd be surprised at how balanced her diet really is. Toddlers need an average of between 1,000 and 1,500 calories per day from one to two years, but they may not eat this amount every day. Instead of worrying about serving your child a balanced meal, try for a balanced *week*. Here are the top sixteen tips for feeding picky eaters, gleaned from our practice and own families:

1. Nibble it. Here is a Sears family favorite. Fill each compartment of an ice-cube tray, muffin tin, or compartmentalized dish with bite-size portions of colorful, nutritious edibles. Call this arrangement a "rainbow lunch." (Remember, feeding young children is a combination of good nutrition and creative marketing.) Be sure to reserve two compartments for nutritious dips. For a younger toddler, try to find a tray with suction cups. But if your child is old enough not to make a mess, just set the nibble tray on his own table. As your toddler makes his rounds throughout the house and by his table, he will stop, nibble a bit, and continue on his way. Teach him to stand by the table while he chews and swallows rather than run around the house with a handful of food or the nibble tray. You can also set the tray on a low shelf in the refrigerator so that he can self-serve. Look for a compartmentalized nibble tray with sliding covers for feeding on the go, such as in the car.

Nibble for two. If your child does not immediately go for the nibble tray, put the tray between you and nibble together. Let your baby see how much fun it is to pick and choose from the colorful assortment displayed before him. Exaggerate your delight in nibbling from the tray by giving your child "it's fun to eat" signals. Our children liked grazing from nibble trays so much that we began grazing with them. See our Nibble Tray at www.AskDrSears.com.

2. Name it. Give the foods in the nibble tray descriptive names that appeal to a toddler:

Avocado "boats" (quarter a small avocado lengthwise)
Little O's (O-shaped cereal)
"Blocks": tofu or cheese
Banana "wheels"
Broccoli "trees" (steamed broccoli florets can be dipped in cheese sauce and called "cheese on trees")
"Sticks" (cooked carrot sticks)
"Moons" (peeled apple slices with or without a thin layer of peanut butter)
Egg "canoes" (hard-boiled egg quartered lengthwise)

3. Dip it. Toddlers love to dip and dunk their food. In fact, dipping less-favored foods, such as veggies, into something tasty is bound to please. Here are some dips to try:

Guacamole (with or without the spices)
Yogurt (plain or flavored with fruit concentrate)
Pureed fruit or cooked vegetables
Nutritious salad dressing
Cheese sauce
Chickpea puree (hummus)

4. Smear it. Toddlers and young children delight in spreading and smearing, so let them smear nutritious spreads (such as avocado, cheese, meat pâté, nut butters, vegetable sauce, and fruit concentrates) onto whole-grain crackers, pita bread, toast, or rice cakes. If you're a neatnik, supervise so that the spreading on the food does not become smearing all over the tray.

5. Top it. Camouflage unfamiliar and less desirable foods with a dollop of yummy toppings: melted cheese, yogurt, cream cheese, guacamole, fruit preserves, hummus, tomato sauce, meat sauce, applesauce, or nut butters.

6. Drink it. If your child prefers drinking to eating, concoct sippable smoothies of yogurt blended with fresh fruit.

7. High-calorie it. Make every calorie count. Encourage your child to graze on nutrient-dense foods, those that pack a lot of nutrition in a small volume. The most nutrient-dense foods are those with healthy fats. Here are our top twelve nutrient-dense foods that toddlers are most likely to enjoy:

Avocado	Oils: olive oil, flax oil
Beans, kidney,	Pasta, whole-grain
and lentils	Peanut butter or nut
Cheese	butters
Egg	Tofu
Fish, especially	Turkey
wild salmon	Yogurt
Oatmeal	

8. Oil it. Healthy oils, such as flaxseed oil and olive oil, are high in healthy-fat calories. For children who really don't seem to eat enough, we advise parents to add a tablespoon of flaxseed oil to their child's diet once a day, for example to a smoothie or oatmeal. Or drizzle some olive oil over whole-grain pasta and marinara sauce. Fish oil supplements are useful too.

9. Sprinkle it. Grind nuts and seeds in a coffee grinder for ten to twenty seconds — this makes these nutritious, yet chokeable, foods safe for preschool children. Add a tablespoonful of these homemade "sprinkles" into oatmeal or smoothies:

Flaxseed meal (ground flaxseeds)
Ground almonds ("crunchies")
Ground sunflower, pumpkin, or sesame seeds

10. Art it. A winner in the Sears family kitchen is zucchini pancakes: whole-grain zucchini pancakes with pea eyes, a carrot nose, shredded cheese hair, and a green-bean smile. Children are more likely to eat what they help create. Use cookie cutters to create edible designs out of dough or slices of bread.

11. Plant it. Plant a garden together. Children are more eager to eat what they help grow.

12. Lap it. Use the lap of luxury. If your child is going through a stage of refusing to get in or stay in the high chair, let him sit on your lap and eat off your plate. As honorary president of the Sears Family Mess-Control Club, Martha has found it helpful to push her plate just beyond baby-grabbing distance and place a few morsels of her food on the table in front of Baby, between Baby and plate. This keeps

**DR. SEARS TIP
No Need to Be a Wimp
About Nutrition**

In their zeal to get their picky eater to eat anything, parents will often become short-order cooks or give in to junk foods instead of "grow foods." How many times have you been over to someone's home only to hear Mother caving in. "Oh, I'm sorry, honey, you don't like the meal tonight? What can I make you?" While you do want to make feeding fun and remove a lot of the parental pressure, there comes an age and stage (around age two) when you want to use what we call the "we" principle: "This is what we're having for dinner!" (See related section on "healthy munching," page 422; immune-boosting foods, page 33; and smart foods vs. dumb foods, page 15.) The earlier you use this principle, the better eater you'll have.

the lap baby's hands out of your plate. We have noticed that babies and toddlers often eat more while sitting on a parent's lap.

13. Dress it. If your child is going through a veggie-refusal stage, play dress-up. Dress up the vegetables with favorite sauces, such as marinara sauce. Use veggies to design colorful faces, such as olive-slice eyes, tomato ears, and a carrot nose.

14. Reverse it. Your child wants pizza for breakfast? Okay! If your child is fixed on eating pizza in the morning and fruit and cereal in the evening, go with the flow. Simply make a healthy pizza using veggie art.

15. Share it. Have a party, invite slightly older children, and serve nutritious foods using some of the above tricks. Seeing how much his friends love to eat may be just the peer pressure your child needs to pick him up out of a picky-eater stage.

16. Psych it. Try reverse psychology. Prepare a meal, sit down to eat, and pretend it doesn't matter whether your child eats. He'll likely join you.

For the child who seems to eat too much or is overweight or obese, see the Dr. Sears L.E.A.N. Program, page 417.

ECZEMA

Every parent cherishes his or her baby's soft, smooth skin. So when it becomes irritated and inflamed, parents want to do everything they can to get their child's perfect skin back. Eczema is the most common skin disorder of childhood, affecting about 10 percent of kids. While some cases are only short-lived, some can last years and continue into adulthood. Here is our guide to everything you need to know to diagnose, treat, and prevent your child's eczema.

Symptoms

Eczema has several different appearances:

Generalized dry skin all over the body. You can feel the dryness as well as see it, and it is usually more prominent on the extremities.

Dry, rough patches with tiny white bumps. You will notice these scattered across the body.

Red, irritated patches. Eczema affects some body parts more than others. In younger children, the inside creases of the elbows and behind the knees tend to be the most severe, followed by the hands and feet. Older children and adults tend to show more trouble on the outside of the elbows and on the kneecaps.

Red, raw, oozing flare-ups. The rash will worsen from time to time, creating itchy and even painful sore areas.

Different Types

Eczema comes in many shapes and sizes:

Temporary eczema. Some previously healthy children may suddenly experience an eczema-type rash for a week or two. These kids generally don't have dry skin or chronic allergies. They just happen to come into contact with something new that causes the rash. (See page 298, Treating the First Episode.) By avoiding the offending agent and treating the rash for several days, this type of eczema usually subsides and only pops up again on rare occasions.

Classic chronic eczema. If temporary eczema persists for more than several weeks, your child may have a genetic predisposition and allergic tendencies to chronic eczema. Such kids usually have dry, easily irritated skin as babies, and the eczema becomes more apparent during childhood. Some kids even begin having troublesome flare-ups as infants.

Circular eczema. Called *nummular* eczema, this is a very mild form that causes several dry, round patches anywhere on the body, with the rest of the skin generally not dry and irritated. Such patches are easily treatable (see below).

Bumpy eczema. This type, called *papular* eczema, manifests as areas of tiny red or white itchy bumps anywhere on the body, and the skin doesn't tend to be dry or irritated as in classic eczema. This is difficult to distinguish from other bumpy rashes. Since most other bumpy rashes are only temporary, the diagnosis of papular eczema is usually made when bumps persist for a couple months.

Causes

Eczema results from the combination of a genetic tendency toward dry, sensitive skin and a susceptibility to allergies.

Dry, itchy, hypersensitive skin. Although most children aren't bothered by the day-to-day wear and tear of soaps, dirt, sweat, heat, clothing, and everything else we come into contact with, the skin of a child with eczema is hypersensitive to everyday life.

Allergies. Children with eczema tend to be allergic to more things than other kids. Exposure to food and environmental allergens causes the skin to flare up into red, irritated patches.

A vicious cycle. These two factors cause continuous daily itchiness. As a baby or child scratches, the skin becomes even more red and irritated. This increases the itching and soreness even more, and the cycle continues.

Treating the First Episode

Because eczema can turn into a long-term and troublesome condition, it's critical to try to identify the offending causes right at the beginning before the situation becomes more chronic and confusing. Ask yourself the following questions to see if there's an obvious and easy cause:

- If breastfeeding, did you just begin eating any major food groups that you'd previously been avoiding?

- Did you just change infant formulas, offer formula for the first time, or wean from formula or breast milk to regular milk?

- Did you just begin giving your baby a new type of food?

- Are you using a new laundry detergent, fabric softener, or dryer sheets?

- Are you washing your baby with a new type of soap or shampoo?

- Is your baby wearing some new outfits that you didn't wash before wearing?

- Did you just go on a vacation where the weather was a lot colder and drier, or hotter and more humid, than you are used to?

- Is your baby suddenly crawling or playing on any new or newly cleaned carpet that could have irritating chemicals or detergents?

- Has your baby recently played on grass for the first time?

Besides trying to determine a cause (if such a simple cause even exists), you can also offer some soothing treatment to calm down the rash before it becomes chronic:

- Massage some baby moisturizing lotion onto the skin.

- Apply an over-the-counter (OTC) hydrocortisone cream twice daily to the affected areas.

- Use an oral OTC antihistamine for bothersome itching for kids two years and older.

If the rash persists for more than a couple of weeks, there are likely some unidentified causes and a genetic tendency toward chronic eczema. You'll now have to move on to some more detailed investigation and treatments.

What You Can Do

Although there is nothing you can do to change your child's genetic susceptibility to dry, sensitive skin, there are many steps you can take to improve skin health, reduce exposure to irritants, track down allergic triggers, and minimize the impact the eczema has on your child's day-to-day life:

Track down food allergy triggers. This is the most important step to improving your child's long-term outlook. If you can determine what foods may be contributing to your child's eczema and eliminate or at least minimize them in the diet, you can create long-term improvement. For some kids, this is even a cure. Experts believe, however, that food allergies only play a role in about one-third of eczema cases, so some of you may not find

this endeavor fruitful. It's still worth a try. Here are seven foods that are responsible for about 90 percent of food allergies:

- cow's milk or milk products
- wheat
- soy
- corn
- nuts
- eggs
- shellfish and some fish

Take these foods out of your child's diet for about one month. Breastfeeding moms need to follow suit. Infants using a milk-based formula should switch to soy and vice versa; if this doesn't help, try a hypoallergenic formula. Allergy testing is also available through your doctor. See page 327 for more details on how to track down food allergies.

Keep the skin moist. For kids with eczema, dry skin is their enemy and moisture their best friend. Keeping the skin moist is probably the most important step in minimizing the rash and breaking the vicious cycle of irritation and flare-up. These steps should be followed every day to keep the skin healthy:

- Give lukewarm baths—hot water can dry the skin.

- Avoid regular soap—most regular soap, whether liquid baby soap or bar soap, can cause dryness. A natural soap mixed with moisturizing lotion and free of perfumes, whether liquid or bar, will enhance skin moisture. These can be found in any drugstore or supermarket.

Try "soak and seal." After your child's bath, pat her skin dry just a bit. Then seal in the moisture with a thin layer of lotion.

- Apply moisturizing lotion after each bath and several times daily. There are numerous brands of lotions available. Choose one that is hypoallergenic, organic, or natural, if possible, and that states on the label that it is for dry skin or eczema.

- Moisturizing oils, such as jojoba oil or coconut oil, can work better than lotion for some kids. Try various lotions and oils until you find what works best for your individual child.

- Buy a humidity gauge and keep the humidity level at about 50 percent. Eczema is worse in the winter and is aggravated by central heating. In your child's bedroom, turn down the heat and use a warm mist vaporizer to humidify and warm the air.

Avoid skin irritants. Here is a list of the most common irritants that affect people with eczema. Figure out which ones seem to bother your child and avoid them if possible:

- Standard laundry detergents can bother some kids. Try one made for infants, or any natural, organic, or hypoallergenic detergent. Do not use dryer sheets or fabric softeners, as these leave residue in the clothing.

- Double-rinse the wash to remove as much detergent as possible.

- Use cotton clothing (organic if possible) and bedding. Synthetic materials can irritate the skin.

- Bathe your child after he plays outside in the grass or bushes or after a hot, sweaty day.

- Install a water filter on the shower head in your child's bath. This will filter out many of the chemicals (such as lead, chlorine, and several others) from the water, which can irritate the skin and contribute to eczema in a small percentage of kids.

- Use PABA-free suntan lotion.

- Avoid scented lotions.

Prevent scratching. This is easier said than done, but it's critical to minimize the itch-scratch-flare-up cycle:

- Keep your child's fingernails and toenails cut as short as possible so that when she does scratch she won't irritate the skin as much.

- Dress your child in long sleeves and pants as much as possible. In hot weather, loose lightweight clothing is usually tolerable.

- In severe cases, place mittens or socks on your child's hands at night to prevent scratching.

Nutritional supplements for eczema. To improve your child's skin from the inside out, add these nutrients to his diet:

- Fruits and vegetables, or a fruit and veggie supplement, can help improve allergic and inflammatory diseases like eczema.

- An omega-3 oil supplement provides beneficial fats to help the skin stay healthy.

- Probiotics taken in liquid, powder, or pill form can help decrease allergies. See page 27.

What Your Pediatrician Can Do

Over-the-counter medications. Medications are very effective at controlling eczema, but it's better if your child doesn't have to rely on them continuously. Focusing on all the above prevention measures should minimize your use of medications. On the other hand, don't be afraid to use these treatments should the need arise. Most kids experience flare-ups from time to time, and using the appropriate treatments right away can lessen the duration and severity.

- Hydrocortisone cream — Use the extra-strength form. Even though this cream is a steroid, it is so mild that it's safe to use at any age. In comparison, some prescription-strength creams are over 100 times more potent. Apply twice daily to irritated areas.

- Oral antihistamines — These are very useful in controlling itching during flare-ups. The most effective one (diphenhydramine) does cause drowsiness, so it's best used at night. The non-drowsy ones are better for daytime use (see Allergic Reactions, page 548).

If you find yourself relying on one or two of these treatments every day for more than two weeks, visit your doctor to see if there is more that can be done.

Prescription medications. There is a lot your pediatrician can do for your child's eczema. If occasional flare-ups are part of your child's condition, and the over-the-counter treatments don't seem to be enough, you and your pediatrician should establish a plan and have prescription medications ready. Here are the most common choices:

- Steroid cream — This comes in low-, medium-, and high-potency forms. It's good to have a low- to medium-strength cream on hand. Apply as directed every day until the flare-up subsides, then for a few extra days for good measure.

- Oral antihistamines — There are several strong ones to choose from. You can start this as well as the steroid cream when needed.

- Non-steroidal anti-inflammatory cream — There is a prescription cream called Atopiclair, that helps with eczema without using steroids. It may not work quite as well as steroid creams but can be used safely over longer periods of time.

- Immune-suppressing creams — Two new creams, pimecrolimus and tacrolimus, work very well at suppressing the allergic reaction within the skin. There have been reports, however, that they may suppress the internal immune system as well. Use these carefully and always with your doctor's guidance.

- Oral leukotriene inhibitors — This type of medication suppresses internal allergies and can work very well in conjunction with any one or two of the above treatments.

Severe cases of eczema may require one or two prescription medications every day. But if the eczema doesn't improve after several months of aggressive treatment, make sure you see an allergist or dermatologist for appropriate allergy testing.

Bacterial infections. Severe cases of eczema sometimes become infected with bacteria that normally live on the skin. This causes red, oozing sore areas that may form a honey-colored crust. Topical antibiotics may help, but oral antibiotics are often needed to quiet these infections (see Impetigo, page 378).

Can Children Outgrow Eczema?

Fortunately, yes. As a child's immune system matures, or the child avoids allergic triggers for years, a child's eczema may improve or resolve altogether. Some kids, however, will continue to struggle with eczema into adult life. There is no way to predict what will happen with each child. The better the disease is controlled during childhood, the better the chance that it may someday resolve.

ERYTHEMA MULTIFORME (EM)

This unusual rash looks almost identical to hives (raised red or white welts and patches, see page 370) but has two distinct differences: EM welts don't itch and antihistamine treatment usually does not make them fade. Doctors aren't certain why EM occurs, but we suspect it is a non-allergic immune reaction to various illnesses or medications. The best way to distinguish between hives and EM is to administer a dose of diphenhydramine (Benadryl; see page 549 for dosing); if the welts fade within the hour, the diagnosis is probably hives (the welts will likely come back after six hours, when the medicine wears off). If the welts don't change it's likely EM. Either way, the rash may fade away quickly within a day or may persist for several days or more. If your child is sick with an illness, then that's likely the cause. If a new or recent medication was given, consider that as a cause and talk to your doctor at the next visit about it. EM is a harmless rash, will eventually fade without treatment, and the precise cause does not need to be determined.

EYES: BLACK EYE

A black eye is caused by bleeding beneath the skin around the eye, usually from a direct blow to the area. The characteristic appearance may take a few days to develop, starting with some mild bruising before escalating into a full-blown black eye. Sometimes a black eye indicates a more extensive injury, even a skull fracture, particularly if the area around *both* eyes is bruised or if there has been a head injury.

What to Do

Using gentle pressure, apply a cold pack or a cloth filled with ice to the area around the eye. A bag of frozen peas works well, too. Take care not to press on the eye itself. Apply cold as soon as possible after the injury to reduce swelling, and continue using ice or cold packs for twenty-four to forty-eight hours.

Danger signs. Although most black-eye injuries aren't serious, there are a few danger signs to watch for:

- Bleeding within the eyeball, called a *hyphema,* is serious and can reduce vision and damage the cornea. With a hyphema, you will see a small rim of red blood where the colored part of the eye meets the white part of the eye.

- Blood in the white part of the eye indicates that the eyeball itself was hit and warrants a doctor visit to check for internal damage to the eye.

Seek medical care immediately if your child experiences vision problems (double vision, blurring), severe pain, or bleeding in the eye or from the nose.

EYES: BLOCKED TEAR DUCT

By two weeks of age, babies' eyes begin tearing. Glands in the eyelids secrete the watery substance in tears as well as an oily component that slows the tears from evaporating. Tears drain into a tiny sac located near the nasal corner of the eyes, then into the tear duct (called nasolacrimal duct), and then into the nose. In around 30 percent of infants, these ducts get plugged. The nasal end of the duct is covered by a thin membrane that gradually breaks open shortly after birth enabling the tears to properly drain into the nose. In some cases, however, this membrane stays closed. In others, the tear ducts are just too narrow for proper drainage.

Even though tears contain natural antibiotics, a general principle of the body is that fluid that gets stuck anywhere attracts germs and gets infected, and blocked tear ducts can cause recurrent eye infections.

Signs and Symptoms

- tears constantly well up in the eyes

- increased tearing running down Baby's cheeks after crying or exposure to wind

- sticky eyes, especially after sleep

- frequent yellow, snotty drainage in the nasal corners of the eyes

What to Do

Blocked tear ducts are harmless and 90 percent of them clear up by one year of age without treatment. Although they are painless and seldom bother babies, they can be a nuisance. To keep those little eyes free of excess gunk:

Wash out the eyes. Clean the gunky tears away with a warm washcloth twice a day.

Massage the tear ducts. Use the tip of your clean pinky finger (with trimmed nail) or a cotton swab moistened with clean, warm water and gently massage the tear duct, recognized by a tiny bump (swollen lacrimal sac) in the nasal corner of the eye. Massage toward the nose in an upward direction at least six times a day or before each diaper change. Massaging puts pressure on the swollen lacrimal sac, pumps the tears into the duct, and eventually pops it open.

Mama's milk to the rescue. A remedy that we have used successfully in our pediatric practice is for mothers to put a drop or two of expressed breast milk into the nasal corner of the affected eye four times a day or apply a drop of breast milk before each massage treatment. Breast milk is rich in natural antibodies that prevent and treat infected tears.

Surgical treatment. About 90 percent of plugged tear ducts will open by one year of age. Of those that don't, most will open by two years. If a tear duct remains plugged after age two, it probably will remain that way indefinitely. Surgical opening can be performed by a pediatric ophthalmologist. There are two different procedures that can be done at different ages:

- Tear-duct probing. This is done in infants twelve months and younger in the doctor's office without anesthesia. The infant is restrained in a papoose and metal probes are inserted into the plugged duct until it opens. It is quite traumatic. The main advantage is that the small risks of general anesthesia are avoided.

- Tear-duct threading. Once an infant is too old to restrain for probing (usually after twelve months of age), this procedure is done in an operating room with general anesthesia. A tiny wire is threaded through the tear duct until it opens. This is much more gentle on the eyes and ducts than the probing.

Deciding when and how to fix the tear ducts is a decision between you and your doctor. Due to the traumatic nature of the probing, and the high possibility that an infant will simply outgrow the problem, we suggest waiting at least until two years of age. If the problem hasn't resolved by then, consider the threading procedure.

EYES: CHEMICAL SPLASH IN EYES

If a chemical splashes into your child's eye, take these steps immediately:

Do NOT let your child rub the eye. This could further damage the eye.

Quickly! Flush the eye with water. Use clean, lukewarm tap water for twenty minutes and use whichever of these methods is quickest while calmly encouraging your child to open his eyes in the water:

Shower. Get into the shower with your child and aim a gentle stream of lukewarm water on the forehead over the affected eye. If both eyes are affected, aim the stream on the bridge of the nose.

Sink. Position your child's head down and turned to the side (with the affected eye

down) so that the eye can be held open under a gently running faucet.

Bathtub. A scared child may do best if he lies down in the bathtub while you pour a gentle stream of water on the forehead so that the water flows into the affected eye.

Remember: Flush for at least twenty minutes and don't let your child rub the eye. If your child wears contact lenses, pause to remove them after several seconds of flushing, then resume the flush. After the flush, wash your child's hands with soap and water.

NEXT! Seek emergency medical assistance. The national poison control center (1-800-222-1222) may be able to help. Be sure to take the chemical container or the name of the chemical with you to the emergency room.

 DR. SEARS TIP
Only Water, Please!

Don't put anything except water or contact lens saline rinse in the eye, and don't use eyedrops unless emergency personnel tell you to do so.

EYES: CROSSED EYES (STRABISMUS)

As you look at those adorable peepers, you may notice that one eye wanders a bit to one side or the other, or up and down. You wonder whether or not your baby's eyes are crossed and if you should worry. Crossed eyes are medically known as *strabismus*. There are six eye muscles surrounding each eye, and each muscle in each eye works in a balanced way so that the eyes are straight. When one or more of the eye muscles do not work together in each eye, one eye appears weaker, or "crossed" or "lazy." If one eye turns in, it's called *esotropia*. If one eye turns out, it's called *exotropia*. And if one eye gazes higher than the other, it is called *hypertropia*.

If the "lazy" or weaker eye is not recognized in early childhood and treated properly, permanent loss or weakening of vision may occur in the affected eye. If both eyes do not focus in a balanced way, a child's vision in the affected eye may be blurred. Because children have a remarkable way of compensating for little anatomical quirks, they conveniently "block out" the vision in the weaker eye and focus on seeing mostly out of the straighter eye. Because of the "use it or lose it" principle, the visual pathways of the brain for the weak eye fail to develop, leading to permanent weakening or loss of vision in that eye, a condition known as *amblyopia*. Amblyopia, usually results from untreated crossed eyes. This is why it's important that you and your baby's doctor recognize strabismus *early* and treat it properly. And the earlier the treatment, the better the result. Strabismus occurs in around 5 percent of children, and it tends to be hereditary. (If crossed eyes are a family trait, be sure to mention this to your doctor and be more vigilant about frequent eye exams.)

DR. SEARS TIP
When in Doubt, Check It Out!

Sometimes the eyes appear straight on routine examination, but you may notice crossed eyes frequently at home. If you notice your child's eyes are crossed (see parent test, below), be sure to mention this to your child's doctor or have a full vision test by a pediatric ophthalmologist.

Temporary crossed eyes of infancy. In the early months, as a baby's eye muscles are developing, the eyes may occasionally cross, especially when Baby is tired (such as at the end of the day). Although most babies have crossed eyes in the early months, with repeated use most of these little eyes straighten perfectly and outgrow this *intermittent strabismus* by six to eight months of age. A study of 170 infants from one to four months with crossed eyes showed that in 27 percent of these infants the eyes straightened out without treatment by seven months of age. The eyes that were only mildly crossed were the ones that usually self-corrected. The eyes that were very crossed were less likely to correct on their own and usually required treatment.

DR. SEARS TIP
Eye *Always* Turned In, See Doctor

An eye that is always crossed is more concerning and needs *earlier* correction than eyes that are only *occasionally* crossed, such as when the child seems tired.

Eyes that appear crossed but really aren't. Sometimes you may look at your infant and her eyes appear crossed, but they are really straight. This is called *pseudo strabismus* and is more apparent than real; that is, some infants have a wide nasal bridge and prominent skin folds over the corners of the eyes near the nose that partially occlude the whites of the eyes, making the eyes appear crossed when they really are straight. As the child grows, more of the whites of the eyes become visible, so the eyes appear less crossed.

How to Tell

Do a home eye exam. Do what we call the "baseball diamond test." Think of the pupil of the eye as the "pitcher's mound" in a baseball diamond. Shine a flashlight or penlight into your child's eyes and encourage him to look directly at the light. If the eyes are straight, you will notice the white dots of reflected light appear in the same place, at the pitcher's mound, in both eyes. If, however, the white dots are at the pitcher's mound in one eye — the straight eye — and first, second, or third

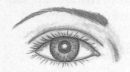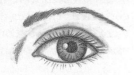

Notice the left eye is turning out and the white dot is off center when it is compared with the straight eye.

base or even home plate in the weaker eye, strabismus may be present, and your child should have a thorough eye exam. Take a series of photos with your baby looking right at the camera. The white dots from the flash should be in the same position in both eyes. In your parent diary, record how often you notice your baby's eyes crossing and if they seem to be getting straighter or more crossed as Baby grows.

 DR. SEARS TIP
Watch for Head Tilt

If you notice your child tilting her head to one side, as if attempting to get an object into focus, take this as a clue of possible vision problems and have your child get a full vision test.

Have your child examined by the doctor. Your child's health-care provider will do some initial screening tests. The doctor will shine a penlight into your child's eyes to see if they are straight in all directions. The penlight test is not always enough to diagnose strabismus. Next, the doctor may do the "cover and uncover" test. The doctor may cover one eye with a small card, observe for eye deviation, and then quickly remove the cover. If both eyes remain straight, this is normal. If, on the other hand, one eye wanders up, down, or sideways, this confirms the diagnosis of strabismus in that eye, and your doctor may then refer your child to a pediatric ophthalmologist for a complete eye exam. Many pediatric offices now have an eye machine, called a *VEP test,* for detecting strabismus.

Treatment

If your child's doctor and pediatric ophthalmologist confirm the diagnosis of strabismus as more than just a temporary maturing stage, the eye doctor will recommend treatments to strengthen the weak eye muscles, usually with patches or glasses. This involves patching the stronger eye to "force" the muscles in the weaker eye to strengthen. Also, by being forced to use the weaker eye, the visual pathways in the brain will develop. Instead of a patch, sometimes glasses or drops are used to effectively blur the vision in the stronger eye to "force" the use of the weaker eye. In more severe cases of eye muscle weakness and for those that don't respond to patches or glasses, surgical correction of the muscle imbalance may be necessary.

It's important for parents to regard crossed eyes as more than just a "he'll grow out of it" quirk. This is a diagnosis that your doctors need to make. True crossed eyes need to be treated as early and as thoroughly as possible to insure the development of normal vision in the affected eye.

EYES: EYELID INFECTIONS

All those little germs that infect the eyeballs can also collect in the glands of the eyelids, causing infections. *Blepharitis* is an infection of the oil glands along the base of the eyelashes. The first sign you will notice is crusty eyes from an accumulation of yellow stuff along the margins of the eyelashes. The inflamed eyelids become swollen and slightly painful and the child may complain of itching or feel that "something is in my eye." The eye may be uncomfortable during blinking, and the affected eye may water more. The eyelashes may stick together with crusty stuff when the child awakes in the morning, but the eyeballs themselves are often not inflamed as with conjunctivitis. The two can also occur together.

How to Treat

- Dip a cotton-tipped applicator in warm water and then in baby shampoo and scrub the crusty areas along the base of the eyelashes.

- Once you remove the crusts, apply an antibiotic ointment if prescribed by your doctor.

If your child gets recurrent infections of the eyelid, do the baby shampoo application one to two times weekly as a preventive measure. See Sty, page 311, for related information.

EYES: PINK EYE (CONJUNCTIVITIS)

Pink eye, known medically as *conjunctivitis*, is an inflammation of the *conjunctiva*, the mucous membrane that covers the white part of the eyeball and lines the inside of the eyelid. Pink eye is a description of the eye, not a diagnosis. Because the inflammation causes the tiny blood vessels in the lining to swell, the eyes turn streaky red. Perhaps it should be called "red eye" instead of "pink eye." Conjunctivitis is one of the most frequent reasons for doctor visits. It is also challenging to diagnose and treat because it has so many causes.

The four clues to note when helping your doctor arrive at the right cause are:

1. What the drainage, if any, looks like

2. How the eyes feel

3. How it began

4. How it responds to treatment

Using these four clues, here are the ABCs of red eyes and how you can figure out which type of infection your child has and when to seek medical care:

Bacterial Conjunctivitis (BC)

Bacterial pink eye is caused when bacteria (usually haemophilus, strep, moraxella, or staph) inflame the conjunctiva, causing the blood vessels to swell (red eyes) and the inflammatory response to produce pus (yellow, goopy eye). With this type of conjunctivitis, the discharge is yellow, green, and yuckier-looking. Oftentimes, the greener the discharge, the worse the bacteria. The eyes are usually worse upon awakening in the morning when they are often crusted shut. *Bacterial conjunctivitis* (BC) is usually the cause of eyes that are matted shut in the morning. The eyeballs tend to be redder with BC than with *viral conjunctivitis* (VC). The rims of the eyelids are also red and swollen. Bacterial conjunctivitis can affect one or both eyes and usually responds quickly, within a couple days, to antibiotic treatment. Unlike other causes, with bacterial conjunctivitis the eyes *look* worse but usually itch less. BC is the most concerning and the most contagious. It is transmitted by exploring little hands touching infected towels, toys, washcloths, and makeup and then rubbing their eyes with the infected fingers. BC makes up around 70 percent of all cases of conjunctivitis in children.

How to treat it. Once your doctor diagnoses bacteria as the culprit, your child will be prescribed either antibiotic drops or ointment to be used at least four times a day. If the "drugs" and "bugs" are the right match, you should see a lot of improvement (the eyes less red and the drainage less yucky) within a couple of days, and those adorable little eyes back to their normal, radiant selves within a week. In addition to the prescription medicine, wash the goop out of the eyes with warm water several times a day, especially to de-crust the eyes upon waking in the morning. To keep your child from sharing his germs with his friends, tell him not to rub his eyes "until the redness is all gone..."

How long will my child be contagious? While bacterial conjunctivitis is highly contagious, it is also highly responsive to treatment. We recommend that you keep your child home from school or daycare for *twenty-four hours* after antibiotic treatment has begun.

DR. SEARS TIP
Drops vs. Ointment

Young children usually show a severe case of eyedrop refusal. Once they see you coming at those already sensitive eyes with that little bottle, eyes close tightly and the protective hands cover them. To avoid the medicine fight, let your child lie flat, relaxed and with eyes closed. Put two drops into the corner of the child's eyes. When he opens his eyes, the drops will seep in. If he doesn't open, you can gently pull down on the lower eyelid to let the drops flow in. Or, ask the doctor to prescribe an ointment, which will gradually melt in. Apply the ointment in the nasal corner of the eyes where the eyelids meet. If your child is cooperative, pull down the lower eyelid and squirt a ribbon of ointment in the pocket. (Tip: put the tube of ointment in your or your child's pocket for a while to warm it up, which makes it easier to apply.) Hold the lid down for at least ten seconds so it melts onto the surface of the eye and not down onto the cheek. Whether to use ointment or drops is a toss-up: some children prefer ointment because drops can sting. Others prefer drops since ointment can temporarily blur the vision.

When to worry. If you notice no improvement in the swelling, redness, or discharge within two to three days, call your pediatrician, since the diagnosis and/or treatment may need to be reevaluated. Depending on the antibiotic used, sometimes the drainage may improve but the redness and inflammation seems to worsen due to an allergic reaction to the solution. Even more urgent "call doctor" signs are swelling, redness, and tenderness above or below the eyeball accompanied by a fever and the child acting generally ill. This means the bacterial infection has spread to the tissues surrounding the eye and, if left untreated, can become a serious infection within the bones and structures around the eye. While this is a rare complication of conjunctivitis, you need to be aware of it. A properly diagnosed and treated bacterial conjunctivitis clears easily with no damage to the sight.

 DR. SEARS TIP
When in Doubt, Check It Out!

Any red eye, especially if only one, that doesn't follow the usual description and isn't showing a lot of improvement with treatment within seven days should be seen by a pediatric ophthalmologist. One of the main reasons is to exclude a herpes infection of the eye, which if left untreated can damage the vision. Suspect herpes infection if the pupil appears a bit cloudy. A further clue is the presence of herpes sores, called *vesicles*, on the eyelids. Again, when in doubt, have an eye specialist check it out.

Viral Conjunctivitis (VC)

This is a less serious but often difficult-to-diagnose cause of reddened eyes. While viral conjunctivitis (VC) can sometimes initially look similar to BC described above, there are usually some clues to tell the difference: the eyes are very red and there is usually no discharge. If there is discharge, it is less yellow, green, and goopy than with a bacterial cause. With VC the eyeballs are very red, but the eyelids are often not as swollen nor are they usually crusted shut in the morning upon awakening.

If you pull down the child's lower eyelid, you can often see lots of tiny nodules in the lining of the eyelid. VC itches more intensely and is very sensitive to light. Nearby lymph glands (such as those in front of the ears) are likely to be swollen. With VC, children often have other symptoms of a viral infection, such as fever and sore throat. Consider VC contagious until the eyes are no longer red, usually from five to seven days. It will often go away without treatment, but antiviral eye medications are sometimes prescribed. Flushing the irritated eyes with warm water or applying warm compresses will usually offer some relief. To ease light sensitivity (called *photophobia*), have your child wear a cap and/or sunglasses.

 DR. SEARS TIP
No Over-the-Counter Eyedrops, Please!

Unless recommended by your child's doctor, we discourage using over-the-counter decongestant eyedrops for any eye irritation for two reasons: they may further irritate the eye, since an inflamed eye is more sensitive to chemical irritants, and they can delay proper treatment or worsen the infection. Bottom line: Either put the right stuff in the eyes or nothing at all.

Allergic Conjunctivitis

Allergies are another cause of red eyes. Clues that your child may have allergic conjunctivitis (AC) are:

• It occurs during allergy season.

• Both eyes are red from swelling of the blood vessels, and the drainage, if any, is more watery and tear-like than yellow and gunky.

- The eyes itch a lot and there are other allergic signs, such as runny nose and sneezing.

- The lower eyelids may be blue and puffy, dubbed "allergic shiners."

Your pediatrician may prescribe an antihistamine eyedrop that blocks the allergic response on the surface of the conjunctiva. These drops can somewhat relieve the redness, itchiness, and watery drainage. Over-the-counter antihistamine eyedrops are also available and work very well. An oral antihistamine can also help. Sometimes decongestant eyedrops are recommended by the doctor to ease the discomfort and swelling of the blood vessels. Flushing the eyes with over-the-counter artificial tears can dilute the allergen effect on the eye and offer some relief. Like VC, children with AC can also be sensitive to light so, again, encourage your child to don a fun hat and to wear protective sunglasses. AC is not contagious, but because the other forms are so contagious, it's best to keep your child out of daycare for at least a couple of days until you decide the problem is allergies. Regarding the contagiousness of conjunctivitis and returning to daycare, pediatric ophthalmologists summarize: "When in doubt, keep them out!"

Irritant Conjunctivitis

Irritants that can cause the blood vessels of the eyes to become inflamed, dilate, and itch are: exhaust and chemical fumes, tobacco smoke, chlorine ("swimmer's conjunctivitis"), contact lenses, and even bright sunlight. In fact, many sun-sensitive children spend most of the summer months with red eyes that, surprisingly, usually don't bother them.

Foreign Body Conjunctivitis

Sand, dirt, or any other little specks can become embedded between the lid and the sensitive conjunctiva. The irritation causes the child to blink more, which rubs the foreign body into the conjunctiva, causing more irritation and inflammation. The diagnosis of foreign body conjunctivitis is usually made when:

- The child expresses that "something is in my eye," even if the doctor can't see it.

- The child has a scratched cornea (the part of the eye that covers the pupil). The doctor can make the diagnosis of scratched cornea by instilling a drop of dye in the eye and examining the cornea with a special light. The scratch takes up the dye and turns fluorescent green, confirming the diagnosis. The doctor might prescribe an antibiotic eyedrop or ointment for a few days to prevent an infection from settling in the scratched area. See Scratched Eye, page 457.

Foreign body irritation of the eye usually causes pain and redness. The good news is that even though the eye is easily irritated and reacts with inflammation, it is one of the quickest tissues to heal. Eye inflammation usually heals within a week; foreign body scratches often heal within a few days.

To flush a foreign body out of the eye, have your child lean over the sink with the affected eye up and wide open. Run a stream of warm water over the eye with your forefinger pulling down the lower eyelid. Usually a few seconds of flushing will remove the foreign body, even though the irritation of the scratch may remain for a few days. If you're uncertain whether a foreign body is still in the eye or the scratch is healing, have the doctor examine the eye using the dye test described above.

See other causes of eye drainage: sinusitis, page 472, and blocked tear ducts, page 303.

With both of these conditions, while the eyes may be goopy, the whole eye is not red, and the child's eyes are usually not uncomfortable.

 **DR. SEARS TIP
Make "Eye-to-Eye" Contact
with Doctor**

We have a policy in our practice not to treat eye problems over the phone. As you can see, because of the many different causes of conjunctivitis (which require different treatments), your doctor needs to examine your child eye-to-eye.

When to Consult a Specialist

While most causes of pink eye resolve easily without complication within five to seven days, you should notify your doctor or see a pediatric eye specialist if:

• The pink eye does not improve after five days of treatment.

• The eye begins to hurt more and have more drainage.

• The child complains of "blurry vision" even after you wipe off the discharge.

• Conjunctivitis occurs during chicken pox or herpes blisters appear around the eyes. These viral complications in the eyes can be serious.

These signs may mean the situation requires a different treatment approach.

EYES: STY

A *sty* is a bacterial infection in the glands at the root of the eyelashes, which grows into a pimple at the edge of the eyelid. It hurts when the child touches it, but usually does not interfere with vision or cause inflammation of the eyeball itself. It may occur with, or following, blepharitis, as described on page 307.

What to Do

Treat a sty like you would any infected pimple:

• Apply warm compresses (such as a washcloth dipped in water as warm as the child can tolerate) for ten minutes at least six times a day. Hot compresses will usually bring the sty to a yellow head so that it is "ripe" to pop and drain by itself. To facilitate the drainage, continue the hot compresses for a few more days. Never try to squeeze or pop any eyelid lump, as this is likely to make it worse. If the head of the sty looks ripe, but it's not popping on its own despite the hot compresses, let your pediatrician do it.

• The doctor may prescribe an antibiotic ointment to apply to the sty and on the surrounding areas around the area of the eyelid.

• The child shouldn't wear makeup or contact lenses until after the sty heals.

Sometimes a sty can form inside the eyelid and grow into a lump, called a *hordeolum.* Or if the sty occurs on the eyelid and becomes a very large lump, it is called a *chalazion.* These are treated just like a sty, but they take longer to heal.

Chalazions initially look like sties but can later turn into a painless lump that can take a few months to resolve on its own. If the lump remains, an eye doctor may need to drain it. Hot compresses will help a chalazion heal. Topical antibiotics are usually not effective.

EYES: UNEVEN PUPILS

The pupil is the dark, circular opening in the middle of the colored iris. Pupils regulate the amount of light that enters the eye. They are naturally larger in the dark and smaller in bright light. Usually the pupils are the same size in both eyes, but in about 20 percent of children they can sometimes be uneven. This is called *physiologic anisocoria,* which simply means normal but uneven pupils. In most children this is a harmless quirk just like uneven arms or legs.

What to Do

• Mention your observation to your child's doctor on your next regularly scheduled visit.

• Bring in some photographs to show the obvious difference in size of the pupils.

• Your pediatrician will do a thorough head-to-toe examination, especially of your baby's eyes.

• If there are no worrisome signs, such as droopy eyelid, abnormal eye movements, or neurological concerns, your doctor will reassure you that this is a normal quirk and

that there will be days when the pupils appear more uneven and days when they appear almost even.

If the doctor suspects an underlying problem in the eyes, the next step will be to have your baby's eyes examined by a pediatric ophthalmologist. Fortunately, the unequal pupils usually turn out to be a harmless quirk.

FAILURE TO THRIVE (FTT)

This isn't really a fair term to use because moms are very sensitive to their babies' growth and weight gain, and we don't like to give the impression that anyone is "failing" here. Babies can "fail" to live up to the growth standards on our established growth charts for a variety of non-medical and non-nutritional reasons. Often it's simply genetics at play, or a fast metabolism that burns off every extra calorie consumed. Here is our guide to understanding failure to thrive (FTT), how you can identify a cause, and what you can do about it.

Signs

FTT is diagnosed in babies who aren't gaining weight at the expected rate over a period of a few months. Usually the length and head size aren't affected (unless the child is seriously malnourished). Here is how a doctor may make the diagnosis:

Falling off the growth curve. Infant growth is measured at each checkup and plotted on a growth curve. A baby that is born large will typically stay on the top half of the weight curve during the first six months of life. A baby that is born slim may be expected to remain on the lower part of the weight curve. Any baby that decreases significantly on this curve over a few months may have FTT. A drop of twenty-five percentile points over two months is a sign that FTT may be an issue (for example, a baby's weight is on the fiftieth percentile line at two months, yet decreases to the twenty-fifth percentile by four months). Even more concerning would be a larger drop (a large baby going from the seventy-fifth percentile down to the twenty-fifth percentile over a two- to four-month period, or a fortieth-percentile baby falling below the fifth-percentile curve a few months later).

Low energy and muscle tone. A baby who isn't getting enough calories will be less active and may show slower motor development. Instead of sitting up in Mom's lap, looking around, waving his arms, and eagerly interacting with everything around him, an FTT baby may be more subdued, not lift and move the head around, and not seem as energetic.

Pale skin tone. An FTT baby may become anemic and have a white or pale skin tone. It's useful to compare the skin color to the rest of the family.

Wrinkly skin. The baby will have loose, stretchy, wrinkly skin, especially on the abdomen.

Low body fat. You probably won't see large rolls of fat on an FTT baby's legs, arms, neck, and belly.

It isn't always easy to know when it's just genetics or true FTT. Some perfectly healthy babies may show one of these signs. Yet, if two or more are present, with poor weight gain, suspect FTT.

Causes

There are several causes of FTT. Some are medical and some are nutritional. However, sometimes a baby is misdiagnosed or unfairly labeled as FTT when there is a perfectly reasonable explanation.

Mistaken Diagnosis

Here are some common reasons why a healthy, thriving baby (who just happens to be slimming a bit) may be unfairly labeled:

Scale error. Sometimes a scale displays an inaccurate reading. Be sure to double-check the weight if you get a low measurement.

Plotting error. It is somewhat common for a nurse to mark a baby's weight (or height or head size) on the wrong part of the growth curve. Have the doctor verify that your baby's marks are placed exactly on the right line for age and weight. Have the doctor go back to the previous two checkup marks and verify them as well. It's important to have an accurate growth chart when evaluating FTT.

Breastfeeding baby. Breastfed babies typically gain weight at the same rate as formula-fed babies in the first few months. But as activity increases around three or four months (kicking, rolling, waving arms), some breastfed babies will slim out a bit. An even more common slimming phase is between six and fifteen months, when crawling and walking begin. Breastfed babies burn off their baby fat more quickly than formula-fed ones (this is probably a good thing). Older American growth charts (compiled from observing many formula-fed babies) didn't allow for this breast-milk slimming, and many breastfed babies would "fall off the curve." Ask your doctor to plot your baby's growth on the new World Health Organization growth chart (see pages 107–110) before a diagnosis of FTT is considered.

Genetics. A slim mom and dad are going to make slim children. The babies don't necessarily start out slim, but they will often go through a slimming phase during infancy if breastfeeding. If this happens, but the baby doesn't show any of the physical signs described above, it isn't FTT. However, it's still important to look for possible causes (see below), though parents and doctors shouldn't be in "worry mode" just yet.

Correct Diagnosis

Once you have ruled out any mistakes in measuring and plotting, and considered the family genetics and breastfeeding metabolism, consider real causes of FTT. Causes can be differentiated into two categories: inadequate intake of nutrition and inappropriate loss of nutrition:

Inadequate nutritional intake. The most common cause is simply that a baby isn't eating enough.

- Formula. Babies on formula should get about two to two and a half ounces of formula per day for every pound they weigh. So a ten-pound baby should get twenty to twenty-five ounces every twenty-four hours. If underfeeding is the problem, the solution is simple. Feed the baby more ounces, more often.

- Breastfeeding. Because we can't visibly count breastfeeding ounces, it's not easy to tell whether Mom's milk supply may be the problem or whether the baby just isn't swallowing enough milk with a normal milk supply from Mom. Mom may feel like she's

making plenty or may have the impression that a baby is eating well and perfectly satisfied after each feed. But sometimes Mom and the doctor can be deceived. A lactation consultant can be invaluable in helping to sort this out. You can also learn more about assessing and increasing milk supply, and evaluating latch and suck problems, in *The Breastfeeding Book*, by Sears and Sears.

- Weak or uncoordinated suck. Sometimes the nerves that travel through the neck that control sucking and swallowing are stretched during the birth process. This can interfere with how effectively a baby can suck, even if it's been a month or two since birth. If your doctor suspects this, an evaluation by an occupational therapist (if bottlefeeding) or a lactation consultant can really help. Seeing a chiropractor (for gentle touch adjustments to the neck) can also restore full nerve function.

Loss of nutrition. Just because Baby may be taking in the milk doesn't mean he is absorbing it all. A baby may have digestive issues or chronic diarrhea that robs him of some calories.

- Formula allergy. See page 331 for suggestions on how to find a different formula if your baby has chronic runny or mucousy stools.

- Food allergies through the breast milk. If your baby has chronic green, runny, or mucousy stools (instead of the classic yellow, mustard-seedy stools a breastfed baby should have) see page 327 to begin taking offending foods out of your diet.

- Chronic medical conditions. Cystic fibrosis is one often overlooked cause of FTT (see page

262). Congenital heart defects are another (see page 355). Your doctor will consider these causes and test for them if needed.

Treatment

Intervention is mostly aimed at looking for a cause and correcting it. If no cause can be found, insuring adequate nutritional intake is key. For a breastfeeding pair with FTT, it's not always an easy decision to begin supplementing with formula. By working with a lactation consultant, you may be able to supplement with pumped breast milk at first. If Baby doesn't begin gaining more weight, formula supplementation (at the discretion of you, your pediatrician, and the lactation consultant) may be needed.

Failure to Thrive in the Older Infant and Toddler

FTT can also develop beyond infancy. Weight gain really varies at this age, and some kids can slim down yet be perfectly healthy. You can use similar guidelines as listed above to help you and your pediatrician decide if there really is a problem. Treatment for the toddler, however, is different because you can now involve solid foods. Overall, if a toddler is a great eater and happily consumes food at every meal and snacks in between, then you know the slim body isn't due to lack of intake. Make sure there aren't any chronic health problems that might contribute to loss of nutrients. It all seems well in these two areas, then you can write if off to genetics and a fast metabolism. If a child is an extremely picky eater, and you feel that lack of intake may play a role, here are some foods that you can offer to maximize fat, protein, and healthy

calories in every precious bite. We call these "grow" foods:

Avocado	Oranges
Beans	Papaya
Blueberries	Pink grapefruit
Broccoli	Poultry
Cottage cheese	Spinach
Eggs	Sweet potatoes
Fish	Tofu
Flaxseed meal or oil	Tomatoes
Lentils	Whole-grain bread
Nut butters	and rice
Oatmeal	Yogurt
Olive oil	

You can also talk with a nutritionist to help count your child's calorie intake and develop various menu items and feeding strategies.

 DR. SEARS TIP
"Grow Food" Smoothies

Make a "grow food" smoothie. Toddlers love smoothies. You can put a lot of these grow foods into a fruit and yogurt smoothie. For example, a tablespoon of flax oil or nut butter is 120 calories, which may be just enough extra calories to help your child grow optimally. (See the Dr. Sears smoothie recipe, page 15.)

FAINTING

Seeing a child faint can be a scary thing for parents to witness, and understandably so! The good news is most fainting spells among children and adolescents are one-time occurrences and are nothing to worry about. Only rarely do fainting spells happen as a result of something more serious.

Causes

Most cases of fainting spells (known as *syncope* in medical terminology) are a result of a natural reflex in the human body. This reflex causes a sudden drop in heart rate and/or blood pressure that results in a brief period of less blood flow to the brain. Since blood carries oxygen, that means that for a very short time the brain is slightly starved of oxygen, resulting in a fainting spell. In most cases, once the child is lying flat, blood flow to the brain is restored and the child regains consciousness shortly. But what can cause this sudden drop in heart rate and/or blood pressure? The most common causes of this are:

- standing up very quickly from a lying or sitting position

- periods of intense anxiety

- exposure to minor traumatic events (such as seeing blood)

- being exposed to intense heat and/or dehydration

- pain and/or emotional stress

- breath-holding among infants and toddlers (This can happen if a child is intensely upset or suffers an injury where he cannot stop crying, which can result in a brief period of lack of oxygen to the brain, occasionally resulting in a fainting spell.)

- low blood sugar, which may occur if the child has gone a long period of time without eating

- prolonged periods of standing

These are common causes of fainting spells that usually are nothing to worry about. The child will quickly regain consciousness and usually not have another episode. Don't rush your child to an emergency room or the doctor's office after a simple fainting spell if you feel one of the above causes is likely. Observe your child and call the doctor if your child doesn't quickly return to her normal self.

When to Worry

Rarely, fainting spells may be a sign of a more serious medical condition. If your child suffers a fainting spell as described below, a visit to the doctor should be made to rule out something more serious. Scenarios that should be more cause for concern include:

Passing out while exercising. This should immediately be evaluated by a doctor, as this may be a sign of a rare, but potentially life-threatening, heart abnormality. If your child or adolescent suffers a fainting spell or loss of consciousness while exerting himself, your pediatrician will perform tests to make sure his heart is functioning properly. If a heart problem is suspected, a visit to a pediatric cardiologist should be the next step. Those who pass out while exercising should be medically cleared before getting back on the playing field.

Repeated fainting spells. Very rarely, fainting spells may actually be a sign of an underlying seizure disorder. If you notice your child having a blank stare prior to the repeated spells, any unusual twitching (before, during, or after), or prolonged drowsiness afterward, testing should be done to see whether your child suffers from seizures.

DR. SEARS TIP
Nutritional Check

Parents, if your teenager complains often of feeling light-headed or dizzy and has an episode of fainting, examine her daily eating and drinking habits. She may be limiting the amount of food she eats or may not be staying properly hydrated. These symptoms may be a sign of poor eating habits, which are very common among adolescents. Of course, if your child has these symptoms, see your pediatrician.

Treatment

Finding the cause of fainting spells is also the best way to treat them. Most cases of fainting are one-time occurrences and no specific cause is ever found. Have your pediatrician perform a thorough history and physical on your child if you suspect a cardiac- or seizure-related condition.

FEET, SMELLY

Smelly feet are a by-product of a sweating quirk called *hyperhidrosis*, or excess sweating. Smelly feet usually accompany sweaty feet, and the child often has sweaty palms, too. If you think about what happens to sweat, you'll understand why you don't want to sniff your child's shoes. When we sweat, the excess moisture produced can easily be rubbed off or evaporate into the air. The reason that sweaty feet smell is that they're covered all day. If you kept gloves on those sweaty hands all day, they would smell like feet. Sweat itself does not have much of an odor (see related section on

body odor, page 197). But when you cover the sweaty soles with shoes and socks, the skin can't breathe and the sweat accumulates. The bacteria that normally live on skin then feast on the sweat, releasing odors. The smell is the by-product of the bacteria feasting on the fatty chemicals in the sweat. Smelly feet may also be caused by athlete's foot (see page 159).

What to Do

Don't worry, be happy. Don't worry and don't let your child see that you are worried. Present this as a harmless, but possibly embarrassing, quirk.

Wash those little feet. Since the combination of sweat and bacteria will produce an odor, the more you wash the feet with ordinary soap and water, the less likely they are to smell.

Air those little feet. Constantly covered moist tissue creates a breeding ground for bacterial growth and consequent odor. Again, this is why excessively sweaty feet smell and hands don't. Let your child go barefoot as much as possible and wear sandals and open-toe and breathable shoes when possible.

Buy cotton socks. Cotton breathes. Loose-fitting, white cotton socks are the most foot-friendly.

FEVER

If your child has a fever, the first thing to do is relax. Don't panic. While fever is usually a sign your child is fighting an infection, most infections aren't serious and will go away on their own. Fever in and of itself isn't a problem. It's simply a sign that the body's immune system is generating germ-fighting chemicals. These natural chemicals elevate the body temperature, and this may help fight off germs. Fever doesn't necessarily mean your child's condition is serious or worth rushing to the doctor or emergency room for an urgent evaluation. Stay home for now and allow us to walk you through what you can do for your child's fever. We will tell you what signs do warrant an urgent doctor visit.

How to Take Your Child's Temperature

The first thing to do is to make sure you are measuring your child's temperature correctly.

What type of thermometer to use. The most convenient and cost-effective way to take a temperature is with a simple *underarm digital thermometer*. These are quick, accurate, inexpensive, and easy to read. Regular glass or plastic thermometers are a less expensive choice for a child who doesn't mind holding still for a few minutes. The main drawback is that they are more difficult to read. We don't recommend ear thermometers for home use because they are expensive, more difficult to use, and may lose some accuracy at higher temperatures.

Where to take the temperature. The underarm is the easiest place to stick a thermometer at any age, so we recommend that route in most cases. Oral temperatures are also fine for older kids who know not to bite down. The only time a rectal temperature is necessary is during the first three months of life. For these young babies, fevers are taken more seriously, so the accuracy of a rectal temperature is a must. For rectal tempera-

tures, insert the tip about one half inch into the anus. For regular glass or plastic thermometers, wait about three minutes before reading. If using a digital one, just wait for the beep.

To add or not to add a degree. Oral temperatures are the closest reflection of how high a fever is. Underarm readings will be about one degree cooler (since it is on the outside of the body), and rectal readings will be one degree hotter than oral. In reality, however, it isn't necessary to add or subtract a degree. The difference really doesn't matter in the long run. When communicating fevers to your pediatrician, just tell him how you took the temperature and let him do the math if he wants to bother.

Rating Your Child's Fever

Normal body temperature	97 to 99 degrees
Low-grade fever	99 to 101 degrees
Moderate fever	101 to 103 degrees
High fever	103 or higher

In general, low-grade fevers are less of a worry. They usually indicate some sort of illness, but probably nothing serious. Moderate fevers indicate that there is definitely an infection and that a doctor should see the child in the next two to three days. High fevers cause parents to worry more and prompt doctors to take the situation more seriously. However, this isn't always the case. A high fever doesn't automatically mean something more serious is going on. Some harmless viruses are notorious for causing high fevers. The degree of temperature isn't the only factor to take into account when assessing a child's illness. We like to evaluate how the child is doing overall, as we discuss below.

Common Causes

Most fevers are caused by viruses, which aren't treatable with antibiotics. Some are caused by bacterial infections, which may, or may not, require antibiotics. Here are some ways you can determine the cause of your child's fever:

Viral Infections

Viruses tend to cause high fevers right from the start, that abruptly subside after one to four days. Rashes, aches, and other flu-like symptoms are also common. Here are some of the most common viruses:

Roseola. This is the most common viral cause of fever in infants over six months. It causes three days of fever (without any other symptoms, except fussiness), then the fever breaks and a lace-like rash appears on the neck and upper torso. See page 448 if you think this describes your baby's illness.

Hand, foot, and mouth disease. This virus causes fever, mouth sores, and sometimes blisters on the hands, feet, and the diaper area. In addition to the fever, other signs of this virus are excessive drooling and refusal to eat. See page 404 for more information.

Viral sore throat. Most sore throat infections during infancy and young childhood are caused by viruses, not by strep bacteria. See page 514 for more.

Viral intestinal infections. Virtually all cases of infant and childhood vomiting and diarrhea illnesses are caused by viruses. See page 278.

Generic viruses. There are numerous viruses that cause fever, aches, rashes, and a variety of other symptoms. These include the common cold, flu, fifth disease, and many others. If your doctor evaluates your child but doesn't find anything that warrants antibiotics, it usually means it's one of these harmless viruses.

Generally, none of these will warrant an urgent call to your pediatrician after hours or a trip to the emergency room. They can wait until the office next opens (except as discussed under When to Worry, page 321).

Bacterial Infections

Bacteria tend to begin with other symptoms of illness (cough, sore throat, and so on), or they may be a secondary infection that develops after a week or two of a viral illness. Fever gradually appears and builds higher and higher over a few days. Most parents seek medical care as the fever gets worse. Here are the common bacterial infections:

Sinus and ear infections, bronchitis, and pneumonia. These are the most common bacterial infections that accompany fever. See their specific sections for more information.

Bladder infection. For older kids and adults, symptoms of this are obvious (see page 191 for more information). But for infants who can't report urinary complaints, it's not easy to tell. Doctors will usually suspect a bladder infection when fevers have persisted for a few days, and no obvious signs of a virus or other bacterial infection develop.

Strep throat and tonsillitis. For kids four years and older, a fever with sore throat is more often caused by a treatable bacteria. See pages 500 and 523 for more information.

These bacterial infections can usually wait until the doctor's office is open to be evaluated, except as directed in When to Worry, below, or in the sections on the specific illnesses.

Treatment

The most important rule is to "treat the child, not the fever." Since fever isn't dangerous (and may even be helpful), you don't have to treat it. The fever will keep your child subdued so he can rest and recover more quickly. Of course, most parents don't like to see their child miserable, so if a moderate or high fever is really getting your child down, here's how to treat it:

Lukewarm bath or cool washcloths. This will help bring the fever down and is a great first step without resorting to medications. Cool liquids can also help and keep your child hydrated.

Medications. Acetaminophen (Tylenol) and ibuprofen (Advil, Motrin) are the two medications used to reduce fever. They also happen to treat any pain that is associated with the illness. They come as infant drops, children's liquid or chewables, and tablets. Acetaminophen also comes as a suppository if needed (called FeverAll). See the dosing chart in the Medicine Cabinet, page 552.

- Acetaminophen can be given every four hours. An initial one-time double dose of acetaminophen can be used for high fevers. This is approved for all ages.

- Ibuprofen can be given every six hours (no double dosing, please). Ibuprofen is also an anti-inflammatory, so it may work better for fevers with body aches and pains. It is

approved for any child three months and older.

- If your child is vomiting or won't keep down any medication, acetaminophen is available in suppository form (FeverAll).

Overlapping fever medications. If one medication doesn't seem to work very well, or wears off too soon, you can safely overlap it with the other medication. For example, if you give your child acetaminophen, but it doesn't seem to do much within an hour and your child is miserable, go ahead and give ibuprofen (or vice versa). If one medication works well initially, but wears off too soon to repeat the dose, you can give the other medication if needed. You can even give them together at the same time. It is better to stick with one medication or the other as a general rule. Don't make overlapping them a habit.

DR. SEARS TIP
Infants Three Months
or Younger

Do not give fever-reducing medications to an infant three months or younger until after you have sought medical care. The doctors must first evaluate how your infant is doing without the aid of meds.

When Not to Worry

The first day or two of fever, even with high spikes, usually doesn't warrant a visit to the doctor (unless accompanied by another sign of severe illness described below). Here are signs that your child's fever is probably just part of a non-urgent illness and you can safely observe and treat your child at home:

- Your child feels ill and subdued when the fever spikes to moderate or high levels, but she perks up when the temperature comes down.

- The fever is overall low grade and your child has no complaints of severe pain or obvious illness that warrant a doctor's attention.

- The fever is accompanied by other obvious symptoms that you can accurately attribute to a non-serious and untreatable illness.

- Overall, your child is feeding well, sleeping well, playing on and off, and interacting with you fairly normally.

DR. SEARS TIP
Follow Your Instinct

If your child's fever fits the above normal descriptions, but your intuition is telling you there may be something serious going on, listen to yourself. It's better to be safe than sorry. There's nothing wrong with taking your child to the doctor and having her tell you it's a harmless virus.

When to See Your Doctor

Here are signs that your child's fever should be evaluated by your doctor in the next twenty-four hours:

- Your child has had fevers of any degree on and off for three days (seventy-two hours).

- Your child has had spikes of high fevers for more than forty-eight hours.

- Your child has other symptoms that indicate a possibly concerning or treatable condition (for example, sore throat, ear pain, or pain with urination).

- Your child is gradually worsening overall.

When to Worry and Seek Care Immediately

Here are signs that your child's fever warrants an immediate call to your doctor's office, an after-hours page to your pediatrician, or a visit to an urgent care facility or emergency room:

Infants three months and younger. Any fever of 101 or higher (no matter how it is measured) in an infant three months of age or younger is considered an urgent situation, since minor infections can quickly become serious in a young infant. Infants six weeks or younger will usually be admitted to the hospital for evaluation. Infants between six weeks to three months old need to be evaluated for infection, but admission to the hospital isn't always necessary.

Meningitis. Any fever associated with signs of meningitis, which include severe headache, neck stiffness, pain when bending the head down and forward, vomiting, or light sensitivity, is urgent.

Kidney infection. Fever with signs of a severe kidney infection — which include fever, mid- to lower-back pain, vomiting, and painful or frequent urination — warrants immediate attention.

Red dots. Fever with tiny red or purple pinpoint dots on the skin that don't blanch (disappear) when the surrounding skin is stretched is serious. See page 443 if your child has a fever and rash to help you identify this type of serious rash, called *petechiae.*

Unresponsive to meds. High fever that doesn't come down a couple degrees after two hours of the treatment measures described here deserves an evaluation.

Febrile seizures. If this happens, call 911 or go to the emergency room. See page 461 for more on febrile seizures or "fever fits."

Irritability. This implies more than simple fussiness. An irritable infant will cry for hours, will show minimal interest or interaction with caregivers, and will be nearly impossible to console. This can be a sign of serious infection.

Lethargy. By this we mean more than your child isn't acting right or just wants to lie quietly in your arms. True lethargy means an infant or child is limp, not responsive to your voice, and won't make eye contact. This obviously means something serious is going on.

FLAT FEET

Flat feet (also known as *pes planus*) is a common condition among children, resulting from underdevelopment of the arch of the foot. In most young children this is a transient, painless, and harmless stage of development. All infants come into this world with pancake-bottom feet. The arch begins to form in most children by three years of age. In some children, the arch fails to develop and the feet remain flat; how flat varies greatly from mild to severe.

Testing for Flat Feet

Your pediatrician — and you — can assess the degree of your child's flat feet by these three simple tests:

The stand-on-toes test. Have your child stand on his toes. If during this test an arch develops, this likely means that the flat feet should not cause further problems.

Pronation test. Stand behind your barefoot child on a hard surface. Imagine a straight line going down the Achilles tendon to the floor (or place a ruler along the tendon to the floor). If the line or ruler is perpendicular to the floor and touches the floor behind the ankle, flat feet seldom bother a child or require treatment. If, however, the line or ruler slants so that the ruler touches the floor near the outer part of the child's ankle, this is called *pronation*, which means the area of the foot where the arch should be rolls inward and touches the floor.

The wet-feet-on-concrete test. Watch your child carefully walk on concrete with wet feet. If there is an adequate arch, the concrete should be dry in the area of the arch. If the feet are flat or pronated, the arch area will also leave a wet imprint.

Sometimes flat feet are due to a malforma-

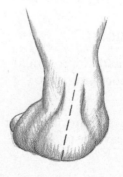
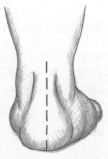

tion of some of the foot or ankle bones. In this case, your doctor may order an X-ray, a CT scan, or an MRI of the feet to examine the bones and ligaments of the feet.

 DR. SEARS TIP
Leaner Child, More
Comfortable Feet

Obesity aggravates the bone-development consequences of pronation and flat feet. If the child is already knock-kneed from "fallen arches," the extra weight to lug around is a double whammy on the ankle and knee joints. We recommend both orthotic and heel cushions while overweight children are going through a weight-management program or until they pass through the normal leaning-out stage of adolescence.

When to Worry

Rarely do you need to do anything for children under the age of three. There seems to be two schools of thought regarding whether or not to treat flat feet between three and four years of age. Most pediatric orthopedists take a conservative approach and seldom treat it. Most podiatrists, on the other hand, tend to recommend orthotics between three and five years of age, depending on the degree of pronation. Over the years we have examined thousands of children with flat feet and, from experience, have sided with the podiatrist camp and become more aggressive in treatment. Based on experience, here are our suggestions:

• Until your child is three years of age, just enjoy those little archless feet. Don't worry, and do nothing.

• Between three and five years of age, if the arch is not developing and your child's feet are becoming *more pronated* (the inside of the ankle rolls inward), it's time to treat.

• If your child is walking awkwardly or complaining of sore feet, ankles, or leg pain, especially at the end of the day, seek treatment. In our experience, a lot of so-called growing pains are caused by severely pronated flat feet.

• If your child is starting to "toe-in" (becoming noticeably pigeon-toed), it's time to treat. Some children will start to toe-in as a natural compensatory mechanism for "making an arch" when they walk. Take this as a clue that the flat feet are interfering with normal walking balance.

The reason that we have become more aggressive about treating flat feet is if the developing child's ankle rolls inward too much it throws the normal axis of weight bearing out of balance, so there is uneven pressure on the inside ankle and knee joints during walking and running.

Treatment

While most mild cases of flat feet require no treatment at all, if your child is showing any of the above signs, consult a pediatric orthopedist or podiatrist about the use of orthotics. These are inserts that fit into your child's favorite pair of shoes and are replaced every couple of years or so as the child's foot grows. Generic orthotics are usually used for ages three to five and are fairly inexpensive. Custom-fitted orthotics are for kids six and older and can cost $200 or more. In our experience, children who really need orthotics enjoy wearing them because they soon notice how much better their feet feel, especially during prolonged standing, walking, or running. Orthotics can be worn in any shoe. Special "orthopedic shoes" are rarely necessary or helpful for children with flat feet. If the doctor feels you don't need orthotics, choose a running shoe with two main features: an adequate arch and a cushiony heel.

FLAT HEAD (POSITIONAL PLAGIOCEPHALY)

The most common cause of a baby developing an unusual shape to the skull is positional plagiocephaly (PP), also known as "flat-head syndrome." The infant skull bones are not fused together to allow for brain growth. This means that external pressures on the skull bones can cause areas of flatness on that beautiful little rounded skull. Studies have shown that the blood flow to the brain and the growth of the brain beneath the flattened areas are normal. So, you don't need to worry that the flat head is keeping the underlying area of the brain from growing normally.

Unlike craniosynostosis (see page 248), flat-head syndrome is not the result of premature fusing together of the skull bones. Rather, it occurs as a result of baby sleeping in one position or consistently on one side of the head. Some babies will favor sleeping with their heads turned to the right or to the left. Because a young infant's skull is so malleable, lying on one side for long periods of time can cause that side to flatten, leading to an abnormal skull shape. Since the inception of the lifesaving Back-to-Sleep campaign (to prevent SIDS), pediatricians have been seeing an "epidemic" of flattened heads (on the back). The good news is that for most babies this is a harmless and temporary cosmetic feature. Infants who have a condition known as torticollis (for explanation, see page 526) may be more prone to PP.

What to Do

Since PP is usually caused by sleeping in the same position and applying pressure to the same part of the skull, the simplest remedy is to encourage your baby to spend equal time sleeping with his head turned to the opposite side.

• If Baby's crib is next to your bed, he will want to turn his head toward you. Each night rotate the crib 180 degrees so that he turns his head toward you on different sides. Or more simply, rotate your baby instead.

• If you notice your baby favors sleeping with his head turned to one side, whenever you pass by the crib gently turn his head while he is sleeping.

• To encourage Baby to turn his head, place safe crib toys on alternating sides.

• If Baby also has torticollis, use the physical therapy exercises outlined on page 527 to encourage equal turning of the neck muscles.

• Take weekly photographs and record the changes so you can share them with your pediatrician.

• Encourage supervised tummy time. The less time Baby spends on his back, the less pressure on the back of the head.

Flat heads are more common in the early months when babies are not as mobile during sleep. Baby's head will gradually round out as he gets older and becomes able to change sleep positions independently, thus distributing pressure equally on the growing skull.

What Your Doctor Might Do

Mention your concerns to your pediatrician and take along your gallery of serial photographs. Let the doctor know if you believe the flattened area has not improved over a few months, especially if you have tried repositioning therapy. The doctor will then do a thorough examination of your baby's skull in an attempt to diagnose whether the flattened area of Baby's head is caused by simple positioning or is secondary to one of two other problems: craniosynostosis (premature fusion of one or more of the sutures between the skull bones; see page 248) or torticollis (see page 526).

DR. SEARS TIP
Look for the "Bald Spot" Clue

Hair that is worn off on the flattened area is a clue that the cause of Baby's flat head is positional.

Besides the above "bald spot" sign, the doctor will look at the overall shape of the head. Studies differentiating PP (also called "positional molding") from craniosynostosis show the following: If the shape of Baby's head is a parallelogram, this is likely to be temporary. If, however, the head is a trapezoid shape, it may be that the irregular shape is due to premature closure of the sutures (craniosynostosis). Look down at Baby's skull from above and determine the shape.

Usually, the doctor will be able to tell the difference between PP and craniosynostosis by looking at and feeling the skull bones. If the diagnosis is uncertain, the doctor may order an X-ray or a CT scan of the skull bones to confirm the diagnosis. If she notices torticollis as well, you may get a referral to a physical therapist for some expert instructions on proper neck stretching.

Does My Baby Need a Helmet?

Usually repositioning therapy is all that is needed to correct PP. But if repositioning therapy was not started until the later months and the head molding is severe, your pediatrician may recommend that your baby be fitted with a helmet or headband that helps mold the head back into a rounded shape. Contrary to popular belief, these helmets don't squeeze the head to help it grow round but rather provide a round space that allows the head to grow into it. Helmets also keep pressure off the flattened area during sleep. Most infants need just a few months of these corrective bands. We have had very good experience with a nationwide company called Cranial Technologies. If the doctor recommends a helmet, visit www.cranialtech.com to find a center near you.

FLU (INFLUENZA)

Your normally overactive four-year-old hasn't seemed quite himself over the past two hours. He has had a runny nose and a bit of a cough. He then begins to complain of a headache and sore throat. Next, his body aches all over and he insists on lying down. You take his temperature, which reads 103.5! His cough gets worse and he starts vomiting. There is really only one bad bug out there that can cause such a plethora of symptoms — the *flu*.

Symptoms

Every parent's biggest worry when a child gets sick is whether it is the actual flu or just a simple cold and cough. Aspects of the flu that really set it apart are the severity of the aches, fever, and feeling of illness, and the huge variety of symptoms and body parts that are affected. The flu will usually cause three or more (or all) of the following symptoms:

- high fever, chills
- sore throat
- headache
- nausea
- vomiting

 DR. SEARS TIP
Swine Flu

In 2009 the world was hit with a surprising new strain of the flu, called H1N1, or "swine flu." While the outbreak initially caused a great deal of unwarranted panic, we soon realized that it was only slightly more serious than the regular flu. Certain groups of people (pregnant women, children, and young adults) were hit harder than would be expected from a flu, and the elderly were largely spared. This new flu hit during the "off season" instead of during the fall and winter. As our nation and the world gains immunity to this strain (either through infection or vaccination), the H1N1 flu will likely blend in with the regular seasonal flu.

- diarrhea
- abdominal pain
- body and muscle aches
- stuffy nose
- runny nose — clear or green mucus
- cough — dry or productive
- irritated, red eyes

What You Can Do

If you think your child has the flu, the first step is to relax. The flu is a virus, so there's no hurry to rush to the doctor to get antibiotics. For symptoms like cough, cold, vomiting, diarrhea, fever, and red eyes, see the specific sections for treatment ideas. Here are some general guidelines to help you and your child get through this illness:

Lots of fluids. Staying hydrated helps keep the mucus running to avoid sinus and ear infection. It also helps decrease aches, fever, and the overall feeling of illness.

Multi-symptom cold medicine. Give children six years of age and older a cold medicine that relieves several of the main symptoms, such as headaches, stuffy nose, cough, and fever. This all-in-one medicine is generally a bit too much for kids under six, however.

Treating specific symptoms. Instead of a multi-symptom medicine, you can also just treat the most bothersome symptoms with a more specific one, such as a pain reliever for fever and aches (ibuprofen is often a better choice than acetaminophen for the aches and pains of the flu; see page 553 for dosing), or a decongestant and expectorant for nasal and chest congestion. Because the safety of over-the-counter (OTC) cold and cough medications is currently under debate for children under four years of age, we don't recommend you use them. An herbal treatment called Sinupret is a great option for supporting a child's, and an adult's, sinus and respiratory systems during a cold or flu.

Extra rest. Nothing helps the body heal like a good night's sleep and a restful day. Sometimes, keeping your child medicated during the day (so he feels like running around and playing normally) is counterproductive. Ease off on the daytime meds (unless he's really uncomfortable) and let your child rest, using appropriate meds at night.

When to See a Doctor

Most children with the flu don't even need to see a doctor, but some kids require evaluation. Here are some guidelines to help you decide if a doctor's visit is warranted:

- Your child has fever for more than four days. While this may still be just the flu, it's best to double-check with your pediatrician.

- Your child has moderate to severe dehydration from vomiting or diarrhea. See page 267.

- You have a gut feeling that your child is unusually ill.

- Your child has a severe cough with chest pain AND shortness of breath. This may mean pneumonia is setting in.

 DR. SEARS TIP
Is It the Flu or Meningitis?

Meningitis can sometimes be mistaken for the flu, and vice versa. Both can cause high fever, headache, and vomiting. The main symptom that helps distinguish between the two is the stiff, painful back of the neck that accompanies meningitis. If your child complains of this and can't look down at his abdomen without significant pain, go to an emergency room or call your pediatrician right away.

Prescription antiviral medications. Your pediatrician can prescribe antiviral medication to help combat the flu. These meds are like "antibiotics for the flu virus." They can do two things: shorten the duration of the illness and lessen the symptoms. To be effective, these medications must be started right at the beginning of the illness. You and your doctor can decide if this treatment is warranted.

FOOD ALLERGIES

Food allergies are one of the most common causes of various health conditions, behavioral problems, and recurrent illnesses. Yet, they are often overlooked. Here is our guide to helping you understand if your child may have food allergies, how to test for them, and how to change your child's diet so you can improve his overall health.

Symptoms

Some symptoms are obvious, such as nasal congestion, rash, or diarrhea, yet food allergies may often trigger more subtle symptoms or problems:

Recurrent infections. If your child is frequently sick with ear, sinus, or lung infections, this may be due to an impaired immune system and mucus overproduction from food allergies.

Skin and respiratory problems. Chronic rashes, eczema, hives, asthma, and nasal allergies can be triggered by food allergies.

Chronic constipation, diarrhea, or abdominal pain. Food allergies will often cause chronic diarrhea, gas, and belly pain. However, sometimes a food group can also cause constipation. This isn't really an allergic reaction; rather, it is a chemical sensitivity to something in the food. Cow's milk products are often a culprit in constipation.

Infant colic and gas. Food proteins will pass into the breast milk from Mom's diet and cause symptoms if an infant is allergic. Infants allergic to cow's milk or soy may react from those types of infant formulas.

Hyperactivity and other behavior problems. Food allergies and chemical sensitivities to various foods can definitely affect behavior and focus. If your child is more than a handful, consider his diet.

The Top Seven Most Allergenic Foods

Thinking about food allergies can be overwhelming for anyone. Testing is available but can be expensive and uncomfortable for a child. It is useful to know the most common allergenic foods. You can try eliminating one or more of these groups for a few weeks and

see if your child's symptoms improve. The following seven foods are responsible for over 90 percent of all food allergies, in order from most to least likely:

- Cow's milk products — milk, formulas, ice creams, yogurt, cheese, butter, sour cream, and any food made with casein or whey proteins
- Wheat — bread, crackers, cereal, muffins, pizza, pancakes, pies, cookies
- Eggs — mayonnaise, meringue, custard, baked goods, French toast, pancakes
- Soy — soy milk, formulas, soy sauce, soy burgers, soy flour, tofu, protein drinks
- Nuts — most likely peanuts (but others are possible), nut butters, cookies or candy bars with nuts, trail mix, foods fried in peanut oil
- Corn — corn syrup as a sweetener, corn meal, cornstarch, popcorn
- Shellfish — shrimp, crab, lobster, clams

Testing

If you have already tried eliminating the most common foods without results, or you don't want to play any more guessing games, it's time for food-allergy testing. Here are the various choices:

Skin testing. This is the most accurate method for children four years and older. It is done by an allergist (most pediatricians don't offer this service). The skin on the back or the arm is pricked with various food proteins, and the reaction is measured. If a child is allergic to that food, allergy antibodies (called IgE antibodies) will detect the proteins and cause the skin to swell up like a bug bite in that area. Any reactions that occur are an accurate reflection of an allergy. However, one drawback to skin testing (especially in kids three and younger) is that a child may be allergic but not show a skin reaction.

Blood testing. This is a better choice for children three years and younger because it is better tolerated (one needle into a vein versus numerous skin pricks) and more accurate for this age group. However, some infants younger than twelve months won't show a reaction to some foods on a blood test, even if they are allergic. There are two types of blood allergy tests:

- IgE testing (called *RAST testing*). This measures the levels of IgE antibodies that are secreted by the immune cells that respond specifically to allergenic foods. If your child is eating an allergenic food, for example, milk, then a certain level of IgE antibodies that will react to milk will be floating around in the bloodstream. The blood test measures the levels of all allergenic foods, and rates the reaction from 1 (barely allergic) to 7 (extremely allergic).

- IgG testing. This is a variation of RAST testing and is an alternative way to assess food allergies (the FDA has not approved it as a way to test food allergies). IgG antibodies are not really an allergic response. They are more of an overall immune system response. It is believed that foods that generate a high IgG response are putting a strain on the immune system, which in turn affects the health of the body, including the nervous system, as a whole. IgG results are rated from 0 (no reaction) to 3. By eliminating the foods that cause a level 2 or 3 reaction, the immune system functions better,

and in turn the body as a whole functions better. It is thought that IgG food sensitivities cause more behavioral, neurologic, and immune-suppressing problems, and IgE food allergies cause more classical allergic symptoms. The accuracy of IgG testing is theoretical right now. In our own office we have found it somewhat useful so far.

No tests are perfectly accurate. The best way to be certain is to observe your child on and off the suspected foods.

Eliminating and Reintroducing Allergenic Foods

Once you have determined what your child is allergic to, take him off all allergenic foods for about two months. Notice what happens to the various allergic, medical, or behavioral symptoms. Once you see some improvement (which hopefully you will!), the next step is to slowly reintroduce the foods one at a time to the diet to see which ones have enough of a negative effect on your child's health to stay off. Of course, if your child only has a few allergies, and you see some wonderful improvements, we encourage you to remain off the foods indefinitely and enjoy a year or two of good health and behavior. If there are numerous allergies, however, it is likely that only some actually affect your child in practical terms. You can determine which foods are the main culprits by reintroducing them. Here are two different ways to do this:

Rotation diets. With this method, you start by reintroducing one food at a time and allowing your child to eat it every four days. After your child has had that food two or three times, add another one, but limiting it to no more often than every four days. Soon your child will be eating several of these foods again but not overloading on them day by day. Watch for any negative behaviors, allergies, or health problems to re-emerge. If they do so, consider one of the most recent additions to be a culprit. By continuing with this method, you will sort out which foods you will need to stay away from for the long term.

Reintroducing one at a time. A more useful way (in our opinion) to observe your child's health during reintroduction is to restart only one food at a time for a few weeks. This allows you to more easily narrow down any reactions to each food.

Milk Protein and Gluten Allergies

So far we have discussed food allergies in general. We would like to put a spotlight onto two specific groups of foods that can have a more profound effect on a child's health if an allergy or sensitivity exists. We refer to *casein,* the protein found in cow, goat, human, and any other mammal's milk, and *gluten*, the protein in wheat and various other grains. (Lactose intolerance, on the other hand, is a sensitivity to the *sugar* in milk.) It is unknown why the casein and gluten proteins are so highly allergenic in some individuals, but eliminating them from the diet can yield some considerable results.

Sources of milk protein. Here are the common milk products that you will need to eliminate:

- cow and goat milk
- butter, cream, sour cream
- cheese, cottage cheese
- yogurt, ice cream

- whey protein
- caseinates (found in hotdogs, for example)

Many prepared, frozen, dried, or canned foods and soups contain powdered milk, cheese, or whey. Baked goods and snacks usually have casein ingredients. Read labels carefully and learn which everyday foods you need to cut from your child's diet.

 DR. SEARS TIP
Say Yes to Yogurt

Many — but not all — children who are definitely allergic to milk as a beverage can tolerate a bit of yogurt for two reasons: First, the culturing process renders the lactose in yogurt more digestible and the proteins less allergenic; and second, many food intolerances are dose related. A couple spoonfuls given frequently may be more intestinal-friendly than wolfing down a cup all at once.

Alternative milk-free foods. Here are alternatives to foods with casein:

- rice milk (Unsweetened is best.)
- almond milk (Unsweetened is best.)
- soy milk (Because soy is a fairly common allergy, try to minimize or avoid this as an alternative to milk.)
- eggs and mayonnaise (Although they are thought of as "dairy products," they don't come from milk.)
- dairy-free yogurt, cheeses, margarines, and ice creams (But check for casein.)
- other non-dairy sources of calcium: calcium-fortified orange juice and cereals,

**DR. SEARS TIP
Casein, Gluten, and Behavior**

Some children with behavioral challenges (autism, ADD, hyperactivity, excess tantrums) have been reported to show dramatic improvement when put on a 100 percent gluten-free and casein-free diet. Such children quickly calm down on this diet. We have seen this work in our own practice. While this doesn't help everyone, it is worth trying.

tofu, molasses, green veggies, sesame seeds, canned salmon, rhubarb, and figs

Sources of gluten. Here are the grains that contain this protein:

- wheat
- oats
- barley
- rye
- semolina
- spelt
- triticale
- kamut

These grains are in most prepared cereals, breads, flours, baked goods, and instant mixes. Reading labels is crucial. Some natural and artificial flavorings, spices, gravies, and dressings may have gluten. If child loves an item and the ingredients are unclear, call the manufacturer.

Alternative gluten-free foods. These foods that do not contain gluten:

- sweet rice
- brown rice
- white rice
- tapioca
- wild rice
- millet
- amaranth
- quinoa
- buckwheat
- bean flours (garbanzo and garfava)
- lentils
- cornmeal
- potato starch
- soy
- dried or canned beans

Starting the Diets

The best approach is to start these diets one at a time. It is easier to go casein-free, so we suggest you start there and allow three to four weeks for it to take effect. After you've concluded whether it's helped, incorporate the gluten-free measures to see if your child benefits even more. It may take up to two months for gluten restriction to show positive effects. If your child's suspected food sensitivity symptoms resolve by just going casein-free, it's probably not worth going off gluten as well.

**DR. SEARS TIP
Check Your Local Health-
Food Grocery Store**

In response to the demand for gluten-free and casein-free foods, most natural foods stores have a section devoted to them. You can find a replacement for pretty much anything.

FORMULA ALLERGY

Most parents will try more than one type of infant formula before they find one that sits well with their baby's tummy. There is a wide, confusing range of formulas to choose from, and many babies will show some allergic reactions to some of them. Here is our guide to figuring out the best formula for your baby:

Symptoms

Every baby is expected to experience some gas, the occasional runny stool, and some minor fussing from time to time. If your baby and his tummy are happy most of the time, you probably have nothing to worry about. But if your baby is experiencing the following symptoms he may be allergic to the formula:

• colicky crying for hours each day (see page 299)

• spitting up large amounts after feeds (see GERD, page 338)

• green, mucousy, runny stools

• large, hard, and painful-to-pass stools (see Constipation, page 240)

• blood in the stools

• chronic rash over much of the body

• chronic nasal or chest congestion or wheezing

Treatment

Change Feeding Techniques

Don't switch formula brands just yet. Some babies simply need an adjustment in their feeding technique. Try these steps first:

Avoid overfeeding. In the first few months, most babies need between two and four ounces at each feeding. If your baby is demanding more, it may be he just likes to suck. Try a pacifier. You may also find your baby does better with smaller, but more frequent, feeds.

Change bottle types. Perhaps your baby is just swallowing too much air during a feed-

ing. This can occur if the nipple flows too fast or with the types of bottles that allow air in. Try a slower-flow nipple or a variety of different bottle types and see if things improve.

Change from powder to liquid. For reasons that are unclear, some babies digest the ready-made liquid formulas more easily than a powder. Before you change brands, try the same brand or type of formula in its liquid form.

Change Formulas

If your baby's troubles persist, here are the steps you can take, in this particular order, to find a good fit for your baby. Each time you make a change, allow one week to look for results before you move on to the next step (unless that change makes everything much worse):

Change brands. If your baby is on a milk-based formula, try another brand of milk-based formula. There are subtle differences between brands that may help. If using a soy formula, try another brand.

Go organic. If using a non-organic formula, try the organic alternative of the same type (milk or soy).

Change to a milk-based "gentle on the tummy" formula. All the major formula companies make a milk-based "gentle," "sensitive," or "comfort" version in which the milk proteins are slightly broken down into smaller proteins. You can make this change whether you are on a standard milk formula or soy.

Change from milk-based to soy, or vice versa. Once you've tried all possible variations within the type of formula you've been using, try a major switch to the other side (soy to milk, or milk to soy).

Try a lactose-free formula. Some companies make a milk-based formula without the milk sugar (lactose). Lactose intolerance is rare in babies, but this is worth a try.

DR. SEARS TIP
Soy or Lactose-Free Formulas: Short-Term Solutions

Soy proteins aren't as ideal for human babies as milk proteins. Lactose sugar is the easiest type of sugar for the human brain to use as an energy source. If soy seems to be the only thing that works for your baby, try switching back again to a milk-based formula after a month or two. As your baby's digestive system matures, he may learn to handle the milk again without much trouble.

Change to a specialized hypoallergenic formula. These formulas use various combinations of pre-digested milk proteins and different sugar and fat sources that are easy on ultra-sensitive tummies. Available brands include Alimentum, Neocate, Nutramigen, and Pregestimil. These are available without a prescription at most grocery or drugstores, as well as from pharmacies or online.

Homemade formula recipes. This is a last resort. If your baby isn't comfortable with even the hypoallergenic formulas, you can try a homemade recipe using goat milk or other alternative milks as a base, then adding a variety of oils, vitamins, and other nutrients. Because these are not FDA-approved complete sources of nutrition, we don't recommend doing this without your doctor's advice.

FREQUENT ILLNESSES

Every child is expected to catch an illness or three every year; an ear infection here, a sore throat there, a little diarrhea from time to time, and the occasional fever. This is part of growing up in a world of germs. However, some children seem to catch more than their fair share. Parents wonder if it's just bad luck or if there could be something wrong with their child's immune system. Here is our guide to approaching the child with frequent illnesses.

Defining Frequent Illnesses

How many illnesses are too many really depends on the lifestyle of the family and the child. On average it is thought that a child should catch about eight colds, flus, fevers, or other routine illnesses each year. That may be true, but it doesn't mean that as a parent you have to accept this fate, especially if you feel it is out of the ordinary for your particular situation. Here are some examples of when to suspect that something more than just bad luck might be at play:

- a breastfed first baby whose parents are never sick and who don't put their baby into any nurseries seems to get sick every month

- a home-schooled child without older siblings who still catches a cold or other illness every month

- a child who has been in child care or preschool for a few years continues to get sick over and over again

- a child in a large family who gets sick far more often than any of the other children

These are all situations that parents may be able to do something about by looking for reasons that might be increasing their child's risk. Rarely, however, a child's illnesses may be due to an immune deficiency, and that is more serious. Such children not only catch frequent routine illnesses but also suffer from recurrent severe illnesses, such as:

- pneumonia

- severe skin infections

- bloodstream infections

If your child has had more than one such episode, talk to your doctor about immune-disorder testing.

Causes

Most cases of frequent illnesses have a reasonable, and preventable, explanation. Here are some of the possibilities you should consider:

Environmental allergies. Some children are allergic to dust, mold, or pollens in the air. These children will often have chronic nasal congestion, which lowers their nasal and respiratory immunity and leaves them more open to catching colds, cough, sinus infections, and ear infections. See page 131 for more information.

Food allergies. While most food allergies cause rashes and intestinal symptoms, two food groups can contribute to more frequent illnesses:

- Cow's-milk products. The chronic nasal congestion caused by this allergy really sets a child up for sinus and ear infections. Consider this cause especially between ages one and two years when cow's milk is usu-

ally introduced. We have solved many frequent illness problems in our practice simply by removing cow's milk from the diet.

- Wheat products (and other gluten grains). Allergy to gluten can cause a variety of allergic symptoms, but it can also actually suppress the immune system.

See page 327 for more information on food allergies.

Enlarged tonsils and adenoids. These immune-fighting tissues at the back of the nose and throat gradually increase in size during the first six years of life, then begin to diminish again. Most children don't even notice, but some will begin to experience congested and obstructed breathing. These enlarged tissues are a magnet for germs and may become repeatedly infected. Having them removed can result in far fewer sinus and tonsil infections. See page 523 for more information.

Careless exposure and improper hygiene. Some children may catch everything that goes around simply because they don't wash their hands, carelessly put every toy or object in their mouths, and attend every playgroup and nursery setting possible. This type of lifestyle, while great for social development, may not be ideal during the winter months if your child seems prone to catching infections. Take an occasional break from the social arena if your child is sick all the time.

Junk-food diet. Don't discount the immune-lowering effects of sugar overload and junk food, or the boosting benefits of fruits, veggies, healthy fats, and overall healthy eating. Take a good look at your child's (and your whole family's) diet if illness abounds in your house. See page 33 for more healthy eating tips.

Prevention

Review the possible causes above and try to correct as many aspects of your child's life as you can. If it's financially possible, take a break from child care. Avoid nursery settings, especially during the winter. Review the list of immune-boosting supplements on page 37. Give these to your child every day for several months to try to break the illness cycle.

FUNGAL INFECTIONS

At some point, almost every child or adolescent will get a fungal infection somewhere on the body. These usually bother parents more than children and are easily treated.

Depending upon the location on the body and the general appearance of the infection, a fungal infection (the medical term is *tinea* infection) may be very easy or very difficult to differentiate from other rashes. Sometimes, a pediatrician may perform a skin-scraping test where skin cells from the area in question are gently scraped off and examined under a microscope. This often reveals whether a fungus is the culprit. The good news is that many fungal infections can be treated with over-the-counter (OTC) antifungal creams. Only more severe infections require prescription treatment. The following is a list of the various fungal infections common among children and adolescents, with tips on treating and avoiding spread of these infections. For fungal diaper rash, see page 543.

DR. SEARS TIP
Are Skin Fungal Infections Contagious?

Yes, they are, but not through casual contact. Repeated or prolonged contact with a fungal rash can transmit the germs, but a child can attend school and playdates without worry to others.

Ringworm

Also known as *tinea corporis*, ringworm is a very common fungal infection among children. It is often transmitted to the child's skin through contact with pets, resulting in a characteristic reddish ring-like rash that can appear on almost any part of the body. This rash often disappears on its own; however, if left untreated, it may spread to other areas of the body. While these rashes are usually not painful or bothersome, their unsightly nature often leads parents to bring the child in for evaluation and treatment.

Ringworm is not always easy to tell from other skin conditions, such as pityriasis rosea, psoriasis, or contact dermatitis. Your doctor may need to scrape the scales and examine them under a microscope to see the fungi. Most ringworm can be cleared with simple OTC antifungal creams or ointments. Only severe ringworm infections require prescription-strength antifungals. If your child has a pet and keeps getting ringworm infections, you should have your veterinarian evaluate your dog or cat for possible ringworm treatment. Ringworm can often be confused with eczema, since eczema can also manifest itself on the body in a ring-like nature. Here's how to tell:

Ringworm	Eczema
• doesn't itch much • location: anywhere except elbows, knees • circular "ring," raised borders with clear center	• itches • location: elbows, behind knees • more flat borders, not always circular, not clear in center

Tinea Versicolor

Another less common fungal infection that can occur anywhere on the body but most often on the face, arms, or trunk is called *tinea versicolor,* which appears as white patches. The patches become lighter in the summer and darker in the winter — hence the name. This type of fungal infection often results from chronic exposure to dampness, for instance from spending a lot of time in pools, reusing damp towels, and sharing towels and washcloths with other people. Tinea versicolor fungal infection often responds to OTC antifungal treatments, but occasionally requires a prescription-strength medication. It differs from vitiligo (see page 535) by its rough feel. Vitiligo (a curious non-fungal quirk of hypopigmentation) is flat and smooth.

Athlete's Foot

Also known as *tinea pedis,* this is a very common condition among active children and adolescents. Fungi love moist, damp, and dark areas, and toes and soles of the feet can become infected with athlete's foot because they are often covered with moist socks and sweaty shoes throughout the day. Athlete's foot is usually very itchy and can occasionally become painful if severe. It also can be notori-

ously difficult to get rid of and may require several weeks of OTC or prescription antifungals. We always advise patients to treat athlete's foot for several days after the area has become completely clear because stopping treatment too early often results in a return of the condition. We also advise a combination of antifungal cream several times a day and intermittent use of foot powders that can help keep the feet dry during the period of treatment.

If your child struggles with recurrent foot fungus, eliminate the culprits that may cause it in the first place. Encourage the use of personal flip-flops in public recreation areas, such as locker rooms, common showers, and around the pool. Sharing shoes with other children should also be avoided. It is also important to thoroughly clean all the shower stalls and bathtubs in the house with bleaching agents in order to kill any fungi. Whenever possible, and if safe, encourage your child to go barefoot or wear sandals or flip-flops to lessen the constant use of shoes and socks. For further discussion on treating athlete's foot, see page 159.

 DR. SEARS TIP
Trash Those Infected Socks!

Another way to help clear up athlete's foot infection is to throw out those old smelly sneakers and socks and purchase new ones. No need to throw out all socks, just the ones that have been around a little too long!

Jock Itch

Known by the medical term *tinea cruris,* this type of fungal infection got its name because it usually presents in the groin area and is often a result of young male athletes wearing jock-straps. The moist, dark environment is a breeding ground for fungus. Jock itch is quite irritating and itchy, as its name implies. It can be notoriously difficult to clear since it is often not possible to avoid the use of a jockstrap during a particular sporting season. To prevent jock itch, encourage your child to remove his jockstrap and sports pants as soon as he is done with the sporting event and then to thoroughly clean the region. OTC antifungal treatment can sometimes take a couple weeks to take effect. Occasionally, a prescription-strength cream is needed. Again, the use of drying powders and anti-itch creams can also be part of the treatment. Make sure you consistently wash your child's jockstrap in order to prevent a buildup of fungus, and buy a new one at least every sports season.

Fungal Infection of the Scalp

Fungus on the scalp is called *tinea capitis*. The fungus invades the hair shafts, causing them to break. This often results in a round bald patch where the fungus resides.

Symptoms. Symptoms of tinea capitis can vary greatly, but may include:

- Scaly or flaky appearance of the bald spot

- Black dots on the bald spot. The small black dots are actually the remainder of hair shafts that have been broken off at the surface of the scalp.

- Itchiness of the affected area

- A red, round nodule, called a *kerion,* forming on the affected area of the scalp

Diagnosis. Your pediatrician may suspect a fungal infection of the scalp based on the characteristic appearance. The doctor may take a sample of the affected scalp and hairs and examine them under a microscope for the presence of fungus. The doctor might also perform a fungal culture, which involves taking a sample of the affected area and seeing if the fungus grows.

Treatment. Successful treatment for fungus infection of the scalp usually requires oral antifungal medications for a period of at least six weeks. Antifungal creams, shampoos, or ointments usually do not effectively treat this condition, although a very mild case may respond to an antifungal shampoo. In almost all cases, the hair slowly grows back following successful treatment.

Is tinea capitis contagious? Yes. Your child can pass this to other children. It is important to talk to your child about not sharing combs, brushes, hats, and so on until she has been successfully treated.

 DR. SEARS TIP
Shampoo Treatment

You can make your child less contagious by washing the hair with a shampoo containing selenium sulfide twice a week until he finishes his oral antifungal therapy.

GASSY BABY

Babies get gas from two mechanisms: swallowing too much air during feeding and producing too much intestinal gas during digestion. De-gasing your baby is accomplished by minimizing these two sources of gas production. Here's how:

Decrease air swallowing when breast-feeding. Be sure Baby has a good latch-on seal by tickling his mouth open very wide so that he latches onto the areola as high as possible above the nipple. The more areola he can latch onto, the less air he is likely to swallow.

Eliminate fuss foods. While there seems to be no scientific rationale for foods in a breast-feeding mother's diet causing gas in her baby, mothers swear it does happen. Foods that have been implicated include dairy products, broccoli, cabbage, wheat, corn, and high caffeine foods.

Lessen air swallowing when bottlefeeding. Be sure Baby's lips are positioned high on the wide *base* of the nipple, not just on the tip. Tilt the bottle forty-five degrees while feeding so the air rises to the bottom of the bottle. Use collapsible "nurser" bags to lessen air collection.

Respond promptly to Baby's cries. Babies swallow a lot of air when crying excessively. If your baby is prone to gassiness, promptly respond to her cries. And certainly don't fall prey to the cry-it-out crowd.

Experiment with various burp positions. Through trial and error you'll notice which techniques get out the most air.

Help the gas pass. Try what we call the *gas pump* position. Lay Baby on his back on your lap with his legs toward you and his head resting on your knees. Pump his legs up and down in a bicycle motion while adding a few attention-getting facial antics. You can also try the *tummy tuck.* Place a rolled-up cloth diaper or use a warm-water bottle enclosed in a cloth diaper under Baby's tummy. Then lay Baby tummy-down on a cushion with his legs dangling over the edge while rubbing his back. See Colic, page 229.

Try the "I love you" abdominal massage. Place Baby on his back on the floor as you kneel at his feet. Do a gentle downward stroke for the "I" on Baby's left side of the abdomen as you press the gas down and out of the descending colon. Then do an upside-down "L" for *love,* moving gas along the middle segment and down Baby's left side. Finally, make an upside-down "U" for the *you* as you stroke again up Baby's right side across the middle segment and down the left side. Be sure to warm your hands.

De-gas baby in a "bubble bath." Massage Baby's abdomen while sitting with her in a bathtub and immersing her tense tummy in warm water. You may notice gas bubbles appear in the water.

 DR. SEARS TIP
General Intestinal Remedy

Remember our rule of twos for any intestinal upset, including gas: feed Baby *half* as much, *twice* as often. Presenting smaller amounts of food to the intestines more frequently allows more complete digestion to occur, so there is less undigested food to ferment and release gas.

GASTROESOPHAGEAL REFLUX DISEASE (GERD) (Acid Reflux, Indigestion)

If your baby seems colicky, spits up a lot, and is a restless sleeper, she might have reflux. Let's follow food from the mouth to the stomach to understand what happens when your baby suffers from reflux. After chewing and swallowing, the food travels down the esophagus into the stomach. Once it has entered the stomach, a circular band of muscle where the esophagus joins the stomach (called the lower esophageal sphincter) contracts and acts like a valve that closes to keep the food and acid-containing stomach contents from regurgitating, or refluxing, back into the esophagus. Sometimes this valve is immature and doesn't completely close. When the stomach contracts, partially digested food and stomach acids reflux back up into the esophagus and irritate (or "burn" — hence the term *heartburn*) its sensitive lining. How much pain the baby has depends upon the severity of the reflux. If the stomach contents reflux just a little way up the esophagus, Baby may hurt but not spit up. But if the reflux is severe enough that the stomach contents come all the way up, Baby may spit up a lot, especially when lying flat. The refluxed stomach contents can also settle in the back of the throat, causing a sore throat, gagging, coughing, erosion of dental enamel, and sour or "acid" breath. During severe reflux the stomach contents can even be aspirated into the lungs, causing wheezing or asthma-like symptoms.

GERD vs. happy spitters. Around 30 percent of all infants spit up a bit, but it doesn't bother them. We dub these babies "happy spitters." These babies are not in pain and they grow normally — this is more of a laundry problem than a medical one. But if the baby does not grow out of the normal spitting-up stage — which most do by seven months — and spitting up is painful and interferes with feeding, sleeping, and growth and development, your pediatrician may diagnose your child with GERD — gastroesophageal reflux disease.

Signs and Symptoms for a Baby

Here are the signs that may indicate your baby has GERD:

- "colicky" baby

- frequent waking in apparent pain

- restless sleep: arches back and squirms a lot, as if "hurting"

- seems to "hurt" right after feeding

- feeding difficulties — either refuses to feed or doesn't feed long enough because he associates feeding with hurting; may arch back and withdraw from feeding or wants to nurse all the time since breast milk can sometimes act as an antacid and Baby associates nursing with comfort

- frequent "wet, sour burps"

- throaty noises — gagging, choking, raspy breathing

- breathing difficulties — frequent respiratory infections, wheezing, stop-breathing episodes

- may be thought to have "baby asthma"

Signs and Symptoms for a Toddler or Older Child

Watch for these signs in your child:

- sour breath

- hoarse voice due to acid irritation of the vocal cords

- frequent ear and sinus infections

- eroded enamel on toddler teeth

- may show inadequate weight gain

- excessive drooling — saliva can act as an antacid and protective lubricant that coats the irritated esophagus

- arching movements and habitual tilting of neck as if having spasms of the back or neck muscles

DR. SEARS TIP
Think GERD, Not Colic

In our pediatric practice we do not use the catch-all term *colic.* Instead, we call it the *hurting baby,* a more accurate term that motivates both parents and doctor to keep searching to find the cause and treatment. Simply labeling Baby "colicky" often misses the right diagnosis. Early in my pediatric practice I (Dr. Bill) was always uncomfortable using the term *colic,* which one of my gastrointestinal professors told me was a five-letter word meaning "the doctor doesn't know." So, in our practice and early writings, I changed the word *colic* to the *hurting baby,* which motivated both parents and pediatrician to search for the reason why Baby is hurting and formulate a treatment plan. After using this approach, I realized in the late eighties that the most common cause of so-called colic is gastroesophageal reflux disease. In 1992 in *The Baby Book* we published the suggestion that parents and pediatricians consider GERD as the root cause of colic. Research over the last twenty years has proven this GERD-colic connection to be correct.

What to Do

A mother in our practice whose infant was ultimately diagnosed with severe reflux once said to us: "I'm going to camp out in your office until you find out why my baby cries so much." Here's a step-by-step guide to both making the diagnosis and helping your baby feel better:

Get the Right Diagnosis

The goal is to figure out whether your baby has GERD and, if so, its severity. Your pediatrician needs your clues not only to make the diagnosis of GERD but to decide if it is minor enough to be treated with feeding and positional changes or if the reflux is severe enough to require antacid medication. You can help the doctor by keeping a GERD diary. In your diary write down:

- signs and symptoms you have noticed (see list above)

- how severe you believe it is

- if the symptoms are improving or worsening

- home treatments you have tried and their results

Tests Your Pediatrician May Do

If signs point to GERD, you and your pediatrician can work out a treatment plan without any testing. If the diagnosis is still in question or your doctor is concerned there may be other mischief going on in the gut, diagnostic tests may be needed, such as:

X-rays or upper GI series. This test is mainly done to be sure there are no abnormalities, such as a partial blockage of where the stomach enters the small intestine or other intestinal quirks. A simple upper GI series is not always sufficient to assess the degree of reflux.

pH probe test. This test can be done as an inpatient or outpatient procedure, or sometimes even at home. One or two thin spaghetti-like tubes are put down your baby's nose and into the esophagus. The other end of the tube is attached to a sensor positioned next to Baby or as a backpack on an older child. The sensor records the pH, or degree of acidity, of the regurgitated material in the esophageal fluid.

DR. SEARS TIP
Be Actively Involved in the Test

To help assess the degree and severity of the reflux, try to note what time of the day your baby has the most severe symptoms, such as crying jags. The interpreter of the pH probe readings will then try to correlate the acid readings with the timing of the observed symptoms.

Endoscopy. In the doctor's office, the outpatient procedure room, or the hospital, a pediatric gastroenterologist will sedate your baby and insert a flexible tube through his nose. This endoscope is attached to a camera, allowing the doctor to see if and how much acid erosion has occurred in the lining of the esophagus and stomach. Although this is the most invasive test, it is often considered the "gold standard" for assessing the degree of reflux. If the lining is only minimally irritated, then a less aggressive treatment approach is warranted. If, however, severe erosion of the esophageal lining is diagnosed, a rigorous and aggressive treatment approach is needed to prevent long-term damage and eventual narrowing of the esophagus.

Gastric-emptying test. Also called *scintography*. Baby is fed a bottle of breast milk or formula containing a very minimally radioactive substance. A computer scans Baby's abdomen and detects how long it takes for the stomach contents to empty. This test can also show aspiration of the refluxed material into the lungs.

Treatment

There are three categories of treatment for GERD:

- feeding changes
- positional techniques
- antacid medications

Practice attachment parenting. (See the Baby B's of Attachment Parenting, page 160.) The four Baby B's of attachment parenting that most help reflux are breastfeeding, baby wearing, bedding close to baby, and belief in the signal value of a baby's cries. Attachment parenting (AP, see page 160) helps babies with GERD in three ways:

- AP babies cry less.
- AP babies enjoy faster digestion.
- AP mothers are able to read their babies' pre-cry or about-to-reflux body language and intervene with positioning techniques.

Avoid the cry-it-out crowd. Remember, babies with GERD cry because they hurt, not because they are "manipulating" you. Uncomforted crying increases pressure inside the abdomen and aggravates reflux. Crying also increases air swallowing and trapped stomach bubbles, which aggravate reflux. We have seen

DR. SEARS TIP
Prolonged Sitting Can Aggravate Reflux

Even though upright, some babies may reflux more when sitting for long periods of time, such as in a car seat or infant seat. Holding Baby more upright and vertical decreases the pressure on the belly and may lessen reflux.

---

babies in our pediatric practice with severe esophageal damage from reflux because well-meaning parents were advised to "let Baby cry it out." Your baby's cry is your baby's language. Also, remember, it's not your fault your baby cries, nor is it a poor reflection of your mothering skills. Respond as sensitively as you can. That's all your baby will expect of you.

Feed Baby frequently. Frequent feeding stimulates saliva production. Saliva lubricates the irritated lining of the esophagus and neutralizes stomach acids. It also contains a substance called epidermal growth factor (EGF),

DR. SEARS TIP
The Reflux Rule of Twos

- Feed your baby *twice* as often.

- Feed your baby *half* as much.

- Encourage your toddler to play "chew-chew" (chew *twice* as long).

The rule of twos is especially important for formula-feeding babies and after beginning solid foods in older infants and toddlers. In our experience, feeding smaller amounts more frequently and slowing down the feedings are effective in easing reflux.

which heals the damaged lining of the esophagus. Also, the less food in the stomach at one time, the lower the degree of reflux, and the faster the food empties from the stomach; so small, frequent meals are best.

Feed Baby a tummy-friendly milk. Breastfeed as often and as long as possible. Breastfeeding helps mothers and babies in the following ways:

- Breast milk empties from the stomach twice as fast as formula.

- Breast milk is a natural antacid, and breast-fed babies feed more frequently.

- During breastfeeding, mothers enjoy a dose of relaxing hormones that help them cope with crying and hurting babies.

- Mother's milk also contains enzymes that aid digestion.

Think of breast milk and breastfeeding as Mom's best medicine for reflux.

Eliminate foods from Mom's diet. Babies with reflux tend to have a higher incidence of allergy to foods in Mother's milk. The usual offenders are cow's milk, wheat, nuts, soy, and corn.

Use a hypoallergenic formula. Babies with reflux may have a double intestinal whammy — food and milk allergies. Formula allergies occur more frequently in infants with reflux. For this reason, if formula-feeding, your pediatrician may advise a "hypoallergenic" formula. Besides being better tolerated by sensitive intestines, some of these formulas are digested more quickly.

Keep Baby quiet after feeding. This is not the time for Dad to play the usual game of tossing Baby around or jostling him on his lap. Jostling Baby can cause stomach contents to splash around and up into the esophagus.

Keep Baby upright after a feeding. Keep Baby both upright and quiet for about thirty minutes after a feeding. Gravity is a refluxer's best friend. Wear your baby in a baby sling for most of the day so that he remains upright at least at a thirty-degree angle.

Burp Baby well. Trapped air bubbles in the stomach aggravate reflux. To minimize air swallowing, burp Baby when you move from one breast to the other. If bottlefeeding, use a collapsible bag nurser to lessen air swallowing and burp Baby after every three to four ounces of feeding.

DR. SEARS TIP
Don't Bottle Prop

Because babies with reflux can regurgitate stomach contents into their throat and gag, choke, or aspirate contents into their lungs, never bottle prop or leave Baby unattended during feeding.

Position your baby for comfortable sleep. Babies with reflux often suffer from painful night waking because when lying flat they don't have the benefit of gravity to help keep the food down. If Baby is a restless sleeper, elevate the head of the crib around thirty degrees using blocks or books. While sleeping on the back is certainly the safest position, babies with reflux will often prefer sleeping on their left sides, the position in which the stomach inlet is higher than the outlet so that gravity helps keep the food down. Special *reflux wedges* to keep Baby propped up during sleep are available at infant product stores.

Pacify Baby. While we generally discourage frequent and extended pacifier use, a pacifier might be helpful to the baby with severe reflux. Frequent sucking stimulates saliva production, which can act as an antacid and soothe the irritated lining of the esophagus.

Dress Baby in loose clothes. Tight diapers and tight waistbands can increase intra-abdominal pressure and aggravate reflux. Also, babies often reflux when lying on their backs during a diaper change. To avoid this, prop Baby up on a reflux wedge during diaper changing.

Don't smoke! Exposure to the nicotine in cigarette smoke increases stomach acid production and opens up the lower esophageal sphincter — both of which aggravate reflux. Not only is smoke bad for Baby, it's bad for Mother. Cigarette smoke can lower the level of maternal prolactin, which helps mothers relax and cope with their hurting babies. Post a "no-smoking" sign in your home and avoid secondhand smoke as much as possible.

Delay solids. If your baby is happy with breast milk or formula alone, no need to increase tummy troubles by introducing solids too soon. Some refluxers improve with heavier foods, such as infant cereal. For others, solid food sitting in the tummy for too long can aggravate reflux. When you begin solids, start with small, frequent amounts and blend them well. If you have a child with reflux, blenders and food processors will be your best friends in the kitchen. If Baby worsens on solids, delay them a few months.

Get support. Consult www.reflux.org. Pediatric and Adolescent Gastroesophageal Reflux Association — PAGER — is a helpful organization of parents with babies who have survived and thrived with reflux.

Reflux tips for toddlers and older children:

• *Raise a grazer.* Continue Dr. Bill's rule of twos above. Let your child nibble on mini-meals throughout the day.

• *Drink the meals.* Fruit and yogurt smoothies blended with vegetables are more easily digested and don't linger in the stomach as long.

REFLUX-AGGRAVATING FOODS

These foods may linger in a child's stomach longer and make GERD worse. They may also pass into the breast milk and irritate a baby's tummy:

• fried foods
• fatty foods
• acidic foods: tomatoes, peppers, citrus fruits, and onions
• gristly meat
• caffeine (Caffeine increases stomach acid production.)
• too much chocolate
• carbonated beverages
• too many spices (chili peppers in excess)
• high-sorbitol fruit juices (Prune, apple, and pear juice may produce intestinal gas and aggravate reflux if your child consumes too much too fast. If your child likes these juices, have him drink them slowly and in small, frequent doses.)

Rapid-transit foods — like smoothies, soups, and low-fat foods — tend to pass through the stomach more quickly.

• *Play chew-chew.* Teach your child to take smaller bites and "chew at least ten times."

• *Don't dine after nine.* Eat dinner earlier and serve a light snack before bedtime. Since reflux is usually worse during sleep, you don't want your child to go to bed either hungry or with a full tummy.

• *Raise a lean child.* Increased intra-abdominal fat can aggravate reflux.

When to Medicate

Most mild reflux can be managed by the parenting style and feeding and positioning strategies mentioned above. But for some infants and children reflux is so severe that suppression of stomach acids is necessary to avoid long-term damage to the esophagus. Before discussing medications, here are a few things parents should think about:

Follow the pills-skills model. (Read the pills-skills model on page 13.) Management of GERD is one of the ailments in which the skills part of treatment really shines. Most refluxers can be managed by self-help skills with a minimum of pills. Remember, pills are in addition to, not instead of, skills.

Pills have side effects. Your pediatrician will put a lot of thought into prescribing antacid medication for your infant or child because acids are necessary for digestion and intestinal health. Besides helping break down food, acids help keep the right balance of bacteria in the lower intestines and can also kill bacteria that may be present in some food. Suppressing stomach acids may allow the harmful bacteria to outnumber the healthful ones and increase the chances of lower intestinal upsets, such as inflammation and diarrhea illnesses.

Types of Medications

Antacids. These are used to treat mild reflux. The main ingredient may be calcium, aluminum, or magnesium, all of which neutralize the acid. Antacids are given three or four times a day just before feedings.

DR. SEARS TIP
Use Probiotics

We routinely give probiotics to children being treated with antacids. Probiotics are the healthful bacteria found in cultured milk products, such as yogurt. Antacids may upset the normal balance of healthful and harmful bacteria in the lower intestines; probiotics can help restore it. (See Probiotics, page 27.)

Motility medications. Also called *prokinetics*, these prescription medicines can both tighten the lower esophageal sphincter and push the food along to the GI tract, increasing the rate of gastric emptying.

H2 blockers and proton pump inhibitors (PPIs). These two medications inhibit the production of acid. The degree of stomach acid suppression depends on the type and dosage of the medicine, which is prescribed according to your child's age and stage of reflux. This is why your diary detailing the severity of the reflux is so important.

Surgery

For children whose growth and development are being compromised by persistent reflux, despite medical and parental efforts, surgical correction is sometimes considered. The most common type is called a *fundoplication*. In this procedure, the band of upper stomach muscle is wrapped either totally or partially around the lower esophagus, which tightens that area and lessens reflux. The partial-wrap surgery still allows the child to vomit. For this reason, it is often the preferred choice. Surgical treatment of reflux is often considered for neurologically impaired children because they tend to have more severe problems with GERD.

DR. SEARS TIP
Eosinophilic Esophagitis (EE)

Children who don't improve on meds may have EE, a severe form of GERD caused by extreme food allergies. It is diagnosed through endoscopy. Ask your GI specialist about it.

GEOGRAPHIC TONGUE

Geographic tongue affects both children and adults. The surface of the tongue resembles a map with areas of reddish plaques surrounded by irregular white borders. It may wax and wane over time, sometimes presenting on certain areas of the tongue and then disappearing only to reappear later on other areas. Geographic tongue may be confused with other conditions in children, such as thrush or burns on the tongue. There is no known cause.

Symptoms

Most children with geographic tongue have no symptoms other than the appearance of the tongue. This condition is considered a painless, harmless quirk. On occasion, children may have the following symptoms:

- burning sensation in the mouth

- difficulty eating

- difficulty sleeping

- increased sensitivity to hot or spicy foods

Treatment

There is currently no known treatment for geographic tongue. The symptoms of geographic tongue generally improve with time. Avoid feeding your child hot or spicy foods if these irritate the tongue.

GROWING PAINS

Just before going to bed your six-year-old says "owie!" as he rubs his thighs and lower legs. He moves his legs a lot, seems restless, and asks for help.

Typical growing pains are a common quirk of active childhood. They hurt but they are harmless. These pains usually come on at the end of the afternoon as your child moans that his legs are hurting and throbbing. While the exact cause of growing pains is not really known, they are real. Your child's legs do hurt. He is not imagining these pains or using them to play on your sympathy. We suspect that growing pains are caused by the overuse of the leg muscles and oftentimes by using the feet and legs in a way they were not designed to be used. Young muscles and bones were designed to run on sand, grass, and dirt, not on concrete, asphalt, and hard gym floors.

Signs and Symptoms

Clues that your child has typical growing pains are:

- Pain typically occurs at the end of an athletic day or before going to bed.

- The child circles the area of the upper thigh or calf muscles but is often vague about exactly where they hurt.

- Pain usually alternates from leg to leg.

- The child does not point to the joints, such as hip, knees, or ankles.

- You don't notice swelling or localized tenderness — called *point tenderness.*

- Movement, such as walking, does not aggravate pain.

- The child does not limp or "walk funny."

- The child is otherwise well.

When to Worry

Clues that these might be more than just growing pains and you should seek prompt medical attention are:

- The child limps.

- Pain is consistently in only one spot for several days or nights.

- You feel a localized area of tenderness and/or swelling.

- The child has associated pain in his back or hurts when bending over.

- The child points to joint areas, such as hip, knees, or ankles.

- Pains are associated with fever, paleness, or other signs of illness.

DR. SEARS TIP
Circle vs. Point Signs

Remember the circling versus pointing sign. If your child is vague and can't localize the pain, worry less. If your child repeatedly points to the pain in the same location, that's a sign for worry.

What to Do

As you do with all chronic pains, keep a growing pain chart, especially charting the severity, frequency, and description. Typical growing pains become less frequent, less severe, and more vague in their description. Growing pains give you an opportunity to reconnect with your child and shine as a home therapist:

- Apply heat, such as a warm towel right out of the dryer or one moistened with warm water.

- Massage the area while you play soothing music and simply talk with your child. A therapeutic touch and a bit of tender-loving care is usually just what your child needs.

- Stretch the muscles by having your child extend his leg and flex the foot upward and downward.

- Offer a warm bath.

- Hydrate your child. After strenuous exercise, dehydrated muscles can hurt. Be sure your child drinks lots of water during and immediately after sports.

- Check the feet. Flat, in-turned (pronated) feet that pound on hard surfaces can throw the axis of weight bearing off balance, stress the muscles, and cause them to hurt. Have your pediatrician examine your child's feet — orthotics may help.

- Use heel cushions. Growing heel bones were not designed to pound on hard surfaces. Get over-the-counter sponge-rubber heel cushions for your child to wear in his running shoes. Try to buy running shoes that have cushiony heels.

Once your child's bones are fully formed, they will outgrow these pains and you will outgrow your worry.

HAIR LOSS

Hair loss, or *alopecia,* in children can have several different causes. Thankfully, they are almost always treatable.

Pulling Hair Out

Hair loss can occur when a child physically pulls her own hair out. This condition is also known as *trichotillomania.* It usually results in irregular patches of hair loss that can occur anywhere on the scalp. These areas are not usually round or oval shaped as with other types of hair loss. Often, trichotillomania develops slowly over time if the child has a habit of pulling or twisting her hair and can worsen if your child is suffering from anxiety or going through a period of stress.

The only successful treatment for this condition is to get your child to break the habit of pulling or twisting her hair. Helping a child through periods of anxiety or stress may also help. With time, the patches of hair loss almost always grow back.

 DR. SEARS TIP
Be a Hair Detective

Observe your child throughout the day if you suspect the hair loss is being caused by the child herself. Children most often pull or twist their hair prior to falling asleep or while watching television or movies.

Physical Damage to the Hair

Children's traction alopecia is caused by direct physical damage to the hair shafts. A young child's hair is much more fragile and brittle than that of an adult. This condition is often seen among girls whose hair has been braided too tightly or undergone large amounts of chemical treatments. Many currently popular hairstyles put too much stress on these fragile hair shafts.

First and foremost, have your doctor make sure that hair loss is due to children's traction alopecia and not something else. Treatment for this condition simply involves handling the hair more gently and switching to a more natural hairstyle. Simply doing this will almost always cause the hair to regrow; however, this process can take several months.

Alopecia Areata

With *alopecia areata,* one or more circular bald spots on the scalp appear. Unlike the scaly appearance of a fungal infection, the skin on the bald spot looks completely normal and is not more sensitive than any other area on the head. Doctors do not know what causes this condition. It may run in families. Alopecia areata is not contagious and is not caused by poor eating habits or stress.

See your pediatrician to confirm a diagnosis of alopecia areata. The only "medical treatment" for alopecia areata is watch and wait. In almost all children the hair grows back within one year. Consult the doctor if this condition is not clearing up or seems to be getting worse after a year.

Telogen Effluvium (aka Normal Newborn Hair Loss)

This is a fancy-sounding term for "normal" infant hair loss. In the first few months of life, some infants seem to be losing hair rather than growing it. Sometimes, a newborn may have more hair on his head at birth than he does three months later! This is a very normal process and occurs as more mature hair replaces fragile and thin baby hair. Occasionally, this can also occur in older children after recovering from an illness due to the fact that hair follicles can go into a resting state during and following a period of illness.

Scarring Alopecia

This is a bald spot on the scalp secondary to some type of trauma, such as cuts or burns to the scalp. Trauma can kill the follicles in the affected area of the scalp, resulting in a bald spot where hair does not grow. If the area of trauma is small, it is usually not noticeable unless the hair is cut extremely short. This bald spot will usually be present for life.

HEADACHES

Headaches are a common addition to a variety of illnesses, such as fever, flu, and sinus infections. But headaches, in the absence of any illness, are fairly rare in young children. Older kids will begin to experience them from time to time as a normal stress of life. Here is our guide to headaches in children of all ages and what you can do about them.

Causes

Some headaches simply occur by themselves, and others are part of an overall illness. Here are the various causes so you can determine the best course of action.

Infectious Causes of Headaches

Cold and flu. Headache is a common part of these routine illnesses. See pages 222 and 325.

Sinus infections. Headaches around the eyes and forehead may be part of a sinus infection. See page 472.

Fever. Fever will almost always cause a headache. In fact, your child's first complaint with a febrile illness may be headache. See page 317.

Strep throat. If your child has a sore throat, fever, and headache, think strep. See page 500.

Meningitis. Severe headache, along with stiff neck, fever, vomiting, and light sensitivity, may indicate meningitis. See page 393.

Non-Infectious Causes

Routine headaches. As children enter puberty, an occasional headache from the simple stresses of life is to be expected every couple months. This doesn't really warrant any cause for concern.

Vision problems. As vision problems begin to set in, so do headaches. This should be the first thing you and your doctor check out if your child has recurrent headaches. A child may not necessarily notice eye strain or minor vision problems.

High blood pressure. This is a rare cause, but is easily checked at the doctor's office.

Low blood sugar. If your child's headaches seem to revolve around hunger or before mealtimes, it may be low blood sugar. This doesn't really need to be tested. You'll just have to stay on top of the healthy snacks.

Migraine headaches. This troublesome condition involves severe, throbbing headaches that last for hours or all day. They are often accompanied by nausea and dark spots in the vision. See page 396 for more information.

Stress. Just as with adults, older kids and teens can get tension headaches. If recurrent and problematic, try to relieve some of the stress in your child's life.

When to Worry; What to Do

Routine headaches are generally not anything to worry about. A little rest in a quiet room and some pain medication (if needed) usually do the trick. Here are some situations, however, that warrant a call to your doctor:

- symptoms of meningitis (see above)

- the "worst headache ever"

- headaches along with other neurologic symptoms such as blurry or double vision, dizziness, or muscle weakness

- severe headache after a head injury

Solving Chronic Headaches

If your child is having unexplained headaches on a regular basis, we suggest you do the following:

- Keep a headache diary. Write down what time of day, relation to meals, severity, what makes it better, what your child is doing at the time.

- See your pediatrician. A vision test, blood pressure check, urine dipstick, and physical exam can rule out any obvious causes.

- See an eye doctor. An eye doctor can detect more subtle problems that a pediatrician would miss.

- See a chiropractor. This may help improve the health and alignment of the neck and spine, which may solve the problem.

- Food allergy testing. Some kids will experience headaches from food allergies. See page 327.

HEAD BANGING

Head banging is a common and usually harmless toddler behavior. An easily frustrated child between two and three years of age who is not yet verbal might convey his frustrations by banging his head. As toddlers are learning to deal with frustration, some choose to meet it "head on."

What to Do

Be reassured that while head banging is upsetting to parents, children seldom hurt themselves. We can't remember an injury in our pediatric practice as a result of this behavior. Yet, as with many behaviors that are upsetting to both parent and child, by helping your child work through the head-banging stage you can shine as a valuable resource.

Track the trigger. List the circumstances that led to head banging. Is your child bored, tired, or in a confined space (such as a crib)? Once you have determined what provokes this behavior, try to intervene.

Try holding time. If your child is going through a head-banging stage, begin each day on a comforting note. As soon as your child gets up in the morning, cuddle for at least ten minutes. If you see he is building up tension during the day, a few minutes of cuddle time can release tension and often prevent the head banging. For some children, head banging can be a sign that they're going through a general disorganized stage of pent-up frustration. They need to be gentled and mellowed, which helps them organize their whole neurological systems. Rock your child in a rocking chair, nap together, and dance to gentling music.

Play show-and-tell. Give your child alternatives by teaching him how to calm himself without hurting himself. Show him how to squeeze his teddy bear or run around in circles. Now your child has safer methods to act out his frustration.

Use distraction techniques. When you see that your child is about to bang his head, quickly interject *stop-behavior* words, such as *go, car,* and *play,* which are cues that trigger a mental picture of a fun activity he likes to do. Try to get his mind off his head and onto a playful activity.

Play the "bump heads" game. If your child seems to like the feeling of bumping his head, stand him in front of you so that your heads are at the same height and *gently* bump foreheads. You can also let him bump against your softer body parts, like your stomach.

Your child will mature out of the head-banging stage. As he becomes more able to express his frustrations verbally and finds less worrisome alternatives, head banging will become just a memory.

HEAD INJURIES

The most important thing to know right away about head injuries is that they are rarely serious. The skull is designed to withstand the hard bumps and bruises of childhood. Although falling from a piece of furniture onto a hard tile floor or tripping and banging the head on a hard surface is sure to leave quite a bump and bruise, the brain inside is almost never harmed. Here is what you need to know when your child bumps his head.

Note: for children who have experienced a concussion during sports or other athletic accidents, please see Concussion, page 238.

What to Do Right Away

First of all, don't panic. If your child senses that you are relaxed, he is more likely to calm down as well. Follow these steps:

Ice. Place several ice cubes and some water into a sealed plastic baggy and hold it to the bump for twenty minutes. This soft, not-too-cold soother will be more easily tolerated against a sore bump than a hard ice pack. Give your child a break for a few minutes, then repeat the twenty minutes of cold again. This will ease the pain and dramatically reduce the eventual size of the lump and speed the healing. We believe it's worth it to force the issue if you have to.

Pain relievers. Your child is sure to have a headache. As soon as your child is calm, take a brief break from icing to administer some ibuprofen or acetaminophen.

Stop any bleeding. If a cut occurred, it will bleed generously because the scalp is richly supplied with blood vessels. Use a towel filled with crushed ice instead of a baggy so that you can use pressure to stop the bleeding. You can examine the wound later, once everyone has calmed down, to see if stitches may be needed (see page 259).

Don't let your child fall asleep for about an hour. Most kids will want to take a nice long nap after all this trauma. It's better, however, to keep your child awake at first so you can monitor his status. Once an hour has passed, a nap is fine.

Check the pupils. Once your child is calm, look at the pupils. As long as they both appear to be the same size, and aren't unusually large or pinpoint, then you can rest assured there is likely no serious injury.

When to Worry

Most routine head injuries don't require a trip to the doctor. However, you should know what serious signs to watch for. Observe your child for the next twelve hours. If your child shows any of the following, a trip straight to the nearest emergency room is probably warranted. You can call your doctor's office while en route.

Loss of consciousness. If your child blacked out, even for a few seconds, this can mean that the force of the bump was strong enough to cause a bruise or bleeding in the brain. A reassuring sign that your child did not black out is that you either heard or saw your child start to cry immediately after the fall.

Difficult to waken. Your child is sure to want a nap, and that's okay. But don't let him nap for more than an hour without trying to rouse him. If the injury happens late in the evening, sleep near your child and set your alarm to go off every two hours. Nudge your child until you at least see him open his eyes and appear annoyed that you woke him. If you have a hard time waking your child, head for the nearest emergency room.

Altered mental status. This means that your child won't focus on you, look you in the eyes, or respond to questions or commands. Complaining of headache and fighting you when you try to apply ice are actually good signs that he is okay.

Vomiting. Many children will vomit once or twice after a big bump on the head, either from crying, coughing, and gagging, or just from the shock to the skull. This is expected. However, if your child vomits three or more times, this could be a sign of internal injury.

Loss of balance. Many children may complain of dizziness. This is expected. But if your child actually loses his balance and repeatedly falls over while walking, go to the emergency room.

Prolonged crying or severe headache. If your child doesn't calm down after about an hour, or complains of a severe headache an hour after medication, it's best to have him checked out by your pediatrician if the office is open, or at an emergency room after hours.

HEARING PROBLEMS

While your pediatrician may inquire about your baby's hearing during routine checkups, it's up to parents to look for clues that their infant or child may not be hearing normally. Be especially vigilant about your child's hearing in the first few years, since keen hearing is necessary for optimal speech development. It's good to keep an ear out for hearing development, especially if your child has had a history of recurrent ear infections or your pediatrician has frequently mentioned that your child has "fluid behind his eardrums." If your child has allergies, for instance, allergic fluid may collect in the middle ear and restrict the movement of the eardrum, leading to speech and hearing delay. The best way to tell if your child hears normally is to keep a speech diary (see Speech Delay, page 488). Children with hearing problems usually show speech delay.

To detect whether or not your child hears normally, develop your powers of observation of how she responds to normal, daily sounds. Use the guide on the next page.

If you have checked several "no" items, it would be wise to have your child's ears examined for fluid behind the eardrum or wax blocking the ear canal. Based upon your child's history, the doctor will decide when and if to refer you to a hearing specialist (an audiologist) for a thorough hearing exam.

YOUR HOME HEARING CHECK			
AGE	**YOUR OBSERVATION**	**YES**	**NO**
2–6 months	• turns eyes toward speaker • quiets to the sound of your voice • turns head toward normal ambient sounds • startles at unexpected noises • enjoys and is calmed by your voice		
6–12 months	• turns toward sound of your voice when you enter the room • turns toward name when called from behind • babbles, as if trying to imitate your voice • seems fascinated and likes to listen to people talking • turns toward familiar voice at normal conversational volume • babbles and seems to enjoy hearing his own sounds • settles to calming music		
1–2 years	• likes imitating your sounds • responds to simple requests: "Go bye-bye." "Get the ball." • responds to simple questions: "Where's Bobby?" "Where's doggy?" • responds to increasingly complex requests: "Get the ball...throw it to Daddy..." • responds to feeding questions: "Do you want more?" • runs toward door when you say "go" • waves when you say, but don't gesture, "bye-bye" • pointing and signing lessens • turns toward your voice on both sides when approached from behind and spoken to in a soft voice from one side and then the other		
2–4 years	• vocabulary increases — at least 2-3 new words a week • asks "why" and "what" questions • points to familiar pictures in a book when hearing them named • notices ambient sounds, such as telephone ringing, knocking at the door		

DR. SEARS TIP
Hearing Test

Schedule a hearing test when the results are likely to be the most meaningful:

• in the morning when the child is most cooperative

• not during a cold or bout with an allergy (may have fluid in the middle ear)

Use these same guidelines when interpreting results of routine hearing tests at school.

The easiest way for parents to tell if their infant or child hears normally is to evaluate how connected and attentive she is at all ages.

Besides the above specific signs, be sure to have your child's hearing tested if you notice your child:

• just doesn't seem connected or attentive (But a warning: We have detected a few children with diminished hearing who actually seemed extremely attentive and watched their parents' faces very closely when they talked. These children were reading lips and facial language but had diminished hearing.)

• seems somewhat dull and uninterested in surroundings

• is using more rather than fewer signs and gestures to communicate

Protect Your Child's Hearing

Besides fluid buildup in the middle ear (see preventing ear infections, page 288, and treating allergies, page 132), too much exposure to loud noises can damage the hearing. Constant exposure can permanently damage hearing. For adults it's easy to tell: If the sound hurts your ears and leaves them ringing, it's too loud. Even though the occasional child may cover her ears, most children just put up with the noise and suffer the damage. Hearing damage can occur from repeated noise levels of 85 decibels (db). To give you an idea of what that means, normal conversation is between 50–65 db; vacuum cleaner: 70 db; hair dryer: 70 db; blender: 100 db; lawn mower: 110 db; power saw: 110 db. The louder the sound, the less time it takes to damage the ears. Noise damage is permanent because it damages the tiny filaments in the ears, called *cilia,* that vibrate in response to sound. The cilia can't vibrate properly, which diminishes hearing. Here are some ways to "ear muff" your child:

• Monitor the volume of audio headsets and iPods. As a general guide, if you are standing a few feet away and can hear the music after the headset is on your child, it is too loud.

• If you're in loud traffic (heavy trucks can generate noises of 85 db), go out of your way to avoid the noisiest sounds.

• Model ear protection. Wear ear muffs or sound-dampening headphones while using a lawn mower, loud power tools, or even a loud vacuum cleaner. You are modeling to your children that they need to protect their ears. Have a smaller pair on hand for your child if she is nearby.

• Avoid sitting close to speakers at rock concerts. In fact, many rock musicians have some permanent hearing loss. If the music hurts your ears, assume it's harmful to your children's ears.

- Use hair dryers at the lowest possible setting, even if it takes longer to dry hair.

- Teach your child to cup her hands over her ears when around loud noises.

- During long airplane trips avoid sitting at the rear of the plane, which is often the area with the loudest noise. If you prefer the rear of the plane (because it's often nearest to bathrooms), you and your child should both wear noise-reducing headsets.

HEART MURMURS AND HEART DEFECTS

Fortunately for parents (and pediatricians), heart problems are not a common occurrence in children. Many heart defects that a baby may be born with actually go away within a year or two. Serious heart problems are extremely rare. Heart murmurs, on the other hand, are fairly common. While a murmur can indicate that there may be a heart defect, most murmurs are just a normal occurrence during infancy. Here is some basic information on heart murmurs and heart defects and how you and your doctor can work together to approach them.

Heart Murmurs

The term *heart murmur* refers to an unexpected humming sound heard when a doctor listens to a patient's heart beat. Usually, the heart makes two distinct sounds when heard with a stethoscope: the familiar "lub-dub" as the heart contracts and relaxes while performing its function of pumping blood to the body. Any sound that is heard in addition to the normal "lub-dub" is considered a heart murmur. Murmurs have many different causes and are actually fairly common in newborn infants and less common in older children. Most are not cause for any concern, and most go away on their own over time.

Heart murmurs are characterized based on several factors, including:

- loudness of the murmur (usually on a scale from 1 to 6, with 1 being the quietest)

- description of the type of sound the murmur makes

- location where the murmur is heard best

- time during the normal heartbeat cycle in which the murmur is heard.

Heart murmurs that are quiet (grade 1 or 2), have a musical humming quality, are loudest just to the left side of the sternum, and occur right between the "lub" and the "dub" are usually considered a normal type of murmur. Various terms for a normal murmur are *innocent, functional,* or *Still's* murmur (named after the doctor who originally described these normal murmurs). About 95 percent of all heart murmurs during childhood are innocent murmurs. They occur because blood flow in the small heart of an infant can sometimes be quite turbulent (as compared to the larger heart of an adult in which there is more room for the blood to flow through smoothly). It is this turbulence that can be heard as a murmur sound with a stethoscope. If your doctor hears an innocent heart murmur, she may decide to simply monitor the heart murmur with routine regular checkups. This murmur usually goes away on its own as your child gets older and the heart grows larger.

When to worry. If an innocent-sounding murmur begins to change in any way, further testing may be required with an ultrasound of the heart (called an *echocardiogram* or *echo*) to make sure there are no actual heart problems. If a newly discovered heart murmur has characteristics that are not typical of an innocent murmur, your pediatrician will probably order the ultrasound to rule out any heart defects.

Any infant with a heart murmur who develops the following signs of heart trouble deserves an immediate ultrasound:

- rapid, labored breathing consistently throughout the day or night (Any baby may have short periods of rapid breathing for several minutes, which is normal.)

- blue coloring of the hands, feet, or around the mouth

- increasing fatigue and shortness of breath during feedings

Older children, adolescents, and teens may have the following symptoms that may suggest a heart defect:

- becoming easily tired

- chest pain at rest or during activity

- increasing difficulty exercising or doing other types of physical activity

- suddenly losing consciousness or passing out during exercise

These are signs that there may be a heart defect that is causing the heart to have to work harder and harder to pump blood and oxygen throughout the body; see your pediatrician right away.

Heart Defects

There are many possible heart defects that can occur during fetal development. Fortunately, most are so rare that there is no reason to include details on every defect in this book. But we would like to share some information on two of the most common heart problems, in case you find yourself suddenly faced with a heart defect in your child. Your pediatrician may suspect your child has a heart defect based on the sound quality of the heart murmur and the presence of any of the above symptoms.

ASD/VSD, or "holes" in the heart. These are the most common heart defects that babies may be born with. Luckily, they are also the least serious and often will correct themselves as the heart grows larger. During fetal heart development, a hole is present in the muscular wall (or septum) that separates the right and left sides of the heart, allowing blood to flow between the two sides (which is necessary during fetal life). At birth, these holes close off as the lungs begin oxygenating the blood and a newborn's circulation changes (the blood no longer needs to pass directly between the right and left sides). When one or more of these holes fail to close completely, a *septal defect* is left. If this defect is in the upper part of the heart, it is called an atrial septal defect (ASD). When it occurs in the lower part of the heart, it is called a ventricular septal defect (VSD).

After birth, blood will continue to flow through this hole and create a humming murmur sound that your pediatrician will hear. The diagnosis will be confirmed with an ultrasound. How serious this condition is depends on the location and size of the defect. Most of these defects are small and close on their own as the child gets older. Larger defects may not close, the murmur sound will persist, and surgery may be required to repair the defect during the first few years of life. A pediatric cardiologist will follow your baby's progress and decide if and when surgery is needed.

Narrow or dysfunctional heart valves. There are four different valves in the heart that open and close allowing blood to flow through the heart and out to the rest of the body. The normal "lub-dub" heart sound is caused by the opening and closing of these valves. If one of the valves is narrow or not functioning properly, a very distinct type of heart murmur will be produced. Valve problems may be present from birth or may develop later in life. An ultrasound is used to diagnose valve defects, and the child would then be followed by a pediatric cardiologist to

**DR. SEARS TIP
Antibiotic Prophylaxis
at the Dentist**

Children and adults with heart defects are prone to a condition called rheumatic fever (see page 502). During dental procedures, invasive testing involving bladder catheterization, or intestinal scoping procedures, bacteria can easily be introduced into the bloodstream. These bacteria have a special affinity for abnormal heart valves or holes within the heart. They will stick there and form a pocket of infection, causing fevers and heart dysfunction. This can be prevented by taking antibiotics at the time of such procedures. Your pediatrician will inform you if your child's heart condition warrants this precaution.

determine if and when surgery may be needed to repair the valve.

Risk factors. Certain newborns may be more at risk of being born with a heart defect. These include:

- infants born with chromosome disorders (such as Down syndrome)

- infants born with other birth defects

- infants born to mothers who took certain medications during pregnancy

- infants whose mothers drank alcohol during pregnancy

- infants born to diabetic mothers or to mothers who developed diabetes during pregnancy

- infants born to mothers who had German measles (or rubella) during pregnancy

- infants born prematurely

HEAT RASH

Heat rash (also known as *prickly heat* or *miliaria rubra*) often arises during the hot, sweaty months of the year. Babies and children are affected more often than adults. It results from a blockage of the sweat glands in the skin. We often see children with heat rash on their return from vacation in a hot and/or humid environment. The combination of heat, sweat, bacteria, and dead skin cells can all play a role in blockage of the sweat glands, and this leads to local redness, inflammation, and irritation.

How to Tell

Clues that it's heat rash:

- Small, red spots resembling tiny blisters may occur over any part of the body. The blistery rash from prickly heat occurs more often on areas that are covered by clothes, such as shoulders, back, torso, buttocks, and thighs.

- The child complains of an itchy or prickly sensation.

- There may be areas of generalized skin redness along with the tiny blister-like red spots over the area of skin affected by heat rash.

What to Do

- If you notice your child beginning to have what resembles heat rash, avoiding excessive heat and humidity will prevent excessive sweating and may prevent the rash from getting worse.

- Dress your child in loose-fitting cotton clothing. Just like diaper rash, the combination of sweat, moisture, and a tight-fitting bathing suit is a setup for the development of heat rash.

- Soothing medications, such as calamine lotion, can help the symptoms.

- If there is an area with severe heat rash, a few days of an over-the-counter hydrocortisone cream can help the itching.

 **DR. SEARS TIP
Air Dry the Rash**

Try to keep the area as dry as possible. Applying cornstarch over the rash can help; it soaks up excessive moisture and helps prevent the rash from getting worse.

The good news is that in almost every case heat rash goes away within about a week. Occasionally, if the child remains in hot and humid environments for long periods of time, it can last longer. Consult your pediatrician if the rash seems to be getting worse rather than improving.

HEAT-RELATED ILLNESSES

There are three potential problems that children and adolescents can encounter in hot weather. These are heat cramps, heat exhaustion, and heat stroke. The following is a brief description of all three, along with tips to treat and prevent them.

Heat Cramps

Heat cramps, which are actually forceful and painful contractions of muscle groups, are a very common occurrence among children and adolescents when they are involved in athletic events in hot weather. Heat cramps can occur in any muscle group; however, by far the most common muscles involved are the calves and hamstring muscles. Heat cramps are usually due to hot weather, dehydration, heavy exertion, or poor physical condition.

Treatment. It is very easy to spot an athlete suffering from heat cramps. She is usually lying on the field holding the back of her legs and unable to stand or move. The good news is that heat cramps are easily treated.

The cramping usually will improve with rest. This is very important as an improper period of rest before resuming activity may lead to further muscle injuries, such as pulled or torn muscles. A child should always rest completely following muscle cramps and should not return to athletic activity until the cramps have been absent for a while. Other important treatments for heat cramps are:

- drinking plenty of water

- massaging cramping muscle

- putting the child in a cool environment

 DR. SEARS TIP
Hydrate Active Muscles

Teach your young athlete to maintain proper hydration habits. Besides lots of water, he should consume a diet high in potassium, which is very important for proper muscle functioning. Diets low in potassium can make an individual more susceptible to heat cramps. Potassium can be obtained through several food sources, including bananas and leafy, green vegetables.

Heat Exhaustion

Like heat cramps, heat exhaustion is also a result of overheating. While heat exhaustion often occurs during periods of intense physical activity, it can also be due to dehydration alone. Very young children and the elderly are most at risk of developing heat exhaustion because these age groups have a more difficult time regulating their core body temperature.

Symptoms. Signs to look for that may suggest your child or adolescent is suffering from heat exhaustion include:

- excessive sweating

- dizziness

- nausea with or without vomiting

- appearing pale

- fainting

- slight fever of 101 to 102 degrees

Treatment. Take the following steps to treat heat exhaustion:

- have your child lie down and rest, preferably in a cool environment

- give plenty of cold water to drink

- ice packs on the forehead, armpits, and groin can help lower body temperature

Occasionally, individuals suffering from heat exhaustion need intravenous (IV) fluids for rehydration.

When to worry. Seek immediate medical attention if your child experiences any of the following symptoms:

 DR. SEARS TIP
Taking an Accurate Temperature

If you suspect a heat-related illness, it is VERY IMPORTANT to measure your child's temperature correctly. You should use an *oral* or *rectal* thermometer only. Do not use ear or forehead thermometers, as these may give falsely low temperatures.

- fever higher than 102 degrees that does not come down within an hour
- LACK of sweat
- severe vomiting
- is acting confused, lethargic, or is unconscious
- seizures

When treated correctly, children and adolescents recover completely from heat exhaustion with no long-term effects.

Heat Stroke

Heat stroke is the most serious type of heat-related illness and is a medical emergency. Heat stroke occurs most commonly in individuals who are exercising heavily in very hot or humid conditions. However, it can also occur in people who are not exercising if they are exposed to conditions that are hot or humid enough. Individuals who suffer heat stroke while not exercising are usually very young or elderly and frail. These age groups have a more difficult time regulating body temperature. Heat stroke in children or adolescents happens most commonly during periods of intense sports activity during the hottest and most humid times of the year.

Symptoms. An individual suffering from heat stroke will usually exhibit the following symptoms:

- has a very high temperature (often higher than 106°F)
- appears delirious or confused
- may collapse and become unconscious
- exhibits seizure activity

- demonstrates a lack of sweating (An individual with heat stroke may not be sweaty at all. However, some athletes who suffer heat stroke after extreme exercise may still be sweating profusely.)
- has warm, flushed skin

If your child exhibits any of these symptoms, call 911 immediately.

Treatment. After calling 911, cool the body's core temperature and replace lost body fluids. If possible, the child should be placed in a cool environment. While waiting for emergency personnel to arrive, use ice packs to cool the body. Placing ice packs in the armpits, groin area, and forehead most effectively lowers body temperature. If cool water is available, immerse the body as much as possible. If available, IV fluids should be started as soon as possible. Once the body's temperature has been lowered and the individual appears to be recovering from heat stroke, observation in a hospital is usually done to monitor for any signs of further problems.

Preventing Heat-Related Illnesses

The good news is that all of the above illnesses can be prevented by taking proper steps. Here are some simple ideas:

- Hydrate, hydrate, hydrate. Water is usually the best thing to help keep body fluids properly replenished. Athletes involved in intense exercise in very hot and humid climates can also benefit from electrolyte-containing sports drinks.
- Salt tablets are *not* recommended, as they can lead to dangerously high levels of body sodium.

- Wear as little clothing as possible in hot weather while exercising. Football players are most prone to heat-related illnesses among athletes. They wear a lot of equipment and practice often begins in the late summer months when the weather is at its hottest and most humid.

DR. SEARS TIP
Sports Drinks—Good or Bad?

There are a large variety of sports drinks available that are marketed toward young athletes. We are often asked, "Which is better, sports drinks or water?" The choice between water and sports drinks depends entirely upon the intensity of the exercise or athletic event, the temperature of the air and the percent humidity, and the duration of the exercise. In mild to moderate exercise, water is usually all that is needed. Some athletes, such as football players or other athletes that are involved in intense, rigorous exercise in very hot or humid environments, may benefit from replenishment with electrolyte-containing sports drinks. Sports drinks are usually unnecessary for athletes exercising at a lower intensity level. Sweetened sports drinks should not be consumed during periods when the child is not exercising or as a water replacement.

- Observe your child at practice. During the hot summer months, make sure the coaches are allowing the athletes to drink as much water as they want.

- Cool down. Be sure that athletes are getting proper rest periods during practice.

HEPATITIS A

Hepatitis A is a fairly uncommon virus that attacks the liver and intestines. It is contracted by eating contaminated food, so it occurs as food poisoning outbreaks in child-care centers, restaurants, or cafeterias. It is a harmless disease in young children but can be tough on teens and adults. Here is what you need to know if your child is exposed or contracts the illness.

There are other types of hepatitis that are very different. Hepatitis B (see page 467) and C (see page 362) are contracted through blood exposure and/or sexual contact and are far more serious.

Symptoms

Signs of hepatitis A vary greatly by age. Most infants and children under age six won't even notice any symptoms. Older kids will experience some uncomfortable intestinal-flu-like symptoms. Teens and adults are hit the hardest, and will have the following signs:

- jaundice (yellow eyes and skin)

- fever

- nausea/vomiting

- diarrhea

- fatigue

- stomach pain

- poor appetite

- body aches

Because these symptoms mimic a regular stomach flu, people often don't realize they have hepatitis A until the jaundice sets in.

Another clue is that the victim will feel much sicker than expected and the symptoms can last for a few weeks. There are no long-term liver problems, and the disease isn't fatal.

Hepatitis A has a very long incubation period — fifteen to fifty days. An infected person will be contagious for one to two weeks prior to feeling any symptoms, and for another two weeks once symptoms begin. The virus comes out in the stools, and if the person doesn't wash his hands after using the bathroom, the virus gets on anything he touches, like food. This is how a restaurant or cafeteria worker may infect the patrons or a caregiver in a group child-care facility may spread the virus from one infected baby to another by changing diapers and not washing hands.

Diagnosis

The illness is diagnosed with a blood test.

What to Do

Fortunately, most young children, and some older children, won't even show symptoms, so overall there isn't much to worry about for kids. Don't page your pediatrician after hours or rush into an urgent care facility if exposed or if you think your child may have the illness. Here is what you should know:

Treatment. There is no treatment for this virus, other than supporting the fever, body aches, and vomiting with medications and staying hydrated.

Containing outbreaks. Once an outbreak is identified, the public health department will usually get involved and interview everyone who was exposed. They will offer you various options:

- If you or your child have previously had the illness, you are protected.

- If your child has had the vaccine (given to all toddlers between ages one and two since 2006) he is protected.

- Anyone who was exposed and hasn't previously had the vaccine or disease can either choose to just go through the disease (a reasonable option for younger children) or get treated with an antibody injection (called immunoglobulin). This injection is effective in preventing the illness if given within two weeks of exposure to the germ. New research also shows that the hepatitis A vaccine, if given within two weeks of exposure, can also prevent the illness.

HEPATITIS C

Hepatitis C is another strain of a virus that infects the cells of the liver. Worldwide, 170 million people are infected, and approximately 4 million people in the United States currently have hepatitis C.

Before 1990, the most common method of contracting the hepatitis C virus was through contaminated blood transfusions. After that, blood donations were routinely screened for the presence of hepatitis C, along with hepatitis B, and other potential contaminants. Since then, rates of contracting hepatitis C through blood transfusions have become almost non-existent. Today, the most common method of contracting hepatitis C is via contaminated needles, usually through needle-sharing among IV drug users. It can also be transmitted via contaminated tattoo needles. Hepatitis C can be transmitted sexually; however, this is much less common than the above-mentioned methods.

Mothers with hepatitis C. A pregnant woman infected with hepatitis C has a less than 10 percent chance of transmitting this virus to her fetus during pregnancy. When a fetus is born to a mother known to be hepatitis C positive, the infant is monitored very closely and tested often in the first several years of life. This is because a newborn who initially tests negative for hepatitis C may go on to test positive within the first few years of life.

Signs and Symptoms

Signs and symptoms of hepatitis C range from no symptoms at all to short-term symptoms of liver disease, including:

- jaundice (yellow eyes and skin)
- fever
- nausea/vomiting
- diarrhea
- fatigue
- abdominal pain
- poor appetite
- body aches

Treatment

There is no cure for hepatitis C. However, there are therapies that can be instituted in order to lessen an individual's risk for developing long-term complications. This includes treatment regimens of interferon and/or chemotherapy, usually lasting a minimum of six

months, and an individual's response is closely monitored during and after treatment. These treatments are highly individualized. If successful, the level of virus in an individual's system will become almost undetectable. All patients with known hepatitis C should be evaluated by a specialist for treatment.

Long-Term Complications

Approximately 85 percent of individuals infected with hepatitis C will go on to develop a state known as *chronic hepatitis C.* Similar to hepatitis B, this can eventually lead to cirrhosis and/or a specific form of liver cancer known as *hepatocellular carcinoma.* About 20 percent of those with chronic hepatitis C will eventually develop one or both of these two often-fatal liver conditions. In fact, hepatitis C is now the most common reason for liver transplant in the United States.

Prevention

Currently, there is *no* vaccine for preventing hepatitis C infection. Hepatitis C prevention is focused upon avoidance of high-risk activities

---

 DR. SEARS TIP
Beware of Body Painting and Piercing

Your teenager comes into the kitchen one day declaring her desire to obtain a tattoo. After what may be a stunned silence when you marvel at how fast she's grown up, it is important that she understand the risks of doing so. It is vital that the artist is state licensed and certified in proper sterilization techniques. Bottom line: Make sure the tattoo artist is certified!

---

that may expose an individual to the virus. This includes avoidance of needle-sharing practices among intravenous (IV) drug users. There are many government programs that assist users in drug treatment, as well as provide clean needles for their use.

HERPES SIMPLEX VIRUS TYPE I (HSV-I)

This virus, also known as oral herpes, is responsible for common "cold sores" in children and adults. By adulthood, 50 to 80 percent of individuals have been exposed to herpes simplex virus type I (HSV-I). HSV-I can affect almost any age group, and is usually transmitted through contact with infected saliva. For information on the sexually transmitted virus (HSV-II), see page 468. If your child is having the first episode of multiple mouth sores and fever, see Mouth Sores, page 404, to determine what type of infection this might be. For single cold sores on the lips, see page 229. For single canker sores in the mouth, see page 210.

Symptoms

Symptoms of an initial infection with this virus can vary greatly. Some children experience only mild symptoms, such as low-grade fever, general fatigue, headache, and mild sore throat. They also usually have small, reddish, and painful sores present on the lips, gums, tongue, tonsils, and back of the throat. Over several days, the red sores tend to develop white spots in the middle of them. Some children have more severe symptoms that may include high fever, difficulty eating,

extremely sore throat and tonsils, and swollen and bleeding gums, along with the very tender sores mentioned above. Initial infection with this type of herpes is usually the most severe. Adults who get their initial infection at an older age tend to have less severe disease. This illness usually lasts approximately one week, but it may take up to two weeks for your child to fully recover.

The saying "herpes is forever" is true. The herpes virus can bury itself in tissues and reside there for a lifetime, and "come alive" when triggered. Herpes usually recurs throughout one's lifetime. Some children and adolescents can have several recurrences per year, while others may experience these much less often. Known triggers for recurrences of oral herpes include fever, stress or anxiety, and even sunburn. Individuals with impaired immune systems usually suffer more frequent and severe outbreaks. The good news is that recurrences are less severe and less frequent as one ages.

 DR. SEARS TIP
Keep the Cold Sores from Erupting

People who are used to getting recurrent cold sores around the mouth often feel tingling a day or so before the sores actually erupt. By applying a prescription antiviral ointment, such as acyclovir, to the area when you first sense "that feeling," you can often prevent the sores from erupting.

Treatment

Unfortunately, there is no cure for any type of herpes. Treatment of oral herpes focuses mainly on symptom relief. Methods can include anti-inflammatories, numbing throat sprays, and over-the-counter cold sore treatments for lip sores. Liquid anesthetic can be applied to very painful areas to help numb them and relieve symptoms. A prescription medication, such as acyclovir, can be used if it is severe.

DR. SEARS TIP
Cool It!

One of the most common complaints parents have regarding children with oral herpes sores is that they refuse to eat because it is too painful to swallow. In addition to the above-mentioned treatments, we recommend sticking to mostly liquid-type diets, such as cold smoothies or shakes. Cold liquids are a natural anesthetic. Avoid acidic or spicy foods. The coolness of a shake or smoothie tends to be easier to swallow than regular food.

Newborn Herpes

Rarely, an adult with oral herpes sores may pass the virus to a newborn baby via saliva and cause a severe infection within the brain.

HICCUPS

Hiccups are a harmless nuisance that occurs at all ages. Babies even hiccup in the womb. Generally, hiccups only bother infants and children if they occur shortly after a feeding. Hiccups are caused by involuntary spasms of the diaphragm, the large muscle draped over the stomach and liver. During a hiccup, the diaphragm goes into spasm and contracts, causing one to take a deep breath. At the same time, the vocal cords snap shut, causing the hiccup sound.

What to Do

While hiccups seldom bother a child, they can be a nuisance if they occur too frequently or last too long. Here is our guide to controlling the hiccups:

Slow feedings. Because the diaphragm is close to the stomach, there is often a connection between activity in the stomach and hiccups. When the stomach distends too fast, it can cause the diaphragm to spasm, leading to hiccups. Try Dr. Bill's rule of twos: eat *half* as much, *twice* as often, and chew *twice* as long.

Reduce air swallowing during bottlefeeding. For infants, swallowing too much air too fast can cause hiccups. Try these tricks to minimize air swallowing:

- To improve the seal on the bottle, make sure Baby's lips are positioned on the wide base of the nipple, not just on the tip.

- Try "nursers" — bottles with collapsible formula bags that minimize air swallowing.

- Tilt bottle to a forty-five-degree angle so air rises to the base of the bottle.

- After feeding, keep Baby upright for at least a half hour to allow swallowed air to rise.

- Burp Baby well halfway through a feeding and after a feeding.

Track the trigger. Keep a hiccup diary. See if you can identify a consistent pattern or triggers of the hiccups and minimize them as much as you can.

Encourage your child to drink liquids.
Have your child slowly sip a glass of warm
water with a tincture of lemon. The theory
behind drinking during hiccups is that stimulating the nerves in the back of the throat
interrupts the nerve cues triggering the
hiccups.

Tell your child to take deep breaths. As
soon as your child feels a hiccup coming on,
get her mind off her tummy and chest. Tell
her to spread her arms out, take a deep
breath, and hold it while she counts to seven
in her head, and then slowly let it out. Hiccup
researchers believe that breath-holding retains
some carbon dioxide that interrupts the
spasms of the diaphragm.

**Have your child breathe into a brown
bag.** Put the bag over your child's mouth and
nose and have her breathe in and out slowly
and deeply through her nose ten times. The
re-inhalation of carbon dioxide may soften the
hiccups.

Distract. To get your child's mind off her hiccups, try distracting her with a favorite game
or activity. However, keep in mind that sometimes too much laughter can trigger air swallowing and aggravate the hiccups.

HIP DISLOCATION IN INFANTS

You may wonder why your pediatrician so
carefully checks your baby's hips at each regular checkup and during the first newborn
exam in the hospital. The doctor is making
sure the leg bone is normally inserted into the
socket of the hip joint. Normally, the leg bone
fits into the socket of the hip bone like a ball-
and-socket joint. Sometimes the ball slips out
of the socket in the few months after birth, or
the hip-bone socket was not tight enough to
hold the leg-bone "ball" at birth, causing the
hips to be dislocated. Doctors pay special
attention to babies who were breech, because
the position of a breech baby in the womb
can keep the leg bone from locating properly
into the hip socket, causing dislocated hips at
birth.

With growth and development of the hip
joint, the ball and socket gradually grow
together into a stable joint. If the ball remains
undetected out of the socket for many
months, the socket grows flat instead of
cupped. The longer the leg bone remains out
of the socket, the tighter the muscles around
the hip joint become, which further limits the
ball-and-socket joint from developing. As a
result, instead of needing a short-term simple
splint, the flattened socket will require major
surgical correction, with uncertain results.

Infant hip dislocation is termed *developmental dysplasia of the hip* (DDH),
encompassing various degrees of dislocation.
This is because the typical signs of dislocated
hips may not be present at birth, but may
"develop" sometime later within a baby's first
year.

DDH isn't common, but the risk goes up if
there is a family history: 12 percent if a parent
had dislocated hips and as high as 36 percent
if both a parent and a previous child had
DDH. The risk of DDH is highest in breech
infants, with the incidence around 23 percent.
Girls have a slightly higher risk. Theoretically,
the maternal hormone relaxin may loosen the
hip-joint ligaments, causing instability in the
hip joint. Dislocation is three times more
common in the left hip than the right, presumably due to the usual position that infants
assume in the womb.

What You Can Do

Here's how you can help your pediatrician be sure your baby's hips are developing normally:

- Inform your doctor if there is a family history of DDH, especially in parents or previous children.

- Be sure the doctor knows if Baby was breech, even if it occurred early on and Baby later turned.

- At newborn and regular checkups, try to relax your baby by nursing and comforting just before the exam. When the hip muscles are relaxed (Baby lying quietly on her back in the diaper-changing position), the exam is easier and yields more meaningful results.

What the Doctor Will Do

You'll notice your pediatrician doing the hip-flexion test at every exam, at least during the first year. While Baby is lying in the diaper-changing position, the doctor holds the upper leg bones and gently flexes and abducts the bone. If the ball of the leg bone pops out of the socket, the doctor will feel a little "clunk." You will notice that your doctor does these tests very gently, since detection of a truly dislocatable hip does not require a forceful flexion.

If the doctor feels that the hips are dislocatable, meaning the ball pops in and out of the socket easily, he will likely refer you to a pediatric orthopedist for further care. The orthopedist may recommend you start with a padded splint (resembling the thickness of two or three diapers) to keep the legs within the hip joints. The older treatment of "triple diapering" to splint the legs in cases of suspected DDH is no longer recommended. In most cases, the orthopedist will recommend the Pavlik harness, which keeps Baby's hips spread open most of the time yet allows Baby to kick freely. This harness keeps the leg bones outward (frog-like) to encourage normal hip-joint growth. In more severe forms of DDH, a pediatric orthopedist may need to place casts around Baby's hips and upper legs to keep the leg solidly within the hip socket for several weeks.

In the early weeks, diagnosis of DDH is totally in the hands of the examining doctor. Prior to four months of age, X-rays of the hips are often unreliable because the hip joints are still primarily cartilage. By four to six months of age, X-rays are more reliable. Even ultrasound evaluation of hip development can be unreliable under six weeks of age, which is why ultrasounds are not a routine part of newborn evaluation. Sometimes a hip exam during the first couple weeks after birth may be "equivocal," which means the leg bone seems to be well located within the hip joint but the doctor may hear or feel some clicks that need to be carefully rechecked. In doctor jargon, a "click" is a "no-worry, but follow carefully"; a "clunk" is a "treat or refer immediately."

 DR. SEARS TIP
Hip Joint Noises Are Normal

Don't worry if you hear a "click" when you spread your baby's legs during diaper changing. These are normal "joint noises" that are also present in the hip, shoulder, elbow, and knee joints. These "benign clicks" usually resolve by one month of age.

Later Signs of DDH

Nearly every case of DDH detected and properly treated in the early months will result in normal hip-joint development. Occasionally the usual DDH clues will not present in some babies, even during the most thorough hip examination. As a result, some cases may go undetected until later signs appear. Here are some clues that indicate you need to seek medical attention:

- Tight hips. You notice Baby's legs are getting harder to spread apart during diaper changing and the muscles in the groin are feeling tighter.

DR. SEARS TIP
Swaddle Wisely!

During my pediatric training, I (Dr. Bill) remember seeing a very high incidence of DDH in Canadian Indians due to the custom of swaddling very young infants for many hours at a time. Prolonged and rigid swaddling, especially overnight, can keep the ball-and-socket hip joint from properly forming. While swaddling is a time-tested baby calmer, we discourage swaddling babies for more than a few hours at a time, especially those that have the above-listed risk factors for DDH. After we published the first edition of *The Baby Book* praising the use of swaddling to soothe a fussy baby, my former professor of orthopedics Dr. Robert Salter, who literally wrote the book on infant hip development, asked me to remove the section on swaddling from our book for fear that parents would overdo it. Bottom line: Swaddling is fine, but not too tight, and not for too long.

- As you are changing Baby's diaper, you notice that one leg is significantly tighter than the other. (Some babies with normal hip joints can temporarily have tight hip muscles that gradually loosen as Baby begins to crawl and walk. Tight hip muscles do not necessarily mean DDH, yet should always be mentioned to your doctor.)

- You notice "asymmetrical creasing" on the inner aspects of the thighs. One thigh has one crease, the other two (this finding is just a clue and may be a normal variant).

- You notice your toddler has a "waddle walk" or "stiff-legged gait."

DDH that develops late or isn't noticed until one year or older often requires surgery to correct it.

HIP PAIN

Because pain in the hips is unusual in children, it is always a "see doctor" complaint.

What to Do

After you've booked the doctor's appointment, begin keeping a diary of all the noticeable signs and symptoms of your child's pain:

- How and when did it begin?

- How does your child describe it?

- Has his gait changed?

- Does he limp?

- Is the pain associated with fever or pain elsewhere, such as in other joints?

- Does it hurt when touched or moved?

- Did your child recently start a new sport or strenuous activity?

- Does he also complain of knee pain?

- Does it hurt to bear weight on the affected side?

- What relieves the pain?

- What makes it worse?

What Your Doctor Might Do

Based on your child's history, the doctor will click into the usual and safest mind-set: "Be sure the child doesn't have any illness that if undetected and left untreated is going to harm the hips." The doctor will examine the hips mainly for swelling and limitation of motion and will do what we call "the frog test." If while lying like a frog your child cannot flex and abduct one hip outward as much as the other and/or it hurts to do so, that is a cause for concern and warrants a deeper evaluation.

Your pediatrician will watch your child walk to see if the hip pain affects her gait. This is followed by a total examination to see if there are any other areas for concern, such as swollen glands, fast heart rate, fever, or signs of inflammation anywhere else in the body.

The doctor will most likely order a series of blood tests and possibly an ultrasound or X-ray of the hip. In addition to the examination, these tests are used to detect and treat the most common causes of hip-joint problems in children:

Synovitis. Synovitis of the hip is an inflammation of the lining of the hip joint, which usually accompanies other signs of a viral illness, such as an upper respiratory infection. Like any other viral illness, most synovitis resolves on its own in time. Your pediatrician may request an orthopedic consultation if there is fluid accumulation in the inflamed hip joint that needs to be aspirated.

**DR. SEARS TIP
Knee Pain? Expect a
Hip Problem**

By some neurologic quirk, the pain fibers that register a problem in the hips register pain in the knee on the same side.

Arthritis. While adult-type arthritis is rare in children, juvenile rheumatoid arthritis (JRA) may begin in the hips. With JRA, seldom is only the hip joint affected; the child often has pain and swelling in the knee, ankle, or elbow joints, accompanied by fever, red rash, and a generally ill appearance.

Hip joint injuries. The ball of the hip joint is prone to two rare, but painful, conditions in children. In *slipped capital femoral epiphysis,* the ball of the leg bone is damaged and slips partially out of the hip joint, either by acute trauma or gradual degeneration, causing pain, decreased range of motion, and a limp. It usually occurs in early puberty and can affect both hips. Diagnosis is made by X-ray and treatment involves manipulating the bone back into place and surgery. Legg-Calvé-Perthes disease is a rare disorder affecting elementary-school-age kids. The ball of the leg bone degenerates for unknown reasons, with symptoms similar to those above. Diagnosis is by X-ray, and treatment involves months in a cast.

HIVES

Hives are raised white and/or red patches or welts of varying sizes. They can be as small as a pencil eraser or as large as a silver dollar (or two). They are almost always caused by an allergic reaction. Hives usually appear suddenly, most commonly on the trunk (chest, abdomen, or back) and spread rapidly to other areas, including the extremities. They rarely affect the face.

Most cases of hives don't need to be checked by a doctor. Here is our guide to diagnosing and treating hives. For information on more severe allergic reactions (swelling of the throat, face, hands, or feet, or difficulty breathing), see page 130.

How to Tell

The easiest way to determine if your child's rash is hives is to simply monitor it for an hour (unless the allergic reaction is making your child uncomfortable). Hives will often fade away from one area and pop up in another, continuously shifting and changing over a few hours. Hives are also usually quite itchy.

Apparent hives can be treated with an over-the-counter oral antihistamine. If the welts subside or disappear completely, then you can be fairly certain it is hives. If the welts do *not* subside, it may be another type of rash called *erythema multiforme* (see page 302).

Causes and Duration

Once you have determined your child has hives, the next step is to figure out the cause. Virtually all causes are allergic, but parents and doctors often can't figure out what the allergic trigger is. Here are the commonly diagnosed causes:

Viral illness. Most cases of hives occur simply because the body is having an allergic reaction to a generic viral illness. Such cases may include fever and other signs of illness along with the hives. Antihistamines should still help minimize the rash, although they won't do anything for the virus.

Food allergy. This is the next most common cause. The usual culprits are peanuts, other nuts, shellfish, or berries. However, virtually any food can trigger an allergy in a child. Think about anything new your child has eaten in the last few hours. If nothing comes to mind, think back further to the day before. If you can't think of anything, don't worry. Often a food culprit isn't obvious. If recurrent episodes continue, a food diary should help you narrow it down.

Medications. This is another common cause of hives, but more so in adults. Antibiotics are the usual culprit, but any new medication can cause an allergic reaction. Stop any new medications your child is taking and contact your doctor. If the medication is an antibiotic, it's best to wait a day or two for the reaction to subside before starting another one, unless the infection you are treating is severe.

Skin irritants. New soap, shampoo, lotion, laundry detergent, new clothes that haven't been washed yet, or close contact with bushes or grasses can cause this rash.

How long do hives last? Hives can last anywhere from a few hours to several weeks. Even after the offending cause is removed, the body can continue reacting. You can also expect the hives to return after each dose of medication wears off. This isn't a sign that the condition is worsening. Hives are not contagious.

 DR. SEARS TIP
Keep It Simple

If none of these causes fit with your situation, don't knock yourself out trying to track down the cause. Treating hives is easy and most cases resolve in a day or two without you ever knowing the cause. If they become chronic or recurrent, then some investigation is in order.

Treatment

Mild cases. If your child only has one or two hives that aren't bothersome, you don't have to do anything. At the most, apply cool compresses and an anti-itch cream. Observe your child for any signs of worsening.

Bothersome hives. If you notice numerous hives right away, it's best to administer over-the-counter oral diphenhydramine (Benadryl) to counteract the allergic reaction before it gets too severe. See the Medicine Cabinet, page 549, for dosing instructions and cautions. There are also a variety of antihistamine creams available at any drugstore. They don't work as well as the oral medication but can be used alone or in conjunction with it. Be sure not to overlap an oral antihistamine with an antihistamine cream if applying cream to numerous areas of the body. This may be too much of the same medication. It is safe to use both if only applying the cream to several areas.

Don't overdo it. You don't have to keep your child loaded up on antihistamines just to keep every last hive under control. It's okay to allow some welts to linger as long as they don't bother your child.

When to Worry

Here are the signs to help you decide whether to go to an emergency room right away or to see your pediatrician in the office:

Severe allergic reaction. Wheezing, throat tightening, difficulty breathing or swallowing, uncontrollable vomiting and/or diarrhea, weakness, light-headedness, extreme paleness, or significant swelling of the hands, feet, or face are all signs of a severe reaction. Go to an emergency room if any of these occur. A shot of adrenaline will probably be given to reverse these severe symptoms. See page 130 for more information.

Moderate allergic reaction. Hives with some swelling of the hands, feet, or face without the other signs of severe allergy can probably be taken care of in the doctor's office with prescription antihistamines and steroids.

Prolonged hives or fevers. If your child is generally well, but you have to administer antihistamines for more than two weeks, it's best to have your pediatrician review the situation. If your child has fevers for a few days or other signs of illness, see the doctor.

HOARSE VOICE

A raspy voice in a child can be worrisome for a parent, especially if your child can only manage a whisper. There are several reasons for a child's voice to go hoarse; some are potentially serious, while others are simply a nuisance. Here is a quick guide to help you pinpoint the cause of your child's hoarse voice; you can then turn to the appropriate pages for further information.

Causes

Croup. This is one of the more common causes of a hoarse voice. Croup is caused by a virus, and there is usually a fever to go along with the barky cough that sounds like a sea lion. Stridor (a whoopy-gaspy sound when your child breathes) is a sign of serious croup. See page 250.

Laryngitis. Similar to croup, but without the severe barky cough or stridor. This is usually caused by a cold virus.

Abscess of the tonsil. This will cause more of a "muffled" voice rather than hoarseness. Often present with fever and sore throat, it will give your child the classic "hot potato voice," meaning his voice will sound like he just took a bite of potatoes that are too hot. This is potentially a serious infection — call the doctor. See Tonsillitis, page 523.

Tracheomalacia. This occurs in young infants. It is caused by a floppy airway: The cartilage that surrounds the windpipe can start off softer than normal, allowing the airway to narrow in certain positions. This is a normal developmental "quirk" in some babies. This doesn't really cause a hoarse voice; rather, it causes intermittent raspy breathing when Baby is lying on his back or when he gets excited. It usually disappears when the infant rolls over, sits up, or calms down. Your baby will outgrow this problem as he gets older, but you should mention it to the doctor at the next checkup.

Allergies. Hoarseness may occur with the other typical allergy symptoms of itchy eyes, nose, or throat. See page 131.

Gastroesophageal reflux disease (GERD). Regurgitated stomach acids may settle on the vocal cords, causing inflammation and thickening of the cords, and result in hoarseness. A clue to this cause is morning hoarseness that often subsides during the day, because reflux usually occurs more at night. See page 338.

Strained voice. Most common in cheerleaders, sports fans, and singers, this problem is caused by overuse of the vocal cords. The hoarseness will usually last one to two weeks.

Vocal cord nodules. This is the most common cause of a persistent hoarse voice in toddlers, children, and adolescents. Also called "screamer's nodules" and "singer's nodules," these are fleshy, benign polyps that grow on the vocal cords, causing them to vibrate more slowly and lower the pitch of the voice. These are nearly always caused by overuse or abuse of the voice. They typically occur in preschool children after they go through a screaming stage. These type of nodules usually disappear with voice-mellowing strategies over a few years. They seldom bother the child, but often bother the parents.

Home Remedies

You will find specific treatment information for many of the above causes by turning to the suggested pages. The following remedies can help your child if the hoarseness is simply caused by a strained voice or laryngitis:

• Gargle with warm water with a little salt added (one to two teaspoons of salt in eight ounces of water). If your child doesn't like the salt water, you can try adding a little honey instead (remember, no honey for children under a year of age).

- Cough drops — these tend to soothe the throat, and help your child *not* talk.

- Resting the voice — the most important treatment for hoarseness is good old-fashioned rest. This might be difficult for the child who is a "screamer" (probably the reason for the hoarseness in the first place). Your child should talk as little as possible; writing notes can be a fun alternative.

- Don't whisper — many people think that whispering is a way of resting the voice, but it actually puts *more* strain on the vocal cords.

- Moist air — run a vaporizer or humidifier in the bedroom.

Call the doctor if:

- breathing is difficult

- any objects might be lodged in the throat

- your child recently choked on anything

- your child is less than two months old

- hoarseness lasts longer than two weeks

Treating Vocal Cord Nodules

If your child's hoarse voice persists for more than a few weeks despite the treatments described above, she may have developed persistent nodules. Here is what we suggest:

Voice training. Professional voice training techniques can be taught by a speech therapist to help your child learn how to talk in a way that rests the vocal cords. After a few

months of this careful talking, the nodules may diminish.

ENT (ear, nose, throat) evaluation. If hoarseness persists for more than several months, you should have an ENT doctor evaluate your child. He can use some special instruments to view the vocal cords to determine the size and severity of the nodules. Surgical correction is an option in severe cases.

HOSPITALIZATION

Leaving the security of her own environment, entering a strange place with strange people, and sleeping in a strange bed can be very traumatic for a child. Illness compounds this anxiety. Or, the child might not understand why she has to be in the hospital if she is not sick (for elective procedures, such as a tonsillectomy). The younger the child, the more hospital-parenting is needed. In this section, we will give you some tips on how to make hospitalization easier on your child.

Ask questions. Be sure you understand the hospital visiting rules and *care-by-parent* policies. What procedures will be done on your child? What type of operation or medical tests will he have? Doctors and nurses realize that fear of the unknown is a problem for both parents and child and are eager to communicate the necessary information to you. You will play many roles in your child's hospital care: parent, nurse, doctor, advocate, translator, massage therapist, and so on.

Prepare your child. If your child goes into the hospital for an elective procedure, tour the hospital a day or so before he is admitted. Read your child a short, simple book about children in the hospital. These books are usually available in the hospital gift shop. The better prepared and the more your child understands what procedures or operation he will have, the less fear he will experience. For example, if your child is having a tonsillectomy, show him pictures of where the tonsils are located. Tell him that he will be put to sleep by inhaling some medicine through a mask placed over his face, and that he might wake up with a sore throat, but that he can eat lots of ice cream afterward to make his throat better. Tell him: "Your tonsils will be removed and placed in a pickle jar and afterward you won't have so many sore throats, won't miss so much school, and you'll be able to breathe and sleep better." Explain to him that he may feel a bit groggy as the anesthesia wears off. Young children often distort information provided about certain procedures or operations, so try to keep it as simple and free of fantasy as possible.

Explore your child's feelings. What are your child's feelings about the impending hospitalization? Ask her to talk about her feelings, even though children seldom do. You will learn a lot about your child's emotions by asking her to draw pictures about what she imagines the hospital will be like.

Stay with your child. The younger the child, the more important the parents' presence and support. One of the biggest breakthroughs in hospital care is that today's pediatric hospitals actually encourage *care-by-parent*. This means you have a rooming-in arrangement, allowing you to sleep on a cot in your child's room. You feed your child, bathe him, care for his simple medical needs (under instructions from your doctor or nurse), and comfort him in periods of pain or stress. Our experience is

that children recuperate faster and have much less fear of hospitals when their parents are intimately involved in their care.

Child-considered hospital care minimizes separation anxiety from parents and eases children into traumatic situations. For example, your hospital may allow you to put on a scrub suit, go with your child into the operating room, and stay with him until the "induction" (the beginning of the anesthesia) has begun and your child is asleep. Then you will be asked to leave.

Be in the recovery room when your child awakens. Ask to be notified when your child is en route to the recovery room. When your child awakens, he is likely to be disoriented and scared. Coming out of the anesthesia is less traumatic if a parent is present.

 DR. SEARS TIP
Continue Breastfeeding

Breastfeeding is the ultimate comforter, and here's where mom-nurse shines. Unless the illness or operation prevents, while your child is hospitalized continue the same breastfeeding schedule you have at home. Realistically, while there may be a slight interruption in this schedule, there are very few medical illnesses that aren't improved by breastfeeding. If your baby is going to be given an elective operation and will require general anesthesia, you may be asked to "refrain from feeding solid foods and breastfeeding after midnight." While this is true for solid foods, newer studies indicate that it is no longer the case for breastfeeding. It is true that the child needs an empty stomach to safely undergo anesthesia for fear of regurgitating the stomach contents and aspirating them into the lungs. Yet, breast milk is absorbed from the stomach so rapidly (within thirty to sixty minutes) that most anesthesiologists now recommend that mothers continue breastfeeding until two to four hours prior to the anesthesia.

Here's a story from the Sears doctors' gallery of memorable hospital experiences: I (Dr. Bill) admitted a nine-month-old for treatment of severe croup. I had notified an ENT specialist to prepare the operating room since it seemed like the baby would need an emergency tracheotomy (a surgical opening into his windpipe or trachea) because his upper airway was so swollen from the croup. Suddenly I had a somewhat unconventional idea. I asked his mother to offer her breast to the baby, through the gap in the croup tent, to relax his inflamed airways and spare him the emergency operation. The baby nursed eagerly, seemingly more for comfort than because he was hungry. Within a minute, he relaxed, as did his airways. His breathing improved, we canceled the operation, and the whole family and medical team breathed better, especially the baby.

Request an early-morning operation. If your child is having an elective surgery (meaning prescheduled, non-emergency), such as a tonsillectomy or hernia repair, request the earliest possible operation in the morning. This enables your child not to have to fast for so long. Children are rapid metabolizers, so their little tummies and bodies need frequent, small feedings. If your child goes to sleep at 9:00 p.m. and doesn't have his surgery until noon, that's too long to go without food or drink. New insights have shortened the interval children are required to go without rapidly digestible soft solids, and your anesthesiologist will discuss these options with you.

Bring along comfies. If your child has a favorite teddy bear or doll he or she sleeps with, bring it along, as well as some favorite books and toys. If possible, surprise your child with some new toys that may get his mind off the discomfort of being in the hospital.

Play show-and-tell. Use all the gadgets around your child's bedside to get her mind off the illness. Explain what the monitors do, what good stuff is going into her veins, and, with the older child, explain what the medical tests measure and what the results mean. Turn the hospital stay into a learning experience for your potential future doctor or nurse.

Be positive and involved! While some children are intimidated by the weird medical garb (such as scrubs and coats), machines, monitors, tubing, and needle sticks, older children may think they have traveled to a science-fiction fantasy land. Even before going to the hospital, tell your child how much better he will feel, how much stronger he will be, and so on — mention all the positive things that will happen. Talk about "all those nice people, like the doctors and nurses, who love kids, are funny, and will take good care of you…and Mommy and Daddy will be right there with you." Present the hospital staff as a chance for your child to meet new friends, or "special friends," that will help her feel better.

Be your child's advocate, politely. A child's illness usually brings out the best in a caring parent, but it may also increase the propensity for actions that may antagonize the medical staff. You are understandably anxious about your child's illness and want her to receive the best care. Both you and your child will have a more pleasant hospital stay if you make a conscious effort to communicate and work constructively with the medical personnel.

Doctors and nurses are proud professionals. If your doctor and nurse feel you have sincere confidence in their ability to care for your child, the hospital experience will be better for all of you.

Parents of hospitalized children often have to take a crash course in public relations. While doctors and nurses are medical professionals who know their subject, you are the parent and you know your child, and she deserves the best resources. If you know something has worked with a previous hospitalization, tell the medical staff. If a certain procedure done by two different people had different effects on your child, let the staff know which one worked best; for example, you might say, "When the nurse put ice on my child's thigh before giving her a shot, it really helped." Ask why each procedure is being done and what effects can be expected. Ask what each medication is for and the dosage. While in the hospital keep a "what works best" diary. This is especially helpful if your child has a chronic illness that may require multiple hospitalizations. After a while you and your child will work out your own personal "what works" list.

Try to stay with your child during a procedure. The doctor or nurse may nicely ask you to "step out" while a procedure, such as placing an intravenous catheter or a spinal tap, is performed. This is a judgment call. On the one hand, it's usually easier on the child to have Mom or Dad there as a natural pain reliever. On the other hand, it can be traumatic on the parents and sometimes can produce anxiety in the people performing the procedure. If you feel it's in the best interest of your child for you to be there during a procedure, mention that the American Academy of Pediatrics (AAP) recommends that parents be able to offer emotional support during painful procedures. Avoid being forced to refuse giving your permission for a procedure unless you are present. There is usually an amicable compromise. If parental presence at a particular procedure is "against hospital policy," you may have to respect this. But if you can be there, radiate a relaxed impression, even if you have to fake it. Your presence should make your child feel less anxious, not more. Ask what you can do to comfort your child, such as rub her forehead, give her something to suck on, or hold her hand.

DR. SEARS TIP
Know the Policy

The degree of parental involvement allowed around the time of surgery may vary from hospital to hospital because of medical or legal concerns. Frivolous lawsuits have forced hospitals to tighten their rules a bit, so we hope you understand their position. Find out the hospital's policy on parental involvement during surgery.

Be the symptom interpreter. Whenever we hospitalize a child, we have this talk with the parents: "You know your child better than anyone else does. Get to know the signs of the worsening condition and notify the appropriate medical staff. You are your child's most trusted bedside monitor." We have had many experiences in which the parent can tell when the child's condition is worsening before the monitor does. For example, one of our parents of a frequently hospitalized child with asthma could often tell and would notify the nurses that her child was about to go into a respiratory attack minutes before the oxygen-monitoring sensor reflected it. You are your child's best body-language reader. Use your experience. Another example is when a child needs certain procedures that cause discomfort. You know when your child has reached the limit of tolerance. While it may be inconvenient for the hospital staff to come back later, it's okay to politely but authoritatively request, "I think she's reached her limit. Would you please come back later? Thank you!"

Room in. Like so many other things, this will be a night-by-night call. The medical staff may suggest, "You're tired. Why don't you go home and rest and come back in the morning." You may ask for a situation like "full rooming-in" where a portable parental cot is placed next to your child's bed. If a short hospital stay is expected, and you believe that you need to spend the night, ask to do so. On the other hand, if the hospital stay is lengthy and the daytime procedures are draining on you, it may be in everyone's best interest for you to occasionally go home and get a good night's rest. Sleep deprivation is a common cause of medical errors. Your child needs your clear judgment.

Feed your child real food. You'd think with the price of the hospital stay your child would get the healthiest gourmet food. It's even more surprising that many of the menus are formulated by the hospital nutritionist. One day I (Dr. Bill) was visiting a child in the hospital who was recovering from surgery. I noticed the diet of white bread, gelatin desserts, high-fructose-corn-syrup-flavored juice, and fiber-less cereal. Astonished, I went home and brought back to the hospital a blender with lots of fruit, yogurt, flaxseed meal, and other "real foods." (See the Dr. Sears healing smoothie recipe, page 15.) The nurses heard the whirring noise coming from the patient's

room. When they asked what was going on, the parent responded: "Dr. Sears is giving him real food." Just at the time in your child's life when he needs healing foods, he's more likely to get hurting foods. By healing foods we mean foods that foster healing by boosting the immune system and speeding tissue growth and recovery. By hurting foods we mean those that do just the opposite. (See examples of healing and hurting foods in the section on feeding your child's immune system, page 33.)

Oftentimes, the intestines slow down during recovery from illnesses or operations in order to divert energy into the recuperating parts of the body, so don't expect your child to eat a whole lot while in the hospital. While the type of food and how it's prepared must be appropriate for the illness and recovery, two feeding tips that will work for most children in the hospital are:

- the Dr. Sears rule of twos: eat *twice* as often, *half* as much, and chew *twice* as long

- The sipping solution: sipping on small amounts of a nutritious smoothie throughout the day is one of the most healing and intestinal-friendly ways to feed a hospitalized child.

Note: Be sure to check with the medical staff before feeding your hospitalized child. There may be certain foods that are contraindicated with a certain illness or medication.

Bring gifts. Nurses have a tough and tiring job. Show your appreciation by showering them with thanks, praise, and gifts. You want to be known as "those nice parents of that little girl in room 223." This is especially therapeutic if you've occasionally had to be the forceful advocate.

IMPETIGO

Commonly mispronounced as "infantigo," this is a bacterial infection of the skin. It usually occurs around the nose, mouth, and chin because these areas are easily irritated by food and nasal mucus, but it can occur anywhere in the body. It appears in the forms of red spots, pimples, or sores, and a honey-colored crust often forms over the sores. Keeping these areas clean and lubricated with ointment during an illness or dry weather can prevent the crust from forming.

What You Can Do

If treatment is initiated promptly, most cases can be cared for without seeing a doctor. Here is what you can do:

- Cut your child's fingernails to avoid irritation caused by scratching.

- Wash the areas with warm water and soap.

- Dab on some diluted hydrogen peroxide (half water), then rinse it off.

- Apply over-the-counter antibiotic ointment.

- Repeat these cleansing steps three or four times a day.

- If the rash doesn't improve, add warm washcloth soaks prior to cleansing. After cleansing, apply a diluted Betadine solution (antiseptic from any drugstore) of about one part Betadine to five parts water instead of peroxide. Allow to dry for two minutes then thoroughly rinse off. Finish with antibiotic ointment.

When to See the Doctor

If the rash doesn't improve or worsens after three days, you should see your doctor. There are two treatment options:

Prescription-strength antibiotic ointment. While it's best to see your pediatrician for this, some doctors might call it in over the phone if the rash doesn't sound too serious.

Oral antibiotics. Sometimes the ointment isn't enough and a course of oral antibiotics is needed. See page 551 for tips on how to minimize antibiotic side effects.

Is Impetigo Contagious?

Yes it is, but only during the crusty phase and only through direct contact with the infected area. Older children who can responsibly avoid sharing food and drinks and keep their hands to themselves can go to school or child care. Frequent hand washing helps. Infants and toddlers who are sure to spread their drool and put their hands everywhere should stay home until the rash is no longer oozing and inflamed. Healing, dry spots are no longer contagious.

INFLAMMATORY BOWEL DISEASE (IBD)

Inflammatory bowel disease (IBD) is a condition that develops from inflammation inside an individual's digestive system. Inflammatory bowel disease affects approximately one million Americans and can affect any age group. Although the disease can begin in early childhood, it most commonly begins between the ages of fifteen and thirty. There are two types of IBD: Crohn's disease and ulcerative colitis.

Crohn's Disease

Crohn's disease and ulcerative colitis are inflammatory bowel diseases that are very similar. Which of these two diseases is diagnosed depends on which part of the digestive system is involved. In Crohn's disease, the most commonly involved area is the small intestine, but Crohn's disease can involve any area of the digestive system — the mouth, esophagus, stomach, colon, or anus.

Crohn's disease can be diagnosed in all age groups, from young children to older adults. The disease usually begins, however, in the teenage years or in the twenties. It does appear that Crohn's disease may run in families.

The cause. Crohn's disease seems to be an imbalance of the body's own immune system (called an *autoimmune reaction*). The digestive system may be exposed to a virus or bacteria, triggering the body's immune system to attack the invader, leading to an inflammatory response in the digestive system. It is thought that the immune system continues this inflammatory reaction after the virus or bacteria has been eliminated, resulting in persistent inflammation.

People with Crohn's disease also seem to have other problems with their immune systems, such as food and environmental allergies, so that allergic reactions may also play a role in this disease.

Symptoms. Possible symptoms, which can vary greatly from person to person, are:

- diarrhea
- recurrent lower abdominal pains
- blood in the stools
- bleeding from the anus
- weight loss
- recurrent fevers
- fatigue
- reluctance to eat
- nutritional deficiencies

Diagnosis. If your pediatrician suspects that your child's symptoms may be due to Crohn's disease, he may take blood and stool samples for testing. Certain blood tests can show evidence of an inflammatory process going on in the body, and stool tests can rule out infections by parasites or bacteria.

If Crohn's disease or ulcerative colitis is suspected, your doctor will most likely refer your child to a gastroenterologist for further testing. This specialist may want to perform two procedures known as *endoscopy* and *colonoscopy* and may also do abdominal X-rays known as an *upper-gastrointestinal series*.

Endoscopy is a test that uses a small tube with a camera at the end. It is placed down through the mouth into the esophagus and stomach. This allows the doctor to visualize these areas for signs of inflammation. The doctor can also take tissue samples for biopsy that will show evidence of Crohn's disease if your child is affected.

Colonoscopy is essentially an endoscopy from the other end of the body — passing a small, thin tube with a camera at the tip through the rectum and up into the colon. Again, this allows for direct visualization of the colon, along with the ability to collect tissue samples for biopsy.

Treatment. While currently Crohn's may not be completely cured, it can be treated so that your child can lead a normal life.

In all types of intestinal ailments, especially Crohn's, the pills-skills model of medical care really shines:

What Doctors Do (Pills)	What Parents and Child Do (Skills)
• make accurate diagnosis • prescribe anti-inflammatory medicines • perform the right GI tests	• keep a careful diary • read about iBod prevention, page 35 • read about good gut health, page 25

Surgery may be performed in small numbers of cases in individuals with severe IBD. Performing surgery will not cure Crohn's disease, but it may help the symptoms. This is usually done only if all other treatment options mentioned above have failed.

Ulcerative Colitis

Ulcerative colitis is caused by inflammation of the inner lining of an area of the digestive tract. The main difference between ulcerative colitis and Crohn's disease is where in the digestive system the inflammation occurs. Unlike Crohn's disease, which can affect any part of the digestive tract from mouth to anus, the inflammation of ulcerative colitis is limited to the colon and/or the rectum.

The cause. Like Crohn's disease, it is thought that the body's own immune system reacts to an invading bacteria or virus, causing inflammation, and that this inflammatory reaction cannot stop itself, leading to the development of ulcerative colitis.

Symptoms. Again, ulcerative colitis shares similar symptoms with Crohn's disease. These include:

- lower abdominal pain

- bloody diarrhea

- loose bowel movements

- bleeding from the rectum or blood in the stools

- nutritional deficiencies

- loss of appetite

- fatigue

- weight loss

- occasional joint pain or skin rashes may develop

See your pediatrician if your child begins exhibiting the above symptoms.

Diagnosis. The process of diagnosing ulcerative colitis is essentially the same as diagnosing Crohn's disease. (See the above section on diagnosing Crohn's disease for more information.)

Treatment. As with Crohn's disease, treating ulcerative colitis is performed on an individual basis. Not every child will receive the exact same treatment for ulcerative colitis. There is no known cure for ulcerative colitis. The main goal of treatment is to help control severe flare-ups of the disease along with the symptoms.

Medication treatment usually begins with using anti-inflammatory medications that will help to control the symptoms. These are used in mild cases of ulcerative colitis. In moderate to severe disease, steroid medications may be used as these have more powerful anti-inflammatory abilities. These are usually used on a short-term basis to control severe flare-ups. In more severe cases, powerful medications that help alter the body's own immune system may be used. Steroids and immune system–altering medications can have many side effects and should be used only under direct care of a treating physician. (See above section on treating Crohn's disease for further tips on other treatments for ulcerative colitis. One important aspect of treatment is to avoid malnutrition or nutritional deficiencies.)

In very severe cases where the above treatments are not effective, surgery may be a last resort. It usually involves removing the affected areas of the colon to improve the symptoms and quality of life.

Flare-Ups

Both of these inflammatory bowel diseases can range from extremely mild to very severe. Your child may have long periods without any intestinal discomfort at all followed by episodes of flare-ups of symptoms. In some people this can be a lifetime cycle of good periods and bad periods. Other individuals may show symptoms for a short period of time and be disease-free for the rest of their lives.

JAUNDICE

Almost every baby turns a little yellow by day 3 or 4 of life, and this isn't necessarily a bad thing. The yellow pigment (called *bilirubin*) that builds up in a baby's bloodstream during the first few days comes from the breakdown of excess red blood cells that the baby built up during fetal development. Once a baby is born, she doesn't need the extra blood cells, and they begin to break apart. Bilirubin is an antioxidant and helps protect the baby from infection. So some degree of jaundice is actually beneficial. Yet, if too much yellow pigment builds up, it isn't good for a baby's brain. Fortunately, the baby's kidneys and liver begin eliminating the bilirubin by day 4 or 5, and the jaundice disappears by day 10 or so. But it's not easy for a parent to know how yellow is too yellow. Here is our guide to understanding jaundice and how you can know when to let your doctor take a look.

When to Worry

Most babies don't show any jaundice until after they are home from the hospital (day 3 or 4). And your first appointment with the pediatrician isn't for another few days. Here is how you can know if your baby is turning too yellow:

Jaundice in the first forty-eight hours. Babies are born a mixture of pink, white, and light brown. If you notice any degree of yellow color in the first two days, this may be a sign that the bilirubin is building up too quickly.

Jaundice of the whole body. The yellow color normally begins in the face around day 3, then moves down to the chest by day 4, then the belly by day 5. At that point, the whites of the eyes will also turn yellow. Then the yellow pigment begins to get eliminated from the body and the jaundice diminishes. If your baby's jaundice progresses down the body faster than this (for example, the eyes and belly seem yellow by day 3 or 4), or if the upper legs begin to show jaundice at any time, see your pediatrician right away.

Increasing sleepiness and poor feeding. All newborns seem to do is eat and sleep. But as the days go by, their level of wakefulness and interest in feeding should increase. Too much bilirubin in the bloodstream can make a newborn drowsy and feed poorly.

Premature babies. Babies born at less than thirty-seven weeks of gestation are more prone to developing problematic jaundice. Have a higher index of suspicion for these babies.

Cephalohematoma. A baby who develops a large swollen area on the head from the delivery is more likely to become jaundiced faster. The swelling is a collection of blood under the scalp, and this trapped blood will leak more bilirubin into the bloodstream.

Treatment

Treatment depends on how high the bilirubin level is, what day of life it is, and whether or not any other risk factors are present. Here is what you can expect over the next few days:

Testing the levels. If you are still in the hospital (as most C-section babies may be), the nurse can use a transcutaneous bilirubin monitor to test the level by simply pressing a little probe against the skin. A blood test is more accurate, however, and is probably what would be done if you have already left the hospital. Treatment should be started if a baby's bilirubin exceeds the following guidelines:

- a level of 12 or higher by twenty-four hours of age

- 15 or higher by forty-eight hours of age

- 18 or higher at seventy-two hours of age

It is also prudent to begin therapy at lower levels than these, depending on the health of the baby and other factors.

Although the above levels are completely harmless to a baby, if they get this high at such an early age it may mean the jaundice is rising too quickly and, if not treated, may eventually reach a harmful range before it starts to level off. This can lead to brain damage. How high is too high? Full-term babies can probably tolerate a maximum jaundice level of around 25 without harm. However, we don't like to let it come anywhere close to there, so we do our best to keep it below 20.

Testing Mom's and Baby's blood types. If a baby has a different blood type than Mom (such as Dad's blood type), this mismatch can cause faster breakdown of Baby's extra red blood cells, trigger jaundice earlier, and build it to higher levels. A blood test can be done to check for this, and if abnormal, more aggressive treatment may be needed.

Bili light therapy. The mainstay of therapy for jaundice is using some special blue lights around the clock to shine on Baby's skin. The light breaks down the pigment into a harmless substance. There are two ways to do light therapy:

- In an incubator with large light bulbs. This can only be done while in the hospital and provides the most effective and concentrated form of light. Baby wears an eye mask.

- Using bili blankets. These can be used in the hospital or at home. The baby wears a blanket that has light strips sewn in.

Babies with very high jaundice levels are kept in the hospital and given the incubator light therapy. Those with levels that aren't so serious can often be sent home with bili blankets and daily follow-up with a home health nurse.

Increase fluid intake. Expanding the amount of fluids within the bloodstream helps dilute the bilirubin, thus lowering the level. Infants with serious jaundice will receive intravenous fluids to help bring down the level quickly. Babies with moderate jaundice can usually get enough fluids through breast milk or formula. Now here's the catch: Breastfed infants usually get more breast milk around day 4 or 5 when Mom's milk fully

**DR. SEARS TIP
Does Breast Milk
Cause Jaundice?**

This is a belief popular among older doctors that is partially true but mostly false. There are two ways that jaundice can be more likely to occur in a breastfeeding infant. One is called breast*feeding* jaundice, in which a baby becomes more yellow due to a delay in Mom's milk coming in. In this case, the breast milk doesn't actually cause the jaundice, but the fact that the baby is breastfeeding, and not getting quite as much milk as a bottlefeeding neighbor just yet, may allow some jaundice to begin. The second scenario is called breast-*milk* jaundice. In this type, a substance in the breast milk actually delays the clearance of the bilirubin out of the baby's system. This isn't common, however, and it doesn't trigger jaundice until a baby is a week old. So, in reality, breast milk itself doesn't cause jaundice in the early newborn period. Breastfeeding moms should continue to give babies what's best. If jaundice persists or increases in the second week of life, talk to your pediatrician about breast-milk jaundice.

comes in. This poses a dilemma for a jaundiced three-day-old. Some hospitals or doctors will insist on formula supplementation as a routine for all jaundiced babies. But this really should be a case-by-case decision. Talk to your doctor about whether or not this is necessary. We find that most of our breastfeeding patients who are on bili blankets at home or in the hospital do just fine without supplementing, as long as Mom has good milk flow starting by day 4.

Prevention

Most babies who go home from the hospital on day 2 or 3 are just starting to show some jaundice. A transcutaneous or blood bili level will often be checked right before you go home and may show a borderline concern. These babies should see their doctors in the office about two days later for a jaundice check. Here is what you can do over the next few days to keep your baby's jaundice under control:

Sunlight therapy. Sunlight does the same thing as the hospital light therapy. Direct sunlight is best, but obviously you can't do too much of that without causing a sunburn. Try these "tanning" tips for your baby:

• Keep the cradle by the window. Let Baby sleep as undressed as possible in a window with the sun shining through the glass. Although the glass filters out most of the effective rays, it will still help some. Even indirect sunlight on a cloudy day helps.

• Feed Baby in the window. Set up a nice chair for feedings in a big, sunny window. Since your body heat will be keeping Baby warm during the feed, he can be completely naked (you may want to keep the diaper on) for maximum sun exposure.

- Go outside. Take three fifteen-minute walks every day outside for some direct sunlight with your baby as undressed as possible without getting cold. This will really help keep the jaundice down.

Frequent feeds. Although you are probably already doing this, try to get your baby to the breast as often as possible. If you feel that your milk isn't really coming in well by day 4 or 5 (see page 52 for signs) contact a lactation consultant to help.

KNEE BUMP, PAINFUL

Your preadolescent — or adolescent — starts noticing and complaining of a painful bump just below his kneecap. This nuisance hurts more after the young athlete exercises, and it feels better after rest. Your child is annoyed and you are worried. Called Osgood-Schlatter disease (OSD) (named after the two doctors who discovered it over a hundred years ago), this growth spurt quirk occurs more commonly in boys and athletic girls. It really isn't a disease, but rather one of those annoying nuisances of adolescent growth spurts. OSD occurs in a localized area where the tendon comes over the kneecap and fits into the cartilage, or growth plate, of the upper shin bone or tibia. Repeated sports activities that involve stretching of this tendon against the growth plate cause painful inflammation and swelling of this area. Dr. Bill remembers having these knee bumps when he was an adolescent and attended a Catholic high school. It hurt very much to kneel in church, and he still remem-

bers the nuns reprimanding him for not wanting to kneel and not believing this painful-knees excuse.

Signs and Symptoms

- There are dime- to quarter-size lumps just below the kneecap in one or both knees.
- These lumps hurt when you press on them, kneel on them, or during athletic events.
- They often hurt more after an athletically strenuous day and sometimes lead to limping.
- The pain is relieved by rest.

What to Do

Reassure your teen that this falls in the category of growing pains of adolescence. He needs to figure out which movements make these areas feel worse and to try to minimize them as much as possible during sports. If the pain and swelling get worse, he may need to change sports. In addition:

- Your child should wear heel pads and shock-absorbing athletic shoes.
- Your child should wear knee pads for contact sports, such as football, basketball, and wrestling.
- Consult your child's coach or trainer to be sure your child has good stretching and warm-up exercises before the sport.
- To minimize inflammation, apply a cold pack to the swollen area immediately after exercise.

- Ibuprofen can be used three times a day for several days to help calm down the swelling and pain.

As with typical growing pains, the majority of children do outgrow these painful lumps once they reach full growth, but occasionally these areas remain somewhat sensitive and tender throughout adulthood.

LEAD POISONING

Lead poisoning usually develops slowly over a long period of time when a child swallows or inhales small amounts of products containing lead. It usually occurs when a child chews on objects containing lead, such as old paint chips or lead-painted toys. Children are usually more prone to lead poisoning compared to adults, as they tend to put things in their mouths. Lead is much more harmful to children because it can cause problems with a child's developing brain and nervous system. The younger the child, the more harmful the effects of lead poisoning.

Symptoms

Symptoms of lead poisoning develop slowly over a long time. The most common symptoms of lead poisoning include:

- decreased appetite and energy level
- difficulty sleeping
- aggressive behavior
- extreme irritability
- headaches
- anemia
- abdominal pain
- constipation
- developmental delays

Symptoms of exposure to a very high toxic dose of lead include:

- severe abdominal pain and cramping
- vomiting
- difficulty walking
- seizures or coma that can lead to death

Common Items That May Contain Lead

- lead-based paint on an old house (Any house built before 1978 may have lead-based paint on its walls.)
- fishing weights
- lead bullets
- toys and furniture painted before 1976
- plumbing, pipes, and faucets in homes whose pipes have been connected with lead soldering
- soil, especially if it is exposed to years and years of car exhaust or old paint scrapings from houses
- paint sets and other art supplies
- pewter eating utensils
- soldering materials, certain pottery glazes
- lead figurines
- painted toys from outside the United States

- exhaust from nearby power plants, especially if coal-burning

- exhaust from nearby freeway truck traffic

 DR. SEARS TIP
Buy American!

Recent concerns over imported toys from other countries have led many parents to be concerned with purchasing toys manufactured outside the United States.

Long-Term Complications

Exposure over long periods of time to low levels of lead can result in the following complications:

- diminished growth rate

- hearing problems

- lower IQ

- problems with attention or behavior

- kidney problems

Treatment

Treatment of low-dose lead exposure over a long period of time involves first testing the blood for the presence of lead. This will show how high the lead level in your child's bloodstream is. Many states have lead screening programs for preschool-age children. Treatment depends on the level of lead in the blood. Low levels of lead are often treated simply by removing the offending agent or agents from the child's contact. The doctor will then retest the level of lead in the blood at a later date to

insure that the level has returned to normal. In cases where higher levels of lead exist, treatment may involve chelation therapy. This involves using agents that bind to the lead in the blood and help the body to excrete it faster.

Your doctor may decide to perform other blood tests if elevated lead levels are found. These may include testing the blood level to screen for anemia, bone marrow biopsy to evaluate lead in the bones, or X-rays of certain bones in the body.

Prevention

- Discard old painted toys or other objects if you are not sure about the paint containing lead.

- Find out whether the plumbing system of your house used lead soldering in construction.

- Have the paint of your house evaluated if you are unsure whether or not lead-based paint was used. This is especially true for houses built prior to 1978.

- If you're worried about lead in your water system, have the lead level of your water tested.

For further questions and advice regarding lead poisoning or exposure, contact the national poison control center at 1-800-222-1222.

LICE

Lice is a very common problem among school-age children. Head lice are tiny insects that live on the scalp and the top of the neck of humans and lay their eggs on the hair shafts. These tiny creatures thrive in environments where there is a lot of close contact among humans. This is why you often hear of outbreaks at school. They can travel very easily from person to person, either through close contact, from touching an infected person's clothing or bedding, or by sharing combs. Head lice can live for over a month, while their eggs (called "nits") can survive for up to two weeks.

DR. SEARS TIP
Lice Can Live in the
Cleanest of Homes

There is often an unfair social stigma attached to head lice infestation. In the past it was thought to be linked to low socioeconomic status or poor hygiene. We now know that such factors do *not* play a role in who does and who doesn't get head lice. Even the cleanest of children can easily be infected with head lice.

Symptoms

- Your child experiences intense itching of the scalp.

- You see tiny white specks at the bottom of hair shafts that look like dandruff but do not come off easily. These are the nits.

- Red bumps on the scalp, neck, or behind the ears due to constant scratching. These may scab and ooze.

Looking for Lice

Head lice and their eggs are very small. Often they are only noticeable upon very close inspection. It is important to examine the scalp thoroughly using disposable gloves. Examine the hair in small sections all the way down to the root, especially the areas around the neck and ears. Use a magnifying glass to help you more easily see the head lice and their eggs.

Treatment

Treatment is almost always recommended if even one egg (also known as a nit) is detected.

Wash those lice right out of the hair. Many times over-the-counter shampoos and lotions can clear up a case of head lice, often with only one treatment. The most effective OTC lotion is called Nix, available in any drugstore. Occasionally, a second treatment is needed approximately seven days later for full clearance. In some cases, however, prescription-strength shampoos are used if the over-the-counter treatment is not effective. We suggest you ask your pediatrician about a new prescription liquid treatment called Ulesfia. It is a mild alcohol solution that is very effective against lice without the strong insecticide chemicals used in most medicated lice products. Because girls typically have longer hair, they are more likely to need additional treatments.

Be a nitpicker. Following treatment with a shampoo or lotion, use a *nit comb* to remove any remaining eggs. A way to make this even more effective is to rub olive oil in the hair prior to using the comb. Doing so will make the eggs easier to remove.

Blow the lice away. Specially designed hair dryers are available in most pharmacies. These can be used following treatment to remove remaining lice and eggs that may still be present on the hair. Using even a regular blow dryer for this purpose can also be effective.

Smother the lice. It's messy, but it works. Apply olive oil, peanut butter, or mayonnaise to the hair. Leave on overnight and wash thoroughly in the morning.

De-louse your house. Wash all clothes, hats, and bed linens that have been in contact with the child since becoming infected. Use detergent and hot water. Lice can live *off* the human body for short periods of time. Rarely, in severe cases of head lice, secondary bacterial infections can develop from the child scratching on the scalp too much. This can cause breaks in the skin that can lead to infection. This occasionally requires antibiotics.

Prevent the spread of lice. The following items should *never* be shared if your child has head lice or if a friend or classmate is suspected of having head lice:

- hats
- combs
- hairbrushes
- bedding
- towels
- clothing

 DR. SEARS TIP
It's Only a Lousy Louse!

Head lice is seldom a medical concern. They do not carry disease and, except for a bit of itching, don't really cause any problems. Schools and daycare centers overreact, hence the name "nitpicker." And they are not a reflection of your home hygiene. Children and their little lice friends can attend school or daycare. "No nit" policies are not necessary!

LIMPING

Limping is a fairly common occurrence among toddlers and young children. Often the cause is obvious, such as a recent fall. But sometimes a child will begin limping one morning for no apparent reason. Here is how you can solve the mystery of the limping child.

Causes

Here are some of the harmless causes.

Recent fall. Perhaps your child stumbled and fell recently and pulled a muscle or sprained an ankle, but it was so mild that you didn't notice and he didn't complain.

Strenuous activity. If your child played hard on the playground, started a new gym class, or jumped on a trampoline, he may have strained something.

Splinter or other foreign body. Check your child's foot very carefully. Even a tiny splinter or piece of glass can cause a limp.

New shoes, or old shoes. A new pair of shoes may cause a blister or red, sore spot. An old pair may be too small. These may even cause a limp when the shoes aren't on.

Slept in a funny position. Some kids will wake with a limp that lasts for a few hours because they slept in an odd position. They may also do this after a long ride in the car seat.

Recent cold or illness. A hip or knee joint can become temporarily inflamed after an illness. See Synovitis, page 369.

As long as you don't notice any of the more serious signs or problems listed below, you can safely wait for about five days before seeing a doctor. These harmless limps almost always resolve on their own (you may need to remove a splinter or two). Of course, it doesn't hurt to get checked sooner just to make sure.

When to Worry

There are some more serious causes of limping that should not wait. Here are the signs to watch for that do warrant a visit:

- *Fever and limp* (with no obvious cause of the fever, such as a cold or diarrhea). This can indicate a bone or joint infection. See your pediatrician that day.

- *Visible swelling.* Examine the entire leg carefully. Swelling may indicate a more significant injury, such as a fracture.

- *Known recent injury.* If your child recently fell from a height, got her foot stepped on, or was hit by something traumatic enough that you think something could be broken, see a doctor that day or the next.

- *Definite pain in one place.* As you move your child's joints and press on every bone in the leg, if you can elicit some pain in only one place, there may be something there the doctor should see within the next day.

- *Limp lasting more than five days.* Even if it ends up being nothing, it's worth checking out.

- *Continuous irritability.* If it's enough to make your child fussy most of the day, it should be checked out by the doctor by the next day.

The doctor can perform a thorough physical exam of the legs to look for any clues as to what might be hurting. An X-ray can be done if any definite pain or swelling is seen or the doctor suspects an injury somewhere. Blood tests can be done if a bone or joint infection is suspected.

LUMPS

Children can have lumps all over their bodies and naturally caring parents get concerned. Here's your crash course in Lumpology 101, a trip through your child's body to learn the cause of these lumps.

Swollen lymph glands. Lymph glands are part of the body's immune system; they make white blood cells and other substances that fight germs. They are usually pea-sized and are most prominent around the nape of the neck, behind the ears, below the jaw, in the armpits, and in the groin. When there is an infection or even a scratch or irritation of the skin near the area of these glands, they swell to several times their size and may be a bit tender to touch. You can even feel these tiny glands in the back of the head and the nape of the neck in babies as young as three months of age. Sometimes as the glands are fighting a nearby infection, they themselves may become infected, such as the glands beneath the jaw following a tonsil infection. Signs that infected glands need medical attention are that the gland is red, swollen two to three times the normal size, and very tender to the touch, causing the child to wince when you gently press on it. Besides antibiotic treatment, your doctor may recommend you gently apply a hot compress on a swollen gland for ten minutes a few times a day. This speeds recovery.

DR. SEARS TIP
Do a Periodic Lump Check

Get used to the "usual" feel of your baby's glands and normal lumps. If you feel or see a noticeable change in these lumps or any of the worry signs listed below, report this to your pediatrician.

Lumps following trauma. Your child bumps his head, and a week or two later you notice a forehead lump. When skin is compressed hard against underlying bone, as it is during a fall, there is often a bit of bleeding under the skin. This blood calcifies into a hard mass, which you feel as a lump. When the fat is squeezed hard, it also calcifies. So, it is common to feel a hard lump where the child fell and the tissue was compressed. These harmless lumps may take as long as a year to disappear. They can appear anywhere on a child's body.

Lumps in groin. Most of the lumps you'll feel along a child's groin are normal lymph glands, which can swell up even when there are sores or scratches on the legs or feet. A large lump, about the size of a thumb, could be an inguinal hernia. (See Inguinal Hernia, page 510.)

Lumps in breast. Pea-sized lumps in the areola, the dark area around the nipple, are a common, harmless quirk that occur in two stages of childhood. Shortly after birth, due to the effects of the hormones that cross the placenta, many infants (boy or girl) have tiny cyst-like lumps under their nipples. These usually subside within a few months. The next breast-lump stage occurs in girls between eight and ten years of age when they begin puberty. Expect pea-sized tender lumps beneath the nipples. In fact, at most eight-year-old check-ups we prepare the child and tell the parents that their daughter may expect tiny, tender lumps around the nipple. These lumps are normal glandular swelling of the budding breast tissue. We tell the child, "These lumps are normal and mean you're starting to develop just like Mom." Breast lumps can become infected; if they become tender, rapidly enlarging, and the child winces when you touch them, best to have them checked by your pediatrician.

Lumps in chest. Try not to be alarmed if you feel a bony, pea-sized lump below Baby's breastbone. This is the normal end of the sternum. Just like navels, there are normal "innies" and "outies." In some infants, especially very lean ones, this end of the breastbone sticks out more. As your baby grows, this lump naturally becomes part of the rest of the breastbone and will be less apparent. No concern or treatment is necessary.

When to Worry

The appearance and feel of a lump can give you clues as to whether or not this is a report-to-the-doctor worry. Generally, a lump that is soft, round, uniform, slightly tender, and moves easily under the skin is a non-worry. But a lump that is irregular, firm, non-tender, and seems fixed to underlying tissue may be more of a concern, and should be checked by your child's doctor. If you're uncertain about a lump, examine it and get a feel for it to see if it changes. Non-changing lumps are less of a worry.

MASTURBATION

While masturbation in adults may mean stimulating the genitals to the point of orgasm, in children it simply means genital stimulation for pleasure. The terms *genital play* and *genital discovery* are really more accurate terms, especially for the preschool child.

Why Kids Masturbate

Genital play is part of a normal phase of children discovering their body parts and the pleasurable feelings that come from them. It can begin during infancy. Because the genitals are richly supplied with sensitive nerves, naturally the child is fascinated by the feelings that come from fondling.

Children will often do this when they are bored or as a comfort measure when something else has been taken away (such as a pacifier). Some might even do it more because they are constantly being told not to.

How to React

How you react to your child's normal genital play sets the tone for later communication when the stakes are higher. Remember, you want him to be comfortable discussing bodily issues with you. You open your four-year-old's bedroom door and discover he's "playing with himself." Don't panic. This is a normal stage of body discovery and does not mean that your child has some sort of psychological problem. Above all, avoid a reaction that conveys to your child that certain body parts are "bad" or that "it is wrong" to touch them. Don't give the message that genital touching is "dirty" or that "it will make you sick." This behavior does not cause any physical harm, and it does not mean your child will grow up to be sexually promiscuous. However, if adults overreact and make the child think it is bad or dirty, it can lead to emotional harm, guilt, or sexual inhibitions.

Track the trigger. What circumstances set your child up for genital play? Is he bored? Tired? Lonesome? Tense? In your diary, note what circumstances seem to prompt genital play.

Distract and substitute. This is a trick that changes the course of many concerning behaviors. If you see your two-year-old "overdoing it" on her rocking horse, distract her from her genital feelings and suggest an alternative activity: "Let's go to the park." Certainly, discourage genital play in public: "We don't 'ride our horse' when Aunt Nancy is around." Give alternative tension relievers. If you feel your child is using genital massage as a tension reliever, offer to give her a back rub instead.

Supervise. If your child is going through a genital-play stage, avoid setups that encourage him to play with other children's genitals. Have an "open door" policy when children are playing together in a room.

Teach privacy. Since you won't be able to completely stop your child's behavior, a realistic goal is to simply control where your child does it. Try to limit it to the bathroom and bedroom. You can say to your child, "It's okay to touch your penis, but please go to the bathroom for privacy." Most kids won't want to leave what they are doing and will stop for that moment.

When to Worry; What to Do

In most children genital stimulation is normal behavior. Like any bodily stimulation, if done in excess it can be concerning. Talk to your doctor if:

- Genital play is becoming increasingly intense and frequent. Excessive rubbing of the genitals, especially in girls, may result in sore vaginal tissues or repeated urine infections. This complication is very uncommon.

- The child withdraws from social activity in order to self-stimulate.

- Genital play is becoming more of a public display. Teach your child the concept of "private parts."

- The behavior continues in public beyond age five.

As your child matures, you should notice the preoccupation with his private parts subsiding a bit and becoming more appropriate for his age.

MEASLES

This viral disease has been almost eradicated from the United States. Only fifty to hundred cases occur each year. Wiser and experienced grandparents may be able to recognize this illness when it occurs, but most young parents (and young doctors) cannot. Here is our guide to recognizing and dealing with measles.

Symptoms

Measles starts off just like most other flu-like illnesses, with fever, runny nose, red eyes, a cough, and possibly diarrhea. Three to four days after these symptoms begin, a striking red, bumpy, and blotchy rash appears on the face and upper body. This spreads down over the rest of the body over the next two to three days. Unusual white spots can also be seen inside the cheeks (called *Koplik's spots*), which are often used to make the diagnosis.

The incubation period is eight to twelve days. A person is contagious starting two days prior to any signs of illness until about four days after the rash first appears.

When to Worry; What to Do

Most children with measles get through without any trouble. There is no treatment. The most important thing to do is to quarantine your child once you see a rash with an illness as described above. The diagnosis is confirmed with a blood test. However, you don't want to expose others by going into the doctor's office or a lab unannounced. Call your pediatrician and discuss how you can best get your child evaluated in a responsible manner. If the blood test confirms measles, the public health department will get involved to make sure the outbreak is contained. Here are a few possible complications that you should watch out for:

Pneumonia. If fever and a bad cough persist more than five days, or your child develops symptoms of pneumonia sooner (see page 434), call your doctor.

Croup. Sometimes the measles virus will cause croup symptoms. Notify your pediatrician.

Encephalitis. This is a rare complication (1 in 1,000 measles cases). Symptoms are similar to meningitis (see below). Go to an emergency room if your child begins having such symptoms.

MENINGITIS

Meningitis is potentially a very serious illness caused by inflammation of the lining covering the brain and spinal cord (known as the meninges). This inflammation is caused by either bacterial or viral infections and can affect children, adolescents, and adults. The two age groups at highest risk for meningitis are infants up to six months of age and adolescents and young adults. Viral and bacterial meningitis may carry with them similar symptoms and are both contagious, but treatments and outcomes are very different.

Viral Meningitis

Viruses can affect any part of the body. Viral meningitis can occur if a virus spreads into the body's bloodstream, which provides a path to the meninges of the brain and spinal cord, leading to inflammation. This does not occur with most viral illnesses; however, it is a possibility.

Viral meningitis is much more common and usually far less serious than bacterial meningitis. The symptoms of viral meningitis can be very mild and resemble the flu. In fact, many cases of viral meningitis go undiagnosed because they mimic other viral-type illnesses.

Symptoms. The symptoms can range greatly from mild to severe. Most cases of viral meningitis resemble the common flu. The five primary symptoms of meningitis are:

- fever
- vomiting
- headache
- sensitivity to light
- neck stiffness

Other symptoms that may indicate meningitis are:

- feeling lethargic
- seizures or convulsions
- irritability
- poor feeding in infants
- jaundice in infants
- a high-pitched cry in infants
- soft spot on the top of Baby's head bulging outward
- weak sucking in infants

With any type of meningitis, those affected will usually have most of the primary symptoms and some of the others. See your pediatrician to rule out this serious illness.

Treatment. If the doctor suspects meningitis, testing may be necessary to rule out the possibility of bacterial meningitis, which is treated much differently from viral meningitis. Children with viral meningitis may need to be hospitalized depending on how severe their illness is and their age. Infants and very young children who are diagnosed with viral meningitis are more likely to be hospitalized because they are more at risk for severe dehydration. Most cases of viral meningitis resolve on their own within seven to ten days, and the patient requires only fluids, rest, and fever-reducing medications to help the symptoms. Almost all cases of viral meningitis require no further treatment. There are a few more serious causes of viral meningitis in children. These include herpes meningitis, which occurs when a newborn is infected by a mother who has an outbreak of genital herpes at birth. The newborn may be infected upon passing through the birth canal. In fact, if a mother is known to have active genital herpes, a cesarean section is performed in order to prevent the newborn from being infected upon passing through the birth canal. Herpes meningitis in the newborn is a very serious and potentially life-threatening condition. Tests can be performed to diagnose herpes meningitis. If detected early and special antiviral medication is given, the outcome is usually good.

Other extremely rare, but potentially serious, causes of viral meningitis include the much-publicized West Nile virus and the bird flu. West Nile virus received much attention several years ago when there were outbreaks in many states throughout the country. Almost all cases were in people over the age of fifty, and children are thought to be a very low-risk group for West Nile virus infection. This disease is spread through mosquito bites and, of course, it is always a good idea to avoid mosquito bites whenever possible. It is important for pediatricians to reassure parents that their children are at an *extremely* low risk for West Nile virus infection.

Again, if your child appears to be suffering from a flu-like illness but the symptoms are getting worse, see your doctor right away.

Bacterial Meningitis

Compared to viral meningitis, bacterial meningitis is much less common, but far more serious. It can affect any age group, but infants up to six months of age, adolescents, and young adults are at highest risk for bacterial meningitis. Every year in the United States there are approximately 8,000 cases of bacterial meningitis, causing about 2,000 deaths annually.

Bacterial meningitis starts as a routine bacterial infection, such as a sinus infection, respiratory tract infection, gastrointestinal tract infection, urinary tract infection, or ear infection. In almost all cases proper treatment and the body's immune system fight off the bacteria and eradicate the infection from the body. Rarely, however, the bacteria can invade the infected person's bloodstream and travel to the meninges (the lining of the brain and spinal cord) and cause an infection there, leading to bacterial meningitis. Many different types of bacteria can cause bacterial meningitis. The type of bacteria usually depends on the age of the person with the illness.

Symptoms may begin as a cold, sinus infection, cough, or virtually any other type of bacterial infection in the body. As the illness progresses, children may begin to show flu-like symptoms. As the bacteria begin to invade the bloodstream and fluid surrounding the brain and spinal cord, the more severe symptoms of meningitis become apparent (see page 393).

 DR. SEARS TIP
Watch for Red Dots

The most severe form of bacterial meningitis (called *meningococcal meningitis*) causes a particular telltale rash called *petechiae,* numerous tiny red dots that look as if someone touched your child's skin with a red felt-tip pen. If your child has symptoms of meningitis, it's critical that you examine for these dots so you know if you have to seek medical care immediately. See page 322 for a detailed description of petechiae.

Children with bacterial meningitis usually appear very ill and symptoms can worsen rapidly. If your child is exhibiting any of the symptoms or the illness seems to be getting much worse, contact your health provider immediately. In fact, if bacterial meningitis is suspected, take your child to the emergency room, as bacterial meningitis requires immediate hospitalization and treatment.

Diagnosis. Laboratory tests are always performed on anyone suspected of having bacterial meningitis. These tests include blood work and a procedure known as a *lumbar puncture* (also known as a *spinal tap*). A lumbar puncture can indicate the presence of bacteria in the fluid around the brain and spinal cord and can also distinguish between bacterial and viral meningitis.

Treatment. Treatment for bacterial meningitis involves first and foremost intravenous antibiotics, which must be administered in a hospital. Doctors may even begin treatment for bacterial meningitis before the final diagnosis is reached because this is such a potentially life-threatening disease. Intravenous (IV) fluids are usually required to prevent or reverse dehydration and steroids may be given to decrease inflammation of the brain and spinal cord. Further treatments depend on how severe the case of bacterial meningitis is.

Complications. The potential long-term complications of bacterial meningitis depend entirely on how early treatment is begun and how severe the child's infection is. The good news is that if diagnosed and treated early, full recovery is expected with no long-term complications. More severe cases of bacterial meningitis may lead to the following long-term problems:

- seizures
- impaired vision
- hearing loss
- learning disabilities
- organ dysfunction, especially the heart, kidneys, and adrenal glands

Multiple organ failure and death may occur in cases of bacterial meningitis that are not promptly diagnosed and treated.

Prevention. Universal vaccination has greatly reduced cases of bacterial meningitis. Infants in the first year of life are routinely vaccinated against the main causes of bacterial meningitis for that age group (Hib and pneumococcal disease). As we discussed earlier, teens and young adults make up the second high-risk population for bacterial meningitis — specifically a strain called *meningococcal meningitis* — especially when they live in close-quarter environments (dorm rooms, military barracks, locker rooms, and classrooms). It is now recommended that everyone between eleven and eighteen years of age receive a one-time vaccination against meningococcal meningitis. If your teen does not receive the vaccine while in high school, it is highly recommended that he does so prior to, or during, college. See page 43 for more on vaccines.

Other important ways to prevent bacterial meningitis involve basic sanitation and hygiene. Decreasing the chances of getting a common bacterial infection, such as a sinus or upper respiratory tract infection, will lower the risk of contracting bacterial meningitis. Be sure to explain to your child the importance of proper hand washing, not sharing utensils, cups, and so on, and being careful not to spread illness if she is feeling sick. When someone is diagnosed with bacterial meningitis, it is often recommended that everyone who had close contact with that person receive oral antibiotics as a precaution.

MIGRAINE HEADACHE

Most children suffer headaches from time to time, usually when they are sick, such as with a cold or the flu. Migraine headaches, once thought to be a problem only among adults, are now being diagnosed more and more in younger age groups. In fact, up to 5 percent of grade-school-aged children and about 20 percent of adolescents and teens suffer from migraine headaches. Preteen and teenage girls are more likely to have migraines than boys are. This is thought to be due to the hormonal changes that a girl goes through during this time. See page 349 for information on non-migraine headaches.

Symptoms

Children can experience many different symptoms during a migraine headache. Some of the most common symptoms are:

- throbbing pain in one spot on the front or side of the head

- nausea and vomiting

- blurred vision

- dizziness or difficulty walking

- fatigue and pale skin color

- flashing lights, tunnel vision, or seeing wavy lines (known as an aura)

- changes in mood

DR. SEARS TIP
Family History

When seeing your pediatrician for the concern of migraines in your child, be sure to inform the doctor if there is a family history of migraines. Up to 70 to 90 percent of children who have migraines have a strong family history of migraines.

Causes and Triggers

The pain from migraines is thought to be caused by dilation (swelling) and constriction (shrinking) of the blood vessels in the brain. Blood vessels do this normally to regulate the blood flow to different parts of the body. However, people with migraines may be more sensitive to these changes. Certain chemicals in the brain seem to play a role in causing blood vessels to swell and shrink. Most migraines have some sort of trigger. There are many different known triggers for migraines, including biological, environmental, and nutritionally triggered. Some of the most common biological and environmental triggers for migraines include:

- bright or flickering lights

- loud noises

- stress

- depression

- anxiety

- changes in normal sleep patterns or not getting enough sleep

- menstruation or changes in hormone levels in the adolescent's body

- changes in the weather or a change in altitude

- strong or unusual odors

- missing meals or being hungry

- intense exercise

In addition, there are many types of food and food additives that are known to trigger migraine attacks. Some of these include:

- processed, canned, or cured meats (ham, bologna, hot dog, sausage, pepperoni)

- certain types of beans

- aged cheese, buttermilk, cottage cheese, sour cream

- onions

- caffeine

- aspartame

- papaya or passion fruit

- nuts and nut butters

- monosodium glutamate (MSG)

- pickled or preserved foods

- sauerkraut

- excessively salty foods

- chocolate or cocoa

Diagnosis

If you are concerned that your child might be experiencing migraine headaches, see your pediatrician. Taking a good history to identify headache patterns, triggers, and duration of the headaches can go a long way toward diagnosing migraines. In fact, many migraine headaches can be diagnosed based on history alone.

Your child's doctor may decide to do a CT scan or MRI of the brain if she is concerned that there might be something more serious going on, such as a brain tumor or blood vessel abnormality. However, these are extremely rare findings in children, and most headaches are due to migraine or other forms of headache and do not indicate anything more serious.

Treatment

When your child feels a migraine attack coming on, you should have her go into a dark, cool place. Have her lie down, close her eyes, and place a cool washcloth across her forehead. If your pediatrician has prescribed a medication to be taken for a migraine attack, taking it at the first sign of a migraine is most effective. For children who only get migraines rarely, taking the above measures and perhaps an over-the-counter (OTC) headache medicine (approved for children) may be all that is needed. If your child gets migraines frequently, or if they are becoming more severe, the doctor may prescribe a daily medication to decrease the number of attacks. He might also refer you to a neurologist for moderate-to-severe cases of migraines. The goal in treating migraines is to:

1. Identify the potential causes

2. Diminish length of time and severity of the attack

3. Decrease the frequency of migraine headache attacks

There are several nutritional supplements on the market that have been reported to lessen the frequency of migraines. These

**DR. SEARS TIP
Don't Overdo OTC
Pain Relievers**

If you find yourself needing to give your child OTC headache medications more and more frequently, go see the doctor. Relying too heavily on OTC headache medications can actually make children and adolescents suffer headaches more often, a phenomenon known as *rebound headache*.

supplements include vitamin B$_{12}$, riboflavin, niacin, and an herbal supplement called *feverfew*. Brand names include MigreLief and Migranal. Talk to your pediatrician about these treatments.

Alternative therapies for migraines. Mainstream medicine can't always find an answer or a cure for a chronic condition. A thorough medical evaluation and treatment plan for migraines sometimes doesn't lead to a resolution of the problem. We encourage you to seek out some alternative therapies to find relief. Chiropractic care, acupressure, acupuncture, or naturopathic medicine can sometimes fix migraines when standard medicine cannot.

Prevention

Although you may not be able to completely rid your child of migraine attacks, there are many different things you can do to control the frequency and severity of your child's migraines. These are:

- Encourage a healthy diet.

- Do not let your child skip meals.

- Give your child healthy snacks if she feels hungry.

- Look for things in your child's life that may be triggering migraines, such as anxiety or stress.

- Look for foods in your child's diet that might be triggering migraines (see the list, page 397). If you can't identify a likely culprit, try eliminating all the foods on the list and see if the frequency of headaches diminishes.

- Work to improve your child's overall mental health.

- Encourage daily exercise (but not too intense).

- Make sure your child is properly hydrated throughout the day.

**DR. SEARS TIP
Keep a Diary**

Whenever we see children in our office for headaches that we suspect might be related to migraines, we always encourage keeping a "headache diary." This means keeping a daily journal of food intake and activities. This is especially important to document on days when a migraine was suffered. Keeping a diary can identify certain foods and/or environmental factors that may be leading to your child's migraines.

Being diligent about trying to identify causes for your child's migraines is one of the most effective ways to treat this condition. In almost all cases of migraine, at least some triggers can be found. While this most likely will not wipe out your child's migraines completely, it can go a long way in improving overall quality of life. Again, see the doctor if your child's migraines appear to be getting worse or if they develop any new symptoms. Further testing may need to be done to rule out more serious causes. Working with a migraine specialist (such as a neurologist) may be required to help manage migraine headaches.

MILIA

Milia are tiny white bumps that appear on the skin of newborns, most commonly on the nose, cheeks, and chin. This is a very common condition. Approximately 40 percent of newborn babies will get them. Some will have a few, others will have many. Occasionally, these may also appear on your baby's gums or the roof of his mouth.

The Cause

Milia are caused when dead skin cells become trapped in little pockets near the surface of a newborn's skin. Skin cells give the milia their whitish appearance. These bumps will slowly slough off over a period of a few weeks and the bumps will disappear.

What to Do

Although milia may be distressing to the parents, no treatment is needed. They will go away on their own within a period of a few weeks, but occasionally may last for up to two months. They do not cause the baby any discomfort and do not lead to any long-term problems.

- Do not put any creams or ointments on the milia.

- Do not attempt to squeeze milia, as this could lead to long-term scarring.

- Do not vigorously wash or scrub the area, as this may further irritate your newborn's sensitive skin.

Patience is all you need.

MOLES

Moles are something we all deal with at some point in our lives. Moles can appear in any age group, although they are more common in adults and adolescents. Occasionally, infants are even born with moles. Moles (also known as *nevi*) are spots on the skin that are usually dark-colored and oval-shaped; however, they can appear in many shapes, sizes, and colors. Moles can appear anywhere on the body. They are usually raised, but may remain flat as well.

Causes

Most moles are caused by exposure to sunlight. Our skin contains special cells called *melanocytes*. These melanocytes are responsible for producing pigment that darkens our skin. When exposed to prolonged sunlight melanocytes may produce more pigment on a certain area of the skin, producing the characteristic darkened appearance of a mole.

Far less common are moles that are present on the skin when a child is born. These moles are known as *congenital nevi*, and they appear in approximately one out of every one hundred newborn babies.

What to Do

Step one is don't panic. In children, moles almost never lead to skin cancer (also known as *melanoma*). However, approximately five hundred children each year are diagnosed with melanoma. Most moles just simply need to be observed at regular checkups. Have your pediatrician check your child's moles for any signs of change. Be sure to have your child evaluated if you notice

DR. SEARS TIP
The A, B, C, D, and E's of Evaluating a Mole

This is an easy way to remember the characteristics of moles that may be more worrisome and warrant a visit to the doctor:

A: Stands for *asymmetry*, which means that the mole does not have a normal round- or oval-shaped appearance or that one part of the mole is shaped differently from the other.

B: Stands for *border*. The borders of most moles are usually round- or oval-shaped. Irregular or notched borders may be a sign that the mole is changing.

C: Stands for *color*. Most moles are only one color, usually dark or light brown. See your doctor if your child's mole begins to contain different colors, such as red, blue, black, or white.

D: Stands for *diameter.* See your doctor if your child's mole begins to grow in diameter. Moles that are less than five millimeters (or about a quarter of an inch) are usually nothing to worry about. Have the mole evaluated if it appears larger than this size.

E: Stands for *evolving*. Any change in size, shape, color, or elevation, or any bleeding, itching, or crusting may be a concern.

any change in the size, color, or shape of a mole. In rare cases, a mole may need to be biopsied or removed if there is a concern.

When to Worry

Moles that are present at birth (also called *congenital nevi*) are more likely to progress to skin cancer, or melanoma, later in life. Again, this is still very rare in children. Be sure to inform your doctor of any moles that your child was born with, as these do need to be watched more closely than moles that appear after the child was born. Your pediatrician may decide to refer your child to a dermatologist at about age ten for a biopsy.

Preventing Moles and Lowering the Risk of Skin Cancer

The following tips can help lower your child's risk of developing moles and may help prevent progression to skin cancer later in life:

- Avoid prolonged exposure to sunlight, especially at midday, between the hours of 10 a.m. and 3 p.m. Choose play areas with some shade cover.

- If your child is going to be outside for more than thirty minutes, encourage the use of long sleeves, long pants, and wide-brimmed hats.

- Avoid prolonged play in areas where the sun's rays may be reflected, such as sand, snow, and water.

- Use high-quality sunscreen if your child is going to be in the sun for more than a half hour. The sunscreen should be SPF 30 or higher and should provide protection against both UVA and UVB. See page 31.

DR. SEARS TIP
Safe Sun Sense

Growing children need vitamin D for healthy bones and bodies. Be a sun-savvy parent — allow adequate sun exposure while preventing sunburn. See page 32 for tips.

Risk Factors for Skin Cancer

Children with fair skin and those with a strong family history of skin cancer are most at risk for developing cancer of the skin. Another important risk factor is frequent sunburn and excessive exposure to sunlight during childhood. This is why it is so important to protect your child's skin early in life. Doing so will greatly reduce the risk for skin cancer as an adult.

MOLLUSCUM CONTAGIOSUM (MC)

If your child has tiny growths on his skin that look like a combination of warts and blisters, he might have *molluscum contagiosum* (MC). These are common, harmless skin lesions caused by the *molluscum contagiosum virus* (MCV). As the name implies, the virus is contagious and spreads easily from child to child. While most children are not bothered by these little wart-like growths, some growths can be itchy and become secondarily infected from repeated scratching. Generally the parental anxiety over these is worse than the growths themselves. Around 20 percent of children experience MC.

How to Tell

They begin as one or two small pimples. Then they grow into rounded pimples and blisters from two to five millimeters in diameter. Some will have a white head on a red base, but most are flesh-colored. If you take a magnifying glass you can sometimes see a dimple in the middle of the bump. They are most commonly found on the chest, arms, and underarm areas.

How a Child Gets Them

Like many viruses, they spread when the child scratches the bumps, gets the virus under her fingernails, and then scratches other parts of her body or another child. They can also spread through sharing towels and clothing and very commonly through contact sports.

What to Do

A wait-and-see approach is generally taken with MC, and they usually disappear by themselves between six months and three years. They tend to rapidly multiply, but as they do, the child gradually builds up antibodies against this virus. The variability in how long they take to go away depends upon how effectively the child's immune system starts fighting them.

Find out how much, if any, they are bothering your child. If they don't itch, aren't infected, and are not a source of irritation to your child, let nature take its course and let the body get rid of them. If, on the other hand, they are bothering your child, in that they itch or he is constantly picking at them or becoming increasingly self-conscious, consider these treatment options:

- To prevent irritation from friction rubs, cover with an emollient.

- To relieve itching, apply a topical steroid ointment twice a day (see Eczema, page 297).

- If they look infected (red, swollen, oozing), ask the doctor for a prescription antibiotic ointment.

- Try this home remedy: Apply a piece of duct tape twice the size of the wart in the morning. The duct tape irritates and thins the top of the wart. Remove the tape before bed, take a clean paper clip, and gently poke the soft center to allow the contents to extrude. Reapply the duct tape each morning and repeat this drainage procedure for several nights. While not as effective as the next suggestion, you could try this home remedy first.

- Finally, there's the "search and destroy" method. If the warts are really bothering your child even after at least a one-year "watch-and-wait" approach, they can be removed by your doctor or a dermatologist. The usual method is to freeze off the warts using a dab of liquid nitrogen. A dermatologist can also scoop the middle out of each wart (if there aren't too many, because it's fairly painful). A new prescription treatment, called Aldara cream, can be effective, but it is expensive. Over-the-counter wart acid can also work.

Usually MCV infections disappear without scarring. In fact, some believe that scarring may be more likely with aggressive treatment. Darker-skinned children are more likely to scar. Permanent scarring rarely occurs.

MONONUCLEOSIS (MONO, EPSTEIN-BARR INFECTION)

This disease is caused by the Epstein-Barr virus (EBV) and is commonly known as the "kissing" disease, since it is commonly passed through saliva among intimate friends or family members. Here is what you need to know if your child, or your teenager's sweetheart, has mono.

Symptoms

Acute phase of illness. Infants and young children often don't show any suspicious symptoms other than a mild fever and generic rash. Older kids and teens will usually be sicker, with the following signs:

- sore throat (usually quite severe)

- swollen neck glands

- enlarged, red tonsils covered with pus

- fever (may last as long as ten to fourteen days)

- generic light red blotchy rash

- fatigue, poor appetite

In addition, the doctor may notice an enlarged spleen (below the stomach on the left side of the abdomen) and other swollen glands, such as the armpits and the groin area.

Chronic fatigue. Less than 10 percent of teens or adults with mono will experience weeks to months of fatigue following the sick phase of the illness. It isn't certain if this is specifically due to EBV or not, as fatigue can also occur after other illnesses as well. If the initial illness was fairly mild, you may not even realize it was mono until fatigue sets in and you see the doctor.

Contagious period. A person is mostly contagious during the initial symptoms and as long as fever lasts, and may spread the illness through coughing and sneezing during that time. Once a child feels better, the virus can still be spread through saliva for several months. Repeated intimate contact is probably needed to transmit the illness. Casual day-to-day contact with peers or family members isn't a risk. The incubation period is one to two months.

Diagnosis

If the symptoms seem obvious to the doctor, she may not order any tests to confirm the diagnosis. However, if your child is significantly ill, some blood work may be done to verify the diagnosis and rule out various other diseases. A *monospot* blood test is the fastest and least expensive way to make the diagnosis. A more accurate, more expensive, and slower blood test (may take several days) called an *EBV antibody panel* can also be done. A complete blood cell count can show a high level of *atypical lymphocytes* (a kind of white blood cell), but this doesn't confirm the diagnosis.

When to Worry; What to Do

Most children get through this illness without any problems. Here are a few things you should know:

Treatment. There is no specific medication for EBV. Treatment is aimed at any uncomfortable symptoms, such as fever and sore throat.

Enlarged spleen and sports. If the doctor feels an enlarged spleen, the child should not participate in contact sports until the spleen is felt to be back to normal (usually about one month) due to the risk of splenic rupture if the child gets hit hard in the abdomen (a life-threatening surgical emergency). Even if the doctor doesn't notice the spleen during the initial exam (it can be missed), it would be prudent to avoid contact sports for one month anyway.

Enlarged tonsils and breathing difficulty. Some children will experience severe snoring and blocked breathing at night due to enlarged tonsils. Oral steroids can be taken for about a week to shrink the tonsils. See the doctor if your child is experiencing troublesome breathing.

Jaundice. In approximately 10 percent of cases of mononucleosis, the virus can irritate the liver, causing mild liver damage and jaundice (yellow skin). This will resolve without treatment, and your pediatrician can monitor the liver's recovery with periodic blood tests.

Allergic rash with antibiotics. Children with mono who take amoxicillin or Augmentin antibiotics because of a suspected bacterial tonsillitis will get an allergic-looking rash due to a unique reaction between EBV, the antibiotic, and the immune system. This isn't an actual allergic antibiotic reaction. This is often how mono is diagnosed: by chance.

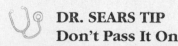

**DR. SEARS TIP
Don't Pass It On**

Your teenager with mono should be instructed not to share drinks with anyone else. Set aside plates, cups, and utensils to be used *only* by the individual with mono. Carefully wash these after each use. This will help lower the risk of transmitting mono to someone else.

MOUTH SORES

Your child has a high fever, is very fussy, is drooling everywhere, and is refusing to eat or even drink her favorite juice. These are common symptoms of sore throat, teething, and ear infections, but one often overlooked cause is mouth sore viruses. Here are some tips to help you through this very bothersome and painful, yet not serious, illness. For information on individual cold sores on the lips, see page 229. For single canker sores within the mouth, see page 210.

How to Tell

Mouth sores are caused by viruses that are transmitted from the saliva of other children or adults. They are very painful and usually come with fever, excessive drooling, refusal to eat (and maybe drink), and extreme fussiness. Here's how you can check your child to see if such sores are the cause of these symptoms:

- You may see sores on the outer lips.

- Gently pull back the upper or lower lips. You may see white or red sores on the insides of the lips or on the front gums.

- Gently pull back the cheeks on each side and examine the inside of the cheeks with a flashlight. You may find some sores there.

- Shine a flashlight at the back of the mouth while your child says "ahhhh" (or is crying). You may see red or white spots in the throat or on the tongue.

- Some viruses also cause small white or red blisters on the hands, feet, or diaper area (see hand, foot, and mouth disease, below).

Two Types of Mouth Sore Infections

There are two different types of mouth sores, and it's useful to try to distinguish which kind your child has because one type is treatable with a prescription antiviral medication:

Hand, foot, and mouth disease (Coxsackie virus). This is by far the most common cause of mouth sore illnesses. It usually affects children ages six months to three years. Symptoms include:

- high fever, often up to five days

- severe fussiness

- severe mouth pain or sore throat

- copious drooling

- refusal to eat or even to drink

- rash: small red or white spots or blisters on the hands, feet, or diaper area, or a red, lacy rash anywhere on the body

Herpes virus. Herpes simplex type I (HSV-I) (unrelated to genital herpes) is a less common cause of mouth sore infections in children. Symptoms are generally the same as for hand, foot, and mouth disease, but there are three factors that can help you and your doctor distinguish this from Coxsackie virus:

- Herpes does not typically cause spots or rash on the rest of the body.

- The mouth sores of herpes are usually more concentrated in the front of the mouth, whereas the sores of hand, foot, and mouth tend to be in front as well as back in the throat.

- In herpes, the gums are usually very red, swollen, and possibly bleeding. This is usually not the case with Coxsackie virus.

Once a child has had this type of severe oral herpes infection once, subsequent mild episodes may occur once or twice each year that only result in a cold sore on the lips (see page 229) or a single canker sore in the mouth (see page 210).

Treatment

There is no treatment that will help Coxsackie sores go away more quickly. Treatment is mainly geared toward minimizing the pain and fever and maintaining hydration. A prescription antiviral medication can be used for herpes virus.

Cold liquids. Popsicles, slushies, or frozen juice (not citrus) can both soothe your child and provide needed fluids during this illness. Cold milk, ice cream, or frozen yogurt can also soothe and provide calories.

Medications. Acetaminophen or ibuprofen can help with the pain and fever. If needed, you can alternate between the two, giving something every three hours. Other meds include:

- *Mylanta/Benadryl/Xylocaine mix.* This is a very effective regimen that will soothe and numb the sores for a short period of time. The first two ingredients are over the counter, but the third is prescription. A pharmacist can mix them for you with a prescription from your pediatrician. This should only be used by children old enough to rinse and then spit it out; the Xylocaine shouldn't be swallowed.

- *Benadryl.* This antihistamine is available over the counter. Because of the risk of oversedation, do not give Benadryl to infants less than one year old.

- *Acyclovir.* This prescription antiviral medication is effective only against the herpes type of mouth sores. If started within the first forty-eight hours of illness, it can shorten the duration and severity. This is one good reason to see a doctor near the beginning of this illness to help you sort out the diagnosis.

 **DR. SEARS TIP
A Little Reassurance**

Most infants and children won't eat any food during the worst few days of this illness. While parents naturally worry about this, in the long run it's okay. Your child may lose weight during this time, but he'll gain it back when he's well! Kids do well on a few days of smoothies (or breast milk/formula for infants).

Is My Child Contagious?

Yes! Both forms are very contagious, mostly via the saliva. When the fever has been gone for two days, and your child is back to her playful, happy self, then she is no longer contagious.

When to Worry

These can be very painful and bothersome illnesses, but they are not dangerous. The expected course is fever, fussing, drooling, not eating, and barely drinking for up to five days. The sores and drooling can continue on longer than this, but they are usually less painful with time. Here are the signs you should watch for that warrant a visit to the doctor:

Dehydration. This is a big worry for parents since kids will seem to go days without drinking much. Most children will get mildly dehydrated, but it is very rare for a child to get so dehydrated that medical intervention is necessary. Just do your best to push cold or frozen liquids, and your child should be okay. See our dehydration information on page 267 to determine if your child is dehydrated enough to see a doctor.

Fever more than five days. If the fever persists or your child is acting unusually ill, see the doctor right away.

Spread of the virus sores. Sometimes a doctor will think a child has an untreatable case of Coxsackie virus, with sores only in the back of the mouth. But occasionally, herpes will begin in the back of the mouth but then spread to the front to infect the lips and gums. If this occurs, treatment with acyclovir can shorten the course of the illness. See your doctor again to consider this treatment.

MRSA: METHICILLIN-RESISTANT STAPH AUREUS

The "superbug" most in the news lately is called MRSA (pronounced "mersah"). Staphylococcus is one of the most common bacteria that live in the lining of the nose and on the skin. You wash it off, it comes back. Usually it resides on the surfaces of the body and does no harm. But, if the skin barrier is broken by a cut or a scratch, these "staph" germs can grow into a sore on the skin.

Once the skin barrier is penetrated, the staph bacteria can burrow deeper into the skin and form a sore resembling a bite; it can go deeper, forming a boil, or an even deeper abscess. If the germ goes unchecked, it can work its way into the bloodstream and cause an overwhelming and possibly life-threatening infection.

DR. SEARS TIP
Don't Squeeze It, Needle It

If your child has a tiny boil (around the size of a chocolate chip), it might be tempting to squeeze it when it has a ripe head. Don't. Not only do you run the risk of transferring the germs to your fingertips, under your fingernails, and then onto other family members, but you also run the risk of forcing the germs deeper into the tissue. Better to have your doctor open it with a sterile needle. Or, if you do not have easy access to medical care, use a sterilized needle yourself. Prick open just the ripe, soft whitehead and apply a hot compress to ease out the pus. Apply antibiotic cream and completely cover it with a bandage as described below.

There is an ongoing drug/bug war in the body. Humans make antibiotics to fight the bugs; the bugs alter their genes to fight or become "resistant" to the antibiotics. In MRSA's case, the bugs won. It is called MRSA (methycillin-resistant staph aureous) because this type of staph has become resistant to the antibiotic methicillin, previously used to treat *Staphylococcus aureus*. But humans have always outsmarted bugs and keep one step ahead of them by making newer and stronger antibiotics to kill these germs.

How to Tell

MRSA can begin like a tiny skin sore that resembles a bite. It then gets crusty, red, and spreads; it looks like a skin infection that doesn't seem to be healing. Family members or friends may have the same type of infection. Initially you may think it's just an insect or spider bite, but it starts looking a bit "angry."

DR. SEARS TIP
When in Doubt, Check It Out!

Any skin infection that doesn't seem to be healing quickly should be checked out by your pediatrician for testing and treatment.

What to Do

If you suspect MRSA, make an appointment with your pediatrician. A doctor will sometimes get a culture of the wound by swabbing the area or draining the boil. Sometimes a nasal swab is taken for a culture if many family members have similar skin sores. This is sent to a laboratory and your doctor will often have the confirmation within forty-eight hours.

Be particularly suspicious of MRSA in boils on the buttocks, especially in infants. The warm, moist, germy environment of the diaper area is a perfect site for bacterial infections, especially MRSA. If your infant develops a boil or an abscess (a bigger and deeper boil), it may be MRSA.

If the skin lesion is small and superficial, your doctor will probably treat it with the topical antibiotic cream mupirocin. If the infection is deeper within the skin, such as an abscess, or there are multiple boils, your doctor may elect to treat your child with oral antibiotics that are, at this writing, effective against most MRSA (Septra, Bactrim, and clindamycin). If your child is acting sick, and the staph infection is deeper into the skin where there is a risk of it entering the bloodstream, your doctor may recommend hospitalization for antibiotics.

Prevention

MRSA, like most germs, is transmitted through skin-to-skin contact. It is most common in crowded settings, primarily hospitals, but also daycare centers, classrooms, sports locker rooms — anywhere people are literally "in touch" with one another. This superbug is particularly contagious in skin-to-skin contact sports, such as wrestling. To prevent your child from getting any type of bacterial infection, especially MRSA, take these precautions:

- Wash hands thoroughly. This is still the most effective way of preventing the spread of staph.

- Don't share skin stuff and personal items, such as towels, washcloths, and uniforms.

- Clean wounds early and thoroughly by washing them with soap and water and applying a prescription antibiotic cream, such as mupirocin.

- Use antibiotics appropriately. It's the overuse of antibiotics that causes bacterial resistance in the first place. (See Antibiotics, page 549.)

Be especially vigilant about the development of skin sores if your child has a compromised immune system or has recently been hospitalized.

DR. SEARS TIP
Cover It Completely!

To keep MRSA from spreading to other contacts, use a bandage that completely seals the area, such as Activ-Flex by Band-Aid. Strip-type bandages, the ones that have open sides, are not as effective as the occlusive type of bandages. When the infected skin area is completely covered by a bandage, your child may attend daycare or school without fear of being contagious. Treat it, cover it, but no need to quarantine it.

MUMPS

This illness recently spread through the United States, with about 5,000 cases in 2007. Most years, however, mumps has been fairly uncommon, with only about 250 reported cases. The MMR vaccine helps keep it that way. Although your child is unlikely to come across mumps, here is our guide on how to recognize it.

Symptoms

Fever and sore throat are the initial symptoms, just like many other illnesses. What makes mumps unique is the swelling of the *parotid glands* (the saliva glands within the cheeks right in front of the ears). The glands will also be tender, and chewing may be uncomfortable.

The incubation period is sixteen to eighteen days. A person is contagious about two days prior to the glands swelling until about five days after the swelling starts.

When to Worry; What to Do

There is no treatment for mumps. The most important thing to do is to recognize the typical gland swelling and then isolate your child. Call your pediatrician to discuss possibly being seen. Here are a few complications to be aware of:

Orchitis (swelling and pain of the testicles). This is a common occurrence in males who catch mumps after puberty and is usually harmless. Sterility is an extremely rare consequence of orchitis. There is no treatment or intervention that will make any difference.

Meningitis. Mumps can cause meningitis symptoms. Go to an emergency room if you suspect this (see page 393).

MUSCULAR DYSTROPHY

Muscular dystrophy is a genetic disorder that causes a gradual deterioration and weakening of the muscles of the body. This disorder can affect many age groups. Some children begin having symptoms in infancy, while others will not show problems until adulthood. There are several different forms of muscular dystrophy, with great variation in severity.

Symptoms

Symptoms of muscular dystrophy may begin to appear in the infant years; however, most children do not begin to have symptoms until after the age of five. Some forms of muscular dystrophy may show no symptoms until the teen or early adult years. In infants and children, some of the most common symptoms of possible muscular dystrophy include:

- stumbling or falling more often than is normal for a toddler or young child

- difficulty standing up

- difficulty pushing objects

- walking on tiptoes most or all of the time

- difficulty climbing stairs

- abnormally large calf muscles (a condition known as *calf pseudohypertrophy*)

- generalized muscle weakness

Most forms of muscular dystrophy are seen only in boys. Although girls can carry the genetic defect, symptoms do not usually present. Remember, symptoms and severity of muscular dystrophy can vary greatly. Some cases are so mild that they go undiagnosed throughout one's entire life. However, most cases will show several of the above symptoms.

Causes

Our bodies make special proteins that help build and maintain muscles. In people with muscular dystrophy, there is an abnormality in the genes responsible for making these proteins. Since the body cannot adequately make the proteins to maintain healthy muscles, the muscles slowly weaken and deteriorate over time.

Diagnosis

If you have questions about your child's muscle strength or any type of abnormal activity, see your pediatrician. He will take a thorough medical history and perform a physical exam. It is also important to inform the doctor of any family history of muscle disorders. There are several types of blood tests that can indicate signs of muscle damage in the body. DNA testing can also be performed by a geneticist in order to look for defects that may point to the diagnosis of muscular dystrophy. Talk with the doctor for more information.

Types

There are two main types of muscular dystrophy that most often affect children:

Duchenne muscular dystrophy. This is the most common form of muscular dystrophy, as well as the most severe. Approximately 1 out of every 3,500 boys is affected. Girls can carry the defective gene, but they do not show symptoms. By age five, boys with this type of muscular dystrophy will usually begin to show symptoms. The most common muscle group that is first affected are the muscles in the pelvic region. As the disease progresses, muscles in the back, arms, shoulders, and legs will also be affected. Most children with Duchenne muscular dystrophy will need a wheelchair by the early adolescent years. Eventually, the muscles that help aid breathing begin to be affected and special ventilators will be required. Sadly, children with Duchenne muscular dystrophy have an average life span of only about twenty years.

Becker muscular dystrophy. This type of muscular dystrophy is similar to Duchenne muscular dystrophy, but it is less common and usually less severe. About 1 in 30,000 boys is affected. Again, girls do not show symptoms of Becker muscular dystrophy. Symptoms are usually not seen until the teenage years. Like Duchenne muscular dystrophy, Becker muscular dystrophy usually begins as muscle weakness in the pelvic region, moving on to the shoulders, back, and less commonly arms and legs. Most children with Becker muscular dystrophy have normal life spans and usually do not require wheelchairs.

There are several other much more rare forms of muscular dystrophy, but we will not discuss those here. Consult your physician for further information.

Treatment

Sadly, there is no known cure for muscular dystrophy at this time. However, doctors and researchers are working very hard toward finding one. The good news is that there are now many types of treatment options that can help slow the disease's progress and improve the person's quality of life. Proper treatment for muscular dystrophy requires a multidisciplinary approach. Several specialists should be involved in the patient's care. Physical therapy and special braces can help maintain muscle tone and strength. A licensed physical therapist should be part of the treatment team to insure proper exercise techniques. Treatment with steroids has been found to slow the deterioration of muscles, which may help

the child walk longer. As the disease progresses and the respiratory muscles and heart begin to weaken, special ventilation may be required. Children with muscular dystrophy are more prone to lung infections that require prompt treatment. Wheelchairs are eventually required for children with the Duchenne muscular dystrophy.

NAIL INJURIES (FINGER AND TOE)

Injuries to fingernails or toenails are extremely painful, and they take a long time to heal. But heal they eventually do. Finger- and toenail injuries are treated the same way. There are a few things you should know to help your child.

Crush Injuries

Crush injuries (something hard falling or slamming onto a nail) should be iced for twenty minutes each hour for several hours, then about three times daily for the next day or two. This helps keep down the swelling. You will see dark red or purple blood under the nail. You need to watch for significant swelling of blood underneath the nail to the point that the nail bed (where the nail disappears into the skin on the back of the finger or top of the toe) is being pushed upward. Here's how you can tell: Look at an uninjured finger or toe from the side, and you will notice the nail bed curves downward as it goes under the skin, and the skin angles upward again (like a very shallow "V"). If the injured nail bed forms a straight line with the skin (no "V") or, even worse, is so swollen that it forms an inverted "V," this painful pressure needs to be relieved, or else the living part of the nail bed (under the skin) may die, and the nail may not regrow. Your pediatrician (or one at an urgent care center) can relieve this pressure by burning a hole through the nail using an electrocautery instrument. It sounds painful, but it's really quite easy and painless. There's no urgent rush; this procedure can wait about twenty-four hours. In the meantime, ice can help keep the swelling down.

Tear or Fracture Injuries

This is perhaps one of the most painful injuries that can happen, and may be part of a crushing injury. In this type, the nail is actually pulled partway out. Part of the finger tissue may be cut or torn as well. This type of wound should be evaluated in an emergency room, as most regular doctors' offices can't devote the time and staff to attend to complicated injuries like these. If the emergency room doctor determines that the nail needs to be fixed, he will numb up the whole finger, push the nail back into position, and sew the nail into place; he may also need to put stitches in any finger lacerations. This traumatic procedure is probably worth it. If the nail is not secured back into place, the nail may not grow back.

Expected Healing Time

New nail tissue that grows in may be thicker and slightly disfigured, and the old injured nail will start to lift away from the finger or toe. This is normal. You can trim away any part of the nail that is inconvenient. Once the injured nail grows all the way out (a month or two), the new nail will probably remain thick and

uneven for a year or two. Eventually, normal smooth nail will start to form again.

NAVEL, PROTRUDING

Some babies have "innie" belly buttons while others have "outies." The appearance of a baby's navel is as variable as hair texture. Whether your child has an "innie" or an "outie" depends on the way the umbilical stump heals, not the way it's cut. In the usual healing process, the umbilical stump shrivels up and gets buried within the "hole" called the navel. Surrounding that hole are two long muscles that extend from the ribs to the pelvic bone. In the early months, you will often feel a one- or two-finger-breadth space between these muscles. As Baby grows, these muscles grow together and the outie may become an innie. If not, there's no harm done. Also, as these muscles grow together, Baby's abdomen becomes firmer, and Baby shows less of a pot belly. Because tiny tissues change so fast, your baby's navel will not look the same now as it will look at the bikini age. As for most baby cosmetic attractions, you'll just have to wait and see. (See related topic, Umbilical Hernia, page 529.)

NECK PAIN AND STRAIN

While neck pain and strain is common among adults, parents don't usually expect their young children to complain of this. Yet, neck pain is not uncommon in kids. Your child may wake up crying and unable to move his neck; he may keep it tilted or turned to one side; he may scream when you try to move his head.

Despite how serious this may sound, it usually is only a harmless muscle or ligament strain. Here is our guide to helping resolve this type of crisis and how to know when something more serious is going on.

Causes

Here are the reasons that your child's neck may suddenly start hurting:

Neck strain. Sometimes a quick turn of the head or sleeping with the neck at an odd angle can cause a sudden and very painful strain on one of the muscles or ligaments in the back or side of the neck. Being in a car accident can also strain the neck (whiplash). The child will keep the head straight or turned to whatever position is most comfortable and will describe a severe sharp pain when he tries to turn his head.

Throat infection. This can cause pain in the front or side of the neck. It's not nearly as severe as a strain, and the child should be able to move the neck around without much trouble. See page 514 for more information.

Meningitis. Many parents naturally worry about this whenever a child has a fever and neck pain. It's important to determine what area of the neck actually hurts. Meningitis causes pain in the back of the neck, and a child won't look down because stretching the neck increases the pain. If it's the front or side, then the fever and pain are probably not meningitis. If the back of the neck hurts, but there's no fever or headache, then it's not meningitis. See page 393 for more information.

Torticollis. This sudden spasm and pain in the muscle that goes from behind the ear to the sternum will cause a child to keep the head tilted and turned to one side. It's similar to a general neck strain, but it occurs in the main muscle responsible for turning the head (as opposed to a strain of a minor muscle or ligament in the back of the neck). The child may point to where the pain is, so you can know which side is tight and in spasm. See page 526 for more details.

Treatment

You can refer to the specific sections in this book that discuss infectious causes and torticollis. For general neck strain, here are some treatment ideas:

Ice. Hold an ice pack to the sore area (your child should be able to point this out) for twenty minutes every hour for the rest of the day. Aggressive icing can help resolve the strain much more quickly.

Ibuprofen. This anti-inflammatory and pain reliever does wonders for neck strain. It does more than just temporarily relieve the pain; it helps the strain heal more quickly. Your child can take it every six hours. Check out page 553 for dosing.

These are really the only two treatments that you need to do. The strain should resolve over the next three days.

When to Worry

As long as the strain is steadily improving, you don't need to worry. Here are some situations that do warrant a doctor's visit:

- Car or sports accident. If your child complains of neck pain after an injury or accident, it's better to see a doctor just to make sure there isn't any injury to the neck bones or spinal cord. It's also useful to get this documented for future liability reasons.

- Neurologic symptoms, such as numbness, tingling, or weakness in the arms or legs.

- Extreme pain. If the pain isn't manageable with ice and ibuprofen, this may indicate a more serious injury.

NOSEBLEEDS

Spontaneous nosebleeds (also known as *epistaxis*) occur at some point in almost every child's life and are one of the more common problems we see. These nosebleeds often seem to appear out of nowhere, usually from one nostril, and can be very alarming to both parents and children. Luckily, in almost all cases, nosebleeds resolve with only minor treatments.

The Cause

Just inside the nose is a collection of tiny blood vessels known as capillaries. These capillaries are located on the middle wall of the nose, called the nasal septum. Because these blood vessels are close to the surface, they pop and bleed when irritated. The three main causes of recurrent nosebleeds in children are nose-picking, nasal allergies, and dry air.

What to Do

Nose-picking is a no-no. The most common cause of recurring nosebleeds in children is nose-picking. Kids may do this as a habit, or because of nasal irritation that is

DR. SEARS TIP
Be a Picking Detective

Since children are unlikely to incriminate their fingers as the culprits, here's a trick we use in our office. Instead of asking children if they pick their noses, we ask, "Which finger do you use to pick your nose?" Before thinking, they quickly hold up the index finger of one hand.

relieved by picking the nose. This can traumatize the blood vessels of the middle wall of the nose, causing them to burst and bleed.

Prevent allergies. Nasal allergies are one of the most common causes of nosebleeds in children. Itchy nasal passages trigger scratching and picking, which causes the already sensitive and inflamed lining of the nasal passages to become more irritated and bleed. Besides distracting those little hands as they habitually find their way to the itchy nose, cut your child's fingernails short and use the following home remedies to keep the nose comfortable so that it doesn't need picking. Start by allergy-proofing the bedroom:

- Install a HEPA or ionic air filter and put a filter on the heating vent in your child's bedroom.

- Remove all possible allergens and dust collectors, such as stuffed or pet animals and fuzzy toys.

- Use hypoallergenic bedding.

- Have a strict no-smoking rule around your child, especially in the bedroom.

- Remember the Dr. Sears classic home remedy for nasal congestion: a "nose hose" and a "steam clean." (See how to, page 20.)

Blame the cold. When a child is sick with a cold, the lining of the nasal passages can become swollen and inflamed. When the nasal passages are in this state, even minor events such as sneezing, coughing, or rubbing the nose can trigger a nosebleed.

Wet and soothe the nose. Dried-out nasal secretions itch and clog and prompt those little fingers to pick them. Run a warm-steam vaporizer: The increased humidity in the bedroom will soften the nasal secretions and make them less irritating and will allow you to turn down the drying effects of central heating. Soothe the nasal membranes by swabbing on lanolin with a Q-tip at bedtime.

The Best Way to Stop a Nosebleed

In most children, a nosebleed can be stopped simply by applying pressure with your thumb and forefinger on the nose at the site where the nasal bone becomes cartilage, approximately halfway down the sides. Gently squeeze the nostrils as well. You will usually need to do this for at least ten minutes in order to prevent the nosebleed from starting again. Have your child sit and lean his head slightly forward rather than tilt the head back. This will prevent blood from draining down the back of the nose and into the throat, which may cause the child to choke on or spit up blood.

If after a ten- to fifteen-minute period of applying proper pressure to the nose, the blood continues to flow freely, try rolling a ball of cotton or tissue the size of the nostril. Moisten it with cool water. Insert this into the side that is bleeding. Apply pressure as in step one. This allows more pressure to reach the site of the bleeding. Leave the cotton in for an hour then remove it *very slowly* so as

not to dislodge the clot and restart the bleeding.

If your child develops any other symptoms, such as looking pale, feeling light-headed, breathing rapidly, or having an abnormally rapid pulse, transport him to a medical facility immediately.

 DR. SEARS TIP
Careful Nose Blowing

Teach your child to blow her nose *gently,* not forcefully, which can trigger a bleed.

Preventing Recurrent Nosebleeds

Nosebleeds can come back soon after the first episode. This is because a clot has formed inside the nose at the site of the bleed. This clot can easily become knocked loose due to sneezing or rubbing or picking the nose.

We usually tell our patients that after getting a nosebleed they should spray a saline or saltwater solution gently inside the nose several times a day. This will rinse out the dry blood and clot. After doing this, apply an ointment, such as petroleum jelly or lanolin ointment, inside the nose. This can prevent a nosebleed from recurring.

Recurrent nosebleeds may be a sign of underlying nasal allergies. Certain nasal sprays and other medications may help control allergy symptoms, thereby controlling nosebleeds. By examining the nose, your pediatrician can usually tell whether or not your child's nosebleeds are caused by allergies.

Recurrent nosebleeds can also be caused by a bacterial infection inside the nose. The doctor will be able to see this on exam. An over-the-counter antibiotic ointment (the same kind you would put on a cut) can be gently pressed up into the nose with a finger twice a day for two weeks. Gently massage the ointment in by squeezing the nostrils together. If this doesn't help, a prescription one may do the job.

When to See an ENT Specialist

If your child continues to have nosebleeds despite the prevention measures above, it may mean the nasal blood vessels are very large and easily irritated. An ENT (ear, nose, throat) specialist can cauterize them to keep them from bleeding again. If this doesn't help, in rare cases recurrent nosebleeds may be a sign of the blood's inability to clot properly. A child with a clotting disorder will usually show other signs along with recurrent nosebleeds, such as:

- bruising easily
- multiple bruises all over the body, even in areas that aren't easily traumatized
- cuts or scrapes that take a long time to stop bleeding
- gums that bleed easily

If your pediatrician suspects a bleeding disorder, blood tests can detect this.

NOSE, BROKEN

The nose is often the first part of the body to get hit during a fall, an accident, or a sports injury. Nasal fractures are uncommon in infants and young children because at that stage the nasal bones are mostly cartilage, and when compressed they bounce back into position without breaking. But a fracture that deforms the structures of the growing nose can, if not properly treated, obstruct breathing later on. In fact, many nasal deformities that are detected in adulthood probably stem from unrecognized and untreated injuries during childhood.

When to Worry; What to Do

When the nose is struck, the cartilage tends to buckle rather than break. The nose flattens and bulges out to one or both sides and causes swelling. At this point parents or other caregivers should immediately:

- Comfort the child.
- Apply ice to both sides of the nose, especially the swollen area.
- Stop bleeding if it occurs (see The Best Way to stop a Nosebleed, page 414).
- If there is no persistent bleeding and the child can breathe through the injured nose, you probably do not need to seek immediate medical attention.

Over the next week, check the following:

- Is the nose straight or crooked when you look at the child straight on? (The bulging of the nasal structures out to one or both sides may still be present.)
- Can the child breathe normally through both sides of the nose?

If there is neither a cosmetic nor a breathing concern, you can still wait a few more days to see if the nose remains straight after the swelling has gone down. If there is any concern about cosmetic deformity or difficulty breathing, seek medical attention.

What Your Doctor Might Do

Your pediatrician will look for cosmetic crookedness or obstruction to breathing flow the same way you did. He will shine a light, called a nasal speculum, up into each side of your child's nostrils to be sure that airflow is adequate on both sides. If the doctor does not detect a cosmetic or airflow problem, the watch-and-wait period is likely to continue. The swollen or flattened nose usually returns to its normal shape within seven days. X-rays are not helpful at this stage because the nasal structures in children are mostly cartilage. If the doctor sees one of the following three things, he will refer you to a pediatric ENT specialist:

1. Cosmetic deformity

2. Obstruction of airflow from the nasal septum being pushed to one side

3. A blood clot (hematoma) on the nasal septum that might be obstructing airflow and may need to be drained

If your child is referred to an ENT doctor, the specialist may wait between a week and ten days to see if the nasal structures realign themselves after the swelling has gone down

DR. SEARS TIP
When in Doubt, Check It Out

It's usually best to have the doctor check injuries to the nose. Since a child's nose grows fastest from ages one to six years, untreated early injuries can lead to later deformities. Even though most of those injured little noses bounce back without any problem, it's wise to always follow the advice "When in doubt, check it out."

before deciding if the nose needs to be repaired. If the nasal structures have not realigned, the doctor may need to "set" the nose under local or general anesthesia.

NOSE, FOREIGN BODY IN

Children tend to stick more than the tips of their fingers in their little nostrils. They also like to poke toy parts (like beads) and foods (like raisins) up into their nose. Clues that your child's nasal discharge may be due to a trapped foreign body are:

- a really stinky odor coming from your child's nose

- a thick, green discharge from only *one* nostril, the plugged one

- no signs of a cold

What to Do

While you can carefully try the following home remedies, it's safer to let the doctor remove the foreign body. Your child's doctor can use a special forceps, suction, or a hook to remove particularly large stuck objects. If you get too aggressive in removing the object, the child can inhale it into her lungs. Even if you decide to have the doctor remove the foreign body, to make it easier try the following:

- A gentle "nose hose" and a "steam clean" (see how, page 20). Sometimes this remedy can loosen the thick secretions enough that the trapped culprit will easily be sneezed out.

- After you've done a "nose hose" and "steam clean," gently try to suck out the remaining discharge, and hopefully the stuck object, with a nasal aspirator (see how to, page 20). Don't use a thin rubber-tipped aspirator that has to be pushed up into the nose to work. This might push the object farther back. Instead, buy one with a wide plastic tip that forms a suction seal on the outside of the nostril.

- Try pressing the side of the clear nostril to close it. Then have your child forcefully sneeze or blow out through her nose. Oftentimes, the foreign body will be ejected.

After the object is removed — either by you or the doctor — be sure to counsel your child not to do this again. Draw a picture of the nose and show your child why nose-picking or putting stuff into the nose can hurt it. Also, it would be wise to continue a "nose hose" and a "steam clean" a couple times a day for several days after the foreign body is removed.

OBESITY: THE DR. SEARS L.E.A.N. KIDS PROGRAM

If your child is overweight (really we mean *overfat*) or obese, we will now help you put together a customized program. We call this the L.E.A.N. Kids Program, named for the four major changes that are necessary to stay lean: Lifestyle, Exercise, Attitude, and Nutrition.

One of the most important "health" words you can learn is *lean.* By *lean* we don't mean thin or skinny, which often isn't healthy. We mean having just the right amount of body fat for your body type. Leanness is associated with a lowered risk of just about every disease you don't want your child to get, such as diabetes, cardiovascular disease, and cancer. Overfatness is a head-to-toe health problem: diminished cognitive clarity, mood disorders, dental problems, vision problems, asthma, cardiovascular problems, high blood pressure, dermatitis, arthritis, and just about every other "-itis" you can think of.

One of the newest discoveries is the finding that extra fat, especially around the middle, which we dub "toxic waist," is a metabolically different type of fat. Excess fat accumulating around the middle becomes like a toxic chemical plant, churning out internal pollutants that literally clog the child's growing cardiovascular system and spewing out inflammatory chemicals that cause wear and tear on nearly every organ of the body, preventing optimal growth. Excess middle fat churns out chemicals that keep your child from metabolizing sugar properly, which not only interferes with optimal growth but causes a lot of "-itis" illnesses and increases the risk of diabetes.

Speaking of diabetes: Parents, we have a problem! The surgeon general ranks childhood obesity as the number one public health concern. We rate childhood obesity as the most serious medical problem we have seen in our nearly four decades of pediatric practice. The good news is that it is also the most preventable one. Here is the step-by-step program for weight management we use in our pediatric practice. It works for all ages, since for a child to stay lean the family needs to stay lean. How many of these steps you need to follow and how conscientiously you need to follow them depends upon how overfat your child is.

DR. SEARS TIP
The L.E.A.N.-Lite Program

Some children are only slightly overfat and need simply a few minor changes, such as eating fifty calories a day less and/or burning fifty calories a day more. This can be accomplished by getting rid of the equivalent of half a cookie a day and/or running ten minutes a day. It's that easy! Losing fifty calories a day translates into a half pound of fat loss a month, or six pounds a year. Adults can also stay lean with this simple L.E.A.N.-lite Program.

Measurements before L.E.A.N. Program	Measurements 3 to 6 months into L.E.A.N. Program
• Height: • Weight: • BMI*: • Waist: • Fasting blood sugar: • Lipid profile: • Insulin level: • Other lab:	• Height: • Weight: • BMI: • Waist: • Fasting blood sugar: • Lipid profile: • Insulin level: • Other lab:
* See page 89 to learn how to calculate body mass index.	

Here's our step-by-step program on how to keep your child lean:

1. Get a Medical Checkup

Schedule a checkup with your child's doctor. Ask for a "long appointment for weight control." Take along a notepad so that you can keep your own personal diary and record the measurements your pediatrician takes. During the medical checkup the doctor will take the measurements listed on the chart above and may order some of the suggested laboratory tests. Keep track of the information before your child starts the L.E.A.N. Program and three to six months into it.

2. Make Goals

We do not call our program a "weight-control program," a "lose-fat program," or any name related to obesity. Children are not only body-image conscious but also performance-oriented. The first question we ask a child is

something like "What would you like to do better, such as run faster, make the soccer team, or play volleyball better?" We then personalize the program: "Suzy's Soccer Program." Have your child list her goals, such as: "My goals are to run faster" and "to have more energy." Ask your child to list her goals in a diary.

DR. SEARS TIP
The No-Gain Goal

Two simple goals that nearly all children can reach are:

• no change in weight for one year

• no change in waist size for one year

We have found that these are the easiest and most achievable goals to set. The child increases in height but not in weight or waist circumference and thereby grows into his ideal weight. We call this process *leaning out*, which is what many children normally do between the frumpy stage of middle childhood and the lean teen time.

3. Make a Signed Commitment

Have your child complete a commitment pledge such as the one below:

I make a commitment to follow the L.E.A.N. Kids Program for at least twelve weeks:

Signed: _____ Date: _____

What physical activities do you most enjoy?

_____

How much physical activity do you average a day?

_____

I will commit to these activities five days a week:

_____

_____

_____

4. Keep a L.E.A.N. Diary

Have your child keep an "instead of" diary and enter at least one "instead of" healthier choice that he made that day, following these examples:

L. (Lifestyle): Instead of eating at our usual fast-food restaurant, we ate at one that had a big salad bar with lots of "grow foods."
E. (Exercise): Instead of playing video games, I played outside for twenty minutes.
A. (Attitude): Instead of worrying about . . . I filled my mind with happy thoughts.
N. (Nutrition): Instead of drinking soda, I drank water.

 DR. SEARS TIP
Eat Real Foods

These three words sum up weight management in a nutshell. We believe that, besides sitting too much, the main cause of the childhood obesity epidemic is that today's children have lost their taste for real, wholesome foods. If parents made this one change in the family's eating habits, the whole family would be leaner: Eat only real foods and no, or very little, packaged foods. This simply means foods that are grown or raised naturally and minimally processed.

The "real foods" diet is the most realistic and easy-to-follow diet you can have for your whole family. Start the real foods diet as young as possible in order to shape young tastes (the three other magic words of weight control) toward appreciating real, wholesome foods. Most of today's children have their tastes shaped toward the artificial fats, sweeteners, colors, and flavors of packaged foods, and as a result many will shun real foods.

In our practice we see that moms who feed their children only homemade foods from infancy throughout toddlerhood have children who grow up to shun junk food and are healthier, happier, and leaner. Children who grew up with the tastes of packaged foods and who shun real foods are sicker, sadder, and fatter.

5. Follow the Traffic-Light Eating Guide

How strict you have to be depends upon how overfat your child is. If your child is truly obese (20 percent over his optimal body

TRAFFIC-LIGHT EATING		
Green-light foods	**Yellow-light foods**	**Red-light foods**
Good for you, enjoy! Eat these grow foods *any time*.	Slow down, not too much! It's okay to eat these *sometimes* as an occasional treat.	Stop and think about a healthier choice! Do *not* eat these foods. They are not grow foods. They're hurt foods.
• All fruits • All veggies • Cheese, low-fat • Eggs • Flaxseed oil or meal • Meat, lean • Milk, low-fat, organic • Nuts and seeds • Olive oil • Salmon, wild • Soy foods, e.g., tofu • Whole grains • Yogurt, organic	• Butter • Cookies, homemade • Frozen yogurt • Fruit juice, 100% • Honey • Meats, less lean • Pasta • Pastries, homemade • White bread	• Beverages with sugar or corn syrup, such as sodas • Cottonseed oil • Dyes, preservatives • Foods with artificial sweeteners • Foods with hydrogenated oils • Gelatin desserts • Marshmallows • Meats, nitrite-containing • Monosodium glutamate (MSG) • Prepackaged or store-bought bakery goods

weight) and has rolls of abdominal fat you can grab, this child should virtually never eat red-light foods and only an occasional treat of yellow-light foods until he reaches his goal weight.

6. Avoid the Three "Bad Words" on Food Labels

During the routine preschool checkup between four and five years of age, we teach parents to tell their children to look for these three "bad words" on the food labels:

- high-fructose corn syrup

- hydrogenated (fortunately, these disastrous oils are finally being phased out)

- any word followed by a number, such as red #40, blue #5

This exercise is a very simple way for children to tell junk food from real food.

7. Feed Your Family Fill-Up Foods

Include foods that are high in protein and fiber, which take up lots of room in the stomach and help children to feel fuller faster so they're less likely to overeat. Snacks should never be carb-only but should always be partnered with one or two of the "friends": fiber and protein. Here's how we explain the concept of "good carbs" and "bad carbs" to our young patients: "A good carb has two friends: fiber and protein. It never plays alone. The two friends slow down the carbs entering the bloodstream. A bad carb, on the other hand, has no friends. It plays alone. Unlike a good carb that has two friends to slow down the sugar rush, it speeds into the bloodstream and the results of this sugar rush can make you tired, jittery, and even fat."

Tasty fill-up foods include vegetables, fruits, yogurt, and nut butters. You can present these foods in a more positive way by calling them "grow foods," which children equate with running fast and growing strong. The concept of eating more "grow foods" helps children believe that healthy eating is cool. It just so happens that real food, "grow foods," or green-light foods (whatever you want to call them) are more filling, so that children seldom overeat them.

 DR. SEARS TIP
Salads First

Beginning a meal with a salad (choose dark greens rather than "see-through" lettuce, or iceberg lettuce) can often satisfy the compulsive overeaters with healthier calories, so they tend to eat fewer less healthy foods during the rest of the meal.

8. Downsize Your Child's Servings

Portion distortion is a real problem for children, since little eyes are larger than little stomachs. Remember, your child's stomach is the size of her fist. Give children smaller plates to make smaller portions look larger. Let children serve themselves. Studies show that children who serve themselves tend to take less food than parents give them.

9. Follow the Dr. Sears Rule of Twos

Teach your child to:

- Eat *twice* as often.

- Eat *half* as much.

- Chew *twice* as long.

The body and the brain have a system that tells the child to stop eating. When the tummy is full, it sends out a signal to the brain saying, "Stop, you've eaten enough!" But the brain may not receive this "full" signal for ten to twenty minutes. Wait ten minutes before serving your child seconds. Your child may then feel full and not want more. Encourage your child to take small bites and talk between bites. Play *chew-chew*. Tell your children to chew each bite at least ten times. Raise a grazer. Studies have shown that people who eat the same foods and the same amounts of calories, but eat them in smaller mini-meals throughout the day, tend to be leaner than the typical three-square-meal gorgers. As you learned on page 38, keeping your child in hormonal harmony stabilizes insulin levels, which discourages the buildup of excess fat. Grazing helps keep this balance.

10. Discourage Mindless Munching

Don't allow your child to eat while watching television. When her mind is off her tummy, she'll tend to overeat. If she does want to snack while watching TV, make it a veggie snack. Take this opportunity to reintroduce veggie snacks that she previously refused.

HEALTHY MUNCHING AT ITS BEST

Here are some healthy snack ideas that will provide protein and healthy fats:

- A handful of raw nuts
- Trail mix
- Peanut butter on apple slices
- Hard-boiled egg
- Yogurt, plain, with nuts and fresh fruit or granola
- Homemade oatmeal/raisin cookies and a glass of low-fat milk
- Edamame (fresh Japanese soy beans)
- Baby carrots dipped in hummus
- String cheese and a piece of fruit
- Cottage cheese and fruit
- Pita bread spread with hummus
- Rice cake with peanut butter and banana
- Parmesan cheese melted on a slice of whole-grain bread
- Blueberries in yogurt
- Popcorn (air popped)
- Celery sticks with peanut butter
- Cherry tomatoes with cheese cubes
- Fruit and yogurt smoothie
- Bean dip and veggie sticks
- Any fruit
- Whole-grain, preferably homemade, muffins
- Cut-up vegetables with salsa and tortilla chips

11. Be Supermarket Smart

The supermarket can be a giant nutritional classroom. As you enter the supermarket, tell your child, "We only shop the perimeter."

"Why, Mommy?" your child might ask.

"Because that's where the 'grow foods' are. Go pick out one yellow veggie, two greens, and three reds…"

Next, go to the bread aisle (our favorite nutrition lesson). Have your child pick up a loaf of white bread in one hand and a loaf of 100 percent whole-grain bread in the other. Ask your child to tell you the difference. You're likely to get an answer such as: "The white bread is lighter and squishy…The whole-grain bread is heavier and feels stronger." Expand on your child's observations by saying, "That's because the white bread is like air bread. It doesn't have any 'grow foods' in it. Whole-grain bread is heavier and not as squishy because it has lots of 'grow foods' in it. Do you want your muscles to feel weak and squishy like the white bread or strong and firm like the whole-wheat bread?" You could even go by the yogurt aisle (goodness, what the food industry has done to healthy food like yogurt!). Play "I spy with my little eyes" on the yogurt label. Let your child pick out an organic yogurt that doesn't have bad words such as "high-fructose corn syrup" and numbered colorings and a list of fillers.

12. Get Kids Moving

No matter one's age, dieting without movement won't work. A habitual sitter stores more calories than she burns, and that's what leads to obesity. We teach parents: "Have a house rule. Moving equals sitting. Each day require your children to spend at least the same amount of time in physical play as they do in front of a screen." Put on a pedometer. This little motivational tool is a matchbox-size meter that clips on the child's belt and records how many steps the child took that day. Make a motivational chart and paste it on the refrigerator showing how many steps the child took that day. Have him try to beat the previous day. For example, day 1 might be 5,000 steps, but by the end of the week the child is up to 10,000 steps. Children like to see their progress prominently displayed.

Encourage your child to work out while watching TV. She can, for example, jump on a mini-trampoline, use stretch bands, or ride a stationary bike while watching TV, or play video games with her feet.

GROWING A LEANER BABY

Here are the two most important steps you can take to begin implanting healthy eating habits into your infant at birth:

Breastfeed. Breastfeed as frequently and as long as you are able. The American Academy of Pediatrics (AAP) recommends that mothers breastfeed *at least* one year; the World Health Organization (WHO) recommends *at least* two years. Yes, we did say *years!* Recent studies show that breastfed infants tend to grow leaner. Several reasons why breastfeeding is good preventive medicine for weight control are:

• The breastfeeding infant is more in control of her feedings—how much and how often she eats. A breastfeeding mother is more likely to watch her baby for feeding cues, since you can't count ounces or encourage Baby to "finish the bottle." On the other hand, the mother of the bottlefeeding baby may be tempted to prod Baby to "finish the bottle."

• The breastfed baby can vary the volume and content of the milk by how he sucks. When hungry, Baby sucks voraciously and gets high-calorie milk. When thirsty or needing only comfort sucking, Baby may get milk with a lower fat and calorie content. Again, Baby controls the calorie content.

• Breast milk naturally changes in fat content as Baby grows—going from "full fat" milk in the early months to "lower fat" milk toward the end of the first year.

• Breastfed babies are natural grazers. They feed more frequently than their bottlefeeding friends, but breast milk is digested about twice as fast as formula. They get used to a different "tummy feel," perhaps being satisfied with a less full tummy, and that becomes the norm for them.

Feed Baby real foods. Make your own baby food as often and for as long as possible. As we said above, this shapes your baby's tastes toward what real food is supposed to taste like. Remember the three magic words of infant feeding: *shape young tastes!*

LEARN MORE ABOUT IT

For a complete in-depth program of weight control for the whole family, try these three resources:

- *Dr. Sears' L.E.A.N. Kids: A Total Health Program for Children Ages 6 to 12.* This 270-page easy-to-read book covers the program in detail.

- Become a Dr. Sears–certified L.E.A.N. coach. You can enroll in a three-day workshop or take the course online.

- The Dr. Sears L.E.A.N. Start Program. This is a healthy-eating and healthy-living program that we put together for the State of California. We use it successfully in our practice and in many of the Boys & Girls Clubs. The program consists of booklets and a DVD, and is especially valuable for pre-school children. These resources can be ordered at AskDrSears.com or at DrSearsLean.com.

OVERUSE INJURIES (aka Repetitive Stress Injuries, RSI)

Pain, tenderness, and swelling of joints are most common during periods of rapid growth, such as during the adolescent growth spurt of ages twelve to fifteen years. The shoulder, elbow, wrist, knee, ankle, and hip joints are most often afflicted. These injuries are caused by both *over*use and *mis*use. Repeated use of a joint without warm-up, rest, or training can lead to inflammation in the bone, muscles, or tendons supplying it. For example, one of the early names for an overuse injury was "nintendonitis," an injury to the wrists and thumbs from playing video games.

Misuse occurs when muscles are used in a way in which they were not intended, and this usually stems from a child not receiving adequate warm-up or training. An example is tennis elbow, or *tendinitis* of the lateral aspect of the elbow joint. If the tennis player is not properly instructed on stretching, warm-up, and training of the muscles and tendons of the elbow joint, tennis elbow is likely to follow. If growing joints could talk, they would say, "Don't overuse or misuse me. Stretch me, warm me, and exercise me gradually, so I'll get stronger and you can use me more. I'll perform better — and I won't hurt."

Overtraining can also cause overuse injuries. Dancers may train one set of muscles more than another, resulting in an imbalance. This causes undue stress on the joint, leading to inflammation. Treatment of these injuries generally involves resting for two to three weeks, icing the affected area for twenty minutes several times each day, taking ibuprofen as needed, and careful resumption of activity as tolerated.

Carpal Tunnel Syndrome (CTS)

Also known as *repetitive stress* or *motion injury*, carpal tunnel syndrome (CTS) is being diagnosed more and more among older children and adolescents. Resulting from repeatedly performing actions that place stress upon the tissues of the wrist, it is known as carpal tunnel syndrome because the specific nerve that is irritated passes through a protective sheath called the carpal tunnel. This nerve is bundled very tightly among the tissues of the wrist, and repeatedly putting stress on the area leads to chronic inflammation and nerve pain.

Common activities that can lead to CTS include typing for long periods of time without taking adequate breaks, overuse of video-game controllers, and certain sports that put a lot of stress on this region, such as weight lifting or cheerleading (stunts and lifts can put a strain on wrists).

The pain of CTS usually develops slowly over time. Severity can increase over weeks, months, or years before treatment is sought. A clue that your child might have CTS is that he complains of a shooting pain traveling from the palm side of the forearm down the wrist into the palm region. Your pediatrician can perform a specific examination technique in order to rule out the possibility of carpal tunnel syndrome.

What to do. To prevent and heal CTS in your child, help her to:

- Avoid or modify the specific activity that caused the injury.

- Take adequate breaks while carrying out the activity in order to give the structures a chance to rest.

- Wear a special wrist brace to aid recovery.

- Take anti-inflammatory medications to provide short-term relief; however, these should only be used as directed and not for long periods of time.

- Get physical therapy if she has a severe case.

- Try alternative treatments, such as acupuncture or massage, which have been shown to be effective among adults. Always discuss alternative treatments with your pediatrician before trying them.

Tennis Elbow

This injury occurs when the tendons on the outer edge of the elbow become inflamed from repetitive use. Although often attributed to improper technique in swinging a tennis racket, it can occur from a variety of wrist motions while using screwdrivers, certain gardening tools, or paintbrushes. The muscles that control wrist and hand movements connect to the elbow, and undue strain on these tendons can result in tennis elbow.

Symptoms. Signs that your child may have tennis elbow include:

- tenderness on the outer aspect of the elbow

- soreness in the muscle within the forearm

- pain that worsens when squeezing or grasping objects with the hand

- aching or stiffness of the elbow joint in the morning

What to do. Your child will likely need to take a break from tennis or the offending activity to allow for a period of healing. To speed up the healing, you can:

- Ice the elbow for twenty minutes three times daily, especially after any necessary activities that cause soreness.

- Take ibuprofen (see dosing on page 553) to reduce inflammation with your doctor's direction.

- Use an arm sling. This can help take the pressure off the arm and limit use of the elbow.

- Make an appointment with a physical therapist or a sports medicine physician to learn proper strengthening exercises and techniques to avoid recurrence of the injury.

A few days of rest and treatment should improve the pain. Resuming the offending activity, however, can cause a recurrence, so your child may need to take several weeks off. See your pediatrician if pain persists despite several days of rest and treatment, or if pain recurs when activity resumes.

Tenosynovitis

Similar to carpal tunnel syndrome, this is a repetitive stress injury that affects a wider area of the lower arm and wrist. Excessive and repetitive strain on the tendons can result in inflammation and pain of this area. The most common type of tenosynovitis is known as *De Quervain's tenosynovitis*. This type of injury is usually not seen until later adolescence or in young adults. Pain is usually present over a rather large area, from the lower arm extending into the thumb region.

Treatment of tenosynovitis always involves avoidance or modification of the activity that caused the injury. Special braces can sometimes help speed healing, along with the occasional use of anti-inflammatory medications like ibuprofen. These should always be taken as directed and should not be taken for long periods of time. Even with the best of treatments, this wrist injury can take weeks or even months to heal.

PACIFIER USE

This popular, peace-inducing plug has been used for decades to ease babies through fussy spells. When to use it and when to discard it are common concerns among parents. Here are the ins and outs of pacifier use.

Do not use one if your infant is breast-feeding. Keep the pacifier out of the breastfeeding baby's mouth for at least the first six weeks. While still learning how to breastfeed, Baby should have only the breast in her mouth. That way, the only nipple a newborn has to learn to use is Mother's. Pacifiers are artificial nipples that may cause nipple preference or confusion. To suck on a pacifier, Baby does not have to open her lips wide. But in order to suck properly from Mother's nipple, she needs to learn to open her mouth wide enough to take in more of the areola around the nipple. If Baby was to suck at Mother's breast the same way she does a pacifier, an uncomfortable nursing nuisance called "tight mouthing" results. Mother will get sore nipples, and Baby may not get enough milk.

Pacifiers also lessen the amount of time Baby spends at the breast, and this can lead to a drop in milk production. We advise breastfeeding mothers to avoid pacifiers until their newborns learn to latch on properly and the milk supply is well established. Studies show that babies who use pacifiers give up breastfeeding sooner than those who don't.

Another reason not to use pacifiers is that frequent nursing helps delay the return of menstruation, a help in spacing pregnancies.

Use your finger instead. When your nursing newborn seems to need constant sucking and your own nipples need a rest, switch to finger sucking. Insert your index finger one and a half inches into Baby's mouth (which is about halfway between the first and second knuckle) with the nail side down. This more closely simulates what the breast feels like in Baby's mouth.

Use a pacifier for the bottle-fed, intense sucker. Babies are born with an intense need to suck and bottle feeding often doesn't provide enough suck time. Besides being soothing for an infant, sucking stimulates production of saliva, which is good for oral hygiene and nature's health juice for the developing intestines. Babies will have an occasional day when they need more oral gratification. We dub them "all-day suckers."

Hold Baby while she is sucking. A rubber pacifier should never replace a real, live person, except for brief intervals when you need to put the baby down. Hours of "zoning out" alone on a "paci" isn't good for a baby's development.

When to Pull the Plug

For most infants, pacifier use is a harmless comforting habit. But the following are situations where you should consider pulling the plug:

When Mother is becoming dependent. How do you know when you're overdoing the pacifier? Clue: When your baby cries and you find yourself, by reflex, reaching for the pacifier instead of reaching for your baby, it's time to pull the plug.

When Baby is becoming too dependent. If you find Baby is reaching for the pacifier instead of reaching for a parent, pull the plug.

When dental problems are occurring. Sucking on a pacifier exerts a lot of pressure and if continued into toddlerhood can lead to overbite and other dental malalignments.

When Baby has frequent ear infections. A study published in *Pediatrics* found that infants who used pacifiers suffered more ear infections. When parents were advised to limit pacifier use, the incidence of ear infections went down. While this is strictly a statistical correlation, it is possible that continuous sucking on a pacifier disturbs the normal functioning of the eustachian tubes, allowing fluid to build up in the middle ear.

How to Pull the Plug

Yes, there comes a time when it's necessary to pull the plug. If your baby has any of the above "whens," here are some hows:

Substitute and distract. Besides your being her human pacifier for a while, give Baby other attachment objects, such as a cuddly doll or teddy bear. When Baby is upset or anxious, occupy her with a fun play activity.

Trade it. Here is the most effective binky-breaking trick that we've used in our practice. Take your child to the toy store and let her pick out a comfort toy to "trade" for the pacifier. Not a bad deal: The pacifier stays in the waste basket in the store and the child leaves with a doll or bear. Experienced toy store clerks are used to this trading game.

Lose it. Make the pacifier less convenient to find. When your toddler starts foraging around the house looking for his rubber friend, distract him with fun activities to get his mind off the plug. Then announce the pacifier is "lost," introduce some novel cuddly toys, and spend more time cuddling with your child.

Trim it. Gradually cut off more of the tip of the pacifier until the child becomes less interested in it.

Invite the "binky fairy." One night the "binky fairy" visits and takes away the pacifier and leaves a more attractive gift.

Enlist peer pressure. Put your child in a group with non-pacifier-using playmates. For the child who is really plugged in, throw a paci-party and have everyone clap as the child throws the pacifier in the trash can.

Wean slowly. If your toddler is truly hooked on the pacifier, gradually shorten the frequency and length of time that she is plugged in. Let her use the pacifier for short periods of time when you feel she really needs it, as you gradually introduce more comforting alternatives.

Remember, weaning from the pacifier, just like weaning from the breast, does not mean stopping cold turkey, but rather moving from one comfort object to another. No matter what techniques you use to pull the plug, you have to simultaneously surround your child with more attachment objects and attachment people.

In a nutshell, regarding the pacifier, use it, don't abuse it, and when the time is right, lose it.

PENIS PROBLEMS

Although the penis usually takes care of itself without any complications, occasional problems may arise over the years. On page 48 we discussed circumcision and how to care for the circumcised penis during the newborn period. The uncircumcised penis usually doesn't require any special care, but some children may experience various problems that we will cover in detail for you. Next, we will describe a few issues you may come across.

Care of the Intact Male Foreskin

For uncircumcised boys, care of the foreskin is very simple and straightforward: do nothing. Doctors used to believe the foreskin should be forcibly retracted during early childhood, but we now know that doing so may lead to the development of scar tissue, risk of infection, and risk of even tighter foreskin down the road. The foreskin will naturally retract on its own when it is ready. Most specialists do not recommend even gentle retraction at all. In the past, it was thought that after age three gradual retraction was advised; however, almost all specialists now refute this, stating that the foreskin will eventually retract on its own. Some foreskins will naturally retract on their own by age three or four; others might take until the early teenage years to do so. Until it begins to retract, only clean the outside with soap and water as part of the regular bath routine.

When your young child's foreskin does begin to naturally retract, usually between two and three years of age, gentle retraction is okay, but never do so more than the foreskin wants to go. Once your little boy's foreskin is retracting, it is time to start teaching him basic care of his penis. This is very simple and involves gentle retraction and cleaning with soap and water as part of the bath. That's it!

We sometimes see worried parents in our office who have noticed a whitish substance underneath their son's foreskin. This is a substance known as *smegma*. It is a completely normal and naturally occurring substance composed of dead skin cells mixed with bodily fluids and can be simply managed by daily gentle retraction and cleansing techniques.

Tight Foreskin (Phimosis)

While the uncircumcised foreskin normally retracts naturally with no help from anyone (age range varies; can be as early as age two and as late as age thirteen; see above), occasionally the foreskin either looks too tight or becomes too tight. Most tight openings are often adequate for urination and need no treatment. But sometimes phimosis can interfere with normal penis function.

When to worry; what to do. Even if the foreskin appears to be tight, your pediatrician will probably recommend a wait-and-see approach, since by four to five years most foreskins will begin to retract more. If the doctor sees that the foreskin is not retracting on its own and may eventually get tight enough to obstruct urine flow, he may advise the following:

- Slowly and gently retract the foreskin as part of your child's daily bath routine. The penis will also do this naturally ten times a day or more with normal erections that stretch the foreskin.

- As long as your child urinates without pain, no need to worry. Watch for signs of obstruction to urine flow.

If you notice the "balloon sign"— the tip of the foreskin balloons out during urination (like a little water balloon filling up with water) — this may mean that the foreskin is too tight. A pediatric urologist should then evaluate your child to determine if surgical correction is needed at this time.

Paraphimosis. This occurs when an apparently tight foreskin is forcefully retracted too far to the extent that it won't slip back into its usual position. The retracted band of foreskin constricts the veins from the penis, causing the whole shaft of the penis to swell so that the stuck foreskin is literally strangling the penis. This is a medical emergency that requires treatment, usually by applying a topical or locally injected anesthetic and manually pulling the constricting foreskin back into place. In rare cases, a partial circumcision needs to be done, followed by a complete circumcision when the foreskin returns to normal.

Infected Foreskin

Called *balanitis,* this is an infection beneath the uncircumcised foreskin that, if severe, can cause enough swelling to obstruct the flow of urine or lead to a urinary tract infection.

How to tell. Signs of balanitis are a very swollen, red, and tender foreskin and a green or yellow discharge. The swelling may be enough to cause a balloon sign during urination, as in phimosis, or your child may refuse to pee altogether.

What to do. If you notice a problem in the early stages of mild redness and swelling, without discharge or difficulty urinating, then warm soaks and antibiotic ointment (described below) may calm down the infection and avoid a trip to the doctor. If your child has all the symptoms of severe balanitis, seek medical care right away. The doctor might culture the affected area or the discharge, if present, to identify the offending bacteria. While awaiting the results of the culture, the doctor is likely to prescribe an appropriate oral antibiotic. In addition to antibiotic treatment, your pediatrician may advise you to:

- Apply an antibacterial ointment, either prescription or over the counter.

- Soak the penis in a warm-water bath to clean out the secretions while *gently* retracting the foreskin.

After the infection has cleared, review with your pediatrician proper care of the foreskin as outlined on page 428. After the normal bath routine of washing the secretions off the glans, be sure to pat the glans dry before letting the foreskin come back. Leaving the glans of the penis too wet can cause inflammation and infection and then balanitis.

If you teach your child appropriate foreskin care, balanitis is very preventable.

Foreskin Adhesions in a Circumcised Penis

After a circumcised foreskin heals, the remaining foreskin should be able to be pulled back to reveal the entire rim around the head of the penis. However, during the healing process, sometimes the raw foreskin reattaches to the head of the penis, partially or completely obscuring the rim of the head. An astute pediatrician will often check this at the first few checkups and can easily retract any potential adhesions before they become firmly stuck. However, often these adhesions go unnoticed for many months until the foreskin is too stuck to easily pull back, and then Dad thinks Baby's penis looks funny because one can no longer see the entire head.

There are two types of foreskin adhesions, with very different treatments:

Simple adhesions. This type occurs when the inner layer of foreskin (shiny red layer, as opposed to the outer normal skin layer) sticks to the head of the penis. This can usually be unstuck by stretching the foreskin down (like an erection); the stuck area will peel away from the head, leaving a raw area that easily heals with Vaseline within a few days. This may be a bit painful, but is fairly simple for the doctor to do. An anesthetic cream applied to the area for thirty minutes beforehand may minimize the pain. For adhesions that cannot be easily unstuck, a prescription hydrocortisone cream can be used with your doctor's guidance.

Skin bridges. This is a more severe type of adhesion in which the outer layer of skin on the shaft of the penis grows onto the head of the penis, forming a "bridge" of skin that stretches into a very noticeable rubber-band-like strand of skin. This type of adhesion cannot be simply pulled back by the pediatrician. A prescription hydrocortisone cream can be used to soften the skin bridge. The penis will then have to be numbed up with an injection or a numbing cream, and the skin bridge will have to be clamped and cut with sterile instruments. An experienced pediatrician who feels comfortable with this technique can do this during the child's infancy. If skin bridges aren't noticed until a child is past age one, it's best to just leave them there and let a pediatric urologist do the procedure when the child is old enough to understand the need to do it.

White Lumps Around a Circumcised Foreskin

Some circumcised boys, especially in early infancy, develop white, pearl-like lumps that collect along the circumcision rim where the foreskin joins the glans of the penis. These result from accumulations of the normal lubricant that collects beneath the foreskin called *smegma.* When the *smegma* becomes trapped in the foreskin, it can form into little white lumps.

What to do. These usually cause no problem and drain on their own as the rim of the foreskin retracts more completely, especially during growth and erections. Sometimes these collections will persist, and your pediatrician may show you how to gently retract the foreskin and rub them off the rim of the penis using a mild soap and warm water. As they are rubbed off, they may leave tiny areas of irritation along the rim, which could get infected. In this case, your doctor may recommend applying a lubricant and/or antibacterial ointment around the inflamed area. As your child grows, these little nuisance secretions will become a part of his past.

Disappearing Penis!

Believe it or not, many years ago our office received a call from a worried mother saying, "His penis disappeared!" No, it didn't really disappear. It was just temporarily covered up by a bunch of fat. In the first year, some babies accumulate a lot of fat around the base of the penis, which sometimes causes a circumcised penis to become buried, only to pop out periodically during an erection and urination. This is a harmless developmental quirk and not a medical problem. As your little boy leans out and those adorable little mounds of baby fat melt away, his penis will reappear. The length and size of the penis during the first year has absolutely no bearing on its later adult size.

PINWORMS

Pinworms resemble tiny pieces of white thread about a third of an inch long. They live and mate in a child's intestines. The pregnant female worm travels down the intestines and out of the anus to lay her eggs, usually at night. All this activity causes the rectum to itch. As the child scratches the egg-infested area around her bottom, she picks up the eggs, which are then transmitted to the child's mouth, to other children, and to other members of the household. The swallowed eggs hatch in the intestines and repeat the cycle. In girls, pinworms may also cause itching in the vagina. The female worms usually die after depositing eggs, so the worms themselves are not transmitted from person to person, only the eggs. Although the worms can only live in people, the eggs can live for a couple weeks on surfaces, such as bed linens, towels, and toys, and can be transmitted from contact with these surfaces.

Signs and Symptoms

- The child scratches her bottom, especially at night.

- She scratches the vagina.

- She has scratch marks around the anus or vagina.

- She squirms while sitting as a way of scratching the bottom.

At night, hold your child's buttocks apart and shine a light on the rectum. You may see tiny, white threadlike worms around the anal or vaginal opening. Occasionally, you can see the worms in the child's bowel movements or on the diaper or underwear when your child awakens in the morning.

What to Do

Don't panic if you see a pinworm. They are irritating but harmless, and there's no need to share your discovery with your pediatrician in the middle of the night.

- If you suspect pinworms but can't see them, try capturing some eggs by placing the sticky side of a piece of tape faceup on a Popsicle stick and blot the tape around the anus and/or the opening of the vagina. This is best done when your child awakens and before she takes a bath or has a bowel movement. Take the tape to your doctor's office or to a laboratory recommended by your doctor. The tape will be examined for pinworm eggs under a microscope.

- If pinworms are diagnosed or highly suspected, your doctor will recommend an over-the-counter or prescription oral deworming medication to be taken by all family members. Be sure you give your child a second dose of medicine ten to fourteen days later to kill the worms that have hatched in the meantime. It's important to treat all family members, otherwise you'll just keep sharing the worms.

- Cut your child's fingernails short and discourage nail biting.

- Remind her to wash her hands and clean her fingernails after using the toilet.

- Discourage your child from scratching her bottom.

- Wash your child's bedding, pajamas, and clothing to kill any eggs that may be lying around. Make sure your child wears clean clothes and underwear every day for several days around treatment to lessen the chance of ingesting any eggs.

(See Rectal Itching, page 447, for more treatment measures.)

PITYRIASIS ALBA

Pityriasis alba is a common skin condition that usually affects children between the ages of six and twelve. Younger or older children may get this condition as well. Children with pityriasis alba have patches of lighter skin, usually on the face, but sometimes on the neck, chest, and arms.

While doctors do not know the actual cause of this condition, it is considered a type of eczema (see section on Eczema, page 297) and is often more noticeable during the sunny summertime months because the non-affected areas of the skin may become darker while the light, patchy areas remain the same color. The light patches may be difficult to see unless you are up close, particularly on fair-skinned children. They are not itchy or painful.

Diagnosis

Your pediatrician can usually diagnose this condition from the classic appearance of the whitish skin patches. There is, however, a similar skin condition that is caused by a fungus known as *tinea versicolor* (see page 336). The doctor can distinguish between the two by collecting a small skin scraping of the light patch, placing it on a slide with a special liquid, and examining it under the microscope. If tinea versicolor is the cause, the fungus may be visible.

What to Do

Treatment is almost never necessary, as this condition improves gradually on its own. It can take several months for the patches to disappear completely. Using a daily moisturizer on the areas may help them go away faster. Hydrocortisone or similar steroid creams can be used; however, this is not usually recommended unless your child's case is severe. You should not use these creams for a period of longer than two weeks unless directed to do so by your pediatrician.

 DR. SEARS TIP
Most Mild Rashes
Are Harmless

If a rash doesn't *itch, ooze,* or *spread,* don't worry, be happy!

PITYRIASIS ROSEA

Pityriasis rosea is a type of skin rash that is fairly common and often seen in older children or young adults. Although the specific cause is unknown, it is thought to be related to exposure to a virus.

Symptoms

Here are the signs to watch for:

- It appears to be more common during the fall and spring months.

- It often begins with a single reddish or brown patch occurring on the abdomen, chest, or back.

- This initial outbreak is followed a few days later by more patches that are usually smaller.

- Patches may be round- or oval-shaped.

- Patches often have a scaly appearance.

- Patches are usually itchy, red, or inflamed. The itching may be very mild or quite severe.

The unique feature of pityriasis rosea is that it begins with a single patch, referred to as a *herald patch*, followed by multiple smaller patchy areas nearby.

Diagnosis

The diagnosis is usually done based on the appearance of the rash alone. If there is any question, or if the rash gets much worse, a skin biopsy might be performed.

What to Do

Mild symptoms usually require no treatment. To soothe the irritation and itching, oatmeal baths, moisturizing lotions, or over-the-counter hydrocortisone cream might be helpful. In children older than two, antihistamines taken by mouth (use only as directed) may help the itching. Sunlight has been shown to help speed healing, but be careful to avoid sunburn.

The rash usually takes at least three weeks to disappear, but it could take up to four months to go away completely.

Is Pityriasis Rosea Contagious?

It is not thought to be contagious; however, doctors do not know for sure. It does not appear to be highly contagious however. Children usually get pityriasis rosea only once.

PNEUMONIA

A common worry for parents when their child has a prolonged or severe cough is whether it might be pneumonia. Here is our guide to recognizing pneumonia and deciding what needs to be done.

Symptoms

Pneumonia usually occurs as a result of bacteria overgrowing within the chest mucus produced during a common cold and cough virus. The infected parts of the lungs can't absorb oxygen, and the child will begin to feel oxygen deprived. Here are the symptoms to watch for:

- Rapid breathing. While it is normal for children to breathe a little faster during a fever, if rapid breathing persists (more than forty breaths per minute) for several hours after the fever is down, this may be a sign of a lung infection.

- Labored breathing. A child with pneumonia will usually have to work harder to breathe in order to take in enough oxygen. You may notice your child raising her shoulders with each breath.

- Grunting. We don't mean making sounds like a little piggy. In medical terms, *grunting* means a humming or groaning sound as a person exhales each breath. This actually allows some air to stay in the lungs longer so more oxygen is absorbed. A child usu-

ally won't consciously do this; it's more of a reflexive coping mechanism for the lungs.

- Nasal flaring. When a child isn't getting enough oxygen, another automatic coping mechanism is that the nostrils will flare open with each inhalation in order to bring in more air.

- High fever and lethargy with a mild cough. Some children with pneumonia may not have much coughing at all. This may make the diagnosis more difficult. If your child is acting unusually subdued and looks much sicker than you'd expect for such a mild cough, have her checked out by the doctor.

- Vomiting. Although this is usually a sign of a gastrointestinal illness, vomiting in the presence of other symptoms of pneumonia should increase the suspicion for infection.

If your child has the above symptoms, see the doctor the same day. Go to an emergency room or urgent care facility if after hours.

What You Can Do

Home treatments usually aren't enough to treat pneumonia. However, the chest-clearing suggestions we make for bronchitis (see page 203) can also benefit the recovery from pneumonia.

What Your Doctor Might Do

Your pediatrician will listen carefully to your child's breathing with a stethoscope and observe for any signs of labored or rapid breathing. Most cases of pneumonia will create some abnormal breath sounds the doctor may be able to hear. However, the absence of any abnormal sounds doesn't completely rule out pneumonia. Some can be undetectable on exam. Here are various approaches to diagnosing pneumonia that the doctor may take:

- Obvious diagnosis. If your child's symptoms are obvious for bacterial pneumonia, the child's color is normal, and the breathing is comfortable enough, and the doctor can hear the infection with a stethoscope, she will probably prescribe antibiotics without further testing.

- Unclear diagnosis. If the diagnosis isn't certain, and the child seems ill, the doctor may obtain an X-ray to confirm the diagnosis and to make sure the infection isn't severe enough to warrant hospitalization.

- Rapid labored breathing and poor color. If a child is really in distress, your pediatrician will probably send you straight to an emergency room for oxygen, breathing treatments, an X-ray, and treatment.

Treatment

Treatment varies depending on the severity of infection. Mild pneumonia may be treated with a simple oral antibiotic. A child with severe pneumonia or labored breathing and poor color often requires hospitalization for a few days for intravenous (IV) antibiotics and oxygen if needed.

POISON IVY AND POISON OAK

Poison ivy frequently causes skin rash in children and adults. Poison ivy is found throughout the United States. The plant has the characteristic appearance of three shiny leaves on a red stem, and it grows in the form of a vine. Remember the old saying "Leaves of three, let them be!"

Poison oak is found mostly on the West Coast and grows as a shrub. Similar to poison ivy, it has three shiny leaves attached to a red stem.

The culprit for the itchy, red rash caused by these plants is actually the oil within the leaves. Upon contact, the oil enters the skin and causes a reaction similar to other types of allergic reaction on the skin. The extent of the reaction varies from person to person. The amount of exposure also plays a role in the severity of the reaction. Poison oak and poison ivy are not usually spread from person to person, but the oils can be spread across other parts of the body through scratching. The oils can also remain on clothes, shoes, and pets, causing re-irritation long after the initial exposure. Burning these plants is not advised because the oils can be spread in smoke and can cause reactions in people exposed to the smoke.

Symptoms

Poison oak and poison ivy produce a raised red rash in patches or streaks at the site of contact. Other symptoms to watch for:

- The rash usually appears within two to three days of exposure and may last more than three weeks.

- The rash is intensely itchy.

- The rash may include large bumps that form into blisters.

- The intensity of the rash varies from person to person and the extent of exposure to the plant.

What to Do

As quickly as possible, wash the entire body thoroughly with soap and warm water. Doing so within thirty minutes of exposure may prevent the oils from entering the skin and can lessen the severity and duration of the rash. Over-the-counter products are available in pharmacies and camping stores that contain ingredients to dissolve the oils of the plants. When used immediately after contact, these can greatly reduce symptoms.

DR. SEARS TIP
Plan Ahead for Poison Ivy

If you are planning a camping trip, carry poison ivy medication with you. Depending on where you are at the time of contact, soap and warm water may not be immediately available.

Following are other important ways to treat and avoid poison ivy:

- Thoroughly wash all clothing and shoes with soap and hot water to clear the oils.

- Stay cool! Heat and sweat can worsen the itching.

- Use a brush to scrub underneath fingernails. This helps prevent spread of the oils to other parts of the body.

- Bathe your exposed animals as soon as possible after contact. People can be infected from exposure to the oil on animals' fur.

- Use calamine lotion and hydrocortisone cream to reduce blistering and itching.

- Use oral antihistamines to relieve itching.

- Try aluminum acetate compresses to relieve symptoms by drying out the rash.

- Try oatmeal bath solutions to soothe itching.

- In severe cases, talk to the doctor about oral or injected steroids to relieve the itching and inflammation and aid in the healing of the rash.

DR. SEARS TIP
Home Remedy

You can make your own oatmeal bath solution. Place uncooked oatmeal in a tube sock and tie the open end around the faucet of your bathtub. Turn on the water. No trip to the pharmacy needed!

PSORIASIS

Psoriasis is a common skin condition that affects people between fifteen and thirty-five years of age. It is usually a lifelong condition that can get better or worse over time.

Symptoms

People with psoriasis usually have irritated, itchy patches of skin on different areas of the body. The flaky, scaly, irritated patches of skin can appear in several colors, ranging from pink to red, often with silver. The patches are often raised. The most commonly affected areas are:

- front or back of the knees

- front or back of the elbows

- abdomen and chest

- scalp

Psoriasis and arthritis. Approximately 30 percent of people with psoriasis may also have symptoms of arthritis. This condition is known as *psoriatic arthritis*.

Causes and Triggers

Doctors are unsure about the specific cause of psoriasis. It is thought to be a type of auto-immune disorder in which the body's immune system treats healthy skin cells as if they are a danger to the body. The resulting inflammatory response leads to classic psoriasis symptoms.

Triggers that are believed to make psoriasis worse include:

- dry air and/or dry skin
- stress
- viral or bacterial infections
- upper respiratory infections
- medications, including lithium, beta-blockers, malaria drugs
- sunburn
- too little sunlight
- excess alcohol intake

Diagnosis

Psoriasis has a very classic and unique appearance, so it is often diagnosed by examination alone. Occasionally, if the diagnosis is in doubt, your doctor may perform a skin biopsy to rule out other conditions. X-rays may be performed if your child is complaining of joint pain.

Treatment

Treatment of psoriasis depends on the nature and severity of the condition. Cases of psoriasis that are mild can often be treated with over-the-counter or prescription medications, such as:

- moisturizing creams and lotions
- steroid creams, such as hydrocortisone, to help control flare-ups
- coal tar creams and ointments
- antidandruff shampoos for psoriasis of the scalp
- oatmeal baths
- medications containing vitamin A
- phototherapy, a medical procedure that exposes patients to low levels of ultraviolet light to help control flare-ups

If these treatments are not enough to control the symptoms, there are newer medications that help diminish the body's immune response. Extremely severe cases of psoriasis may also be treated with immunosuppressive medications. Talk to your pediatrician for more information regarding these new treatment methods.

 DR. SEARS TIP
Go Fish!

Omega-3 oils are anti-inflammatory foods, so they are very good for the skin. Daily supplementation with omega 3s containing DHA and EPA (specific types of omega 3s) may help keep the skin moist and prevent flare-ups.

When to Worry

Complications of psoriasis may include:

- secondary bacterial infections from severe flare-ups (Your doctor may prescribe antibiotics.)

- severe or worsening arthritis

Psoriasis can be very difficult to treat, depending on the nature and severity of the disease. The main goal is to prevent flare-ups and to find effective treatments for flare-ups as they occur. (See also tips for general skin care, page 29.)

PUBERTY PROBLEMS—EARLY OR DELAYED PUBERTY

Early Puberty

Early puberty in children is known in the medical field as *precocious puberty*. This condition may be seen in both sexes, but it is more common in girls than in boys. The medical definition of early or precocious puberty is when girls begin to show signs of starting the changes of puberty before eight years of age, and boys before the age of nine. This can be a challenging problem both physically and emotionally for the children as well as their parents.

Signs and symptoms. If you notice the following in your child, these may be signs of early puberty:

In girls before the age of eight, these signs include:

- development of underarm or pubic hair

- developing breasts, tender lumps around nipple

- onset of menstruation

- a very rapid growth spurt

- developing body odor that resembles the body odor of an adolescent

- beginning to have acne on the face or other parts of the body

Signs to look for in boys before the age of nine include:

- developing underarm hair, facial hair, or pubic hair

- unusual deepening of the voice

- enlarging penis and/or testicles

- a very rapid growth spurt

- developing body odor that resembles the body odor of an adolescent

- beginning to have acne on the face or other parts of the body

Note: Early body odor and/or acne without any other signs and no early growth spurt probably does not indicate precocious puberty.

Children entering early or precocious puberty may show any or all of the above signs. However, some children show what is known as *partial precocious puberty*. This occurs when a young child shows some signs of early sexual development, but then these signs disappear and normal development continues. In some instances, very young girls develop small breast buds at a young age that disappear as they get older. Of course, if you notice any changes in your child that are mentioned above, consult your pediatrician.

NORMAL PUBERTAL DEVELOPMENT: TANNER STAGES

Doctors use these five stages of development to describe the normal progression of puberty:

TANNER STAGES FOR GIRLS:

Tanner Stage	Breast Tissue	Pubic Hair	Other
1	None	Fine light hair	
2 Avg. age 11	Small breast bud appears beneath enlarging areola	Sparse, slightly pigmented hair along labia	Clitoris enlarges, labia darken
3 Avg. age 12	More breast tissue beyond border of areola	Coarse, curled hair connects above labia	Underarm hair, acne
4 Avg. age 13	Areola projects out from breast; distinct breast shape	Adult-type hair but not on thighs	Menstrual cycles begin
5 Avg. age 14	Adult breast contour	Adult-type hair spread to thighs	Fully mature genitalia

TANNER STAGES FOR BOYS:

Tanner Stage	Genitalia	Pubic Hair	Other
1	Infantile	Fine light hair	
2 Avg. age 12	Scrotum thins and reddens; testicles slightly larger	Sparse, slightly pigmented hair at base of penis	
3 Avg. age 13	Penis lengthens; testicles grow larger	Coarse, curled hair spreads upward	Voice breaks; growth of muscles
4 Avg. age 14	Penis enlarges, including glans (head); scrotum darkens	Adult-type hair but not on thighs	Voice changed; underarm hair; acne
5 Avg. age 15	Adult-size penis and testicles	Adult-type hair spread to thighs	Facial hair; muscles continue to grow

Causes. In many cases of early puberty there is no known underlying medical cause. This is, however, more true for girls than boys. Boys who enter puberty too early (before the age of nine) are more likely to have an underlying medical condition.

In rare cases, entering early puberty is caused by the following medical conditions (again, these are very rare):

- brain tumor or other problem with brain structure

- infection of the brain (known as meningitis)

- injuries to the brain suffered during head trauma

- problems with development of the ovaries in girls or the testicles in boys

- problems with the thyroid gland

- problems with the glands in the brain responsible for producing sex hormones

See your child's doctor if your child is showing any signs of early puberty or sexual development. If the doctor suspects there may be an underlying medical problem, tests can be done to confirm this. These may include:

- blood tests to measure hormone levels in the body

- MRI scans of the brain

- ultrasound of the ovaries or testicles

- special X-rays of the child's wrists that can compare the age of the bones to the actual age of the child. In early puberty, some children's bones age faster than the children themselves.

DR. SEARS TIP
Obesity and Early Puberty

Children who are overweight are at higher risk of entering puberty too early because excess body fat often produces excess estrogen. This is yet another reason why maintaining a healthy weight in your children is important.

Treatment. If your pediatrician is worried that your child may be entering puberty too early, he may refer you to a pediatric endocrinologist who specializes in treating precocious puberty. The main goal of treatment is to stop or reverse the child's sexual development until she reaches an age where it is appropriate to begin puberty. In the rare cases where early puberty is caused by an underlying medical condition, treatment for that condition is an important part of your child's care (such as treating a brain tumor). As we discussed above, however, most cases of early puberty have no underlying medical explanation. Most cases of confirmed precocious puberty without any underlying medical cause are treated with special hormones called *LHRH analogs*. These hormones block your child's body from producing the sex hormones that are responsible for early puberty. This treatment is usually continued until your child's doctor feels it is an appropriate time for your child to enter puberty. This usually is between the ages of eleven and twelve for girls and between twelve and thirteen years of age for boys.

Long-term complications. If left untreated, precocious puberty can have several long-lasting effects. Girls and boys who enter into puberty too early usually will not achieve their full height potential as compared to their peers. This can have long-term emotional and psychological effects. There can also be dramatic social consequences for a child who starts developing too early. They may be teased by their peers and may suffer emotionally and psychologically because they feel "different from everybody else."

It is good news to know that when properly treated (as discussed above), the vast majority of cases of early puberty can be corrected and the child will go on to develop into a normal, healthy, and well-adjusted adult.

Delayed Puberty

This is an issue that some adolescents and parents deal with when children enter their middle teen years. Adolescents may notice their peers' bodies changing in ways that their own bodies are not. As you can imagine, this may be a cause of great concern for the adolescents and the parents.

Signs and symptoms. Children entering into adolescence should be evaluated at their routine checkups to be sure their physical development is proceeding normally. The most common signs that your child may be experiencing delayed puberty include the following:

For girls:

- failure of breasts to begin developing by the age of thirteen

- lack of developing pubic hair by the age of fourteen

- failure to begin menstruating by the age of sixteen

- a span of more than five years between when the breasts begin to develop and periods begin

For boys:

- no pubic hair by the age of fifteen

- failure of the testicles to begin enlarging by the age of fourteen

- a span of more than five years for the genitals to reach full enlargement

These are very strict guidelines to follow, but each child's individual sexual development is unique. As you can see in a typical eighth-grade classroom, there is an extremely wide variation among the sizes and shapes of normal adolescents' bodies.

For girls, puberty can begin between the ages of eight and thirteen; for boys, puberty can start between the ages of nine and fifteen. As you can see, this is an extremely wide range of ages, and all are within the normal range of sexual development.

Causes. Most cases of delayed puberty are what is known in medical jargon as *constitutional delay*. This is medical speak for being a late bloomer. This type of delayed puberty usually does not require any type of treatment other than reassurance for the adolescent that there is nothing wrong with his or her body. Constitutional delay, or being a late bloomer, usually runs in the family. Brothers, sisters, cousins, parents, aunts, or uncles may also have gone through the same thing. Late bloomers will reach their full adult height and develop into fully mature adults, although possibly at a slower rate than their peers.

However, in rare instances there are medical problems that may cause delayed puberty. Some medical conditions that may result in delayed puberty include:

- Children with long-term medical conditions like diabetes, asthma, or kidney problems may also suffer from delayed puberty.

- Problems with the pituitary gland (responsible for producing sex hormones) or thyroid problems can lead to delayed puberty.

- Poor nutrition can lead to delayed puberty.

- Females who are extremely athletic may experience a delay in menstruation.

- Children with chromosome abnormalities, most commonly *Turner's syndrome* in girls and *Klinefelter's syndrome* in boys, show delayed sexual development.

 ### DR. SEARS TIP
Be Aware of Anorexia

Girls who appear to be unusually thin, malnourished, or seem to be overly obsessed with their weight and how much food they eat should be evaluated for their risk of anorexia (see page 142 for details on anorexia). This can also occur in boys. Delays in menstruation (for girls) and sexual development may be a sign of an underlying eating disorder.

If your pediatrician suspects that your adolescent's lack of sexual development is something more than just being a late bloomer, she may order tests to rule out a more serious cause. Testing may include:

- blood tests to check levels of sex hormones and thyroid hormone

- tests to check for chromosome abnormalities

- special X-rays of the hands and wrists to assess the "bone age" to be sure the bones are developing normally

- MRI or CT scans of the brain if a pituitary or other problem is suspected

Any abnormal tests should be immediately referred to a pediatric endocrinologist for further evaluation and treatment.

Treatment. Treatment depends on whether there is an underlying medical explanation for any delay in puberty. Often, once an underlying cause is found and treated, puberty then begins progressing normally. Most cases of constitutional delay or simply being a late bloomer are not treated. The adolescent is simply reassured that he will "catch up with everyone else." A pediatric endocrinologist might administer short courses of sex hormones to "jump-start" a child's sexual development, but only if there are no other underlying and treatable medical conditions and the delay in puberty is causing great emotional or psychological distress in the individual. This would be performed at the discretion of the medical specialist.

Long-term complications. In the vast majority of cases of delayed puberty, there are no long-term complications, and the child reaches full adult height and development. Treating any rare underlying medical condition causing the delayed puberty usually results in normal development. One of the main complications of delayed puberty is psychological or emotional damage that an adolescent may go through if his body is not changing like everyone else's. Once a more serious medical condition is ruled out, it is important to be supportive and reassure your adolescent that there is nothing wrong with his body and in the long run he will mature just like everyone else.

RASHES

Every child develops some sort of rash during childhood, and virtually all rashes are harmless in the long run. The most important thing is to understand when a rash is serious and needs urgent evaluation and treatment. Once you know that no immediate action is needed, you can take the time to evaluate the rash and determine its cause. Here is our guide to understanding and treating childhood rashes.

Recognizing a Serious Rash

The single most important type of rash you need to be able to recognize is called *petechiae* and/or *purpura*. This occurs when blood vessels within the skin layers rupture and leave red, pinpoint-size dots (petechiae) or larger red or purple blotches (purpura). This type of rash is important to recognize because it can be caused by a very serious bacterial infection that requires prompt treatment. Urgent evaluation is warranted.

The key to differentiating this rash from all other types of red and purple dots is that these don't blanch; when you place a finger on each side of the spot and stretch the skin in opposite directions away from the spot, the spot does NOT fade away. Virtually all other types of spots, from chicken pox to heat rash, will blanch, or fade almost to normal skin color, when stretched or pressed.

Another key feature of petechiae and purpura is that they are *within* the skin. You won't feel any bump on the skin when you run your finger over them. Most other types of spots will feel bumpy.

So, since you are probably reading this page because your child has a mysterious rash, take a moment right now to make sure it isn't petechiae or purpura. Once you have done that, you can breathe a sigh of relief and casually work through the rest of this section to determine what *is* causing your child's rash.

If you feel your child's rash fails the "blanching test" and he may have petechiae or purpura, it is extremely important to have this evaluated as discussed below:

When NOT to worry about petechiae or purpura. Just to offer you a bit of reassurance, sometimes this kind of rash occurs for no serious reason at all and is perfectly harmless. For example, if your child has been repeatedly vomiting or having severe coughing fits, the pressure in her face might have built up high enough to cause little ruptures in the skin vessels of the face. If you *only* find these spots on the face and nowhere else on the body, then you probably have nothing to worry about. If your child generally feels well and has no fever, see the doctor the next time the office opens.

When to worry. Anytime you see such spots anywhere on the body besides the face (not just one tiny spot, but several), call the doctor. If your child has a high fever, a severe headache, is lethargic or extremely irritable (see the symptoms of meningitis, page 393), and has these spots, go straight to an emergency room. If your child isn't acting very ill and has no fever, meningitis is unlikely and an emergency room visit may not be necessary just yet. See your pediatrician right away. Blood tests will be done to evaluate why your child's skin vessels are bleeding so that appropriate treatment can begin right away.

Common Childhood Rashes

Here are the most common childhood rashes. While none of these require urgent medical attention, some do warrant prompt home treatment:

Normal newborn rashes. During the first two months of life, most newborns have a rash called *seborrheic dermatitis*. These red bumps, pimples, and splotches are usually on the face and upper body but can occur anywhere. This harmless "baby acne" clears up without treatment and your baby will be ready for his first portrait sitting by two months.

Hives. These are raised, itchy, white and/or red patches or welts of varying sizes. They can be as small as a pencil eraser or as large as a silver dollar or two. They are almost always caused by an allergic reaction. Hives usually appear suddenly, most often on the trunk (chest, abdomen, or back), and they spread rapidly to other areas, including the extremities. They rarely affect the face. Hives will often fade away from one area and pop up in another, continuously shifting and changing over a few hours. An easy way to diagnose hives is to treat them with an over-the-counter oral antihistamine. If the welts subside or disappear completely, then it is almost definitely hives. For more detailed information on hives, see page 370.

Eczema. This results from a combination of dry, sensitive skin and an allergic reaction to something in the diet or the environment. It often starts on the inside of the elbows and behind the knees, but it can begin anywhere on the body as dry, or sometimes moist, skin-color or red, slightly rough patches. There can be just one patch or dozens, and they are usu-ally quite itchy. See page 297 if you feel your child may have eczema.

Generic viral rashes. There are dozens of viruses that can infect children and cause rashes. Some of these are fairly common and easy to recognize, such as chicken pox, rose-ola, and fifth disease, which are discussed below. However, most other viral rashes all look similar and generally can't be distinguished from one another. Fortunately, since these are all harmless and untreatable, an exact diagnosis isn't usually necessary. It's enough to simply determine when a child has a generic viral rash. Here's how to recognize these:

- The rash can have a variety of appearances: A red lacy spread-out pattern, scattered tiny pimples, larger red spots, and even hives.

- Viral rashes usually (but not always) begin on the trunk and spread out to the extremities.

- Fever will usually be part of the equation.

- General aches and not feeling well is common.

- Viral rashes (except chicken pox) are usually not itchy.

Most viral illnesses with rashes are contagious from the day before the illness begins until the day after the fever goes away. The rash may linger for a week or so, but it is not contagious once the child feels well again.

Chicken pox. This is the most easily recognizable rash. It begins with several red bumps on the trunk that look like insect bites. More spots will appear throughout the first day. By day 2, the first spots will have changed into small blisters filled with clear fluid (as opposed to insect bites, which get bigger but generally don't blister). More of the initial red bumps will appear on the second day. By day 3 you will see three different types of spots: the initial red bumps spreading out onto the extremities and face, small blisters that used to be red bumps, and finally crusts as each blister opens and drains. It is this variation day by day that makes chicken pox recognizable. Don't rush to the doctor on day 1 expecting her to be able to give you an exact diagnosis. If your child has a fever and some itchy red bumps, assume he's contagious and keep him home. By day 2 or 3 it will be obvious whether or not it's chicken pox. See page 215 for more details on diagnosis and treatment.

Fifth disease. This rash is caused by the parvovirus. It is characterized by bright red cheeks that look like they've been slapped. After one or two days, this facial rash subsides and a generic viral rash (described above) appears, sometimes with fever, runny nose, cough, and general body aches. Once the facial rash is gone, the illness is indistinguishable from other generic viral diseases. There is no treatment for this illness, and it will pass after several days without any problem. The only issue to be aware of is that pregnant women in their first trimesters who are exposed to this virus can experience some complications with the fetus. Contact your obstetrician.

Roseola. This is perhaps the single most common cause of fever and rash during infancy and toddlerhood. Caused by a herpes virus (not the sexually transmitted or oral one), this illness begins with about three days of very high fever and virtually no other symptoms (besides feeling crummy from the fever). Just when parents and doctors start to get worried, the fever fades and a generic viral

rash appears. That's when the diagnosis is usually made, not from the way the rash looks, but rather from the timing of it compared to the fever. This virus will pass without any specific treatment. The only thing to do is follow the proper fever treatment and precautions on page 317.

Impetigo. Commonly mispronounced as "infantigo," this is a bacterial infection of the skin. It appears as red pimples that enlarge and form a crusty oozing layer of pus. It usually occurs around the mouth and nose but can show up anywhere on the body. See page 378 for details.

Cellulitis. This is a bacterial infection within the deeper layers of the skin (as opposed to impetigo, which is on top of the skin). It is often triggered by a cut or insect bite that allows bacteria to get into the deeper layers. It appears as red, warm, and swollen skin that gradually spreads out in all directions. See page 213 for more details.

Contact dermatitis. This red, itchy, bumpy, and sometimes oozing rash can result from skin coming into contact with an irritant. Poison ivy and poison oak fall into this category. The rash generally appears hours or days after contact with the suspected irritant. As a child scratches, the irritating substance can be spread into lines of rash. See page 243 for details.

Prickly heat rash. This unsightly, but harmless, rash occurs numerous times in every infant's and toddler's life. Heat rash appears as numerous tiny red pinpoint bumps around the neck and upper trunk, usually after a particularly hot day or sweaty experience. Simple cooling measures should take care of it. It can be a daily occurrence during hot weather. See page 357 for more information.

Erythema multiforme. This uncommon rash looks identical to hives (page 444) but won't respond to antihistamines. See page 370.

Summertime rashes. During the summer the combination of heat, sweat, suntan lotion, chlorine in pool water, sand, grass, and everything else a child comes in contact with when it's hot and sunny mix together to cause a generic red bumpy rash. This type of rash is diagnosed simply by ruling out all other causes of rash. It's really a combination of prickly heat rash and contact dermatitis. If it doesn't bother your child, just leave it alone and wait for summer to end. If it's itchy or irritating, over-the-counter anti-itch creams can help minimize the discomfort.

Swimmer's itch and sea bather's rash. These occur from swimming in the ocean; tiny marine animals cause numerous little stings that turn into itchy bumps. There are two types: One occurs only in areas covered by swimsuits (because the little critters get trapped in there); the other occurs only on skin *not* covered by swimsuits. Treatment involves oral antihistamines and topical hydrocortisone (a prescription strength may be needed).

Scabies. This is thought to be the itchiest rash known to mankind. It is caused by a tiny mite (microscopic insect) that burrows down into the skin and causes an itchy bump or patch. Scratching can spread the culprit along straight lines to form a string or line of raised itchy red rash. See page 453 for details on diagnosis and treatment.

Scarlet fever (strep throat rash). This rash is caused by an immune reaction to the strep bacteria as it infects the throat. It appears as hundreds of tiny, red, pinpoint bumps all over the trunk that feel like fine sandpaper. The presence of this rash doesn't mean the strep throat infection is any more serious than regular strep without a rash. It actually makes the diagnosis of strep throat easier. See page 500 for details.

Insect bites. These itchy bumps come in a variety of shapes and sizes. They are generally diagnosed through three criteria: there are usually only a few at any one time, they tend to grow larger over several days, with a visible bite dot in the center, and they itch. See page 186 for more details.

Facial drool rash. Although this is a harmless rash, it can be very stubborn and bothersome to parents because it detracts from their baby's natural beauty. It is distinguishable from facial impetigo in that it lacks the crusty oozing. You can minimize this rash with a lanolin ointment (like Lansinoh) from a drugstore. It is likely to come and go for many months during the early years.

Ringworm. Despite its name, this rash is caused by a fungus, not a parasitic worm. It shows up as a red, raised round ring with fairly normal skin in the center. It can vary in size, and may grow larger if left untreated. There is often only one spot or rash, but it can spread out and is sometimes itchy. The only way to distinguish it from a patch of eczema is by the normal skin in the middle of the ring; eczema patches are often rough and raised over the entire round patch. See page 335 for more details.

Scalp rashes. Various forms of scalp rashes occur throughout childhood. See page 337 for details.

Pityriasis patches. These are small white, red, or brown round patches that occur anywhere on the body. They may itch. See pages 432 and 433 for more details.

Autoimmune diseases. This class of diseases is caused by a person's immune system reacting to her own body. The exact cause of this phenomenon is unknown and the various autoimmune diseases are too complicated to list here. It's worth mentioning, however, that any chronic, red, non-itchy rash that is accompanied by recurrent unexplained fevers, joint and muscle aches, swelling of the hands, feet, face, or joints, frequent illnesses, chest pains, or unusual fatigue may be indicative of an autoimmune disorder.

Treatment

Sometimes even the most observant parent or doctor can't determine what a particular rash may be. It doesn't hurt to try several different types of treatments to see which one helps the most. This may allow your child to be rid of a bothersome rash without ever really knowing what it was. Try these remedies:

- Moisturizing lotion — this may soothe and heal irritated skin.

- Antihistamine cream — this type of over-the-counter anti-itch cream can provide some fast relief.

- Hydrocortisone cream — this mild over-the-counter steroid cream can improve almost any raised, red, itchy, or irritating rash (except for bacterial infections).

- Antifungal creams — these over-the-counter creams are very safe to use and harmless even if the rash is not due to a fungus.

You can try two or three creams at the same time, each applied to a different area of the rash, to see which one works best.

If any rash seems to worsen with treatment, stop immediately and have your pediatrician take a look (unless you were just there and she is as stumped as you are!). Let a dermatologist have a go at it if necessary. (See also general skin care, page 29.)

RECTAL ITCHING

Is your child always scratching his bottom? Here is our guide to rectal itching.

Causes

The four most common causes of rectal itching in young children are:

- pinworms (see page 431)

- food allergies (see "Target Sign," page 197)

- fungal infection, usually following antibiotic treatment (see antibiotic side effects, page 551)

- bacterial infection

Bacterial infection. A common cause of a persistent, red, raised, circular, and itchy rash with pimples or pustules scattered around the anus is a bacterial infection, usually strep or staph bacteria. Suspect this if:

- The rash persists with no treatment.

- The rash is looking worse: more swollen, more red, sometimes it even bleeds.

- Treatments such as diaper and antifungal creams are not working.

- Other causes have been ruled out.

If your pediatrician suspects a bacterial infection, the appropriate antibacterial cream will be prescribed.

What to Do

Besides diagnosing the cause, try these general home remedies:

- Have your child sit in a baking soda bath (add half a cup baking soda to warm bathwater).

- Apply a diaper ointment to the itchy area several times a day and especially before bed.

- Trim those little fingernails as short as you can. Scratching can intensify and spread the infection.

ROSEOLA

This common childhood illness is caused by herpes virus type 6, which has nothing to do with genital or oral herpes; it simply happens to be in the herpes family. The symptoms of roseola are clearly defined: three days of high fever followed by a generic viral rash. The rash commonly begins behind the neck and on the upper back. It looks like flat red spots or bumps. It can spread to the face, chest, and abdomen, and occasionally out to the extremities. The rash is not itchy and it requires no lotions or any other treatment. It lasts anywhere from a few days to two weeks. Some children won't have any rash at all — just high fever. Although the fever can be uncomfortable, there is no harm in the long run.

Roseola is transmitted like a common cold. A child is contagious from the day before fever until about two days after the fever is gone, even if the rash continues. The incubation period is about ten days. There is no specific treatment for the rash, only for the fever (see page 317).

Diagnosis

Parents and doctors can't determine that an illness is roseola until the fever breaks and the rash appears. The diagnosis is made after the fact. Because the first symptom is only fever, the doctor will look for other obvious causes of fever, like an ear or throat infection. If none are found, and there are no other symptoms that could explain the fever (like cough, nasal congestion, diarrhea), then the doctor determines the fever is likely caused by a virus. For children between six months and three years of age, roseola would be the most likely virus.

If a doctor doesn't see the child until the rash appears, then the three-day history of fever followed by rash makes it obvious. Some children will then go on to develop a runny nose, cough, vomiting, or diarrhea as well.

When to Worry

There really is no need to worry with roseola unless the fever is worrisome — see our section on fever on page 317.

ROTAVIRUS INFECTION

Rotavirus infects the gastrointestinal tract of infants, children, and adults, leading to nausea, vomiting, and diarrhea. It is a major public health issue, responsible for three million cases of diarrhea and about 55,000 hospitalizations of young children each year in the United States. Death from rotavirus is rare in America, but worldwide the virus causes more than half a million deaths every year.

The virus is present in the stool of people with rotavirus infection. Infants and children can become infected if they touch an object or another person that has been contaminated with stool containing rotavirus and then touch their mouths, thereby ingesting the virus. The virus is highly contagious. Outbreaks are frequently seen in facilities with lots of infants and children, especially daycare centers, children's hospitals, and households with many kids. Most commonly, the virus is spread when children and caregivers do not wash their hands often enough, especially after using the bathroom or before eating. Little hands contaminated with rotavirus often touch little faces, creating an easy path for the virus to travel. Rotavirus is present in an infected person's stool before he begins having symptoms and for weeks after the symptoms resolve, making it very difficult to prevent spread. Children can catch rotavirus more than once, although the first episode is usually the worst.

Symptoms

Following are symptoms of rotavirus:

- fever

- nausea

- vomiting

- frequent, watery diarrhea

- abdominal cramps

- signs of dehydration (see below)

- may have cough or runny nose

Infected children may have any or all of the above symptoms. Children under five years of age can have severe cases. Older children may have only mild symptoms or none at all. Adults are usually only mildly affected.

Signs of dehydration:

- thirst

- lethargy

- dry mouth and tongue

- irritability and/or restlessness

- sunken eyes

- dry skin

- fewer than three wet diapers in a twenty-four-hour period

- fewer trips to pee in the bathroom, in potty-trained children

(See page 267 for more details on how to assess your child's level of dehydration.)

Diagnosis

A stool test can be done to confirm rotavirus infection. This is usually only done in severe cases to determine if something else might be going on. Your pediatrician may test your child's blood, stool, or urine to see if the symptoms are due to other causes.

When to Worry

The main reason to seek medical care is if the vomiting and diarrhea cause moderate to severe dehydration. See page 267 for information on how to assess the degree of dehydration and when to seek emergency medical care. Most cases of rotavirus don't require an emergency room visit, but a trip to your pediatrician may be needed.

Treatment

Because it is a virus, antibiotics cannot treat rotavirus. The mainstay of treatment is to keep children hydrated. Treatment depends upon how severe the symptoms are.

Mild diarrhea. In children with only mild diarrhea and no signs of dehydration, normal eating can continue, but these kids should receive more clear fluids. Do NOT give sugary drinks like fruit juices or soft drinks, as this will make the diarrhea worse. Water, electrolyte solutions, and sugar-free Popsicles are good choices. Breastfeeding or formula should continue and be encouraged. Call your pediatrician if symptoms worsen.

Diarrhea with symptoms of mild to moderate dehydration. Consult your doctor. The key to treatment is, of course, rehydration. Offer over-the-counter oral electrolyte solutions. Diluted white grape juice also works. If you are breastfeeding, continue. A temporary change to a lactose-free or soy formula can help the diarrhea resolve more quickly. Once dehydration has been corrected, begin to introduce bland BRATY foods back into the diet. If your child is tolerating these, she can go back to eating normally. (See more diarrhea treatment tips, page 277.)

Diarrhea with vomiting and mild to moderate dehydration. Again, rehydration is the key to treatment. Encourage clear liquids — electrolyte solutions are especially important. Again, continue breastfeeding. In a vomiting child, liquid should be given in small, frequent

---

BE A BRAT!

The so-called BRAT diet offers a good mnemonic term for remembering the bland foods.

B: Bananas

R: Rice

A: Applesauce

T: Toast

In our office we often add plain, organic yogurt (a rich source of intestinal-healing probiotics), so the term would be BRATY.

---

amounts to avoid making vomiting worse. Bland foods can be given once fluids are tolerated. Call the doctor if symptoms of dehydration are getting worse.

Severe diarrhea and vomiting with severe dehydration. Call the doctor or go to the hospital immediately. Severe cases of

---

 **DR. SEARS TIP
Dehydration Risks**

When I talk to a parent about a child who may have rotavirus, I always ask: "Is it coming out of one or both ends?" Diarrhea or vomiting alone does not usually cause severe dehydration. However, a child that has it "coming out of both ends" (meaning vomiting and diarrhea) is more at risk of becoming dehydrated. The second question I always ask is: "Is he keeping liquids down?" This is a good sign. Again, in a vomiting child, it is important to give smaller, more frequent drinks. Let your pediatrician know if your child has vomiting, diarrhea, or both.

rotavirus infection often require hospitalization for intravenous (IV) fluid rehydration. Infants younger than six months of age and those with severe vomiting and diarrhea who cannot keep oral fluids down are at highest risk for hospitalization. Small infants can become dehydrated very quickly because of their size. Children four and older are rarely hospitalized; the emergency room rehydration usually does the trick.

Prevention

You can lower the risk of rotavirus infection, but the fact is most people will get rotavirus at some point in their childhood. Taking the following steps can help prevent rotavirus:

• Frequent handwashing — especially after using the bathroom, after handling food, and before eating — can lower the risk of infection. Hand sanitizers also work.

• Breastfeeding can prevent the infection, or at least minimize the symptoms, if exposed.

• Children with rotavirus should stay home from daycare or other children's groups until diarrhea has resolved.

• Make sure caregivers wash their hands after changing diapers.

• Make sure your child gets the rotavirus vaccine. This is the single best method of preventing rotavirus infection. It is given orally in three doses at age two, four, and six months and is part of the recommended first-year vaccine schedule. (See vaccine section for more information, page 43.) The vaccine dramatically reduces your child's risk for severe rotavirus infection; it has been found to prevent 75 percent of all rotavirus cases and 98 percent of severe

cases. Talk to your pediatrician for more information.

RSV: RESPIRATORY SYNCYTIAL VIRUS

RSV (respiratory syncytial virus) is the most common cause of lower respiratory infections and the leading cause of hospitalization in babies under age one. RSV is mainly prevalent during the late fall through early spring months. Each year approximately 125,000 children are hospitalized in the United States with RSV, and it is responsible for around 500 deaths annually. Because it's highly contagious, nearly all children are exposed to RSV during the first two years of life.

Symptoms

Initially the symptoms of RSV may be similar to those of a common cold:

• low-grade fever

• runny nose

• cough

Most children three years and older won't have any other unusual symptoms. Infants and toddlers, on the other hand, often develop asthma-like symptoms because the virus is much more irritating to the lungs than a regular cold virus. Symptoms include:

• audible wheezing

• rapid breathing (normally a baby may take about twenty-four breaths per minute; during RSV this may increase to forty to sixty breaths per minute)

- labored breathing (with each breath you may notice Baby's nostrils flaring and the neck and stomach caving in)

- out of breath during feedings

Prevention

All infants. Basic precautions for all infants are prudent during the late fall and winter months, including:

- avoid large group daycare if possible

- avoid church nurseries

- don't pass the baby around among groups of friends

- ensure anyone who holds your baby isn't sick with a cold

- leave any playgroup functions where you notice children with cold symptoms

- avoid cigarette smoke

RSV can live up to twelve hours on toys and hands, so frequent hand washing is very helpful when playing with other children. Of course, you can't live in a bubble. But you can limit your child's exposure as best you can.

Premature infants. Premature infants, especially those with compromised lung function, are at much higher risk of suffering severe symptoms and requiring hospitalization for aggressive treatment. For this reason, specific preventative medical therapy is recommended for such infants with an injected medication called Synagis during the first late fall and winter season of life. This medication is a manufactured antibody that neutralizes the virus. It is injected into the muscle in the same manner that a vaccine is administered. The antibodies circulate around the infant's

bloodstream for about a month, and if the infant is exposed to RSV, the antibodies will fight it off. It is given once a month from October or November through March or April (this varies year by year) to keep the antibodies circulating throughout the entire RSV season. Virtually all insurance plans cover this treatment as long as the infant meets the criteria. It costs about $1,000 per injection. Because this treatment is so expensive, only premature babies with certain criteria qualify for Synagis:

- infants with either chronic lung disease or significant congenital heart disease (with congestive heart failure, pulmonary hypertension, or cyanotic heart disease) who are less than two years of age at the start of RSV season (October)

- premature babies born prior to twenty-eight weeks who are less than twelve months old at the start of RSV season

- premature babies born between twenty-nine and thirty-two weeks who are less than six months old at the start of RSV season

- those born between thirty-two and thirty-five weeks who are less than three months old at the start of RSV season *and* who have one or more risk factors that would make it more likely for them to catch RSV, such as having older siblings, attending a group daycare, or being exposed to cigarette smoke

- certain infants born prior to thirty-five weeks who have congenital abnormalities of the airway or neuromuscular disorders

Criteria for Synagis treatments change every year. Ask your pediatrician if your premature baby qualifies.

What the Doctor Might Do

Diagnosis. RSV is generally a clinical diagnosis based on the infant's symptoms. Nasal secretions (collected by flushing saline into the infant's nose and suctioning it back out again) can be tested for the presence of the virus. This is usually only necessary for hospitalized infants in whom the diagnosis needs to be certain.

Treatment. As this is a virus, antibiotic treatment does not help. The same supportive treatments that are done for regular coughs and colds (see page 222) can help an infant get through RSV. For infants who have problematic wheezing with rapid, labored breathing, an inhaled muscle relaxant medication called *albuterol* can be given through a nebulizer machine every four hours to help open up the lungs and relax the breathing. This is the same medicine that a child with asthma would use (see page 151). Some infants with RSV only need one or two treatments each day for a couple days; others may require it every four hours for several days or longer. Every child is different. For reasons unknown, some infants don't respond to albuterol treatments at all. Your pediatrician will help you decide how to proceed based on how your infant responds to the first treatment in the office. Steroids may be used in severe cases.

Recurrent Episodes

If your infant gets RSV, it's possible that the lungs will react in an asthmatic manner to other cold viruses that may come along during the next few years. You may need to pull out that nebulizer machine again and again. Fortunately most children outgrow this tendency and stop wheezing with colds by the time they are five years old. A small percentage of infants with RSV will go on to have long-term asthma.

SCABIES

This skin infection is caused by a microscopic mite named *Sarcoptes scabiei*. This mite occurs worldwide and can infest any age group.

The scabies mites burrow into the top layer of skin to lay their eggs. Scabies can easily pass from person to person, usually from skin-to-skin contact. The mite can also be spread through shared clothing, towels, and bedding. Mites can live for two to three days on non-living materials, such as towels and toys. When living on human skin, however, mites can live for more than a month. Scabies outbreaks are more common in crowded institutions such as:

- child-care facilities
- schools
- households
- hospitals
- nursing homes

Symptoms

Scabies usually appears as a specific type of rash on the body and has the following clues:

- Skin irritation initially appears like pimples or flea bites. These rashes pop up at the sites where the mites burrow into the skin to lay their eggs. These can appear anywhere on the body, but most commonly occur between the webbing of fingers and toes, wrists, armpits, penis, breasts, elbows, buttocks, navel, and shoulder blades. As the mites burrow under the skin, the rash later looks like a half-inch-long raised line.

- The rash is intensely itchy.

- The pimple-like bumps or blisters may break and become scabbed.

- Itching can occur all over the body, not just where bumps are.

- Itching tends to be worse at night.

- Sores on the body can get worse if they become infected with bacteria.

- Symptoms may take four to six weeks to appear following someone's first contact with scabies.

- A child who has been infected with scabies in the past may develop symptoms after only two to three days of reinfestation.

- There are usually fewer than ten bumps on the body.

- Severe infestations with up to hundreds of bumps may occur in people with weakened immune systems and the elderly.

Diagnosis

Your pediatrician may be able to diagnose scabies just by looking at the rash, because the bumps often have a very characteristic distribution on the body and a specific burrow-like appearance, and they *itch intensely.* The doctor may scrape off a small amount of infected skin and examine the scrapings under a microscope for mites and/or their eggs. However, even if no mites or eggs are seen under the microscope, that does not completely rule out scabies.

Treatment

Scabies MUST be treated by a doctor. Your pediatrician will prescribe a special cream or lotion to be used. It is very important to follow all the instructions completely. It is applied over the *entire* body except for the face, mouth, and eyes. It is extremely important to leave the lotion or cream on for at least eight to twelve hours before washing it off. Leaving it on for a shorter amount of time will not treat the scabies fully. Even when instructions are followed completely, the treatment often needs to be repeated seven to ten days later.

DR. SEARS TIP
Don't Wash Your Hands!

Yes, you heard us right! After applying the lotion over your child's entire body from the neck down, DON'T wash the lotion or cream off your own hands. Scabies mites love to live in the webbing between your fingers. Washing the cream or lotion off your hands after you apply it to your child may leave you at risk for scabies.

Besides a prescription, here are some other ways to treat scabies:

- Close contacts and household members should be treated at the same time as the infected individual, even if they are not showing any symptoms.

- Sexual partners must be treated at the same time.

- All bedding, clothes, towels, and anything else worn by the infected person must be washed in hot water and dried in a hot dryer. Any blankets or items that cannot be washed can be set aside for three days in the garage. The scabies can't live longer than that without a warm body to feed them.

- A secondary bacterial infection can develop in the rash from the intense scratching and may need to be treated with prescription antibiotic cream.

- Oral antihistamines may help the symptoms of itching.

- Hydrocortisone cream may help itching.

- An infected person is usually no longer considered contagious a few hours after receiving treatment.

- Pregnant women and younger children may be treated with milder prescription medications.

- Treatment is considered successful when no new rash or bumps appear on the body, but itching can persist for two to three more weeks following treatment.

- Call the doctor if new scabies bumps and rashes crop up following treatment.

Children can return to school once the overnight treatment is done.

Prevention

If you or your child has been in close contact with someone who has scabies, there is no 100 percent surefire way of avoiding them. However, there are ways you can lower your chances:

- Practice good hygiene, particularly frequent hand washing, especially before meals.

- Encourage daily baths or showers.

- Wear clean clothing.

- Avoid sharing clothing or bedding with others.

Even with the most intense efforts, scabies is easily transmitted from person to person. The good news is that it is very treatable.

SCOLIOSIS (CURVATURE OF THE SPINE)

While everyone's spine curves somewhat, some spines curve too much and in the wrong direction. *Scoliosis* is a lateral curvature of the spine. Excessive curvature of the upper spine in the forward direction is called *kyphosis* (hunchback) and excessive curvature of the lower spine is called *lumbar lordosis* (swayback). A slight degree of scoliosis (around 10 degrees) is harmless and usually causes the child no pain or problems. If left undetected and uncorrected, more severe curves (30 degrees or greater) can restrict ribcage movement and compromise breathing and cardiovascular function. Most scoliosis is *idiopathic,* meaning it has no particular cause. This type of scoliosis usually becomes apparent during the preadolescent growth spurt that commonly begins around age eleven. Rapid growth of the spine during this time will make any curve in the spine more noticeable. Mild scoliosis can become significantly worse over just a few years. So it's important to recognize subtle scoliosis early on in the growth spurt so proper measures can be taken to minimize the curvature during adolescence.

Scoliosis can also be *congenital,* meaning the child is born with curvature of the spine, secondary to a maldevelopment of some of the vertebral bones. *Neuromuscular* scoliosis means the muscles on one side of the body are stronger than the other, so that the stronger muscles pull the growing spine toward that side. *Leg-length discrepancy* (one leg is longer than the other) can cause the whole pelvis to tilt and the spine to curve. This type of scoliosis seldom causes the child any harm unless the leg-length discrepancy is greater than an inch.

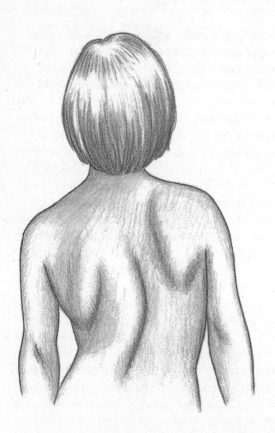

How to Tell

Although your pediatrician will examine your child's back for excess curvature during routine checkups (especially beginning at around age eight years), you can also do the assessment at home.

Try the forward-bend test. Have your child stand straight in front of you, facing you, with his shirt off, feet together, knees straight, arms dangling, and bend gradually forward, slowly lowering the head and bending almost far enough to touch the toes. Stand in front of your child and get your eyes level with his back. Look for one side of the back (the "hump") being higher than the other. This test can also be performed with the child sitting on a table, which eliminates the appearance of the secondary curvature of the spine from a leg-length discrepancy that you would see while examining your child standing. While your child is still bent over, walk around and view the hump from the back and the side. If you notice uneven shoulder blades or an uneven waist, have your pediatrician check it out.

Check for leg-length discrepancy. Have your child stand with both feet together and place your index fingers against the hip bones at her waist. If you notice your fingers are not at the same level, one leg is likely to be longer than the other. If you see this "pelvic tilt," estimate the difference between the height of your two fingers (e.g., half inch, one inch), then place a book of the same width under the child's questionably shorter leg and see if the curvature of the spine straightens out on retest.

When to Worry; What to Do

If you suspect curvature of the spine, be sure to have your pediatrician check it out. She can estimate the degree of scoliosis using a device called a scoliometer (similar to a carpenter's level). If the doctor agrees that there is a curvature of the spine, either idiopathic or secondary to leg-length discrepancy, the next test your child may need is an X-ray examination called a *scoliosis series*. An X-ray is necessary for two reasons:

1. To determine the precise degree of scoliosis

2. As a baseline so the doctor can assess the severity of the curvature on subsequent X-rays

If the scoliosis is significant, usually over 10 degrees, your pediatrician may refer your child to an orthopedist to work out a treatment plan. Most idiopathic scoliosis corrects itself after children go through adolescence. But in a small percentage, the curvature may progress rapidly during the growth spurt of adolescence, which is why vigilant orthopedic follow-up is necessary.

Scoliosis screening is now frequently done in schools. It's an important part of the physical examination. If the curve is less than 20 degrees, an orthopedist will usually recommend watchful waiting (and avoiding backpacks with loads greater than 10 percent of the child's weight). If the curve is over 20 degrees, the orthopedist may recommend a back brace. While the back brace won't straighten the spine, it keeps it from getting worse, particularly through the growth spurts, and may keep the child from needing surgical correction. Surgery is necessary in severe scoliosis where the curvature is greater than 40 degrees.

DR. SEARS TIP
Help Your Doctor Make the Diagnosis

While idiopathic scoliosis usually causes the child no pain or limitation of movement, some forms of scoliosis, particularly if there is an underlying spinal bone deformity, may cause the child to have recurrent back pain. Since "back pain" is unusual in children, be sure to mention this to your doctor. Recurrent back pain in children nearly always merits at least an X-ray of the spine to be sure that one of the lumbar bones has not slipped out of place.

SCRATCHED EYE

Scratched or poked eyes can be a big worry for parents, and quite painful for children. Yet they aren't always an emergency. There are two types of eye scratches. One causes pain and requires treatment and the other does not:

Cornea scratches. Here is how to tell if your child has a scratch over the cornea (colored part of the eye):

• Pain. A cornea scratch causes significant pain during blinking as the inner surface of the eyelid rubs across the scratch. Even a tiny scratch will hurt. Keeping the eye closed usually feels okay.

• Feels like sand in the eye. If you look around the eye and under the eyelid and don't see a foreign body, but your child insists he feels something there, think cornea scratch.

• Visible dull spot. The surface of the cornea is usually smooth and shiny. While you won't be able to see a tiny scratch, you may be able to notice a dull scratch line or spot on the cornea if large enough.

- Red eyes. The severe pain will cause the whites of the eyes to turn very red and irritated.

Scratch in the white of the eye. There are no pain nerves in the whites of the eyes. If your child was scratched or poked in the eye, but doesn't complain of any pain, then the injury probably occurred in the white area. No treatment is necessary for this type of scratch.

Diagnosis

Corneal scratches can be diagnosed by your pediatrician or at an urgent care center with a *fluorescein* eye exam (a painless, yellow solution that is placed into the eye). The doctor will shine a special light (the kind that makes white clothing light up in dark rooms) into the eye, and any scratches on the cornea will show up bright yellow.

If you suspect your child has a corneal scratch, it's best to have the eye examined instead of just calling the doctor for treatment over the phone. Large scratches are more likely to become infected, take longer to heal, and may become a chronic problem. So it's useful for the doctor and you to know what you are dealing with up front. If your child gets a scratch in the evening or night, call the doctor for an eyedrop prescription to start that night, then see the doctor first thing in the morning.

Treatment

Corneal scratches usually heal within one to three days without any treatment. However, they can become infected during that time, so prescription antibiotic eye ointment or eye-drops must be used for two to three days. Corneal scratches that do become infected won't heal well and can affect long-term vision.

It's also a good idea to keep the eye closed and rested to minimize irritation to the scratch. Older kids and adults can wear an eye patch to help. Younger kids who won't tolerate a patch don't need to wear one; the eye will heal without it.

You should have a follow-up eye exam with the doctor in three days to make sure the scratch has healed. If it persists, the doctor will refer you to an eye doctor for ongoing care to make sure it eventually heals.

SCREAMING

Screaming peaks between one and two years of age for two reasons:

- Toddlers like to try out their voices and are amazed at the loudness and power of the sounds they make.

- They also enjoy the effect of their "sirens" on their audience.

What to Do

Once a toddler discovers how much power she has in her voice, it can become ear-piercing. Here's how to mute your little screamer:

Track the trigger. As with the other annoying behaviors of toddlerhood, such as biting and hitting, record the circumstances that provoke screaming and mellow them as much as you can.

Use your nice voice. Toddlers will try on whatever sound gets them the best response. The more she screams, the softer your response should be, so that the child learns that she'll most likely get what she needs by using her softer "nice voice."

"We only scream on the grass." Try this trick we used to mute our little screamers. As soon as your child begins to scream, quickly interject in a cheerful voice, "We scream only on the grass," and quickly usher your little screamer outside to release his stored-up sounds. "Outside voice has to go outside!"

Once your child becomes fluent in language and social gestures and figures out that a "nicer voice" is more effective, screaming will pass. Consistency will help it pass sooner.

SEIZURES

Seizures or convulsions are one of the scariest situations a parent can confront. Fortunately, most seizures only last a few minutes, and the child is fine afterward. Once things have calmed down, the search for a cause or a reason begins. Here is our guide to helping you understand seizures and how your pediatrician and a neurologist will guide you through them.

If your child is having a seizure for the first time, you should put this book down, call 911, tend to your child, and get emergency services. Most of the time no urgent treatment is needed, but it's better to be safe during the first episode.

Signs

Some seizure episodes are obvious: rhythmic jerking of the arms and legs, stiffening of the whole body, eyes twitching from side to side. This is what most people usually picture when they hear the word *seizure*. However, most seizures in infants and children aren't so cut-and-dried. Most cases we see in our office are more subtle and we must spend a lot of time sorting out if what the parents witnessed even was a seizure. In order to understand if your child's episode was a seizure, it's helpful to know what types of twitches and movements are *not* seizures:

Normal twitches of childhood. Here are some situations that you don't have to worry about:

• Twitching while falling asleep. It is very normal for infants and some children to have whole-body twitches five to ten times as they drift off to sleep. Some infants will only twitch one arm or leg briefly.

• Startle movements. Young infants will suddenly spread their arms wide in a startle reflex.

• Leg kicks. It is also normal for babies to have rhythmic, involuntary kicking movements in their legs from time to time.

• Muscle spasms. Some infants will show rapid spasmodic twitches of the chin, arm, or leg at random times for a few seconds.

• Infant or child continues to talk or interact during twitches, which would be unusual during a seizure.

Signs of possible seizures. Here are some clues that your child's movements may be seizure related:

• Rhythmic movements. Some seizures are jerky movements that continue in a rhythm every second or so.

- Stiff spasms. Other seizures may be more like stiff, trembling spasms.

- Prolonged movements. Any rhythmic jerky movements or spasms that continue for more than thirty seconds are probably a seizure.

- Infant or child is unaware and out of it. During a seizure, a child will usually not really be aware of what is going on around him.

- Child falls into a deep sleep afterward. This is called a *post-ictal state,* and is a sure sign that what just happened was a seizure.

If your baby or child begins having suspicious movements, and they occur predictably enough that you can get them on video, do so. This will really be useful to the doctor.

Causes

The first thing all parents want to know is why their child had a seizure, and if it will happen again. Although there are some known causes that will be tested for, most of the time all results are normal and an answer can't be found. Here are the possible causes:

- Fever. Sometimes a high fever due to a routine illness can cause convulsions. These febrile seizures are evaluated and treated differently than non-febrile seizures. See page 461 for more information.

- Meningitis. Some cases of meningitis (see page 393) will have seizures. Fortunately, most cases of seizures are not caused by meningitis.

- Brain tumor. This is the one cause that is on every parent's mind. Tumors are an extremely rare cause of seizures.

- Low blood sugar. This is a somewhat common cause.

- Electrolyte imbalance. Various electrolyte levels (calcium, sodium, magnesium, potassium) can sometimes be too high or too low, which can trigger a seizure.

- Stroke. Another very rare, but serious, cause.

- Metabolic problem. Some infants are born with defects in their metabolism that allow certain proteins or acids to build up. This will often trigger a seizure.

What Your Pediatrician (or Emergency Physician) Might Do

The most important thing to do (besides giving medication to stop the seizure if it is still occurring) is to rule out any urgent causes that require immediate correction. Here are the steps the doctor might follow:

Febrile seizures. If your child has a fever (or had one that day), the doctor will probably treat this less seriously because it isn't as much of a worry. He will make sure there isn't any serious or treatable infection going on. See page 461.

Recent medical history. The doctor will ask many questions about the past few days to see if there was any unusual event that might have been a trigger.

Physical exam. A thorough exam is important to look for any signs of infection, recent trauma, or neurologic problems.

Blood testing. The doctor may do some blood work to rule out any easily correctable electrolyte problems.

If no cause is found, and all tests are normal, most doctors will take a wait-and-see approach. Many children who have one seizure will never have one again. There's a saying in medicine: "The first seizure is free," meaning that other than looking for any immediate cause, most doctors agree that no further evaluation is warranted right away.

Recurrent Seizures

A small percentage of children will go on to have another seizure days, weeks, or months later. Now a further evaluation is warranted. Here's what your doctor will probably do:

EEG test. An EEG, or *electroencephalogram,* measures the electrical activity throughout the brain, looking for any areas of minor or continuous seizure activity. Numerous electrodes are taped to the child's head and you sit with him in the EEG lab for about an hour. This test can be ordered by the pediatrician or family doctor while a referral to a neurologist is under way (an EEG can be obtained much faster than a neurology appointment in most places).

Neurology appointment. Usually a neurologist will take over further testing and decide what, if any, tests or treatments need to be done. Further testing options include MRI of the brain, more extensive blood work, and a more detailed twenty-four-hour EEG.

Seizure medications. Unless a correctable cause of the seizures is found (in most cases one isn't), an anticonvulsant medication will probably be prescribed if your child has had two or more definite seizures, especially if the EEG shows underlying seizure activity within the brain.

Outgrowing Seizures

Fortunately, many kids outgrow their seizure disorder, stop having seizures, and come off the medication. After a child is seizure-free on a medication for about a year or two, most neurologists will allow you to stop your child's treatment and see if the seizures return. In most cases they don't.

SEIZURES, FEBRILE

Convulsions experienced by infants or small children during a fever are known as *febrile seizures.* When a child experiences a febrile seizure, she will often lose consciousness, and one or more of her limbs will begin to shake or convulse. Febrile seizures can last for as little as a few seconds to more than fifteen minutes; most last less than two minutes. Febrile seizures are fairly common. Approximately one in every twenty-five children will have a febrile seizure in her lifetime. About one-third of children who experience a first febrile seizure will experience additional febrile seizures during their lifetime. Most febrile seizures occur in children between six months and five years of age. After this, children typically outgrow them.

The exact mechanism for the development of a febrile seizure is unknown, and we don't know why some children with fevers get febrile seizures and others do not. Febrile seizures usually occur when a child has a rapidly rising rectal temperature greater than 102 degrees and generally within the first day of a child's fever. Remember that even if your child does have a fever greater than 102 degrees, the risk of having a febrile seizure is relatively low.

Are Febrile Seizures Harmful?

A febrile seizure is a very frightening experience for parents. The good news is that the overwhelming majority of febrile seizures are not harmful. A frequent question we get from parents is "Will the febrile seizures increase my child's risk for epilepsy or brain damage?" There is no evidence to suggest that febrile seizures cause brain damage of any kind. And, about 98 percent of children who suffer from febrile seizures will NOT go on to develop epilepsy. However, a small percentage (between 2 and 5 percent) may develop epilepsy later in life.

It is important to inform your pediatrician whenever your child suffers a febrile seizure to insure that there is nothing more serious or potentially life-threatening going on, such as meningitis or another serious infection, as seizure can be a symptom of more serious illness.

Risk Factors

There are several things that may increase your child's susceptibility to febrile seizures. These include:

- history of frequent, high fevers
- family history of febrile seizures
- first febrile seizure occurred before fifteen months of age

Diagnosis and Treatment

Most febrile seizures are observed by parents or caregivers. By the time a child is seen by a doctor, the febrile seizure has stopped. Your pediatrician or emergency room physician may want to perform tests to rule out any other serious infections, such as meningitis. Once other causes of the seizure have been ruled out, most cases require no further treatment. Children with febrile seizures generally do not need to be hospitalized. However, children with prolonged febrile seizures or other signs of infection should be hospitalized for further evaluation and treatment.

What to Do

- Stay calm.

- Place the child on the floor to prevent falls during the seizure.

- Do not restrain or try to pin down a child who is experiencing a febrile seizure, as this can lead to further injury.

- If possible, remove any objects, such as food, from the child's mouth and place him on his side to prevent choking during the seizure.

- NEVER place any object inside a child's mouth during a seizure. Objects in the mouth can be broken off and lead to choking.

- Call 911 so that emergency medical personnel can arrive to assist your child if the seizure doesn't stop shortly. Fortunately, in most cases the seizure lasts only a minute or three, and by the time the ambulance arrives there isn't any emergency care needed. But it's important to have professional help on hand just in case. The ambulance will likely take you and your child to the nearest emergency room for evaluation. Call your pediatrician as well to let him know what is occurring.

Prevention

Prevention among children who are prone to febrile seizures can be difficult. Using fever-reducing medication, such as acetaminophen or ibuprofen, can help lower the fever. It has never been proven that using fever-lowering drugs lowers a child's risk for febrile seizures, but it is a good idea to use these medications in fevers greater than 101.5 degrees in order to make the child more comfortable and prevent a fever from rapidly getting higher. Occasionally, children who are especially prone to febrile seizures may be prescribed anticonvulsant medication (a rectal suppository) to take for when they are experiencing a prolonged fever.

The good news is almost all children will outgrow febrile seizures by the age of five.

SENSORY PROCESSING DISORDER (SPD)

Sensory processing disorder (SPD) is a newly recognized developmental disorder in which the brain has difficulty accepting various sensations and turning them around into appropriate behavioral and motor responses. Children are exposed to numerous sensations on a daily basis: the feeling of certain clothes against their skin, loud noises in crowded rooms, odors and textures of various foods, swinging and spinning movements on playgrounds, and sticky hands during various art and craft projects. While most children experience these sensations without a second thought, the central nervous system of a child with SPD will be overstimulated by some or all of them and won't know how to appropri-

ately react to them. The result is a constant influx of irritating sensory input that the brain can't process correctly. With time and maturity, the child may eventually begin to filter out and handle this better, but SPD can create some developmental challenges along the way because the child doesn't interact appropriately with the world around him. Fortunately, SPD is treatable. Early recognition is important.

Symptoms

Signs will vary according to the age of the child:

SPD in infants

- has colicky symptoms

- is bothered by certain articles of clothing and tags

- sleeps restlessly

- has need for constant motion

- resists being held in a cradle position

- may not like being swaddled

- becomes overwhelmed by loud crowds and noises

SPD in toddlers

- extreme tantrums

- refuses to wear shoes or socks that don't feel "right"

- refuses to walk barefoot in sand or grass

- won't wear clothing that doesn't fit correctly

- bothered by tags on clothing
- has developmental delays in balance and coordination
- has finicky eating habits; refuses certain food textures

SPD in preschoolers

- won't engage in activities that involve bouncing, spinning, or swinging
- shows hyperactive and fidgety behavior
- has immature social development
- has obsessive-compulsive tendencies

The consequences of SPD vary greatly. Many children simply mature and begin to handle sensations properly and don't have any challenges at all. Some, however, will continue to struggle, and once they reach school age they have some difficulty understanding the subtle nuances of social behavior and interaction with their peers. This can result in social developmental immaturity that begins to be noticed by other kids.

Treatment

SPD is usually diagnosed by a pediatric occupational therapist. These are found in children's hospitals, university medical centers, state-funded developmental therapy programs, and private centers that treat various developmental disorders. Any parent who suspects her child might have SPD should get an evaluation right away. SPD can exist alone or be part of a more significant developmental disorder such as autism.

Treatment involves specialized occupational therapy techniques that are designed to gradually

---

READ MORE ABOUT IT

In *The Autism Book,* Dr. Bob covers SPD in more detail, including various alternative medical approaches to treating it. Even when autism isn't involved, many of the treatments designed for autism may improve SPD as well. Visit www .TheAutismBook.com for more information.

---

expose a child to the offending sensations. In this way, the child learns to handle them appropriately. Exercises vary according to the child's individual age and needs. Therapy should be guided by an occupational therapist who is specifically trained in sensory integration therapy. Because SPD is a newly recognized disorder, some traditional occupational therapists are not trained to treat it.

For more information, visit www .SPDfoundation.net.

SEXUALLY TRANSMITTED DISEASES (STDs)

Sexually transmitted diseases (or STDs) are becoming more and more common among the adolescent and young adult population. Here is a brief discussion of the various types of STDs, when to suspect your teenager may have one, possible complications, and treatments.

Chlamydia

Chlamydia is the most common sexually transmitted disease in the United States today. More than one million people in this

**DR. SEARS TIP
Talk to Your Teen, Early**

Talk to your preteen or adolescent about sex and any serious consequences. It is important not to take a judgmental attitude. It is enough to review the dangers listed here. Note that "safe-sex" practices are not an absolute guarantee. Above all, the Pill and use of a condom cannot protect a person's heart.

country get chlamydia every year. It is caused by infection from the bacteria *Chlamydia trachomatis*.

Symptoms in women. About 70 percent of women with chlamydia may have no symptoms at all. This is why all sexually active females *must* be screened for chlamydia and other STDs. If women do have symptoms, they include:

- burning upon urination
- discharge from the vagina
- pain while having sex
- rectal pain
- abdominal pain

Symptoms in men. Men who are infected with chlamydia are more likely to have symptoms than women. However, up to 25 percent of men with chlamydia infection have no symptoms at all. Symptoms among men include:

- clear, cloudy, or yellowish discharge coming from the penis
- sensation of burning upon urination
- testicles that may be tender to the touch
- rectal pain or discharge

Diagnosis. Again, all sexually active females should be screened for chlamydia and other STDs during their annual Pap smear and, of course, if they are ever having symptoms. The doctor can test for chlamydia infection by obtaining a sample of the discharge in males or females. Some tests use urine samples. It is also important to obtain samples from any and all sexual partners.

Treatment. Since it is a bacterial infection, a variety of antibiotics effectively treat chlamydia. Sexual partners should also be treated at the same time to avoid the possibility of re-infection. A follow-up test after treatment is completed may be done.

Prevention. Using safe sexual practices is of the utmost importance. *The most effective form of prevention is through abstinence.* Condoms must be used every time, and stable monogamous relationships must be encouraged. People at highest risk for chlamydia are those with multiple sex partners who do not practice "safe sex."

Long-term complications. There are several potential long-term complications of this disease, especially in women. These include:

- pelvic inflammatory disease (PID)
- salpingitis: inflammation of the fallopian tubes that can lead to long-term scarring of the fallopian tubes, possible infertility, and ectopic pregnancy (which can be fatal if not detected early)

Chlamydia infection can also cause complications in newborns who are born to women infected with chlamydia at the time of delivery. Complications can include severe eye infections or chlamydial pneumonia as the infant comes into contact with the chlamydia bacteria upon passing through the birth canal.

Gonorrhea

This STD, also known as "the clap," is another bacterial infection transmitted sexually. It is caused by the *Neisseria gonorrhea* bacteria and is the second most common STD in the United States, affecting around 700,000 people a year. The bacteria can be passed from one person to another through vaginal sex, oral sex, or anal sex.

Symptoms in women. Women may have few or no symptoms at all, or they may have very severe symptoms. Possible symptoms include:

• burning or painful sensation while urinating; infected women may urinate more often

• discharge from the vagina

• pain during sexual intercourse

• pain in the lower abdominal area in severe infection

• sore throat if gonorrhea was transmitted through oral sex

• fever

Symptoms in men. Again, symptoms vary widely from no symptoms at all to severe symptoms, including:

• urinating more often or feeling the need to urinate more often

• burning and painful urination

• painful penile discharge that may appear white, cloudy, or yellow

• testicles that may be tender or slightly swollen

• sore throat if the gonorrhea infection is passed through oral sex

Talk to your pediatrician if your adolescent is experiencing any of these possible symptoms. This can sometimes be a tricky proposition, as teenagers are often reluctant to admit they are participating in sexual activity.

Diagnosis. Samples of any discharge from the penis, vagina, rectum, or throat can be tested. Urine can also be tested. Because it is possible to have more than one type of STD at the same time, people with gonorrhea may also be tested for other STDs, including chlamydia and human papillomavirus (HPV).

Treatment. Gonorrhea infection is treated in a similar fashion as chlamydia. Since gonorrhea is a type of bacteria, certain types of antibiotics are used for treatment. The doctor will decide upon treatment depending on how severe the infection is. It is also very important to test all sexual partners to be sure they do not have gonorrhea. Early treatment with antibiotics is important in order to lower the risk of long-term complications.

Prevention. The only sure way of avoiding gonorrhea infection is through abstinence. Also, it is important to explain that it is possible to transmit gonorrhea through oral contact. A stable, monogamous relationship lowers the risk greatly. Using a condom with every partner, every time, is very important.

Long-term complications. There are several potential long-term complications of this STD. Among women, long-term complications are similar to the complications from chlamydia infection (mentioned above). Untreated or poorly treated gonorrhea infection can lead to infertility and ectopic pregnancy. This occurs through permanent scarring of the woman's fallopian tubes. Other potential complications among women include:

- pelvic inflammatory disease (PID)
- long-term problems with pain during sex

Possible long-term complications in men:

- long-term problems with urination
- narrowing of the urethra, leading to possible fertility problems
- formation of an abscess around the ureter
- kidney failure

Gonorrhea infection can occasionally become a body-wide infection. This is known as *bacteremia* and can be potentially life-threatening and require hospitalization. Gonorrhea can even infect the joints of various parts of the body, especially the knees.

As with chlamydia infection, a newborn can be infected with gonorrhea upon passage through the birth canal of a woman who has a gonorrhea infection. Complications can include severe eye infection (known as gonococcal conjunctivitis), pneumonia, and sepsis, a blood infection that can be fatal.

Hepatitis B

This is a virus that attacks the liver. Although most adults who catch hepatitis B get through it without any long-term problems, a small percentage will suffer permanent liver damage, liver failure, and become lifelong hepatitis B carriers. It is transmitted through unprotected sexual intercourse, by sharing intravenous (IV) drug needles, and rarely by blood transfusions, contaminated tattoo needles, or ear-piercing equipment. Infants who catch

hepatitis B from their mother during the birth process and children who catch hepatitis B through accidental blood exposure are very likely to suffer chronic liver failure. Hepatitis B is very different from the fairly benign hepatitis A, which is an intestinal illness caused by food poisoning (see page 361). There is also a hepatitis C, which is covered on page 362.

Symptoms. Some people who contract the virus don't notice any signs at all. Those who do may show a wide variety of symptoms with varying degrees of severity:

- jaundice — yellow eyes and skin
- abdominal pain
- poor appetite
- fatigue
- vomiting

Diagnosis. Hepatitis B is diagnosed with a blood test.

Treatment. There is no treatment to help a person through the initial phases of the liver disease. Once a person has recovered (*if* he recovers) and becomes a chronic carrier of the virus, chemotherapy medications are somewhat effective in limiting further liver damage and may eliminate the virus completely.

Prevention. "Safe" sexual practices (or *abstinence!*) and not sharing IV drug needles (or not using any drugs at all!) are the two primary ways to prevent exposure to the virus. Identification of hepatitis B–positive pregnant mothers, so that proper treatment can be given to the newborns to prevent transmission of the virus, is critical. The hepatitis B vaccine is given to all infants to prevent accidental infection during childhood and to offer protection once sexual activity begins. If your older child has never had this vaccine, talk to your pediatrician about getting this three-shot series at your next appointment.

Herpes Simplex Type II (HSV-II)

There are several types of herpes viruses, but the only one that is an STD is herpes simplex type II (HSV-II), or genital herpes. For information on oral herpes simplex type I, see page 364.

Symptoms. When someone is exposed to genital herpes infection for the first time, symptoms usually begin as fever, headache, fatigue, and muscle aches, lasting up to a week. Several days after these symptoms begin, painful red sores begin to appear. In women, they often appear on the external genitalia, including the labia, inside the vagina, and often the cervix. In men, they usually appear on the head or shaft of the penis and occasionally on the scrotum, thighs, and buttocks. These sores are extremely painful and often drain. They last for several days, up to two weeks, and slowly crust over. Some individuals show no symptoms.

Unfortunately, like its cousin oral herpes, genital herpes recurs over time. The first year of infection usually has the most recurrences. Some people can experience ten or more outbreaks in the first year. Patients often report feeling tenderness, pain, and a burning sensation in the genital area one to two days prior to outbreak of the herpes lesions. Outbreaks can also be associated with triggers such as illness, stress or anxiety, and a weakened immune system. Women also are more at risk for outbreaks during their menstrual periods.

Diagnosis. Genital herpes can be diagnosed with testing. Often samples from the painful areas are collected and a viral culture can be performed.

 DR. SEARS TIP
Children with Herpes

Any child diagnosed with genital herpes must be evaluated for signs of sexual abuse.

Treatment. There is no cure for genital herpes. Antiviral medications have been developed that can lessen the severity and length of herpes outbreaks. Two methods of treatment for genital herpes have been devised. One method focuses on beginning antiviral medication at the first signs of an outbreak to lessen the severity of the disease, and the other involves daily suppressive therapy with an antiviral medication. This has the benefit of reducing the number of outbreaks, as well as reducing the risk of transmission to one's partner. Talk to your pediatrician for more information on treatment of genital herpes.

Prevention. Intercourse should never take place if one partner has an outbreak. Parents, talk with your teens about what genital herpes is and its lifelong consequences. The only surefire way to avoid herpes is *abstinence* from genital and oral sex. Increasingly, cases of genital herpes transmitted through oral sex have been documented. Genital herpes can infect the oral cavities the same way it infects the genital area, and is becoming more and more common. If your teen is sexually active, stress the importance of "safe" sexual practices and avoidance of high-risk sexual behaviors, such as multiple sex partners. It is sobering to note that some studies have shown that the majority of individuals are infected with genital herpes when their partners showed no signs or symptoms of an outbreak.

Neonatal Herpes

This rare but serious and potentially fatal disease of the newborn period is caused by herpes simplex type II, or genital herpes, but a small percentage may be due to herpes simplex type I, or oral herpes. Newborns are usually infected during passage through the birth canal. Occasionally, the fetus may be infected while still in the womb. If you are pregnant or thinking of becoming pregnant, it is very important to tell your obstetrician if you have a history of genital herpes, a partner with genital herpes, or a history of potential exposure.

Symptoms. Many infants who are infected with herpes virus are born prematurely and have low birth weights. Initial symptoms may be non-specific and may include irritability, lethargy, fever, or poor feeding. Any infant with the above symptoms should immediately be evaluated, and most likely hospitalized. Symptoms then usually progress to the appearance of herpes lesions on the skin, eyes, and inside the mouth. Seizures may occur within days of initial symptoms. Untreated, neonatal herpes can progress to a body-wide infection involving multiple organ failure.

Diagnosis and treatment. If a newborn exhibits symptoms indicating possible neonatal herpes, immediate hospitalization is required along with extensive testing. A viral culture will be performed of multiple body fluid sites, as well as tests for other serious types of disease. Treatment usually involves intravenous antiviral medications. Women who are known to be infected with herpes are sometimes treated with oral antiviral medication in their last trimester of pregnancy.

Complications. Complications of this disease can include:

• seizures

• muscle spasm

• blindness

• learning disabilities

• coordination difficulties

Both parents should give thorough sexual histories during their first prenatal visit. If any STD is present, parents should be counseled on safe sexual practices and condom use during pregnancy. All women in labor with active herpes infections must deliver their infants by cesarean section, which will lower the chances of the infants being infected.

HIV (Human Immunodeficiency Virus)

Human immunodeficiency virus (HIV) is a very serious and complicated disease. Due to the constantly changing information regarding treatment of HIV, we have decided not to include specific details on HIV in this book. Prevention is similar to the various other STDs. For the most up-to-date information on HIV, visit www.cdc.gov.

Human Papillomavirus (HPV)

Human papillomavirus (HPV) is a group of several viruses that can infect humans. Certain types of HPV can cause genital warts, while other types have been found to lead to cervical cancer in women.

Genital warts are transmitted when an infected individual comes into sexual contact with another person. They are often visible on the penis or outer portions of the vagina.

Risk factors. Anyone who engages in sexual intercourse is at risk, particularly men or women with a history of multiple sexual partners. It is now known that when a woman is exposed to high-risk types of HPV during sexual contact, the virus can invade the cells of the woman's cervix. Approximately 90 percent of the time, a woman's natural defenses will clear the HPV infection. In about 10 percent of cases, the HPV infection can lead to abnormalities of the cells of the cervix. Over time, this can lead to cervical cancer. Women are usually infected with HPV by men who are carriers of the high-risk type but don't show any symptoms of infection.

Diagnosis. After becoming sexually active, women should get yearly Pap smears in order to detect the presence of HPV infection. Along with traditional Pap smears, many doctors are now testing women for high-risk types of HPV. Regular Pap smears are important in order to detect abnormalities before they turn into cancer. Virtually all visible warts in the genital area are from HPV. A doctor can test the wart to determine if it's a high-risk type of HPV.

Treatment. Therapy depends on where the HPV is found:

• Genital warts. There are several treatments for genital warts. The most common therapy is podophyllin applied topically by the doctor or the patient himself. Other topical treatments include various acids or freezing. Electrocautery, laser surgery, and

READ MORE ABOUT IT

Read about the HPV vaccine and the Hep B vaccine in *The Vaccine Book* by Robert Sears.

surgical excision can also be done. Recurrence of warts near the treatment areas is fairly common.

• Cervical HPV. If an adolescent or adult is found to have HPV infection along with an abnormal Pap smear, further testing and treatments may be needed. These include biopsy of the cervix and possible removal of the abnormal cells of the cervix.

Prevention. HPV infection is preventable through several methods. Condom use can reduce the risk of infection. Also, avoiding high-risk sexual activities, such as beginning sexual intercourse at a young age and having multiple sexual partners, can lower one's risk of infection. Abstinence works best.

The latest breakthrough is that a vaccine against HPV has been developed. The vaccine has been approved for men and women between the ages of nine and twenty-six, and is given in a three-shot series. It is hoped that vaccinating all young people against HPV prior to exposure to human papillomavirus will drastically reduce the number of abnormal Pap smears in women and thereby the incidence of cervical cancer.

Syphilis

This STD is less common than the ones mentioned above, but the rates of syphilis have been steadily increasing. Syphilis is caused by a bacteria called *Treponema pallidum*. The age group most at risk for exposure is sexually active adults between twenty and twenty-nine years of age. However, syphilis is occasionally seen in younger people. It is spread through sexual contact.

Symptoms. Initial symptoms of syphilis are usually nothing more than the presence of one or more painless sores (called *chancres*) a few weeks after exposure. These sores are usually present in the groin region and/or inside the vagina of females and are usually gone within six weeks. The patient usually has no other symptoms. If left untreated, syphilis will progress through life. See long-term complications below.

Diagnosis. There are several blood tests that can be performed to test for syphilis.

Treatment. Syphilis is very treatable when diagnosed early. Because it is a type of bacteria, antibiotics are used. Injected penicillin is still the most effective treatment and usually only one treatment is required.

Prevention. "Safe sex" practices (condom use with each partner) dramatically lowers the risk of syphilis. Abstinence is 100 percent safe.

Long-term complications. If left untreated in the initial stage, the disease can progress through two more stages. The second and third stages of syphilis can take decades to develop, and symptoms are usually not seen until later in life, including nervous system, heart, blood vessel, skin, and bone problems. Talk to your pediatrician if you'd like more information.

Congenital Syphilis

This is a very unfortunate medical condition that occurs when a pregnant mother infected with syphilis passes it on to her fetus through the placenta during pregnancy. This is life-threatening for the fetus. About half the fetuses infected with syphilis in the womb die during the pregnancy or shortly after birth if not treated. Mothers who are infected earlier in the pregnancy tend to have more complications in their babies than those who are infected later in the pregnancy. Thankfully, this condition is rare today. Women in the United States are screened for syphilis during pregnancy.

Symptoms in newborns:

• poor weight gain, also known as "failure to thrive"

• large amount of clear discharge from the eyes

• extreme irritability

• small, red-spot rash on the palms of the hands and soles of feet

• expanding rash that can spread to the face, genitalia, and anus

• pneumonia

• abnormally shaped or small nose

Symptoms in infants and toddlers:

• bone pain, often in the arms and legs

• swelling of the joints

• refusal to move arms and legs due to the pain

• abnormally shaped teeth

- loss of vision

- diminished hearing or deafness

- scars on the skin due to the rash

Diagnosis. As mentioned above, all pregnant women in the United States are tested during pregnancy for syphilis. In children with suspected syphilis, other testing will be performed.

Treatment. There are very effective treatments if syphilis is diagnosed early. Pregnant women who test positive for syphilis will receive penicillin during their pregnancy. This will treat the fetus as well and drastically reduces the chance that syphilis will be passed through the placenta to the fetus. When detected and treated early, infants have an excellent long-term prognosis. After birth, affected infants will also receive penicillin treatments to eradicate the germ.

Long-term complications. If treatment is delayed or not given at all, there are several long-term complications. Among these are:

- severe hearing loss or deafness

- blindness

- multiple deformities of the facial structures and bones

DR. SEARS TIP
Learn More About It

Educate yourself about STDs, then educate your children in an open fashion. STDs can cause a lifetime of medical problems and regrets. There is good information available online through the government's website at www.cdc.gov.

- mental retardation and other neurological abnormalities

- abnormalities of the teeth

SINUS INFECTIONS

Sinus infections typically don't occur in infants and toddlers because children don't develop sinus spaces around their nose and eyes until they are a few years old. They are, however, a common occurrence among children and adults. Here is how you can diagnose and treat your child's sinus infection.

Symptoms

Sinus infections typically don't just come out of nowhere. They usually occur as a complication of a prolonged cold. A cold virus creates nasal congestion and mucus production. As the mucus sits in the sinus spaces, the bacteria overgrow and create thicker, greener

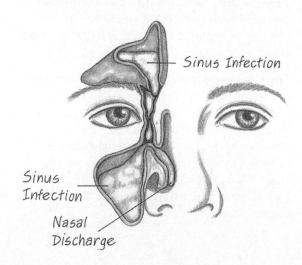

Sinus Infection

Sinus Infection

Nasal Discharge

mucus and irritate the facial bones and tissues surrounding the sinuses. Here are the symptoms to watch for:

- thicker, greener nasal drainage after one to two weeks of a common cold

- headaches, especially around the eyes and forehead

- tenderness when pressing on the upper cheeks and around the eyes

- pain in the upper teeth or jaw (the sinuses are right above this area)

- fever may or may not be present

- in the absence of the above bothersome symptoms, any green nasal drainage that persists for more than three weeks

- chronic cough with nasal drainage for more than a month

Some common cold and flu viruses can hit hard and create these symptoms right at the start, yet it is unlikely that any bacteria have had enough time to create a true bacterial sinus infection until one or two weeks have passed. So don't be too quick to rush into the doctor thinking your child needs antibiotics right away.

DR. SEARS TIP
Antibiotics? Just Say Wait!

Several years ago medical researchers discovered that most sinus infections will resolve after a few weeks without antibiotics. With antibiotic resistance on the rise, the American Academy of Pediatrics (AAP) created a new policy recommending that doctors do not prescribe antibiotics for sinus infections during the first few weeks of symptoms (unless a patient is significantly ill).

Home Remedies

Treatments for a sinus infection are the same as for a regular cold on page 222: nose hosing, steam cleaning, and supportive natural remedies or over-the-counter (OTC) medications. For a bothersome sinus infection, here are a few tips:

- Decongestant medications and pain relievers (ibuprofen or acetaminophen). This is a great combination to relieve sinus headaches and pressure. Current guidelines as of the publishing of this book state that children under four years of age should not use OTC cold and cough medications.

- Nasal flush. Instead of simply using a saline mist or steam to clean the nose, follow our sinus flushing suggestions on page 21 every day to really experience a nice cleanout.

- Herbal remedies to support sinus and respiratory health. In our office we have found that Sinupret, an herbal remedy for the sinus and respiratory systems, can be of benefit to kids and adults. Check out www.SinupretForKids.com.

When to See a Doctor

Because antibiotics probably won't be prescribed during the early weeks of the illness, there's no hurry to rush into the doctor's office. Many patients come into our office after just a few days of symptoms "to see if it's a sinus infection." The truth is, it doesn't matter in the first week or two whether it's a bacterial sinus infection or just a long cold, because the treatment is the same at this stage. Plus, the doctor can't directly visualize the sinuses to see if they are infected (like she can the ear or throat), so she might not be certain anyway. Therefore, don't waste your time and money with an early visit. Here are the two situations that do warrant an appointment:

- Severe symptoms, such as fever, headache, and facial pain with green nasal drainage, that persist more than five days at any time during the illness. If your child is significantly ill, your doctor will prescribe antibiotics.

- Prolonged green nasal congestion that lasts for more than three weeks. If you've given the home treatments a valiant effort, and your child continues to suffer from sinus symptoms, see your pediatrician.

A sinus infection is rarely a reason to go to an emergency room or urgent care facility. It can usually wait until the doctor's office next opens. When antibiotics are prescribed for a severe sinus infection, expect a fourteen- to twenty-one-day course. The usual seven- to ten-day course may not be long enough to really clear out the infection. And don't rely on antibiotics alone; continue your usual home treatments and natural supplements to augment drainage and healing.

SLEEP APNEA

Obstructive sleep apnea (OSA), also called *obstructive sleep apnea syndrome* (OSAS), is a commonly overlooked cause of inadequate, restless sleep, and consequently of poor alertness and behavior. OSA is usually caused by an obstruction in the nose or throat severe enough to interfere with breathing — either blocked nasal passages or swollen tonsils and/ or adenoids. When the airways are partially obstructed, the child will partially awaken and be startled from lack of air. Because he's scared, he gets an adrenaline rush, which further revs up the nervous system and interferes with sleep. The muscles that normally keep the airway open during the day become relaxed during sleep, narrowing the airway at night. The air passing through these narrowed airways causes a vibration of the respiratory passage tissue, producing snoring. Because the airways are partially obstructed during sleep, the child does not go through the normal stages of light and deep sleep and, therefore, does not enjoy good-quality sleep, although he may seem to stay asleep. Poor-quality sleep at night carries over into poor behavior and learning the following day.

Signs and Symptoms

- Loud snoring. Children with OSA will usually snore almost as loud as adults. When you can hear the snoring from down the hall, this should be your first clue that OSA may be a problem.

- Mouth breathing. A child with OSA will probably breathe through her mouth most of the night (as opposed to the normal comfortable nose breathing that most kids do). You may also start to observe more mouth breathing during the day as well.

- Gasps and pauses in breathing. The child may snort and gasp a lot while sleeping. The typical child with OSA breathes normally during the day but has noisy and irregular breathing at night with frequent ten- to fifteen-second pauses followed by a loud and heavy "catch-up" breath.

- Turning and twisting a lot during sleep and sleeping in unusual positions. A child with OSA will tend to twist her neck and body to figure out the position in which she sleeps best, either on her tummy, back, side, or with her neck extended and mouth wide open.

- Early-morning troubled sleep. Because OSA occurs mostly during REM (rapid eye movement) sleep, and the greatest amount of REM sleep occurs in the early-morning hours, OSA may be worse during the few hours before your child normally wakes up. This is important because the early-morning hours are when parents are least likely to hear or observe their child's troubled breathing during sleep.

- Excessive daytime tiredness. The lack of restful sleep may leave your child feeling more tired during the day.

- Otherwise unexplained behavior problems. A tired child will be grumpy. Think about OSA if your snoring child is a handful behaviorally.

- Poor school performance. Without adequate rejuvenation overnight, the brain won't be able to focus during the day.

 DR. SEARS TIP
Suspect OSA with ADD

OSA is a commonly overlooked cause of ADD (attention deficit disorder) or ADHD (attention deficit hyperactivity disorder). Be sure to evaluate your child's quality of sleep if he receives the ADD label.

What to Do

If you suspect your child has OSA, your pediatrician should evaluate your child. But before you make an appointment, do a home study.

Home study. You can make your own observations and collect your own data on your child by doing the following:

- Observe your child's sleep. During the late evening, sit and watch your child sleep for a couple hours. Observe for mouth breathing, pauses in breathing, gasping, and restless sleep. You can also set your alarm for the middle of the night and observe for a short time to get a better idea of how persistent the problems are throughout the night. Keep a written log of how many pauses and gasps you see over how many minutes each night.

- Make a video of your child's sleep patterns. Usually your child's doctor or an ENT (ear, nose, throat) specialist can make the diagnosis, or at least have a high degree of suspicion, just by looking at your child's sleep patterns on the video. The doctor will mainly be looking for the sounds and sights of breathing difficulty.

ENT exam. Schedule an exam by your child's doctor or an ENT specialist. Be sure to take your sleep log and video with you. The doctor will evaluate your child's airway, starting with the nose, and focus on the tonsils and adenoids. By listening to your child's history, examining your sleep log, and watching the video, the doctor can usually make the diagnosis and prescribe proper treatment. If tonsils and/or adenoids are the problem, they should be in a pickle jar. If it is unclear whether or not the sleep apnea is harmful enough to require surgical treatment, the doctor may recommend the next step:

A sleep study. *Nocturnal polysomnography — sleep study* for short — is the gold standard in diagnosis and assessment of OSA. Your child would stay overnight in a sleep laboratory. (Tell your child it's like a hotel room with a lot of video cameras.) Using leads that are taped on the head and chest, your child's sleep patterns will be recorded, mainly to see if he has the normal in-and-out pattern of light and deep sleep. A small, painless clip will be taped to one of your child's fingers to measure the percentage of oxygen in his blood during the night. The sleep study measures how much your child's blood oxygen drops during obstruction. An electrocardiogram (ECG) will also be performed. A thorough evaluation of the physiologic changes that occur during sleep is very important. Persistent, untreated OSA can not only weaken a child's overall growth and learning but also overstress the heart. A sleep study is the most accurate way to diagnose simple snoring that needs no treatment or OSA that requires removal of the obstruction.

Abbreviated sleep study. If spending the night in a sleep laboratory is not appealing, your pediatrician may recommend a naptime sleep study, which is an abbreviated study of the blood-oxygen and sleep patterns during a two- to three-hour nap. However, naptime sleep studies are only reliable if they show positive results. A "normal naptime sleep study" does not necessarily exclude the possibility of OSA at night. The doctor would probably then recommend doing a more thorough overnight sleep study.

If your child's OSA is due to tonsils and/or adenoids, your pediatrician will probably recommend that these obstructive tissues be taken out as soon as possible. (See information on tonsillectomy, page 525.) In addition, you can help your child breathe and sleep better with the following home remedies:

- Air purify the bedroom (see page 135).

- Use a "nose hose" and "steam clean" to clear nasal passages (see page 20).

- Treat nasal allergies (see page 131) and eliminate allergenic foods.

- Adjust the child's sleep positions to best relieve obstructive breathing. (The sleep specialist who performed the sleep study can advise you on these positions, based upon the results of the study.) Older children and adults with OSA sometimes need to sleep with a special facial mask designed to keep the airways open. This is called *continuous positive airway pressure (CPAP)*.

 DR. SEARS TIP
Take OSA Seriously

If you suspect your child's poor sleep, behavior, or school performance may be due to OSA, be sure you and your pediatrician do a thorough evaluation and find the right treatment. In our experience, many behavioral and learning problems can be attributed to OSA, but the diagnosis can be missed.

SLEEP PROBLEMS

"How do I get my baby to sleep through the night?" is one of the most common questions pediatricians get. It is also one of the most difficult ones to answer. Here are ten time-tested ways to help your whole family get a more restful night's sleep.

1. Develop a Healthy Sleep Attitude.

Instead of *putting* your baby down to sleep, think of parenting your baby to sleep. You cannot force a baby to sleep. Think of your role as creating restful conditions that allow sleep to overtake Baby so that he goes to sleep more willingly and stays asleep as long as he needs to. Remember, the ultimate goal of your nighttime parenting is to instill in your baby a healthy sleep attitude: that sleep is a pleasant state to enter and a fearless state in which to remain. Here's an excerpt from Martha's parenting journal: *Once I changed my attitude toward my baby's night waking, it became much easier. When Peter awakened for a middle-of-the-night nursing, we would snuggle together, just the two of us, with no interference from the busy world. I learned to value this special closeness that, I knew, would pass all too soon.*

2. Establish a Consistent Bedtime Routine.

While you cannot force your baby to sleep, you can set the conditions that encourage sleep to overtake your baby naturally. Babies who have reasonably consistent bedtimes and going-to-sleep rituals usually sleep more predictably at night. Keep experimenting with different bedtime rituals until you find a recipe that gets you and your baby the most restful night's sleep. We like to use the less rigid term *routine* rather than *schedule*. Babies are creatures of habit. A regular bedtime routine will help your baby fall asleep more easily. Bedtime routines set the stage for sleep. In psychology, bedtime is known as a "setting event." A rou-

tine sets you up to expect the usual consequence. When Baby begins the night with a set routine, such as rocking, wearing down in a baby sling, walking around the house, taking a relaxing bath, hearing a bedtime story, getting a back rub, or whatever ritual works, she is set up to expect that sleep will follow this routine. A bedtime routine helps your child learn to associate the sequence of events with feeling relaxed and sleepy. This pattern of association becomes established in Baby's mind.

DR. SEARS TIP
Enjoy "Wearing Down"

Here is a Sears family sleep tip that we have used with all of our babies: Shortly before the consistent and predictable bedtime you strive for, put your baby in a baby sling and stroll around the house while listening to soothing music. Your walking and swaying motion will eventually lull Baby to sleep. See page 236 for tips on how to use a sling safely.

3. Anticipate Your Baby's Sleep Signs.

You can't force a baby who is not sleepy to sleep. Make a sleepy-time chart to help you anticipate Baby's "ready for sleep" signs: droopy eyelids, eye rubbing, cranky behavior, and slowing down in activity. Every evening for a week, write down the time when Baby seems sleepy. After a week, analyze the information on your chart. Does Baby seem sleepy around the same time (plus or minus twenty or thirty minutes) every evening, say between 7:30 and 8:00? Record this in your sleepy-time chart. Try this for naptimes, too. Getting to know your baby's ready-to-sleep signs helps you develop a consistent bedtime with fewer hassles. Sleepiness comes in cycles. If Baby's eyelids start drooping at 7 p.m., but you ignore these need-to-sleep signals until 7:30, you've missed your window of opportunity, and Baby may stay awake for another hour.

4. "Move" Baby to Sleep.

Babies love to be rocked or walked to sleep. This isn't all that surprising, since Baby was used to being rocked in the womb. Remember when your baby slept in the womb when you were moving but seemed to be awake and moving when you wanted to sleep? Rocking or walking not only relaxes Baby, it also relaxes frazzled moms and dads. Rock back and forth at approximately sixty beats per minute, the average heart rate your baby was used to listening to in the womb.

As you're walking while wearing Baby, sing and gently pat her on the bottom. These soothing moves, calming sounds, and loving touches will help Baby drift off to sleep. Ease Baby out of the sling or out of your arms when she is in a deep sleep. Trying to put her down before she is completely asleep invites a protest. You can tell when Baby is in a deep sleep and ready to be put down into her bed by watching for the *limp-limb sign:* When Baby's arms and legs are completely relaxed, like a rag doll, and her usual fisted hands are open and relaxed, you'll know she's in a deep sleep.

5. Feed Baby to Sleep.

The sucking rhythm, Mother's warmth and closeness, and warm milk filling the tummy will help Baby drift off to dreamland. If breastfeeding, try the technique we call "nursing down." It not only soothes a fussy baby, but helps relax a tired mommy. Lie down on your side with your baby on your bed. Place a pillow behind your lower back, between your legs, and under your head. Put Baby on his side and pull him close to you to nurse. Nursing down is a great way to nap with your baby or enjoy an early bedtime together. Once Baby is in a deep sleep, ease him off your breast and sneak away, or put him in his own bed. The different ways Baby goes off to sleep are called "sleep associations." Get Baby used to many sleep associations. If Baby is put to sleep the same way all the time, he will learn to expect that. Besides Mother breastfeeding baby off to sleep or Father bottlefeeding off to sleep, get Baby used to other ways, such as wearing down (mentioned above), going to sleep with soft music on, rocking in the arms of a caregiver, or simply being put down when drowsy and patted off to sleep.

6. Set the Stage for Baby to Go to Sleep and Stay Asleep.

Try these tips for a sleep-inducing environment:

Comfortable sleepwear. Be sure that Baby's pajamas are comfortable and soft, such as cotton. Many mothers in our practice have reported that their babies seem restless when they put them in irritating, synthetic sleepwear.

Comfortable temperature and humidity. A comfortable temperature for sleep is around seventy degrees and a humidity of around 50 percent. A warm-mist vaporizer helps keep the temperature where Baby sleeps consistent and prevents dry air from drying out Baby's nasal passages. Babies are less likely to awaken when the temperature in the bedroom is consistent.

Dim the lights. When it's time for bed, start dimming the lights around the house, especially where Baby sleeps. Going from light to darkness stimulates the brain to release the sleep-inducing hormone melatonin.

Sing, sing, sing. Humming lullabies is a great way to get your baby off to sleep. Sing or hum in a low voice with no sudden shifts in pitch, tempo, or volume. The monotony of the melody may induce Baby to sleep.

Clear Baby's nose. Babies who can't breathe well can't sleep. Clear your baby's nose well before bedtime. (See "nose-hose" technique, page 20.)

Clear the air of irritants. If your baby does have a stuffy nose a lot, suspect allergies. To make Baby's bedroom as allergy-free as possible, remove fuzzy blankets, down comforters, and dust-collecting fuzzy toys. Use an air

NIGHTTIME PARENTING TIPS FOR DADS

Here are some nighttime fathering tips from the Sears family men that not only help your baby sleep but help you shine in the eyes of your tired wife:

Try the neck nestle. As soon as Baby shows the usual ready-to-sleep signs, hold or rock Baby with Baby's head nestled in the crook of your neck so that your voice box and chin bones are against Baby's skull. Then sing or hum a droning song, such as "Old Man River" or our favorite: "Go to sleep, go to sleep, go to sleep, my little baby. Go to sleep, go to sleep, go to sleep, my little boy." Use a traditional lullaby melody; add your own words.
The lower-pitched male voice and the deeper vibrations of the male voice box and cheek bones during humming and singing are likely to lull Baby to sleep. Babies hear not only with their eardrums but with the vibration of their skull bones.

Try the warm fuzzy. Drape Baby skin-to-skin on your chest. Exaggerate the rise and fall of your chest during deep breathing while humming. As soon as Baby is in a deep sleep, ease him into his own bed.

Wear your baby. Put Baby in a sling and wear him around the house until he is in a deep sleep and then ease him out of the sling into his bed.

Bring Baby to Mommy. Babies under six months old wake up at least a couple of times a night for feedings, especially if breastfeeding. When Baby does awaken for a feeding, instead of simply rolling over and pretending to be asleep, offer to get out of bed and bring Baby to Mommy for a feeding and then return Baby back to her bed. If Mommy doesn't have to get out of bed, she is likely to get back to sleep more easily. Remember, *nursing* means "comforting." Only mothers can breastfeed, but fathers can also "nurse."

Add the finishing touch. To help Baby learn other ways of falling asleep besides breastfeeding, let Dad be the parent in charge when Baby is finally ready to nod off. After Mom finishes breastfeeding and Baby is drowsy but not fully asleep, gently hand Baby over to Dad to walk or wear Baby down to sleep.

Let Mom sleep in. On weekends, holidays, and other days when neither you nor Mom has to go to work, take your infant or child out for some daddy-child time after first waking and feeding in the morning. Let Mom sleep in while Dad cares for Baby — out of the house.

filter. As an added nighttime perk, the "white noise" of the air filter may help your child sleep. Rid Baby's bedroom of airborne irritants, such as cigarette smoke, baby powder, hairspray, and animal dander (see page 136 for more on allergy prevention in the bedroom).

7. Relieve Teething Pain.

Babies start teething around the middle of the first year and experience the night-waking discomfort of teething for the next year and a half. A wet bedsheet under Baby's head or drool rash on the cheeks and chin, swollen and tender gums, and a slight fever are tell-tale signs that teething may be what's disturbing your baby's slumber. (See Teething, page 509.)

8. Use Cue Words to Coach Baby to Sleep.

The more sleep associations you can imprint into Baby's mind, the better. Sleep associations are words, sounds, or an environment that Baby associates with going to sleep and staying asleep, many of which we have already mentioned. Repeating cue words and other sounds that Baby associates with going to sleep will often help Baby get back to sleep. Say these cues as the last sounds Baby hears

BEWARE OF SLEEP TRAINERS

Be discerning about using anyone else's techniques to get your baby to sleep, especially those of sleep trainers who tout variations of the old "cry-it-out" methods. Remember, sleep is not a state you can force upon a baby. Nighttime parenting means setting the stage where Baby is comfortable going to sleep and staying asleep. We have two problems with the usual rigid sleep-training advice:

1. Sleep training can desensitize parents to the cues of their baby. The sleep-training regimens that involve Baby crying it out are biologically incorrect. (See an in-depth discussion on page 252.) It's easy for someone else to advise you to let your baby cry it out. She is not there at 3 a.m. Most mothers we have interviewed about the cry-it-out method of sleep training tell us, "I just can't do it." That's because mothers are biologically wired to respond to their babies' cries, not ignore them. Consider what science says. Studies show that when a baby cries the blood flow to mother's breasts increases, accompanied by Mother's biological urge to pick up and comfort her baby. Mothers are made that way. Sleep trainers should not interfere with this beautiful biological design.

2. Sleep training can cover up hidden causes of night waking. Sleep trainers claim that Baby is waking up because of "poor sleep habits." This is often true, which is why most of the tips we have given you are designed to help Baby develop good sleep habits. But be careful about that assumption, as it can keep you and the doctor from uncovering hidden medical causes of night waking. The most common of these is gastroesophageal reflux (see GERD, page 338). Another hidden medical cause of night waking is food allergies. Nighttime is scary for little people, so be careful about using methods that don't feel right to you.

before drifting off to sleep. Use these same words again when she awakens in the middle of the night: *sleepy-sleepy, night-night, happy nappy, shhhh.* The time-tested *shhhh* that mothers naturally do has a biological basis. It is similar to the sound of uterine blood flow that Baby was used to in the womb. When Baby starts to awaken, quickly issue reminders: "Shhhh . . . sleepy-sleepy" to let Baby know it's not time to get up yet.

9. Promote Restful Days.

Restful days provide sleepful nights. Try a trick called "cluster feeding," which means feeding Baby more frequently during the day in order to tank him up so he sleeps longer at night. Wear your baby in a soft baby carrier at least three hours a day. Proximity promotes calmness. A baby who is more rested and less anxious during the day is likely to be less anxious at night. Mellowing fussy tendencies during the day carries over into a more restful night. If you work outside the home and away from Baby many hours during the day, your baby might wake up more at night. That's because he wants to make up for missed touch — and sometimes nursing — time at night. This is why it helps to be sure your caregiver gives your baby as much touch time as possible during the day.

10. Decide Where Baby Should Sleep.

A question pediatricians often get is "Where should my baby sleep?" The answer is usually based upon the pediatrician's own personal parenting experience, or it could be influenced by confusing information in the literature. Our answer: Wherever all family members sleep the best is the right arrangement for you — and this may change at different stages in your baby's development. Consider these options:

DR. SEARS TIP
Get Behind the Eyes
of Your Baby

How to respond to your baby's nighttime needs (letting her fuss a bit to try to self-comfort, going to her immediately, nursing, singing, and so on) is often a dilemma for new parents, especially now that many sleep-training books have found their way into parents' bedrooms. Here's an absolute foolproof way to help you respond appropriately. When your baby awakens and you're confused about what to do, immediately put yourself behind the eyes of your baby and ask yourself, "If I were my baby, how would I want my parents to respond?" You'll always get it right. If you were a baby, would you rather wake up in a dark, quiet room, alone, disoriented, behind bars, and be forced to cry it out back to sleep, or wake up securely close to familiar people you love and be quickly comforted back to sleep?

A crib in parents' room. At least during the first year, babies should sleep in the same room as the parents. In fact, the American Academy of Pediatrics (AAP) recommends this policy. Remember, nighttime is scary for little people, and separation anxiety is normal during the first year or two, especially at night.

A bedside co-sleeper. This is a crib-like bed that attaches safely and securely to the parents' bed. It puts Mother and Baby within arm's reach of each other for easy comforting and nursing, but Baby and parents have their own separate sleeping spaces. We recommend the Arm's Reach Bedside Co-sleeper for parents who choose this arrangement. (See www .ArmsReach.com.)

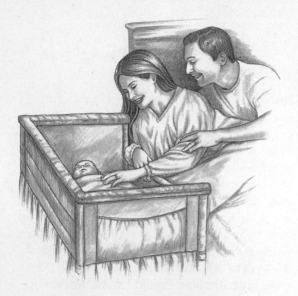

READ MORE ABOUT IT

We believe that instead of discouraging sleeping with your baby, it would be wiser for medical professionals to teach parents how to do it safely. For parents who truly believe that their baby belongs in their bed, here are two resources that will help you share sleep with your baby safely. These two books also tell you what science says about the health benefits of sharing sleep with your baby:

- *The Baby Sleep Book: The Complete Guide to a Good Night's Rest for the Whole Family,* by William, Robert, James, and Martha Sears

- *Sleeping with Your Baby: A Parent's Guide to Cosleeping,* by James J. McKenna

In parents' bed. What a pity that such a natural custom practiced the world over has become so controversial and scientifically confusing! At this writing, there is controversy going on about the science and safety of babies sleeping in parents' beds, and a thorough discussion is beyond the scope of this book. On the one hand the AAP discourages bed sharing because of a very small risk of suffocation in bed-sharing infants. On the other hand this risk is eliminated by strict adherence to safe-sleep guidelines in *The Baby Sleep Book.* The foremost sleep researcher in the world, Dr. James McKenna, professor of anthropology and director of the Mother-Baby Behavioral Sleep Laboratory at the University of Notre Dame, has published studies demonstrating that co-sleeping is the safest place for a baby and suggesting that the incidence of SIDS is actually lower in bed-sharing infants.

A final sleep-well message from the Sears family: Enjoy those precious moments of nighttime parenting. Your baby will eventually sleep through the night. All those middle-of-the-night moments in your arms, in your bed, and at your breast last such a short while, but the messages of your love and availability will last a lifetime.

SMOKING: DANGERS OF SECONDHAND SMOKE

We believe smoking around children is child abuse. Every year in the United States, it is estimated that 30 to 40 million children and adolescents are exposed to secondhand smoke. Tobacco smoke contains hundreds of chemicals known to be toxic or to cause cancer in humans. These include benzene, formaldehyde, arsenic, carbon monoxide, and many others.

How Secondhand Smoke Harms Your Child's Health

Exposure to secondhand smoke has been linked to many health problems in infants and children:

- Infants whose mothers smoked during pregnancy and after birth are more at risk for sudden infant death syndrome (SIDS).

- Mothers who smoke during pregnancy are more likely to give birth to babies with low birth weights.

- Secondhand smoke increases infants' and young children's risk for bronchitis, pneumonia, and ear infections.

- Children exposed to secondhand smoke are more likely to develop asthma, allergies, and other respiratory conditions.

- Secondhand smoke increases a child's risk for cancer.

- Exposure to secondhand smoke has been linked to poor school performance and behavioral and cognitive problems in children.

Remember, there is no "safe" level of secondhand smoke exposure among children. Any amount of secondhand smoke can cause the health problems above.

How to Avoid Exposure

Here are some ways to reduce or eliminate your child's risk of secondhand-smoke exposure:

- STOP SMOKING, STOP SMOKING, STOP SMOKING! If you or anyone in the household smokes, they must quit. Quitting may be difficult, but isn't your child's health worth it? If you, your spouse, or another family member has tried to quit in the past, talk to your doctor about ways to quit smoking.

- NEVER smoke while pregnant. If you are thinking about becoming pregnant, quit smoking right away.

- NEVER allow anyone to smoke while in your car, even if your child is not present. Smoke can linger in the fabric long after the smoking has stopped.

- NEVER take your child to a restaurant or any other setting where people may be smoking. We would advise against eating in any restaurant that has a smoking section.

- NEVER allow anyone to smoke in your home.

- Find out if your child's babysitters or caregivers smoke. If so, hire someone else. Smoke stays on hair and clothing.

- Talk with your child about the dangers of smoking. If you are watching a TV show or a movie where somebody is smoking, use that opportunity as a good teaching moment. Let your child know that the person who is smoking is damaging his health and the health of others.

- Be involved in your teenager's social life. Find out if he has friends who are smoking or if he is at risk for starting to smoke.

- When staying in a hotel, always stay in a non-smoking room.

Remember, there is no "safe level" of secondhand-smoke exposure. Children are more susceptible to the toxic substances in secondhand smoke than adults are. Even though you

DR. SEARS TIP
Take It Outside

Parents often ask us, "Is it okay if I smoke outside my house where my child cannot be exposed to secondhand smoke?" We always tell these parents they need to quit. However, if they must smoke, smoke outside the house. It is important to know that smoke does not just float around in the air. It gets into a smoker's clothes and stays on the smoker's hands, fingers, mouth, lips, and hair. Smoke can remain on these items for long periods of time, well after the smoker is back indoors among the children. If you must smoke, change all your clothes after smoking, wash any areas of your skin that came into contact with the cigarette or smoke — mainly hands, fingers, and lips. This will limit the amount of secondhand smoke that may have remained on your clothes and body.

may not see it, secondhand smoke can be very harmful to your child's little lungs.

SNORING

Snoring in most children is just a noisy nuisance, but it could also be a clue to an underlying medical problem.

Snoring is the sound produced by air passing through vibrating soft tissues of the airway, similar to the musical sound produced by a reed instrument. Newborns are naturally noisy breathers because their airways are small and narrow and they produce lots of bubbly secretions in the nose and throat. The air passing through these puddles of mucus causes noisy breathing. As babies grow, their airways grow. They become better able to swallow their throat secretions and the stage of newborn snoring and noisy breathing gradually lessens.

What to Do

As a general guide, if the snoring is not interfering with your child's sleep or breathing, don't worry. But since snoring might be a clue to some underlying structural problems or clogging in your baby's airways, consider these steps:

Tell your doctor about Baby's snoring. At your next routine checkup, mention that your baby "snores." Your doctor will pick up on this cue and carefully check your child's airways to be sure she has none of the following structural problems:

• Deviated nasal septum. Sometimes the nasal septum (the bone that divides the two nasal passages) is pushed to one side, obstructing airflow in one of the nostrils. The child compensates by inhaling more air through the unobstructed nostril, accounting for noisy breathing.

• Large tonsils and/or adenoids. Your doctor will check your child's tonsils and adenoids to see if they are large enough to obstruct your child's breathing (see related section, Sleep Apnea, page 474).

• Laryngomalacia. Your pediatrician will watch the front of your infant's neck as he breathes. Sometimes the cartilage that surrounds the trachea or windpipe is soft in the early months, causing the trachea to partially collapse when your child takes a deep breath. What the doctor sees is the normal dent in your baby's neck just above the breastbone caving in a bit when Baby inhales. As your infant grows, the cartilage becomes stronger and this windpipe quirk subsides.

Watch for nasal allergies. Your pediatrician will look into your baby's nose and check for signs of nasal allergies (the nasal structures called turbinates would be swollen and the airways partially plugged with secretions). (See allergies, page 131; and "Nose-Hose" and "Steam-Clean" techniques, page 20.)

Change sleeping positions. Observe which sleeping positions cause the most snoring. Rotate positions, such as tummy sleeping (for infants over a year), side sleeping, or back sleeping. Record in your diary in which position your child sleeps most comfortably. Mention this to your pediatrician. The main medical decision you and your pediatrician need to make is whether your child's noisy breathing, or snoring, is interfering with her quality of sleep. If there is any suspicion that this is happening, the doctor may order a sleep test called a *polysomnogram* in which your child's sleep patterns are recorded by a special instrument. A simple test can be done in the child's own bedroom. If a more elaborate polysomnogram is needed, it would have to be done in a sleep laboratory (available at most major hospitals). Here's where your diary helps: If according to your observations over time you notice that your child's noisy breathing is compromising the quality of his sleep, a thorough sleep study may be needed. (See related topic, Sleep Apnea, page 474.)

SOILING PANTS

The typical story goes somewhat like this: "My five-year-old son is getting lazy about his bowel habits. His underwear is always soiled. I scold him, but he tells me, 'Daddy, I just don't know when I have to go.'" Sound familiar?

Pants soiling, medically known as *encopresis*, is a common nuisance as those little bowels are growing up. Pants soiling is much more common in boys — males at all ages pay less attention to their bodily signals — and is more a mechanical and maturity problem than a psychological one.

Causes

First, we want you to understand the four main reasons why children soil their pants:

Busy little bowels. Little boys with little bowels are forgetful. They get so engrossed in a game that they tune out their urge-to-go signals.

Lazy little bowels. A child is standing in line or playing a game and doesn't want to lose his place or stop the game to go through all the trouble of getting undressed, redressed, and back into the game. So he ignores his signals.

Embarrassed little bowels. A child is in a classroom and may be too shy to ask to go to the toilet, especially in front of his playmates. This is why you want to teach your child that toileting, like eating, is a normal part of life: "Mommy and Daddy go to the toilet every day, and so do your teacher and your friends."

Blocked little bowels. You may be surprised that even though the bowel movements "run out," the underlying problem is often chronic constipation. What you see in your child's stinky underwear is what the bowel pressure has forced to leak by the constipated stool.

What to Do

Use this bodily nuisance as a teachable moment to achieve two purposes: first, to show your child that you are a valuable resource and can help him overcome uncomfortable and embarrassing situations, and, second, to help your child learn about an important part of his body. By the end of this session, your child will probably know more about intestinal health than any other child his age. You can adjust the following ten recommendations according to your child's age and stage of maturity.

1. Have the bowel talk. Play show-and-tell. Draw a picture of the bowels and explain to your child where poop comes from: "The left-over stuff from your food collects in your bowels and you call it poop. The poop starts out about the size of a small hot dog. Along the walls of your bowels are little nerves that can tell when your bowel is full. These tiny nerves send a signal up to your brain. The bowel then says to the brain, 'Brain, I'm full.' The brain says, 'Go to the toilet.' These are your got-to-go signals. Suppose you're too busy playing and you don't do what the brain says. Eventually, the brain and bowels stop talking to each other. They stop being friends. The brain says, 'If you won't listen to me, I'll stop talking to you.' So, you don't know when you've got to go. Then the poop starts growing, sometimes even as large as a baseball. When your poop gets big like a baseball, it hurts to poop, which then makes it harder and more difficult to poop. Because it hurts to poop, you don't want to poop. The bowel is like a muscle. If the baseball keeps growing, it stretches the muscle and the muscle gets weak. Then you're really in trouble because two things happen: the nerves get weak and stop talking to the brain even more, and the muscles then get so weak they can't push the poop out.

"Also at the end of your bowels, where the poop comes out, is a muscle called the doughnut muscle. This doughnut muscle gets smaller to keep the poop in. It also gets so weak that it can no longer hold the poop in so you leak and go into your pants. Honey, you're right, you often don't even know you have to go because your doughnut muscle and your bowel muscle don't talk to the brain anymore. What we have to do are four things:

1. Get your brain and bowel talking to each other again.

2. Get your got-to-go signals going again so you know when you have to go.

3. Get your doughnut muscle stronger again.

4. Get your poop down to hot-dog size rather than baseball size."

 **DR. SEARS TIP
Be a Teacher, Not
a Disciplinarian**

You want your child to see you as a resource for learning about bowel problems in an informative, helpful way, not a punitive one.

You want to break the messy cycle: chronic constipation s-t-r-e-t-c-h-e-s the bowel muscles and the doughnut muscle. Your child loses sensation of the urge to go and *leaks* — but doesn't feel it or smell it because he's become so accustomed to it, which makes him more constipated, losing more bowel sensation.

2. Have an evacuation plan. If your child has been pants soiling for more than several months, chances are he is so chronically constipated and his bowel muscles are so weak that you need to begin with a good cleanout. Have your pediatrician check your child. The doctor can often feel golf-ball-size stools in the child's lower abdomen (in addition to a weak doughnut muscle) by doing a rectal exam. If the doctor feels your child is severely constipated, you may need to begin this whole plan with an enema for a few days followed by laxatives for a week. Your child's doctor can prescribe these (see laxatives and enemas, page 242).

3. Feed misbehaving bowels. What goes in at the top end greatly affects what happens at the bottom end. Raise a little grazer. Try the Dr. Sears rules of twos: eat *twice* as often, *half* as much, and chew *twice* as long. If more complete digestion takes place at the top end, there is less wear and tear and residual at the bottom end of the bowels. (Depending on your child's level of comprehension, you can draw a picture of a smaller amount of food in the stomach that is all chewed up into smaller portions so more of it gets used up before it "makes poop.")

4. Water little bowels. Remember, one of your goals is to help your child be more comfortable going. Be sure he drinks at least an ounce of water per pound per day. If the stools sit there too long, the intestines steal back the water, and the stools get even harder, which is just what you don't want. Tell your child, "The more water you drink, the easier it is for your poop to pass." Extra water is especially important if your child has a high-fiber diet (fruits, vegetables, and whole grains). A high-fiber diet without extra water can actually make constipation worse.

5. Smoothies soften stools. In our medical practice, we use the "sipping solution" for alleviating constipation and many other intestinal malfunctions. Make your child a smoothie that contains at least three stool-softening ingredients:

- flax oil, 1 tablespoon (a healthy laxative)

- yogurt, 8 ounces (the healthy bacteria in yogurt are good for intestinal health)

- fruits, such as blueberries, mango, papaya, pineapple

Other special ingredients could be high-fiber grains, such as a tablespoon of psyllium husks, wheat bran, or ground flax seeds.

6. Salad softens stools. Get your child to eat lots of high-fiber salads containing greens, garbanzo beans, kidney beans, sunflower seeds, and olive oil.

7. Move—your bowels! Move your body to move your bowels. If your child sits too much, intestinal contents just sit there, too.

8. Schedule toilet sitting. After breakfast, lunch (if not at school), and dinner, encourage your child to sit on the toilet for at

**DR. SEARS TIP
Don't Dangle the Feet**

When your child's sitting on the toilet, let his feet rest on a footstool. Dangling tightens the doughnut muscles and makes it harder to let loose. Remember, your child needs all the help you can give him. Tell your child, "Propping your feet up on a footstool relaxes your doughnut muscle and makes it easier to go."

least ten to fifteen minutes. This habit takes advantage of the body's own biological bowel clue called the gastrocolic reflex. When the upper intestines get full, the lower intestines get the message that it's time to empty.

9. Put the best "bugs" in the bowels. Chronic constipation leads to generally poor intestinal health. Healthy intestines contain millions of healthy bacteria called *probiotics*, like those naturally found in yogurt. Healthy bacteria crowd out the harmful ones that oftentimes grow in the bowels during chronic constipation. (See probiotics, page 27.)

10. Help your child clean up after himself. Encourage your child to take responsibility for soaking the mess out of his pants before putting them in the laundry. Present this not in a punitive way, but as a simple matter of fact that he needs to take responsibility for his bodily behavior.

As you can see, pants soiling is primarily a mechanical problem, but it can become a behavioral one. Your child may be embarrassed when other kids say, "Here comes Stinky!" especially when "Stinky" doesn't feel it or smell it because he's become so accustomed to it. The embarrassed child then withdraws, hides his soiled underwear, and becomes even more embarrassed. This is why it's so important to address the problem before it escalates. You want your children to be comfortable coming to you with any embarrassing problem. Your kids are going to have lots of embarrassing problems down the road, but here's an opportunity to give them the message "No matter what problem you have, I will help you solve it." This way, they'll be comfortable telling you anything. When you help your child make a project out of a problem, you've turned the problem into an opportunity for you to connect with your child. (See also Constipation, page 240.)

SPEECH DELAY AND LATE TALKERS

Just as there are normal late walkers, there are normal late talkers. There are two phases of speech development: *receptive* language (meaning how much your child understands) and *expressive* language (meaning how much he says). Receptive language reflects the child's hearing and understanding abilities. If your toddler has normal receptive language, meaning he understands simple requests, then you don't need to worry. It is typical for parents to volunteer during their toddler's checkup, "He understands everything but says very little." Many toddlers still use body language to express what they want. Remember, speech is what a child verbally says, but language includes gestures, signing, and all kinds of body language. You want your child to be comfortable communicating in all ways, not just by talking. Late talking is more common in boys than girls and is often dubbed the "Einstein syndrome," because this genius was reputed to be a late talker.

Normal Speech Milestones

Language development varies greatly among children. The milestones below describe the minimum number of words most toddlers should know at various ages. If your child isn't quite meeting these marks, it doesn't mean you necessarily need to worry. You should discuss your child's progress at your next checkup.

- one year — one to two words

- fifteen months — five words

- eighteen months — ten words

- two years — fifty words, two-word phrases, about half understandable to a stranger

- three years — four-word sentences, relates stories, three-fourths understandable

When to Worry

Besides not meeting the above milestones, here are some other factors that should lead you to see the doctor:

- Your child has a history of frequent ear infections.

- You are concerned about your child's hearing.

- Your child has poor social skills.

- There is a delay in other milestones, such as walking.

What to Do

Keep a speech diary. As with other developmental milestones, progress is more important than timing. As long as your toddler is adding about one word a week and uses two-word phrases by age two that gradually expand into intelligible sentences by age three, you don't need to worry. If, however, your child "plateaus," meaning does not add a lot of new words over a three- to six-month period, you should consult your pediatrician or a speech pathologist to see if there is a developmental problem (such as Autism, page 167) that may cause delayed language or an anatomical challenge (such as tongue-tie, misshaped palate, or uncoordinated mouth and tongue muscles) that may cause disarticulated speech.

Raising a Good Communicator

Read with your child. Look at picture books together. Ask him questions about the pictures: "Where is the ball?" Use a concept we call "expansion"— expand a word into an idea. For example, if while you're reading your child asks, "What's that?" you answer, "That's a bird." You then add: "Birds fly in the sky." You have not only answered his question but have also given him a word-associated idea — that birds fly in the sky. When you're reading a book together, point to various pictures and ask your child questions, such as: "Where's the dog?" "Where's the boy?" Encourage your child to find the pictures and point to them. In this way he learns to associate the sound with the picture.

Look for teachable moments. Speech development is caught and not taught. Research has established that child-initiated interaction is more meaningful than parent-initiated interaction. Look for openers. Suppose you are walking through a park and your child points to a dog. Start talking about how "dogs run, jump, bark." Your child is likely to mimic these sounds. If your child points up at the sky and utters "buh" for *bird,* add the correct sound. "Yes, that's a bird. Let's look for more birds." Using the toddler-initiated opener, keep repeating the words your child is interested in.

Play body-part games. Toddlers enjoy traveling around their body and naming their body parts. Ask your child where his eyes, nose, and belly button are. Encourage him to point to them. Besides a brief anatomy lesson, you're teaching him the correct words for his parts.

Be a narrator. As you go through your child's daily rituals, such as bathing and changing, provide a running commentary: "Now we put on a diaper," "Now we put on your shirt," and

DR. SEARS TIP
Pointing Is Okay

Don't worry if your child is a persistent pointer. Many late talkers use pointing and sign language to get what they want. If your child points at the cookie jar and grunts "uh ook," take her cue and put it into words: "Tell Mommy what you want! Do you want a cookie?"

so on. As you are dressing or doing chores around the house, talk about what you're doing, as if you're narrating a story. There is a little person with big ears and a developing language center processing every word he hears. Infants of chatty parents tend to be more talkative toddlers.

"I need your eyes; I need your ears." Teach your child to engage with you when you are talking. It helps for children to associate sounds with lip movements and facial gestures.

Use the KISMIF principle. *Keep It Simple, Make It Fun.* For the beginning talker, usc short sentences with exaggerated, drawn-out vowels, such as "Goooood baaaaby!" Keep the speech lively. Toddlers are more likely to use words that are associated with animated facial gestures. Toddlers love signing, such as "Wave bye-bye to Grandma" as you wave your hands. To keep your child riveted on your speech, talk in a sing-song way and exaggerate key words.

Ask questions. Children enjoy listening to a higher-pitched voice. Asking questions will naturally raise the pitch of your voice and encourage your child to respond. "Does Suzy want to go outside and play?"

Sing-sing-sing. Singing uses more language centers in the brain than words alone do.

SPRAINS AND BROKEN BONES

Virtually every child is going to sprain an ankle or a knee, or fall and hurt an arm or a leg. Fingers and toes can get bumped and broken, and elbows and wrists can easily be injured. The main questions that need to be answered in such cases are whether the body part is sprained or broken and whether an X-ray is warranted. Once that is determined, proper treatment can be applied.

The term *sprain* means that one or more ligaments in a joint have been overstretched or partially torn. Ligaments are tough tissue fibers that connect one bone to another. For example, the ankle ligaments connect the ends of the leg bones to the foot bones. When the ankle is twisted or bent too far, the ligaments are stretched, resulting in a sprain. When the whole ligament is torn, the injury is called a *torn ligament*, like those that occur in season-ending knee injuries in athletes.

Broken bones are called *fractures*. There is a common misconception that the word *fracture* means a bone is only partly broken. The truth is, any break in any part of a bone is called a fracture. There are many varying degrees of fracture; the more severe the fracture, the longer it takes to heal.

Here is what you need to know when your child gets hurt.

Ankle Injuries

It stands to reason that the ankle joint is the one most commonly injured in childhood since it is the one that is most used — and abused. Upon examining your child, the doctor will diagnose not only the area of the sprain but its severity. Most children and adolescents sprain ankles by suddenly in-curving the foot and overstretching the joint ligaments. Ankle sprains are more likely to occur in children who play sports involving running, jumping, and sudden changes in direction, such as basketball and gymnastics.

Record the details. Your role as your child's home doctor is to provide your child's pediatrician with a written, running commentary of everything you recall about the injury, such as:

- How the injury occurred. For example, did your child injure herself while jumping off the monkey bars or playing basketball?

- The first symptom you and your child noticed. With ankle sprains the child feels immediate pain followed by swelling, tenderness, and often a bluish discoloration.

- How your child described the immediate sensation. If the young athlete described a sudden "pop" or "snap" and sudden pain, this may be a clue to a more severe tear.

- How limited your child is in moving the injured foot. Does it hurt when he bends it in a certain direction?

- Where it hurts. If your child circles the whole ankle, it may indicate a different type of injury than if he points to one "owie" spot with his pointer finger.

- Whether it hurts to stand on it. Don't push your child to stand on it if he refuses; your pediatrician can assess this in the office.

- Whether it's gotten better or worse between the time of injury and the time of the doctor's exam.

These are all clues that will help the doctor make the right diagnosis and prescribe the correct treatment.

Go to the doctor's office. After reviewing your child's history (which you wrote down and brought with you, right?) don't be surprised if your pediatrician first examines the normal ankle. The doctor does this for two reasons: (1) To calm the anxious child with a manipulation of the foot that doesn't hurt and (2) To get an idea of the anatomy of the child's normal ankle, so as to compare it with the injured one.

The doctor will then examine the injured ankle to determine the likelihood of a fracture. Suspecting a fracture and determining when to get an X-ray is a case-by-case decision. Explaining the nuances of this decision is beyond the scope of this book.

You may notice that the doctor takes childhood or adolescent sprains of any joint very seriously. Here's why. At the end of each bone is a growth plate, seen in X-rays as a line between part of the end of the bone and the rest of the bone. This area continually fills in with new bone and is what causes the child to grow. Unlike a fully grown adolescent or adult, when a child sprains a joint, the attached ligaments can dislodge the growth plate from the rest of the bone. If this is not properly diagnosed and treated, the injured growth plate may malfunction and interfere with the growth of that bone. This is why your doctor may take an X-ray or refer your child to an orthopedic specialist. In addition to a sprained ligament, a fracture at the end of one or more of the ankle bones may be likely.

Treatment. Any type of ankle fracture should be referred to an orthopedic specialist. Treatment will depend on the type and severity of

**DR. SEARS TIP
RICE It!**

Applying the right type of first aid to any injured body part that might be sprained or broken can greatly help the healing. Use the following acronym:

Rest: The child should not bear any weight on an injured leg or lift with a hurt arm until the doctor has had a chance to evaluate it. Keeping all stress off an injured bone or joint during the first forty-eight hours can significantly speed healing.

Ice: Apply an ice pack: on for fifteen minutes, off for fifteen minutes, for the first few hours. Ice not only provides relief from pain and swelling but also promotes a reflex dilation of blood vessels, encouraging all the natural healing nutrients in the blood to rush to the site of the injury. Continue icing for two to three days (at least four times a day) or according to the doctor's advice.

Compress: Wrap the injured joint (if possible) with an Ace bandage to lessen swelling, but not too tight. The combination of the wrapping and the ice should minimize any pain and swelling.

Elevate: To lessen pain and swelling, have your child sit and sleep with the injured ankle above the level of the heart. A pillow under the ankle while sleeping really helps.

the fracture. For an ankle sprain, your doctor will outline a treatment plan that is aimed at:

• relieving the pain and swelling

• getting your child "back on his feet" in an appropriate amount of time

• preventing any long-term injury that could interfere with use or growth

The treatment plan will basically be a continuation of the "RICE" steps above:

• Rest. Be sure your child understands the importance of not bearing weight on the injured ankle. Crutches can be rented or purchased from a pharmacy. The more days that pass without any weight bearing, the faster it will heal. After about three days, allow your child to test the ankle. Once she can bear weight without any pain, allow her to carefully walk around without overdoing it. Continue to use crutches for significant walking periods (such as at school) until your child is able to walk around for extended periods without pain.

• Apply an ice pack as described above for the first three days.

• Keep the ankle wrapped with an Ace bandage. You may need to unwrap it during icing.

• Keep the ankle elevated at every opportunity for the first two to three days.

• Unless advised by the doctor, don't apply heat for at least twenty-four hours and until the swelling has started to diminish. Heat increases swelling. Later on in the healing process heat will also increase blood flow, which promotes healing.

DR. SEARS TIP
Preventing Joint Injuries (Ankle, Knee, and Hip)

Encourage your child to stay lean. The more overweight your child, the more likely he is to injure these joints. When climbing stairs or walking up a hill, the weight on the ankle and knee joint is four times what it is when simply standing.

Tell your child to go slow. If your child tries out for a new sport, caution her against overusing the muscles and joints too fast. It takes a few weeks of training to build stronger bones and muscles, which is why sprains and fractures are most likely to occur at the beginning of the sport.

Don't forget rehabilitation. When do you think your child is most at risk for re-injuring the joint? The answer: within a few weeks after the first injury. A logical principle of muscle and bone health is "If you don't use it, you'll lose it." While the child's joint was immobilized to promote healing, the surrounding muscle weakened. So, the muscles and the entire joint are more prone to re-injury right after the child resumes mobility.

When you get the doctor's okay to begin muscle- and joint-strengthening exercises, take your child swimming. It is the perfect rehabilitation exercise for joint injuries because the joint moves without excessive weight bearing.

Collarbone Injuries

The collarbone (also known as the *clavicle*) is the bone that connects the *sternum*, or breastbone, to the shoulder blade, or *scapula*. The collarbone plays a role in shoulder and arm movement. Collarbone fractures can occur in a newborn during a difficult vaginal delivery or at anytime during childhood or adult life from a traumatic impact injury.

Symptoms. Symptoms that indicate your newborn may have broken his collarbone during delivery are:

- painful crying while moving the arm (such as when dressing the baby or rolling the baby over)

- decreased movement of the affected arm

- slight movement of the fractured area when the doctor presses it

- a grape-size lump over the fractured bone several days after injury (this is a normal overgrowth of cartilage during the healing process)

Symptoms that may indicate your child has suffered a broken collarbone include:

- shoulder pain

- difficulty moving the arm or shoulder

- swelling and/or bruising in the area of the collarbone

Causes. The way broken collarbones occur depends upon age group:

- In newborns, broken collarbones are usually the result of the tight squeeze as the infant passes through the birth canal, especially with a difficult labor. This is usually detected during routine newborn examinations.

- In children and adolescents, broken collarbones usually occur as the result of a fall, particularly if the child breaks the fall with an outstretched arm or falls directly onto the shoulder.

- Athletes often injure or break their collarbones as a result of being hit or tackled or falling. This is a common injury among young football players.

Treatment. Treatment depends on age group as well:

- Newborns. Because collarbone fractures are not uncommon in newborns and they are quite easy to detect on exam, a doctor typically won't do an X-ray to confirm the diagnosis. Treatment simply involves loosely binding the baby's arm in a horizontal position across his upper abdomen by folding the lower part of his shirt or outfit up over the arm and safety-pinning the edge of the shirt to the chest area of the shirt. This acts as a loose sling to keep the arm in a comfortable position while it heals over the next few weeks. It is not designed to keep the arm tightly bound or still. You should allow the baby to move his arm several times each day to avoid stiffness.

- Children. If a broken collarbone is suspected in a child, your doctor will take X-rays to see if there is a fracture. Most broken collarbones require only an elbow sling to keep the arm and shoulder in place. One of the more common slings is known as a "figure eight" splint in which a bandage is wrapped around the collarbone and under the arm, then around the back of the neck and over the opposite collarbone and under the arm. This more complicated sling bandage is usually done only if the fracture is so severe that one end of the bone has broken through the skin or in

cases where the fractured bones are severely separated from one another. In very rare cases, a broken collarbone may require surgery to realign the broken bone.

Most broken collarbones in older children heal completely within twelve weeks when properly treated with a splint. In younger patients, the healing time may be shorter than six weeks. Activities such as throwing a ball, lifting heavy objects, driving, etc., should only be undertaken if the activity does not cause pain. A child who suffers a collarbone fracture may have a painless bump at the fracture site that persists for months or years.

Elbow, Pulled (Nursemaid's Elbow)

Pulled or dislocated elbow is the most common elbow injury in young children. Imagine the following scene: You're walking along a busy street holding your child's hand and suddenly he throws a tantrum and tries to dart away from you. He yanks one way and you pull the other way. Or, it could be a danger-preventing reflex: The child starts running out into the street and gets yanked by the arm out of harm's way.

Then you notice two signs: Your child won't use his arm, and the arm hangs limply and painfully at his side. Your child's elbow is probably dislocated.

Signs and symptoms:

- The arm hangs limply.

- The child may hold the affected arm across his chest, as if making a sling.

- He is unwilling to use the injured arm.

- He may hold the arm slightly flexed and the hand palm-side down.

- He may experience slight pain, though swelling or severe tenderness around the elbow joint is unlikely.

Why pulled elbow occurs. The ligaments that hold the upper and lower arm bones in the elbow socket are much more flexible in toddlers and preschool children. A quick yank on the lower arm can cause the larger bone (the *radius*) to pop out of the socket. As the child grows, the ligaments become less elastic, making dislocated elbows unusual in children over the age of seven.

What to do. Take your child to the pediatrician, who will be able to relocate the elbow with a simple maneuver. Sometimes the

child will favor the affected elbow for a couple hours, which is why we often put the child's arm in a sling for a day to let the stretched ligament heal. You can make a

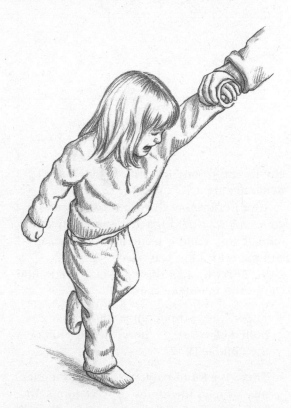

Don't lift or yank your child by her arm. Lift her shoulders instead.

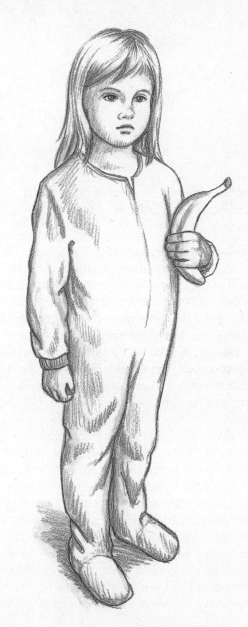

A dangling arm is typical of a pulled elbow.

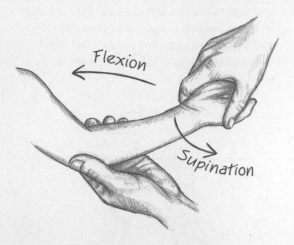

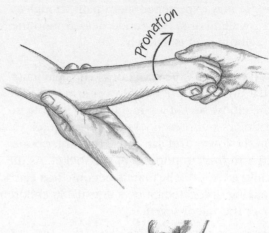

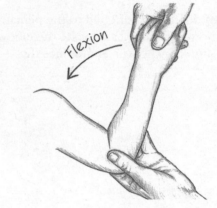

simple sling out of the child's T-shirt by pinning the lower front of the shirt up over the arm.

Do-it-yourself maneuver. Once your child gets a dislocated elbow, it's likely to recur in normal play. Since it may occur when access to medical care is limited, have your pediatrician show you how to pop the elbow back in so you can do it next time, or follow these steps (see illustration): First, cup your child's elbow in one hand and take hold of the wrist with the other. Then rotate your child's forearm to a hand-up position (called *supination*). Sometimes this maneuver alone will relocate the elbow. If not, while supinating the forearm, flex (bend) the elbow until your child's palm is almost touching his shoulder. While doing so, gently squeeze both sides of the elbow joint with your thumb and fingers and you should feel the arm bone "pop" back into the elbow joint. You will know if the maneuver was successful because your child will begin moving his arm normally. If this maneuver does not properly relocate the elbow, try the same move but pronate your

child's arm (rotate inward or palm down) while flexing it.

After performing this maneuver, observe your child playing for a few minutes to determine if your child is using his arm normally and the relocation was successful.

Never try to treat this yourself if your child shows the following signs:

- The history is not compatible with a pulled elbow (e.g., there was no yank or the child fell).

- There is a lot of pain, swelling, and tenderness around the elbow or wrist joints. In this case, the child may have an underlying

DR. SEARS TIP
Lift Smart

Always lift your child from the torso under *both arms* and instruct other caregivers to do likewise. Never pull on only one arm.

fracture that needs to be professionally treated. If your child naturally holds his arm in the position of comfort, you can help him by fabricating a sling until you can seek medical attention. An X-ray will confirm the problem.

Finger and Toe Injuries

Fingers and toes bear the brunt of stub, jam, and slam injuries. Fortunately, most such events don't require a trip to the doctor. Here is the information you need to help you decide the best course of action (for nail injuries, see page 410).

Is it broken or just sprained? In practical terms, it often doesn't matter for any of the four digits (not including the thumb or big toe). Breaks in a finger or toe usually don't need a cast anyway, so you don't really need to know whether or not it is broken. First, you ice it for about twenty minutes every hour for the rest of the day. Then you simply buddy tape it (see details below) and let it heal over a few weeks. If it feels almost better in just a few days, then it probably wasn't broken. Having said that, some finger injuries do need a specific type of splint and careful orthopedic follow-up. So it may be best to see your doctor to help you decide if an X-ray is in order, especially if any of the following scenarios occurred:

- Thumb or big toe. If you think your child may have broken one of these (based on

the severity of the impact or the degree of pain and swelling), you should see a doctor.

- Bent at an angle. If the finger or toe is bent at a funny angle (use your child's opposite hand or foot to compare), then this type of break may need special treatment.

- Broken joint. If the pain and swelling are worse over a joint, this might need to be X-rayed. Some joint fractures require special treatment.

- Deep laceration. If you think your child might have broken a bone, and there's more than just a simple small cut involved, see a doctor that day. This type of injury can easily become infected.

- Can't bend it. Despite the pain, your child should still be able to bend most minor fractures. If she can't, this may indicate a more significant injury.

- Athletes. If your child is involved in sports or is very active and likely to re-injure a hurt finger, it is best to get an X-ray. If fractured, a cast can be applied to speed up the healing so the child can return to sports more quickly or to protect the finger if your child is going to continue participating in the sport while injured.

- Finger was bent or pulled during injury. Some fractures to the fingertip, such as when catching a ball or having a finger caught in a sports jersey, do need a special splint to heal well.

Treatment. Minor and straight broken fingers and toes take a few weeks to heal, but heal they do, and without a cast. Buy some paper tape and wrap the injured finger or toe together with the largest adjacent digit (called buddy taping), but do not wrap the thumb or large toe without a doctor's advice. Your child shouldn't keep his fingers straight; he should allow them to bend slightly. Once a day untape the fingers and tell your child to cautiously bend and stretch them to avoid any tightness.

Knee Injuries

Knee sprains are very common and usually resolve without any special treatment besides rest and ice. However, knee injuries can be confusing to parents because of the possibility of a ligament injury or tear, and it isn't easy for a parent to determine the extent of an injury without seeing a doctor. Here is our guide to the various types of knee injuries and how you can decide whether your child should see the doctor.

Knee sprain. A sprain occurs after a minor twist or hyperextension of the knee, and one of the ligaments (the fibrous tissue that holds the bones of the knee joint together) is mildly stretched. Symptoms include minor pain with bending or attempting to stand and tenderness and swelling over the injured area. The child should still be able to move the knee in all directions and walk with only mild to moderate pain. Proper treatment right away can minimize the degree of pain and swelling and speed healing.

The most important step is to immediately begin "RICE" procedures:

- Rest. Try to avoid putting any weight on the knee. Use crutches for a day (if available) or assist your child when he walks. Complete avoidance of weight bearing on the knee for the first twenty-four hours can help a minor sprain heal quickly. Limping

around on a sprained knee will increase the swelling and irritation and prolong healing.

- Ice. Apply twenty minutes of ice to the entire knee, then take a twenty-minute break. Continue icing for twenty minutes on and twenty minutes off for several hours, then decrease to twenty minutes out of every hour for the next twenty-four hours (or as often as is practical).

- Compression. When not icing, keep the knee wrapped in an Ace bandage.

- Elevation. Have your child sit with his leg raised on a pillow in front of him whenever possible. This helps decrease the swelling and inflammation.

- Pain medication. Ibuprofen (see dosing chart, page 553) will help with pain and inflammation and giving three doses each day for two or three days can help speed recovery.

When to worry. A sprain should begin to feel somewhat better the next day, with continued improvement and resolution of all symptoms within three or four days. If this isn't the case, it may be a more serious ligament injury (see below).

Ligament injury. If one of the knee ligaments is stretched too far, torn, or completely snaps, then the degree of pain and swelling will be more immediate and severe. The knee will feel unstable and may give way during weight bearing. An orthopedic doctor can often distinguish between a sprain and a ligament injury by carefully examining the knee; however, an MRI is needed to make a definitive diagnosis.

Besides a period of initial RICE and ibuprofen, your child will likely need to:

- use a knee brace for several weeks or longer.

- undergo physical therapy sessions for a number of months.

- undergo surgical repair if therapy doesn't adequately re-strengthen the ligaments.

Torn meniscus or cartilage. The meniscus is the tissue that cushions the knee joint and allows it to work smoothly. Cartilage is where the bones rub together. Injury to these tissues may not be as painful or cause as much swelling initially, but chronic or recurrent pain will persist and the child will feel popping or grinding in the knee joint. The torn tissue will be seen on an MRI. Treatment is often surgical.

Fractured kneecap. This uncommon injury occurs when a child falls directly on the kneecap. The degree of pain is quite severe, especially when pressing on the kneecap. It is diagnosed with an X-ray and surgical repair is often needed.

Wrist Injuries

Wrist injuries are common among children because the wrists often bear the brunt of a child's weight during a forward fall. It's important to determine whether a wrist injury is just a sprain or a fracture. If not properly treated, an injured joint can lead to problems down the road.

Wrist sprain. An awkward fall on the wrist or other accident can result in a sprain of the wrist—an injury to the tendons and/or ligaments. These structures connect muscles and bones and can become inflamed, swollen, and painful when injured. Clues to a sprain are:

- Your child complains of generalized pain in the area of injury.

- You may notice swelling around the painful area.

- The pain may worsen when your child moves the wrist.

Wrist sprains can take a few weeks to heal. Keep your child from doing too much stressful activity with the wrist, as this may prolong healing time. Sprain injuries usually don't require a doctor's visit, but if in doubt, have your doctor check it out when the office next opens.

DR. SEARS TIP
Sprain vs. Break

Point tenderness is your clue to a possible fracture and merits an X-ray. If your child points to one spot consistently and whines when you press there, suspect a *broken bone*. If your child is *vague* about the location and *circles* the area instead of pointing to it, and you can't pinpoint the exact area of pain, suspect a *sprain* rather than a break. When in doubt, have your pediatrician check it out.

Wrist fracture. Active and rambunctious children and adolescents often take hard falls, which can certainly lead to wrist fractures. Activities that can lead to this type of injury include skateboarding, snowboarding, or any type of sport where, on falling, a child has to break his landing with his hands. Any accident where wrist fracture is a possibility should prompt a same-day pediatrician's or urgent-care evaluation. Delays in diagnosing and treating wrist fractures can lead to permanent disability or immobility of the wrist.

During the first few years of life, the wrist bones within the hand are usually too small to be fractured. However, as the bones grow, they become more susceptible to injury. During a fall onto outstretched hands, the two bones in the forearm (the *radius* and *ulna*) are remarkably easy to fracture where they connect to the hand. With a wrist fracture, children will often complain of severe pain and swelling of the wrist.

DR. SEARS TIP
Broken Bones Can Become Shorter Bones

At the wrist end of the arm resides the *growth plate,* specialized bone tissue cells that rapidly multiply and make the bone longer. If these are injured, bone growth could be compromised. You will notice the doctor "tapping" on the growth plate areas to check for pain and swelling.

With a fracture, the pain is usually most severe at one specific point, whereas in a strain/sprain the pain is more spread out. Your pediatrician can perform a wrist examination in order to determine whether an X-ray is necessary to rule out a wrist fracture.

Treatment involves casting or bracing of the wrist for four to six weeks in order to keep it in one position to allow the bones to heal.

DR. SEARS TIP
Be Prepared for a Bump

Don't be surprised or alarmed if you feel a lump months after the fracture has healed. You are feeling bone remodeling as part of the normal healing process.

STREP THROAT

Strep throat is an infection of the throat caused by a type of bacteria known as *group A streptococcus*. There are many types of streptococcus bacteria, but this one in particular causes strep throat. It is the most common bacterial infection of the throat, and is seen most often in children five to fifteen years of age. It is much less common in preschool and younger children.

Kids get strep through person-to-person contact, usually through saliva or nasal secretions. The germs can spread easily in areas where there is close contact, such as in households and classrooms. Even being exposed to tiny droplets of moisture that are released from the breathing passages upon sneezing or coughing can easily spread strep. Shaking hands with an infected person is another common way strep is spread.

Symptoms

It can sometimes be difficult to differentiate strep throat from other infections of the throat. Most sore throats are caused by viral infections and do not respond to antibiotics. Only your pediatrician can say definitively if your child has strep.

Children with strep throat may have any or all of the following symptoms:

- sore throat

- difficulty swallowing

- red, swollen tonsils and throat

- white patches on tonsils and throat

- "strawberry" tongue — taste buds are inflamed and red

- swollen and tender lymph nodes in the neck

- headache

- fever

- chills

- loss of appetite and nausea

- abdominal pain

- rash

- muscle aches and pain

- joint stiffness

- nasal congestion

- neck pain

Symptoms begin *two to five days* after exposure, a shorter incubation than most germs, and often have a very rapid onset, with fever commonly being the first symptom. As you can see from the long list of symptoms, diagnosing strep can sometimes be difficult. And given the range in severity the symptoms can have, some people might have very mild or almost no symptoms at all while others will have severe symptoms, which makes diagnosis that much harder.

What to Do

If you suspect strep throat, or if your child has been in close contact with another child diagnosed with strep throat, see the doctor right away. Until your child is seen by a doctor, you should keep her away from other children as much as possible. Your pediatrician will take a history and examine your child's throat. Sometimes the appearance is "obvious strep." A test, known as a *rapid strep test,* can be done in

the office; the doctor takes a throat swab and tests the sample. This takes approximately five minutes and is around 95 percent accurate in diagnosing strep. However, in some cases the rapid strep test will miss true cases of strep. A negative rapid strep test should be followed by a throat culture. This involves taking another throat swab and placing the contents of the swab on a special culture that will grow strep bacteria if present. This test takes forty-eight hours to complete and is considered the most accurate. A negative throat culture can almost completely rule out strep as the cause of your child's symptoms.

Treatment

If strep throat is confirmed, it should be treated with antibiotics, even if your child seems to be feeling better. Sore throats from strep will usually improve on their own; however, treating with antibiotics is still necessary because:

- Your child is still contagious even after her symptoms are improving. If she is treated with antibiotics, she will no longer be contagious twenty-four to forty-eight hours after beginning treatment. Children can be contagious for up to twenty-one days when not treated with antibiotics.

- Symptoms will be alleviated faster with antibiotic treatment.

- Treatment with antibiotics prevents complications of strep throat, covered below.

As more and more bugs become resistant to drugs, occasionally strep does not respond to the usual milder antibiotics. If your child has not improved within two to three days, contact your pediatrician.

DR. SEARS TIP
Complete the Course!

It is *very* important to complete the whole course of antibiotics. If treatment is stopped too soon, even if your child is feeling better, strep throat can return.

In addition to taking the antibiotics properly, the following can help strep heal:

- Be sure your child gets plenty of liquids to prevent dehydration.

- Cool water and Popsicles soothe a sore throat.

- Bland soups and special teas designed for sore throats can help soothe the throat as well.

- Saltwater gargles can help the pain.

- Ibuprofen can help reduce the pain and inflammation of strep throat, as well as reducing the fever.

DR. SEARS TIP
Easy on the Sore Throat

Avoid acidic beverages when your child has strep throat. These include orange juice, lemonade, grapefruit juice, and others that can worsen the throat irritation.

Do not send your child back to school if she is still running a fever or is still contagious. Schools have different policies as to whether they let children back twenty-four or forty-eight hours after beginning treatment for strep throat. Talk to your school administrator about your school's policy. Remember to start probiotics with the course of antibiotics (see Antibiotics, page 549).

Complications of Untreated Strep

The following are complications that can occur if strep goes untreated.

Abscess. Rarely, a throat infection will spread into the surrounding neck tissues and cause a large, infectious swelling in the neck called a peritonsillar abscess. A large mass will be evident on the side of the neck, and the child may have trouble swallowing or even breathing. This requires immediate evaluation in the doctor's office or an emergency room and intravenous (IV) antibiotic therapy.

Rheumatic fever. Very rarely the strep bacteria will enter the bloodstream and travel to the heart, where it adheres to one of the heart valves. The bacteria can form a small mass of infection on the valve, which interferes with heart function. Symptoms include chest pain and shortness of breath, along with persistent fevers. Anyone with these signs with a known strep infection should go to an emergency room right away. Treatment involves aggressive IV antibiotic therapy.

Glomerulonephritis. This fancy word simply means inflammation of the kidneys. This isn't an actual strep infection in the kidneys. Rather, it occurs when the immune system creates antibodies to attack the strep, but the antibodies inadvertently attack the kidneys as well, causing them to temporarily stop working. Blood in the urine (either red or cola-colored) is a sign of this complication and hospitalization may be required.

Scarlet fever. This isn't actually a complication of strep. It is simply an allergic-type immune reaction to the bacteria, resulting in a red, pimply, rough-feeling rash throughout the body. Scarlet fever is really no more dangerous than basic strep throat, although a child may feel more ill. There is no treatment for this rash, other than antibiotic treatment for the infection.

Prevention

Teaching your child good hygiene practices is important in preventing strep. Frequent hand washing is a good idea, especially during times when there are known strep throat outbreaks at school. Tell your children to cover their mouths when coughing or sneezing and wash their hands afterward. If your child has strep, keep her eating utensils and toothbrush separate from everyone else's.

If your children seem to be passing strep throat around more frequently, one or more of them might be *carriers* of strep throat. A carrier harbors strep bacteria in his or her throat but does not have symptoms. Carriers are capable of passing strep to others. Treating carriers with antibiotics can eradicate the bacteria from their throats and help break this cycle of re-infection. Occasionally, children who get repeated strep infections year after year might need to have their tonsils removed.

 DR. SEARS TIP
Toss the Toothbrush!

If your child gets strep throat, buy a new toothbrush and have her start using it two days after starting the antibiotics. If the same toothbrush is used, bacteria are still present on the bristles and can re-infect your child after the round of antibiotics is completed.

STUTTERING

Beginning talkers usually go through a stage of development called *normal dysfluency.* As toddlers learn to talk, they frequently hesitate or repeat words and syllables, such as: "I-I-I want…," "When-when-when…Mommy come home…," "Ca-ca-ca…can I have a cookie?" They often use hesitation syllables, called fillers, as they change words and thoughts: "er," "uh," "um," and they get especially dysfluent when they are tense, tired, excited, anxious, in a hurry to speak, speaking about new or complex topics, or feeling pressured to answer a question. Dysfluency is particularly common with tongue-challenging sounds like "L" — "li-li… like." The young language learner is unaware that he is not talking "correctly." Tiny talkers enjoy experimenting with various sounds and sequences, and this is perfectly normal.

When to Worry

The following are clues that your child may have more than just normal dysfluency and may need some speech therapy:

- Your child shows behaviors that she is uncomfortable speaking, such as blinking, head bobbing, and avoiding eye contact.

- You notice no improvement over a period of six months from the time the stuttering began. Your child becomes increasingly stuck in speech and repeats the beginnings of words three or more times: "ki-ki-ki… kitten."

- When stuck on a word, your child often replaces normal vowel sounds with "uh" — "Buh-buh-buh…bicycle" or "Cuh-cuh-cuh…cat."

Our number one speech therapy advice is that a child must first be comfortable *speaking* before worrying about speaking *correctly*.

What to Do

Keep a speech diary. If you notice gradual improvement over a period of six months and your child is becoming more fluent, this is most likely normal dysfluency, not stuttering, and does not need therapy. Identify what we call tense-talking triggers. Does your child stutter when she is tired, anxious, nervous, hurried, or when talking to strangers? A tense mind can lead to a tense tongue. If, however, she is stuttering at other times and there seems to be no improvement over six months, consider speech therapy.

Make talking fun. As we've said above, it's important that children feel comfortable speaking before they have to focus on speaking correctly. The young language learner is unaware that he is not talking "correctly." He simply enjoys experimenting with various sounds and sequences. Let him experiment without feeling judged or pressured to speak correctly. Above all, don't call attention to the fact that he "stutters" or "speaks incorrectly."

Talk eye to eye. Teach your child to be comfortable with body language while talking. If her attention wanders while she talks, draw her into you by addressing her by name and saying, "Sally, I need your eyes; I need your ears."

Be a careful listener. Children speak more clearly if their listener believes what they have to say is important.

Children become more fluent when they speak about their favorite subjects. Invite your child to talk about something she loves. Let her know that she is fun to listen to and you love to hear her stories. Again, no judgment about the "correctness" of her speech.

Listen patiently. Children who feel rushed are more likely to become dysfluent. If your child stumbles during a sentence, ignore it. Keep your usual attentiveness and eye contact and patiently wait for him to finish. Above all, resist the temptation to finish your child's speech or hurry him to the end of the sentence. Let him make "mistakes" as he tries out different sounds.

Speech is caught, not taught. Instead of correcting, simply repeat the sentence "correctly" yourself and let your child hear how it's supposed to sound. Speak slowly and distinctly, and give her a chance to mimic your speech patterns. You can ease in gentle "corrections" with a well-timed "slow down" or "tell me again."

When to Take Your Child to a Speech Therapist

If your child is becoming less comfortable talking, better to get help earlier rather than later. You want your child to be comfortable talking and communicating as she enters school, because stuttering can be a target of ridicule. Take your child to a speech therapist if:

- Your child is over three years old and according to your speech diary you haven't seen any improvement over six months.

- You sense that your child is becoming increasingly uncomfortable talking.

A certified speech therapist can tell you if your child is still going through a stage of normal dysfluency or if there really is a problem. A speech therapist can also advise you on how you can help your child at home and can give you a list of playful speaking games. Finally, a well-trained speech therapist can spot an anatomical problem, such as tongue-tie (see page 521) or tongue thrusting, that is interfering with your child's normal speech. She can teach your child how to use her tongue properly.

DR. SEARS TIP
Sing, Sing, Sing

Singing is a fun way to give your child "speech therapy." Singing teaches children how to use their tongues and vocal muscles properly. It is relaxing and fun, and allows a child to elongate vowels and other sounds. Wouldn't your child rather take "singing lessons" than see a speech pathologist?

LEARN MORE ABOUT IT

For helpful information, contact the Stuttering Foundation of America (1-800-992-9392); www.stutterSFA.org.

SUDDEN INFANT DEATH SYNDROME (SIDS)

The sudden, unexplained passing of a baby during sleep has always been a fear in the back of every parent's mind. While we still don't understand exactly what causes this tragedy, parents no longer need to feel helpless. In light of new research, there are some steps that parents can take to lessen their worry and lower the risk for their baby. The following are three practical steps that have been proven by research to reduce the risk of SIDS:

1. Don't allow smoking around your baby, pre- or postnatally. One of the most significant risk factors for SIDS — and one that mothers can do something about — is smoking when their babies are in the womb or in the same room. Exposure to cigarette smoke more than doubles the risk of SIDS. Suppose you were about to take your baby into a room when you noticed a sign that read: "Warning! This room contains poisonous gases of around 4,000 chemicals, some of which have been linked to cancer and lung damage and are especially harmful to the breathing passages of young infants." Certainly you wouldn't take your baby in there. But that's exactly what happens when mothers take their babies into rooms frequented by smokers. Also, smoking interferes with natural mothering. Mothers who smoke have a lower level of the hormone prolactin, which not only regulates milk production but increases the mother's awareness of the health of her infant.

2. Place your baby to sleep on her back, not her stomach. The "Back to Sleep" campaign of the past decade has reduced the rate of SIDS by as much as 50 percent, from a rate of 1 in 1,000 babies in 1995 to 1 in 2,000 in 2005. Research shows that arousability from sleep, an infant's built-in protective mechanism, improves when babies sleep on their backs rather than their tummies. Also, when sleeping facedown a baby may press her head into the mattress and form a pocket of air around her, leaving her to rebreathe her own exhaled air, which has diminished oxygen. A baby's breathing system seems to work best in the back-sleeping position.

3. Breastfeed your baby. In 2007 the federal Agency for Healthcare Research and Quality (AHRQ) published an analysis of over 9,000 medical studies on breastfeeding and infant health. One of their conclusions was that breastfed infants are 36 percent less likely to die of SIDS. Theoretically, breastfeeding may lower the risk of SIDS because breast milk contains brain-building substances, or "growth factors," that may enhance neurological development, especially development of the respiratory control center. Breast milk is kinder to tiny airways because it doesn't contain allergens. Breastfed babies seem to have better arousability from sleep. Also, breastfeeding seems to improve breathing/swallowing coordination.

What to Do

For the reasons we have listed above, try your best to get Baby to sleep on her back. Even though back sleeping does lower the risk of SIDS by around 50 percent, this statistical correlation does not at all imply that your baby is at greater risk of SIDS if she sleeps on her tummy. Some SIDS researchers believe that babies will naturally assume the sleep position that allows them to sleep and breathe the most comfortably during the night. This could

READ MORE ABOUT IT

For a deeper understanding of how you can prevent SIDS, read *SIDS: A Parent's Guide to Understanding and Preventing Sudden Infant Death Syndrome*, by William Sears.

be the reason why some babies twist and turn at night. In some babies, back sleeping allows stomach acids to reflux up into the esophagus, causing painful night waking. If your baby refuses back sleeping, you might have your health-care provider evaluate her for possible GERD (see page 338).

What about back-sleeping-promoting wedges? The American Academy of Pediatrics (AAP) and SIDS organizations discourage the use of wedges and props that are touted to keep babies sleeping on their backs. These props have never been proven safe or effective in reducing SIDS.

SUNBURNS

Even though parents and children should adhere to our sun-protection precautions on page 31, it's inevitable that a child will suffer a sunburn or three over the years. Here's what you can do if (or when) this occurs:

If the sunburn is bad enough to blister: This is a second-degree burn — see Burns, page 205. Prescription burn cream can help.

If it's red and painful but not yet blistery:

• Apply cool compresses, such as a washcloth soaked in cool water. If the burn is on the torso, let your child wear a T-shirt soaked in cold water.

- Apply an aloe vera gel to both soothe and soften the skin; this can prevent peeling.

- Give ibuprofen twice a day for two to three days (see page 553) to help with pain and decrease redness and swelling.

- Hydrate your child well. Burned, peeling skin dries out. Give your child at least an ounce of fluid per pound a day.

SUNGLASSES FOR CHILDREN

The age group that most needs sunglasses is the least likely to wear them. Infants and children are actually at increased risk for sun damage to the eyes because their relatively large pupils allow more damaging ultraviolet light to get in. Excessive ultraviolet (UV) light "oxidizes," which means causes wear and tear on the retina and other tissues of the eye, increasing the risk of two problems later on in adulthood: cataracts and macular degeneration. As children grow and reach teen time, the lens of the eyes is able to screen out more damaging UV light.

Picking sunglasses for those little peepers: Ophthalmologists recommend you look for glasses labeled "blocks 99 percent of UV rays" or "meets American National Standards Institute requirements." Above all, avoid toy sunglasses, especially the really dark ones. These can actually be more damaging, because the pupils dilate and let more UV light enter. If your child refuses to wear them, don some funky ones yourself and your child will likely want to copy. For added eye protection, teach your child never to look directly at the sun,

and get him used to wearing baseball caps or hats that shade those growing and sensitive eyes.

SWIMMER'S EAR (OTITIS EXTERNA)

Swimmer's ear is an infection of the lining of the ear canal, as opposed to a middle ear infection (see otitis media, page 285), which is an infection behind the eardrum. The lining of the ear canal contains glands that normally secrete a protective, waxy coating that is both water repellent and acidic, and this can retard invading germs. The water from swimming and diving can wash away this protective coating and provide a warm, damp environment that is a setup for germs. A child is more likely to get swimmer's ear from warm water or polluted lake water, which contains more germs, than from colder or chlorinated water.

Symptoms

The following are clues that your child may have swimmer's ear:

- The ear begins to itch or hurt shortly after swimming.

- Pain begins a day or two after swimming and quickly worsens.

- There is smelly drainage from the ear canal that resembles mucus from the nose.

Try the Dr. Sears earlobe-pull test: Pull on the earlobe or press down on the small flap of tissue that covers the ear canal — this compresses the inflamed ear canal. If your child winces or complains of pain, it is likely he has swimmer's ear.

How to tell swimmer's ear from middle ear infection. A middle ear infection usually follows or is accompanied by cold symptoms, such as nasal discharge, eye drainage, and a low-grade fever. Middle ear pain is usually worse at night when a child is lying down and the earlobe-pull test is usually painless. Sometimes an infection in the ear canal can develop following a middle ear infection if the infected fluid from the middle ear ruptures through the eardrum and infects the ear canal. In this case, you may see fluid draining from the ear canal, but your child "feels better" because the eardrum has ruptured, relieving the pressure on the middle ear. (See related section on middle ear infections, page 285.)

Prevention

Don't bother with earplugs or cotton balls; they are usually ineffective. They not only leak, but press trapped wax farther back into the canal. Here are some effective ways to prevent swimmer's ear:

• Don't allow your child to swim in polluted water.

• Don't let your child put his head underwater in a hot tub. This creates the conditions for an outer ear infection.

• Show your child how to tilt and shake his head to one side and then the other side after swimming to encourage drainage from the ears. Pulling up and back on the ear while your child tilts his head straightens the canal and helps the water drain out.

• Make a wick by rolling a small piece of tissue between your thumb and forefinger and gently insert it about a half inch into the ear canal to absorb the remaining water.

• Try drying the ear canal by carefully holding a hair dryer at a *low setting* a few inches away from the ear for about thirty seconds.

Immediately after your child swims, try this home prevention, which we have used in our practice for several decades:

Mix equal parts of white vinegar and water. The vinegar contains acetic acid, which is a germicidal and restores the normal germ-inhibiting acid environment that was washed out of the ear. Have your child lie down, and then gently pull the ear up and back to straighten the canal. Using a dropper, apply at least five drops of the vinegar solution in the ear. Leave them in for a minute, then let them drain out. Repeat in the other ear. Apply this white vinegar rinse after each swimming session.

If this doesn't prevent infections, you can change to a mix of half vinegar and half rubbing alcohol. This may work better. You can also buy a swimmer's ear prevention solution in a drugstore.

Treatment

The best "treatment" is prevention using the above measures. But if your child develops swimmer's ear:

• Increase the use of white vinegar/water solution to four times a day. Don't add the rubbing alcohol at this point — it will sting too much.

• If the pain persists (and especially if it worsens), or you see gunky and foul-smelling discharge, have your child's ears checked by a doctor. Prescription antibiotic drops, pain-relieving drops, and/or cortisone drops may be needed to relieve the pain and swelling and treat the infection.

- Acetaminophen or ibuprofen can help with pain relief.

- It's best that your child not swim for a few days until the infection begins to clear up.

TEETHING

Teething is perhaps the most harmless, yet bothersome, challenge for young babies and their parents. Weeks of fussing and nights of frequent waking can really take their toll. We see many fussy, drooling, ear-tugging infants brought into our office by parents who are worried that the babies might be sick. When we can't find anything wrong and write it off to teething pain, parents feel a mixture of relief that all is well and annoyance that their baby "tricked" them into coming to see the doctor.

 DR. SEARS TIP
Is It Teething or
an Ear Infection?

Most babies pull on their ears when teething in an attempt to find relief from the headache and jaw pain. Babies also pull on their ears when they have an ear infection. Ear tugging from teething pain is the number one cause of unnecessary doctors' visits. Here's how parents can tell the difference: A baby with an ear infection will also have cold symptoms (nasal congestion and cough) and often a fever over 101 degrees. Any infant who is pulling on his ears without cold symptoms is probably just teething.

Symptoms

Although the first teeth usually don't break through until six months of age, pain from teething can begin as early as three or four months and will continue on and off for the first two years of life. Signs include:

- excessive drooling

- intense chewing and biting

- increased night waking

- visible swelling of the gums

- fussing for no other discernible reason

- low-grade fever (lower than 101 degrees)

- loose stools

- cough from saliva collecting in the throat

Treatment

Here are our favorite time-tested remedies for teething pain:

Anything cold. A frozen teething ring, frozen banana, frozen wet washcloth, an ice cube placed in a baby sock, or a cold metal spoon are all convenient ways to numb aching gums.

Medications. Acetaminophen and ibuprofen (see dosing charts, pages 552 and 553) are effective ways to suppress teething pain, but they shouldn't be overused. We recommend that parents save them for nighttime when nobody is getting any sleep and not use them more than seven nights in a row.

Teething gels or drops. These are solutions that are rubbed onto the aching gums. We do not recommend anesthetic gels that numb the gums. While these work well, they do have the drawback of numbing the entire inside of the mouth and tongue, which may bother the baby more than the teething pain. Natural teething remedies are also available at drugstores and health-food stores that include ingredients like clove oil, natural licorice herbs, chamomile, and homeopathic belladonna. These are very safe and effective alternatives.

TESTICLE PAIN AND SWELLING

Pain and/or swelling of the scrotum and testicles can cause great concern among boys as well as their parents, and understandably so. There are several causes of these problems; some require immediate medical attention, while others do not. Here's a rundown of the most common causes of these symptoms among the pediatric and adolescent male population. It is important to note that any boy complaining of pain in his scrotum or testicles should immediately be evaluated by a physician.

Epididymitis

The *epididymis* is a structure that lies directly next to each testicle. *Epididymitis* is an inflammation of the epididymis. It is most common in patients aged fifteen to thirty years of age and is occasionally seen in younger boys. In teenagers and young adults, the most common cause of epididymitis is sexually transmitted diseases (STDs), usually chlamydia or gonorrhea. In children, epididymitis is usually caused by bacteria such as *E. coli*, which also cause bladder infections. Young children who are diagnosed with epididymitis may have underlying structural abnormalities of the bladder or urethra. Your

doctor will perform a urine test in order to identify the specific type of bacteria causing the infection.

Symptoms. The most common symptom of epididymitis is a *gradual* onset of pain and swelling in the scrotum. The patient may also experience painful or burning urination, more frequent urination, or sudden and abnormal urges to urinate. Fever and chills as well as a urethral discharge may also be present. Symptoms vary widely in severity, with some boys experiencing few or no symptoms.

Treatment. Your pediatrician will perform a complete examination of the scrotum, testicles, and penis and will analyze a sample of your child's urine. If the diagnosis is in doubt, the doctor may order further imaging studies. Often an ultrasound will show evidence of epididymitis, and might need to be done, especially in younger children, in order to rule out any possibility of testicular torsion (see page 512). If epididymitis is diagnosed, the doctor will prescribe an antibiotic. In addition, your child may require bed rest if the pain is significant, along with scrotal support and elevation, which can ease the symptoms. Icc packs and anti-inflammatories, such as ibuprofen, may also be used. Occasionally, a child may experience recurrent episodes of epididymitis. Consultation with a urologist and further testing is required to check for underlying structural abnormalities of the bladder, ureter, or urethra.

Inguinal Hernia

During development of the male fetus, the testicles are inside the abdominal wall. As development continues in the womb, the testicles, along with their spermatic cord, travel through an opening in the abdominal wall and down through a special tube into the scrotum. In most cases, this process is complete prior to delivery. Later in life, a weak point can develop around the hole that the testicle passed through on its way to the scrotum. This can result in what is known medically as an *indirect inguinal hernia*. Portions of the small intestine can pass through this weak point and follow the same path the testicle did down into the scrotum. This results in a gradually swollen scrotal sac; it occurs more commonly in adult men, but children can develop hernias, too.

When to worry. Hernias usually develop very slowly and are generally painless. Parents and children are often completely unaware of the presence of hernias when they are diagnosed on routine physical exams. The longer it goes undiagnosed, the more noticeable it can become, as more of the intestines begin passing into the scrotum. Many people walk around with these types of hernias for years without any problems, and the intestinal contents can usually be pushed back into the abdomen. Complications arise when the intestine gets stuck in the scrotum, a condition doctors call a strangulated hernia. This is a surgical emergency. Pain associated with hernia is usually evidence of strangulation. Any hernia that becomes painful should immediately be seen for surgical evaluation.

What the doctor will do. During your child's routine exam or sports physical, when the doctor examines the penis and testicles and asks your child to "cough," he is checking for the presence of a hernia. Hernias are often diagnosed at a very early stage on routine physical exams, before the patient even realizes he has one. The doctor will carefully check to make sure the hernia is "reducible," meaning that the intestinal contents can easily

be pushed back into the abdominal wall. Very small, easily reducible hernias are usually approached with a watch-and-wait mind-set. Your pediatrician may order a surgical consultation if a hernia is present. Which hernias should be treated surgically and which should be simply monitored closely is an area of great debate. Successful surgery will usually prevent the hernia from getting worse or strangulating. Of course, as mentioned above, any hernia that becomes painful should receive immediate surgical evaluation.

Hydrocele

This most commonly occurs in newborn infants. During fetal development, the testicles begin inside the abdominal wall and descend into the scrotum through a special tube. This pathway usually closes off by the time a baby is born, but occasionally this tube fails to close completely and fluid from the abdominal cavity can leak through the opening into the scrotum. This can cause the male infant's scrotum to swell. This often worries parents, but hydroceles usually do not cause the infant any pain. Your pediatrician will rule out any other more serious causes of the swelling on the routine newborn examinations. While they may look like hernias, hydroceles are soft, nonreducible, and pass the "positive light test": Your doctor will press a penlight gently against the swollen area. A hydrocele will light up; a hernia will remain opaque.

Treatment. Most hydroceles go away on their own within a few months, as the tube that remained open slowly closes and the fluid in the scrotum is slowly reabsorbed into the body. Only rarely will a hydrocele remain after the first few months of life. If this occurs, it does put the child at a higher risk for inguinal hernia. Surgery may be needed to correct the defect in the tube if it persists, the swelling gets worse, or a hernia develops. The vast majority of hydroceles go away on their own.

Orchitis

Orchitis describes inflammation of the testes with no other structures inside the scrotal sac involved. This condition most commonly arises secondary to infection with the mumps virus. Since routine vaccination for mumps began, cases of orchitis have dropped dramatically. Several other types of viruses have been associated with orchitis, and a bacterial infection can also cause orchitis, but orchitis is rarely seen in doctors' offices anymore.

Symptoms. Symptoms are similar to those of epididymitis and include gradual onset of scrotal pain and swelling, along with possible painful and frequent urination. The patient will also likely experience symptoms of mumps, including fever, muscle aches, and a general feeling of malaise. Orchitis usually develops several days after the beginning of a mumps infection. Symptoms of mumps vary widely among patients. Some patients experience few or no symptoms at all. Orchitis occurs in 20 to 40 percent of adolescents and teens who suffer from the mumps. (See Mumps, page 408, for more information.)

Treatment. Your pediatrician will perform an examination of the scrotum and testicles and obtain a history. If mumps infection is suspected, the doctor may do a blood test to confirm this. If the diagnosis is in doubt, further testing along with consultation with a urologist may be needed. Mainstays of treatment for orchitis due to viral causes are bed rest along with support of the scrotum, ice packs, and anti-inflammatories. Almost all cases of orchitis resolve completely, although sterility can occur in 7 to 13 percent of males affected with mumps orchitis. If a bacterial cause of orchitis is found, treatment with antibiotics is needed.

Testicular Cancer

Although rare, testicular cancer does occur in males between the ages of fifteen and thirty-four. One of the symptoms of testicular cancer can be sudden swelling or collection of fluid inside the scrotum. Testicular pain may also be present, and a lump or enlargement of the testicle might be felt. Your pediatrician can rule out testicular cancer through a thorough examination along with further studies, such as ultrasound. Talk to your pediatrician for more information regarding testicular cancer.

Scrotal swelling and/or testicular pain should immediately be evaluated by your pediatrician. Although most cases are nothing to worry about, potentially serious complications can occur. See your pediatrician if your child experiences these symptoms.

Testicular Torsion

This is a relatively rare, but call-doctor-immediately problem. The spermatic cord is attached to the testicle and is responsible for supplying blood to the testicles. Because the testis hangs freely in the scrotal sac, it can twist on itself. When twisting occurs, the blood supply to the testicle can get cut off. This can ultimately result in death or damage of the testicular tissue, possibly leading to problems of infertility.

Symptoms. Here are clues to the diagnosis:

- The child experiences a sudden onset of constant scrotal or testicular pain, usually following activity or trauma to the groin.

- There is swelling, tenderness, and red or blue discoloration high in the affected scrotal sac.

- Nausea and vomiting occur.

- The child has pain on walking.

- The child flexes the leg on the affected side.

- The twisted testis retracts higher.

Initially, testicular torsion may be difficult to tell from scrotal pain and swelling following a kick in the groin. With the latter cause the pain and swelling gradually lessen, but with testicular torsion it continues. If there is any doubt, a surgeon may need to explore the area.

What the doctor will do. The pediatrician will perform a careful examination of the testicles and scrotum. If torsion is strongly suspected, immediate surgical evaluation is required because any delay in treatment may result in loss of the testicle. While waiting for the surgical evaluation, the doctor may order an ultrasound of the scrotum in order to evaluate blood flow to the testes. If torsion is diagnosed, immediate surgery should be done, preferably within six hours of the start of pain. The surgeon will manually untwist the cord and usually perform a surgical procedure known as *orchiopexy,* which will anchor the testis in place and prevent recurrent twisting. Occasionally, the affected testis is no longer viable because of a lack of blood supply and must be removed. Fertility problems are unlikely, because males with one testicle can still be fertile. The twisted cord may untwist on its own, but if this occurs, close follow-up

DR. SEARS TIP
Hold the Food

With testicular torsion, not only will your child hurt so much that he won't want to eat, but you should hold the food so that he's ready for surgery.

with possible repeat ultrasound should be done in order to insure proper blood flow.

Torsion of Appendix Testis

The *appendix testis* is the name given to the structure that lies on the top portion of each testicle. It is a leftover remnant of development of the fetus and serves no function. The appendix testis is prone to twisting upon itself and is a common cause of scrotal pain in children. Torsion of the appendix testis occurs most commonly in boys six to thirteen years of age.

Symptoms. The most common symptom of this condition is pain in the scrotum. The pain normally has a more gradual onset than the pain of testicular torsion. Occasionally pain may develop more rapidly. The intensity can also vary widely from mild to severe. Other symptoms of testicular torsion such as tenderness, swelling, nausea, and fever are usually absent. These symptoms can often distinguish this type of torsion from the more serious testicular torsion (see page 512).

Treatment. Your pediatrician will perform a full examination of the scrotum, testicles, and penis. Depending on the results of the examination, further testing may be required. An ultrasound is usually performed to rule out testicular torsion. Once torsion of the appendix testis is diagnosed, treatment consists mainly of pain control. This includes ice, reduced activity, and support of the scrotum. Anti-inflammatories can also provide some pain relief. In rare cases, the pain can be so severe that surgical removal of the appendix testis may be necessary. The pain from this condition usually resolves within one week. Occasionally, it may persist for several weeks.

Testicular Trauma

Obviously, pain and swelling of the scrotum and testes can result from trauma to the area. As any man will attest, trauma to the testicular area results in extreme pain for a short period of time. Depending on the degree of trauma, pain may be short-lived or last for several minutes.

Treatment. Put ice chips in a sock and place the ice pack in the child's underwear or jockstrap. This will help the pain and diminish the swelling. Monitor closely to insure that symptoms resolve. Evaluation by your doctor is required if the pain persists for more than an hour or if the swelling worsens. (See testicular torsion, page 512.)

Varicocele

This is another potential cause of scrotal swelling. Whereas a hydrocele is caused by leakage of abdominal fluid into the scrotum, a *varicocele* is caused by enlargement of veins inside the scrotum. The scrotum contains a very elaborate blood supply, involving many veins. These veins have one-way valves on the inside of them to keep the blood moving back to the heart. If these valves aren't working well enough, a backup of blood can occur in the veins of the scrotum, causing the veins to enlarge. This is the same way that varicose veins develop in the legs of adults.

Varicoceles typically cause *painless* scrotal swelling. They are most common in men between the ages of fifteen to twenty-five and usually occur on the left side. We see many young men with varicoceles in our office who think they have a mass on their testicles and are worried about testicular cancer. You should have your child evaluated if any mass is felt or suspected around the testicles. Your pediatrician can perform an examination to determine whether symptoms are due to varicocele or another more potentially serious cause. If the diagnosis is still in doubt following physical examination, ultrasound of the testes will be performed.

Treatment. If the varicocele is small, and the patient is having no other symptoms, a wait-and-see approach will be taken. If, however, the varicocele continues to enlarge or the patient begins having other symptoms, such as discomfort, surgical repair may be needed.

THROAT INFECTIONS

Sore throat is a common complaint. Usually the throat itself isn't even infected; it simply hurts as part of a general flu, cold, cough, or viral illness. Sometimes, however, a specific throat infection does occur. Here is our guide to diagnosing and treating sore throats and throat infections.

Causes

Generic viruses. Sore throats are usually caused by cold and flu viruses. The throat itself won't necessarily appear red, but throat pain can be quite considerable.

Specific throat viruses. Some viruses do specifically infect the throat, causing swollen lymph nodes, enlarged tonsils, and a red, painful throat. Often, viral canker sores appear. The most common such virus is called *Coxsackie virus*, which can also cause canker sores throughout the mouth and little blisters on the hands and feet, a condition known as hand, foot, and mouth disease (page 404).

Strep throat. This is the classic bacterial throat infection. The throat will often show dark red spots on the palate, red swollen tonsils with white discharge, and swollen lymph nodes. It's important to treat strep throat with antibiotics to avoid complications. (See page 500.)

Tonsillitis. Sometimes other types of bacteria besides strep can infect the tonsils, causing redness, swelling, and white discharge. Tonsillitis also responds to antibiotics. (See page 523.)

Allergies. These are known to cause sore throat in some kids. Symptoms may include itching as well. If a child has a chronic sore throat but no symptoms of illness, suspect allergies. (See page 131.)

Laryngitis. This is usually caused by a virus infecting the vocal cords and throat. (See page 371 on hoarseness for more information.)

When to See a Doctor

The main question that parents, and doctors, must answer when a child complains of sore throat is whether or not it is strep. If left untreated, the strep bacteria can spread to the heart and kidneys and cause some very serious complications. Fortunately, this is fairly uncommon. It is safe to wait a day or two, until your doctor's office opens, to get testing and treatment. Other bacterial causes of sore throat usually don't need to be treated.

Strep throat. Here are signs that your child should see the doctor and get tested:

- Sore throat is your child's main symptom.

- The throat appears red, especially with blood-red spots on the palate.

- The taste buds may be inflamed and dark red, making the tongue look like a strawberry.

- Pus is evident on the tonsils.

- Headache and abdominal pain are present.

- The pain is worse on swallowing.

- Your child is three years of age or older. Strep is fairly uncommon before then.

- It is late fall or winter, when strep is more common.

- Your child has a fever. Although fever can also mean a viral illness, if there is *no* fever, strep is less likely.

If your pediatrician suspects strep throat, a throat swab can be performed to test for it. See page 500 for more information on diagnosis and treatment of strep throat.

Viral sore throat. If the following describes your child, he probably has a virus and doesn't need to go to the doctor:

- There is no visible redness or pus.

- Other viral symptoms such as cough, runny nose, and diarrhea are present.

- There is no fever.

- Visible white canker sores appear in the mouth or throat.

- The pain is worse while coughing, but not troublesome while swallowing.

- The pain is worse in the morning, but resolves after drinking liquids and getting started with the day.

If you aren't sure, or are worried, it's best to have a doctor check your child.

 DR. SEARS TIP
Sore Throat in the Morning

Non-strep sore throats usually hurt more in the morning and improve as the day progresses. If your child wakes up feeling sore, give him a drink and start the day as usual before you assess how he is really feeling. If it's strep, he won't improve. If it's viral or non-infectious, he'll probably complain less once he gets into normal daily activities.

Treatment

Whether the infection is viral or bacterial, pain relief is usually needed. Here are some effective ways to soothe your child's sore throat:

- Pain-relieving medications such as acetaminophen or ibuprofen can be used. In cases of severe pain, alternate both. See pages 552 and 553 for dosing.

- A warm saltwater gargle (for older kids) is a great way to temporarily ease the pain. Use one half to one teaspoon of salt in eight ounces of water.

- Throat lozenges and anesthetic throat sprays can also help.

THYROID PROBLEMS

The thyroid gland is located in the front of the neck and produces hormones that help regulate our metabolism. *Hypothyroidism* results from a diminished ability of the thyroid gland to secrete enough thyroid hormone. Overproduction of thyroid hormone, called *hyperthyroidism,* is virtually unheard of in children.

Causes

The most common type of hypothyroidism arises mostly in adults. However, it can also be seen in children and adolescents. This type of hypothyroidism is called *Hashimoto's thyroiditis.* This condition is thought to arise from the process of the body's own immune system attacking the thyroid gland. It is not known exactly how or why this happens; however, viral illnesses have been implicated in the progression to Hashimoto's thyroiditis. When this occurs, the thyroid gland begins producing less thyroid hormone. Other less common causes of hypothyroidism in adults and children are:

- surgical removal of the thyroid gland

- radiation exposure of the thyroid gland

- inflammatory conditions

There is a rare birth defect known as *congenital hypothyroidism*. This is seen in 1 out of every 4,000 babies. Thankfully, most states now screen for congenital hypothyroidism as part of the normal newborn screening process.

Symptoms

Symptoms include:

- fatigue

- weakness

- intolerance to cold

- weight gain

- depression

- constipation

- brittle fingernails

- brittle hair

- joint or muscle pain

- irregular menstrual periods in women

- slurred speech

- extreme drowsiness

- hair loss

- delayed growth

Patients may have any or all of the above symptoms.

Treatment

If your pediatrician suspects hypothyroidism, blood tests will be performed to measure the amount of thyroid hormone in your child's body. If a patient is found to be hypothyroid, a daily dose of thyroid hormone in pill form is usually all that is needed to correct hypothyroidism. The doctor will most likely start at a low dose of thyroid hormone and slowly increase it until the proper dosage is achieved. This thyroid hormone replacement may be needed for the patient's entire lifetime.

TICK BITES

Ticks are insects that live in tall grasses, fields, areas of heavy brush, and woods. Once ticks are on the skin, they travel to moist, warm locations on the body, such as in the hair, armpits, or groin, and attach themselves onto the skin to suck blood. Ticks vary greatly in size. Some are so small they are hard to see, while others may be as large as a thumbtack.

Most ticks do not carry disease. There are several diseases, however, that can be transmitted to humans through tick bites. These include:

- Lyme disease

- Colorado tick fever

- Rocky Mountain spotted fever

- Tularemia (rabbit fever)

The Best Way to Remove a Tick

If you discover a tick on your child's body, and you are near a medical facility, have a healthcare professional remove the tick for you. However, if you are in the wilderness and far away from any medical help, here's the best way to remove a tick:

1. Using tweezers or your fingernails, grasp the tick at the head or jaws.

2. Pull the tick straight out in a slow and steady motion.

3. Check to make sure there are no remaining body parts, such as jaws or head, left in the skin.

4. Using soap and water, thoroughly clean the area of the tick bite.

5. Monitor your child closely for any signs of illness.

**DR. SEARS TIP
Don't Destroy the Evidence**

After removing the tick, place it in a closed jar and save for a couple of weeks. We recommend this for two reasons: First, inspecting the tick can insure that you removed all its body parts. Second, if your child does begin showing signs of a tick-borne illness, it is helpful to the doctor to know what type of tick it was.

NEVER use any of the following methods to remove a tick:

- Do not try to burn the tick with a match or a lighter.

- Do not attempt to smother the tick in alcohol, oil, or Vaseline.

- Do not twist the tick when pulling it out.

Symptoms of Tick-Borne Illness

A child with a tick-borne disease will often develop symptoms within one to three weeks following a tick bite. Symptoms to look for include:

- fever

- headache

- neck stiffness

- muscle or joint aches

- swollen lymph nodes

- weakness

- flu-like symptoms

- round target-shaped rash spreading out from the location of the bite

- spots spreading over the body

- paralysis or muscle weakness

- heart palpitations

- chest pain

- difficulty breathing

If your child exhibits any or all of the above symptoms following a tick bite, seek medical attention immediately. When detected in time, tick-borne illnesses can be effectively treated.

Preventing Tick Bites

When he is walking in areas that may harbor ticks, insist that your child wear long pants, a long-sleeved shirt, and a hat. Keep the shirt tucked into the pants. Pull socks over the outside of pants to prevent ticks from crawling up the legs. Encourage your child to wear light-colored clothes, as this makes it easier to spot a tick. Spray tick repellant over the clothes.

**DR. SEARS TIP
Frequent Tick Checks**

Have frequent tick checks when on vacation in areas where you or your child may be exposed to ticks. Carefully examine clothes and skin for ticks. At the end of the day, or upon returning home, have all family members remove their clothing and inspect their skin surfaces. Pay special attention to the scalp, armpits, and groin areas.

TOENAILS, INGROWN

Even toenails have growing pains. If you've ever had an ingrown toenail, you know it can be quite painful as well as hard to get rid of.

Most ingrown toenails occur at the big toe. Occasionally, the thumbnail or fingernail can ingrow. The outside edges of the nail grow inward underneath the skin. Over time, this can cause a breakdown in the normal skin barrier that prevents infection from developing. The area where the nail is growing inward can slowly cause an inflammatory reaction as bacteria begin to invade the soft tissues underneath the skin. Unless treated, this infection can often get worse and lead to such complications as abscess or a spreading skin infection known as *cellulitis*. If you suspect that your child is developing an ingrown toenail, the symptoms will include redness, pain, and swelling on the sides of the nail.

Treatment

Treatment for an ingrown toenail depends on how severe it is:

- Soak the toe several times a day in warm water with Epsom salts.

- Apply OTC antibiotic ointment after each soak.

- Have your child wear open-toed sandals.

- Your pediatrician may gently try to lift up the edge of the toenail in order to prevent it from becoming worse. He may advise you to do the same at home.

- The doctor may prescribe an oral antibiotic, if needed.

- If it appears that the above-mentioned treatments may not be enough, the doctor may decide to remove part of the toenail. This is normally done by first injecting the toe with an anesthetic in order to prevent pain. When done correctly, the patient feels little or nothing in the way of pain during the procedure. The doctor will then raise the toenail off its bed using forceps and use scissors to cut part of the toenail off. The rest of the toenail may or may not fall off, but not to worry, the nail will grow back! This almost always prevents recurrence of the ingrown toenail.

Prevention

- Purchase shoes that are not too tight, and make sure your child is not wearing shoes that are too small for her.

- Avoid narrow-toed shoes, such as high heels and dress shoes. If toes are constantly crammed into too small a space, this makes ingrown toenails more likely.

- Encourage your child to wear open-toed sandals whenever it is safe to do so.

- If you notice that an edge of your child's toenail is becoming ingrown, or if she starts complaining of pain, redness, or tenderness in that area, it is a good idea to try to gently and carefully lift the edge of the nail upward using a nail file once or twice every day. This may lift out the area of the toenail that is beginning to become ingrown and may prevent it from getting worse. You should only do this if the infection is not severe. If you are uncomfortable doing this, your pediatrician can do it.

DR. SEARS TIP
Use a *Square* Cut Rather Than a *Round* Cut

Proper grooming habits of nails, especially of the big toenail, are very important. Avoid cutting the big toenail in a crescent-shaped pattern. Cut it straight across from one end to the other so that the edges of the nail grow over the skin rather than into it. The edges of toenails that are cut in a curved fashion are more likely to continue growing downward and become ingrown.

TOE WALKING

Most toe walking is a normal and temporary quirk as many toddlers go through the toe-standing stage between one and two years. Beginning walkers like to experiment with different ways of standing, walking, and running, so they experiment with toe walking. Once the child realizes this is an uncomfortable way to stand or walk, the toe walker gradually puts his feet on the ground.

Causes

There are three main causes of toe walking:

• Most cases of toe walking are caused by simple curiosity and immaturity that will pass without any intervention.

• Some cases are caused by a tight Achilles tendon that may require stretching (see below).

• Rarely, toe walking may be part of a larger developmental problem with other signs of developmental delay.

When to Worry; What to Do

Keep a diary. Record how often your child toe walks and if it's getting more or less frequent.

If the following describes your child, you shouldn't worry:

• Child does not persistently toe walk, and sometimes the gait seems perfectly normal.

• When sleeping or lying on the floor relaxed, the child's feet are not pointing forward.

• You can easily flex the foot up and down without having to apply a lot of pressure.

If any of the following are true for your child, see the doctor:

• The toe walking lasts all day so that the child is always walking like a ballerina.

• The feet remain flexed forward even when your child is sleeping or relaxed.

• The Achilles tendon and lower leg muscles seem tight when you force-flex them.

What the Doctor May Do

Your pediatrician will do three things:

• Watch your child walk.

• Flex the foot to see if the Achilles tendon is naturally loose and to see if your child can stand flat-footed.

• Assess your child's overall development, muscle tone, and coordination and provide further help and testing if needed.

If the Achilles tendon or the lower leg muscles seem tight, the doctor may refer you to a physical therapist who will show you Achilles tendon–stretching exercises you can do at home. Around ten times a day, simply flex your toddler's foot toward the front of the leg. Sing songs and make these exercises a fun game rather than a medical chore. You can even make this part of your diaper-changing routine. For an older child, have him face a wall and lean into the wall while keeping one foot at a time flat on the floor with the knee bent toward the wall.

TONGUE-TIE

Tongue-tie (also known as *ankyloglossia*) is a common condition in children. During fetal development the cord of tissue, called the *lingual frenulum,* that connects the base of the tongue and the floor of the mouth slowly recedes toward the back of the tongue. After birth, the short tongue lengthens as Baby grows, thus stretching the frenulum. Sometimes this cord remains attached to the front of the tongue. In most cases, tongue-tie does not cause a problem and self-corrects. But sometimes it can cause sucking difficulties for the breastfeeding infant and later speech problems for the child.

Signs and Symptoms

The following are signs that your child might have tongue-tie:

The tight tongue is heart-shaped. Observe for what we call the "heart sign." While Baby is crying or at another time when Baby has her mouth wide open, see if the tip of the tongue

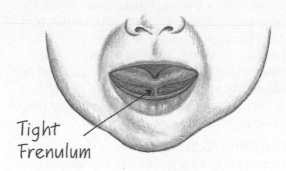

Tight Frenulum

is so tightly attached to the front of the mouth that the tongue assumes a heart shape, with the tongue-tied area looking like the top crescent of a heart. This heart sign is a clue that should be mentioned to your pediatrician at your baby's first checkup, or even sooner. Next, observe the tightness and thickness of the frenulum. Some tongues look tight, but the frenulum is a thin membrane. These tongues are less of a worry since they usually stretch and self-correct. If, however, the frenulum appears so thick that when you put your little finger underneath the tongue you can't stretch it upward, that's more of a sign. Also, the tip of the tongue normally extends past the lower gum when Baby is smiling, laughing, and relaxed. If the tongue doesn't extend past the lower gum to lick the lips but instead forms a trough at the tip, the tongue may be too tight. Also, look for the "humpback tongue" sign: If the back of the tongue lifts up while the front of the tongue remains tied to the floor of the mouth, this may indicate it is too tight.

Baby has a sucking problem. If early in the newborn period you find Baby is not latching on well, your nipples are getting sore, your milk supply is insufficient, and Baby's weight gain is inadequate, these are clues that the tongue is so tight that Baby cannot latch on properly to suck enough milk out of your breasts. Another clue is if breastfeeding hurts. Also, because tongue-tied babies have to work harder to suck, they tire more easily. And tongue-tied babies tend to frequently "fall off" the breast during a feeding. As well said by La Leche League: "The tongue is the major player in breastfeeding."

Difficult toddler talk. If your two- to three-year-old is having increasing articulation problems, and your child still looks tongue-tied, your pediatrician may refer you to a speech pathologist who will analyze your child's tongue movements during normal speech. If the tongue-tie is the culprit, the next referral is to an ENT (ear, nose, throat) specialist for a clipping.

DR. SEARS TIP
When in Doubt, Clip It Out

There are two kinds of pediatricians when it comes to evaluating and treating tongue-tie: the "wait-and-see-ers" and "the clippers." We are "clippers." This is based upon thirty-five years of experience during which we learned to appreciate how often breastfeeding difficulties are due to tongue-tie and also how many babies don't "grow out of it." A ten-second procedure can give Baby years of Mother's good milk and possibly help the child talk more easily.

What the Doctor Can Do

While it sounds like a big deal, it really isn't. I (Dr. Bill) remember a mother driving a couple of hours for a tongue-tie consultation because her doctor made the right diagnosis but wanted to send Baby to an ENT specialist who was going to "hospitalize Baby" to "clip

the tongue"! This wise mother wanted a second opinion. I looked at the baby and agreed with the pediatrician's diagnosis (but not the referral). When Baby opened her mouth wide, I quickly grabbed the tip of the tongue with a piece of gauze (sometimes if the mouth is open wide enough holding the tongue is not necessary) and took a one-second "snip." The procedure was painless and bloodless. I still remember the amazed mother exclaiming, "Is that all there is to it?" Yes, that's all there is to it. After the procedure, Baby can go to the breast immediately for comforting. Mothers often sense the improved latch-on right away. Sometimes clipping the frenulum yields a couple of drops of blood, but this quickly stops and doesn't bother Baby. We believe that not being able to suck enough milk, or having to work very hard to get it, would bother a newborn baby much more than having the frenulum clipped.

The benefit of doing early clipping is that in the first month or so the frenulum is mostly thin and membranous and not as richly supplied with blood vessels. It is easier to clip and the procedure is less bothersome to the baby. The longer the tongue-tie is left unclipped, the more muscular the tether can become, and the more extensive and difficult the procedure will be. If you wait a few months to a year, the frenulum thickens and becomes more vascular, and the procedure becomes more complicated, requiring sutures or cauterization to control the bleeding.

Tongue-tie is probably one of the most underestimated and undertreated problems in early infancy. If Baby could talk he would probably say, "Get that thing out so I can suck and talk right!"

Once upon a time, conventional wisdom was to leave tight tongues alone and they would gradually loosen up. This more conservative approach was prevalent before breast-feeding made its comeback, since tight tongues don't bother bottlefeeders. Now that more women are breastfeeding, more doctors have to be tongue-tie savvy.

TONSIL AND ADENOID ENLARGEMENT

The importance of tonsils and adenoids has long been a subject of debate. The fact that they are lymph-gland tissues, which make infection-fighting blood cells and immune-boosting substances (and they are strategically located around the throat and airways, where most germs enter the body), leads doctors to suspect that they do help a child fight off germs and should only be removed if they are harming the child's health. The tonsils are marble-sized tissues located on both sides of the throat. You can usually see them when your child opens his mouth wide. The adenoids are located above the tonsils behind the *uvula* (the flap of tissue that hangs down from the back of the palate). *Adenoids* can usually only be seen with a special light. Because the adenoids are located behind the nasal passages, when they are swollen the child has difficulty breathing through the nose. When the tonsils are swollen, the child has difficulty swallowing. Generally, both the tonsils and the adenoids become swollen during an infection.

The tonsils and adenoids generally get bigger until the child reaches age six, then gradually shrink thereafter. They seem to be largest and most bothersome when your child is most prone to upper respiratory infections during the preschool years.

DR. SEARS TIP
Know Your Child's Tonsils

Get used to your child's normal tonsil size. Have her look up at the ceiling, open her mouth wide, and say or sing "aah" or "eeh" and hold that sound for at least five seconds while you look.

Should the Tonsils and/or Adenoids Be Removed?

The three main criteria used to determine whether your child needs a tonsillectomy and/or adenoidectomy or whether a watch-and-wait approach is more appropriate are how much these tissues are disturbing your child's:

* eating
* sleeping
* growing

How parents can help in the decision. Here's where your parent diary really shines. Record the following information:

* Are the enlarged tissues interfering with your child's sleep, and how?
* Does your child have difficulty swallowing?
* How frequent and severe have tonsil infections been?
* How often does your child need antibiotic treatment?
* Does your child have frequent ear infections? Swollen adenoids block the normal drainage of the eustachian tube, the tiny tube that connects the middle ear with the

throat and allows fluid and mucus to drain out of the middle ear during a cold.

- How much are the infections interfering with your child's growth and development? Is she missing school? Does she have a poor appetite?

When looking at your diary, the doctor or ENT specialist is trying to make two decisions: How much are these tissues bothering your child, and is the situation getting better, worse, or staying the same?

DR. SEARS TIP
Trouble Sleeping—
Get Them Out!

If your child is suffering from obstructive sleep apnea (OSA), the tonsils and/or adenoids must come out. For more on OSA, see page 474.

TONSILLITIS

Since the tonsils seem to be the first line of defense against germs entering the throat, they seem to get infected a lot, especially during early childhood.

Symptoms

Clues that your child might have tonsillitis are:

- sudden onset of snoring, noisy breathing, and difficulty sleeping

- complaints of sore throat

- difficulty swallowing

- raspy, throaty voice

- fever and generally feeling uncomfortable

- swollen, tender lumps beneath the jawbones

- enlarged, red tonsils covered with a thick, white film

- stinky breath

What the Doctor Will Do

Red, swollen, pus-covered, painful tonsils in a sick child with fever and swollen neck glands is usually a "no-brainer" for the doctor. This combination of symptoms almost always indicates bacterial tonsillitis, and a ten-day course of antibiotics is usually warranted if the child is acting considerably ill. If a child isn't feeling too bad, the tonsils aren't too swollen, and the pus is minimal, this may indicate a less serious viral sore throat (see page 514) and a wait-and-see approach may be taken. If the doctor suspects strep bacteria may be the cause of the tonsillitis (dark red spots on the palate and "strawberry tongue"— see page 500), a throat swab strep test may be done so that if other family members or close friends come down with symptoms, it will be known that strep is going around, and the strep can be promptly treated.

One confounding factor with tonsillitis is that some cases may actually be the mono virus, and not bacterial at all (see page 402). Mono can cause all the same tonsil symptoms, fever, and swollen neck glands. Five additional clues that suggest mono tonsillitis instead of bacterial are:

- The tonsils are completely covered with pus. This screams mono. In bacterial tonsillitis, the pus is more scattered in patches.

- There are other swollen glands in the armpits or groin area.

- An enlarged spleen is felt on the left side of the abdomen below the ribcage.

- The child has a light red blotchy rash.

- The child has had an allergic reaction to antibiotics. If the doctor treats your child with amoxicillin or Augmentin for bacterial tonsillitis, the mono virus will react with the antibiotics to cause an allergic-looking red, pimply, or blotchy rash throughout the body. If this occurs, your doctor should do a blood test for mono, instead of just labeling your child allergic to that antibiotic and switching to another.

 DR. SEARS TIP
Clinical Clue

How your child acts is more significant than how the throat looks. Your child will likely act more sick when the fever is very high and perk up when the fever is down. This is a good sign. The doctor will rely on your input as to whether your child is getting better or worse overall.

What You Can Do

Besides the doctor's treatment, here are some home treatments for a sore throat and tonsillitis:

- Feed your child a soft, non-irritating diet to ease the painful swallowing.

- Try the "sipping solution" — smoothies, ice cream, frozen yogurt, Jell-O, and Popsicles. To avoid the dehydration that is associated with a fever, be sure your child sips on fluids throughout the day.

- Encourage your child to suck on ice chips to ease throat pain or eat frozen yogurt or ice cream; put a cup of his favorite yogurt in the freezer and let him munch on the frozen, soothing yogurt all day long.

- Homemade soups, like Mom's chicken soup, are usually a favorite.

TONSILLOLITHS

One day you look into your child's throat and see a pea-sized white lump lodged in the tonsils or beneath the flap of skin between the back of the throat and tonsils. Your child has been complaining of a weird sensation in his throat, and you've noticed stinky breath. The white lump you are seeing is called a tonsillolith or "tonsil stone."

Tonsil stones are an accumulation of all the stuff (dead skin cells, postnasal drip, etc.) that collects in the back of the throat. Over time the body seems to neatly package all this junk into a little white ball. These stones seem to settle in the nooks and crannies of the tonsil areas.

How to Tell

Clues to suspect your child has one or more tonsil stones are:

- stinky breath

- complaints of uncomfortable swallowing

- complaints that "something is in my throat"

What to Do

No need to run to the phone to call your pediatrician. You can make an appointment at your convenience. Tonsil stones often form after a prolonged period of postnasal drip from a sinus infection or a lingering cold. The best ways to prevent tonsil stones from forming are:

- by preventing and treating postnasal drip

- for the older child, by gargling with salt water and scraping the back of the tongue as part of daily dental hygiene

Sometimes these stones will dislodge over time with the above throat-hygiene measures, but if they are bothering your child, they can be removed either by your pediatrician or an ENT (ear, nose, throat) specialist. The doctor sprays a local anesthetic in the throat and grabs these little white stones with forceps. In very cooperative children, we have removed these in our own office without a topical anesthetic. It's a good feeling for both doctor and patient to see the little white stone on the end of the forceps, and the child feels instantly better. We ask the child if he'd like to put this little stinky white thing in his scrapbook. The parents usually decline!

TORTICOLLIS

Torticollis (meaning twisting of the neck) is a spasm of the *sternocleidomastoid* (SCM) muscle, the large muscle that runs from the skull bone behind the ear down alongside the neck into the joint between the collarbone and the breastbone. This muscle is the main one involved in tilting and turning the neck.

Signs

Doctors will often notice torticollis during one of Baby's first checkups, but it's useful for parents to be aware of the signs so you can point it out to the doctor:

- Baby will hold his head tilted toward the shoulder of the tight-muscled side.

- Baby will prefer to keep his head turned away from the tight side.

- The SCM muscle feels tight.

- Baby resists you turning his head toward the tight side.

For example, a baby with a tight right-side SCM muscle will have his head tilt toward the right shoulder while preferring to turn his head toward his left.

The Cause

Torticollis seems to be caused by trauma to the sternocleidomastoid muscle. The injured muscle goes into spasm, becomes tighter, shorter, and pulls the back of the head to that side. Trauma was once considered to be due to an unusual position Baby assumed in utero — perhaps Baby was twisted a certain way or there was uneven pressure on one of the SCM muscles. Babies with torticollis have a higher incidence of other positional problems, such as turned-in feet and hip dislocations.

Another likely theory is that the muscle was stretched during delivery, a type of sprain. There may have been bleeding into the injured muscle, which healed as fibrous tissue, accounting for the apparent shortening and firmness of the muscle and the characteristic lump that many parents feel in the neck. The shortened muscle goes into spasm and pulls the back of the neck toward one shoulder, causing the chin to point to the other shoulder.

How to Tell; What to Do

While some babies just like to turn their necks to one side, with torticollis it's always to that one side, and it's tilted, not just turned. The shortened muscle on the affected side feels harder, as if it's in spasm. Also, when you try to rotate Baby's head to the other side, it meets a lot of resistance.

Mention your concern to your pediatrician, who will not only examine your baby's neck to confirm the diagnosis but also look for other positional quirks, such as in the hips, legs, and feet.

DR. SEARS TIP
Child Tilting Head—
See Doctor

Head tilt in an older infant or toddler may be a clue that a child is turning the head to accommodate for vision problems, such as a lazy eye.

Treatment

Because the problem is a contracted, stiff muscle, the treatment is to gradually stretch the affected muscle. The doctor will show you how to do two types of exercises: those that require you to stretch Baby's neck muscle and those that encourage Baby to stretch it herself. Try these tips to teach Baby to use the weaker muscles:

- Approach your baby from the unaffected side. This will encourage her to turn her head in that direction. Making baby sounds or shaking a favorite toy while you approach her will often cause her to want to turn her head in that direction, and this will help strengthen the unaffected muscle group.

- Do shoulder-to-shoulder stretching. With each diaper change, hold both sides of your baby's head and rotate the neck so the chin approaches each shoulder. Start with just a little rotation and gradually increase the rotation until the chin can just about touch the shoulder.

- Teach tummy time. Tummy time is very important for infants with torticollis. Periods of between fifteen and thirty minutes a few times a day on the tummy can dramatically improve neck strength and flexibility. Hold a toy above her to encourage her to turn her neck toward the toy.

- When you place your little one to sleep, turn her head toward the unaffected side. This will help keep the affected side from becoming too tight.

- Carry Baby in the football hold (the diaper area straddled over the palm of your hand and her head in the crook of your elbow). Turn her head outward, away from the affected side.

- When going for a stroll around the house or outside, carry Baby forward-facing. Turn her slightly away from the more interesting attractions so that she has to turn her head toward them and stretch the affected muscle.

Because the head will always spring back after stretching exercises, try to do these as frequently as possible as part of your daily play-with-Baby routine. Do the shoulder-to-shoulder stretching at least after every diaper change.

Your pediatrician may refer you to a physical therapist who will show you SCM stretching exercises. While it's true that you'd want the physical therapist to do most of the stretching in the tight muscle, we have always taught parents to also do the shoulder-to-shoulder stretch so that both neck muscles receive a bit of stretching therapy. In a nutshell, physical therapy focuses on stretching the head and neck away from where the muscle is pointed. The muscle pulls the head to the side and down and slightly rotates the neck to the opposite side. Your stretching exercises will do the opposite: rotate the head to the affected side and up.

 DR. SEARS TIP
How to Best Use Therapists

We use a lot of therapists in our pediatric practice, and here's what we've learned: It becomes a hassle to have to go to the therapist once or twice a week for many months. For most, but not all, ailments, use the therapist primarily as a consultant. Go for a few sessions and have the therapist teach you how to do the exercises at home. That way you can use your travel time to do more home therapy and you can tailor the therapy for when Baby is in the right mood. Having to stretch a baby's muscle who is upset and tight all over is not going to get the best result. Sometimes you have to be politely assertive, saying, for example, "The drive is so hard on my baby. Could I come for just a few sessions and you show me how to do the exercises at home?" Both home therapy and regular progress checks with the therapist are wise.

Most infants regain full motion of their neck within three to six months of physical therapy, and it often takes only a few weeks to a month to see an improvement. If the torticollis is discovered within the first two months, it will usually be fully corrected by the age of one year, providing the physical therapy exercises are performed routinely. If, despite rigorous physical therapy, the condition has not corrected itself after the age of one year, the doctor may discuss other treatment options, such as surgical correction. Occasionally surgery must be performed in order to lengthen the affected muscle group. This is necessary in only a small number of cases of torticollis.

Torticollis in the Older Child

Torticollis that occurs in the first few weeks or months is called *congenital torticollis* because it is thought to be due to trauma to the SCM muscle pre-birth or during birth. *Acquired torticollis* happens in the older child and is secondary to an injured muscle or inflammation of the tissues surrounding the muscle. One of the most common causes is inflamed lymph glands alongside the muscle, secondary to a viral infection or sore throat. With this type of torticollis, also known as "wryneck," the head is tilted *away from* the affected side and the child experiences some pain in the affected muscle. Turning away from the affected side seems to offer relief from the pain or irritation.

This type of torticollis usually resolves without any treatment once the underlying irritant heals. Sometimes a moist, warm compress will help relieve the pain in the affected muscle. In fact, it's better not to try to stretch inflamed muscles.

UMBILICAL HERNIA

A baby's "outie" navel that gets larger during crying or straining is called an *umbilical hernia*. The term *hernia* means "protrusion of the bowel through an opening." These may range from marble to golf-ball size.

The Cause

When the fetus is in the womb, the umbilical cord passes through the abdominal wall into the fetus's body, supplying blood to the fetus. After the infant is born and the umbilical cord falls off, the muscles of the abdominal wall begin to close around the area of the belly button. An umbilical hernia can develop if these muscle layers do not completely close shortly after birth.

Sometimes the space between the abdominal muscles is large enough to let the underlying bowel protrude a bit against the thin abdominal wall, especially when Baby cries or strains and increases the intra-abdominal pressure. These painless and harmless hernias nearly always seal off by themselves by two years of age as the abdominal muscles grow together. Rarely do they require any treatment. Occasionally, the hernia occurs in the muscles above the navel. This type of hernia is less likely to heal unaided and may need minor surgical closure later. Umbilical hernias are more common in African-American babies and in premature infants. While there is some evidence that the practice of "strapping" (applying adhesive tape over large hernias, such as those that protrude more than a half inch) may hasten the healing, most pediatricians recommend that parents leave these "outies" alone.

When to Worry

Rarely the intestinal tissue that protrudes through the hernia opening can become stuck or strangulated and need immediate surgical repair. This warrants a trip to the emergency room. In the thousands of umbilical hernias we have seen over thirty-five years in pediatric practice, we have seen this complication occur only once. Signs of a strangulated umbilical hernia are:

- Baby is in intense pain.
- The protrusion is harder than usual.
- The protrusion can't easily be pushed back in as usual.
- The protrusion is discolored.
- It is very painful to your baby when you touch it.

You don't have to worry that you will miss these signs, as they are obviously different from a typical umbilical hernia.

VACCINE REACTIONS

Vaccines are a very important aspect of disease prevention in our country. Unfortunately, some children will have a reaction to the shots. Thankfully, most reactions are fairly mild and harmless. Very rarely, a child may experience a more severe reaction. In this section we will discuss the mild and expected vaccine reactions and how you can treat them. We will also share how to recognize a more severe reaction.

Expected Vaccine Reactions

Most babies are expected to show at least some reaction to their vaccines. Here is a list of what you may see happen, and how you can alleviate your baby's discomfort.

Fussiness. This is the most common reaction. Most babies will experience pain from the injection, then muscle soreness for hours to days because the vaccine solution may irritate the skin or muscle. This will cause varying degrees of crying.

Fever. This is fairly common. Many babies will experience a low-grade fever. Some may show a high fever for a day or two. This occurs because the immune system is reacting to the vaccine.

Redness and swelling at the site. Some children will show mild redness and swelling from the injection.

Persistent bump at the injection site. This occurs in some children when a pocket of calcium from an internal bruise remains behind after the blood dissolves away. It will resolve after a month or two and is harmless.

Rash. Two vaccines, MMR (mumps, measles, rubella) and chicken pox, are well known for causing a generalized rash throughout the body about a week after the shot. This is a normal immune reaction to the vaccine and is not contagious.

Severe swelling and redness of the upper arm or leg. Less commonly a child will experience more extreme swelling of the entire upper part of a limb where vaccines were given. This is a mixture of irritation from the vaccine ingredients and an allergic reaction. You can keep the reaction under control with the measures below, but this may be an indication not to repeat that vaccine.

None of these reactions really warrant an after-hours call to your pediatrician. Let the doctor know how your baby did next time you are in the office.

DR. SEARS TIP
Don't Overmedicate

If your baby is having a difficult vaccine reaction, such as high fever and extreme fussiness, it's useful to treat with ibuprofen. However, don't administer the medication around the clock. Let it wear off from time to time so you can monitor how your baby is doing. You don't want to hide a severe reaction. If your baby reacts badly enough to need around-the-clock meds for several days, this may be a warning that you need to proceed more carefully with the next round of shots.

Treating and Preventing Expected Reactions

Before the shots. Here are some steps you can take before your baby gets shots to prevent these uncomfortable reactions:

- Bring a plastic baggy with ice cubes to your appointment and ice the areas where the shots will be given for a few minutes to numb the nerves.

- Breastfeed your baby while the shots are being given to distract from the pain.

- Give your baby a pacifier dipped in sugar water (or your finger if you don't use a paci); this reduces the pain response.

- Give your child (three months and older) ibuprofen about thirty minutes prior to the shots to decrease pain and inflammation.

Acetaminophen can also be used at any age, but may not be as effective.

After the shots. Here are some ways you can ease the pain and discomfort after the shots are given:

- Ice the areas for five minutes after the shots. You can continue icing on and off for a few days if you see any redness or swelling in the shot locations. This is especially useful for severe swelling reactions.

- Ibuprofen or acetaminophen can be continued for a few days if needed for fever and fussiness. Don't routinely give these for no reason; only use them if needed.

- Arnica is a homeopathic remedy that can be given by mouth or rubbed on the shot areas to decrease swelling.

- Diphenhydramine (Benadryl) can be given in cases of severe swelling or any other signs of an allergic reaction.

When to Worry

Rarely, vaccines can cause serious reactions. These are thought to occur in about 1 in every 100,000 doses, although precise statistics on this aren't known for sure. Such reactions include seizures, inflammation and swelling of the brain (called encephalitis), various nerve dysfunctions, sudden fainting or shock, severe allergic reactions, autoimmune reactions, and various body organ dysfunctions. We don't know how to predict or prevent these reactions. Fortunately, they are extremely rare.

If your child has one of these severe reactions, see your doctor right away, or call 911 if it's an emergency.

DR. SEARS TIP
Don't Ignore Extreme
Fussing and Fever

A somewhat rare reaction that occurs from time to time is *encephalitis*. This occurs when the vaccine components irritate the nervous system and cause inflammation within the brain. The brain itself may swell slightly and become slightly red (if you could see it). The baby will have high fevers and extreme irritability for a few days. He may have prolonged periods of intense screaming. After a few days the reaction subsides, the inflammation and swelling go down, and the baby returns to his normal happy self. Although this is definitely no fun to go through, virtually all babies weather it without any residual problems. Ibuprofen can be given every six hours as needed to minimize the inflammation and fever as much as possible. However, if the same shots are repeated all together again, *this reaction could be worse the next time around and neurological injury may result*. We suggest you talk with your pediatrician about spreading the shots out over more than one visit next time to minimize the risk.

For more detailed information on vaccines and vaccine reactions, see *The Vaccine Book*, by Robert W. Sears.

VAGINAL CONCERNS

Like the penis of a male infant, the vagina in a female infant is usually a self-maintaining organ with only a few medical problems. But there are some normal quirks that parents of little girls need to be aware of. Here are the most common ones:

Vaginal Bleeding in Newborns

Because of the leftover maternal hormones, it's normal for some newborn baby girls to have a few days of slight vaginal bleeding during the first few weeks. This is basically a mini-menstrual period. As the effects of the maternal hormones wear off, this is the last "period" she will experience for the next ten or more years.

Vaginal Discharge

Normal, physiologic vaginal discharge. During infancy and toddlerhood vaginal secretions begin, which keep the membranes from drying out. Usually discharge looks like and has the consistency of egg white and is nearly odorless. Medically known as *physiologic vaginal discharge* (*physiologic* is medical jargon for "normal"), some little girls will make more discharge than others, and it's very common to notice these egg white secretions on little panties. Expect this to increase during pre-puberty and adolescence. While this discharge is normal, if it does bother your child, try the tips on page 533.

Discharge from vaginal infections. Germs, especially yeast, grow in a moist, warm, dark environment. The vagina is therefore a perfect environment for infections such as yeast, or candida. *Candida* is the most common vaginal infection at all ages. Clues that your child may have a vaginal yeast infection are:

- The discharge is thick and white, somewhat like cottage cheese. It may have a slightly moldy odor.

- You notice some redness.

- It commonly occurs a week or two following antibiotic treatment.

- Your child complains of itching.

Although bacterial infections as a cause of vaginal discharge are unusual in small children, they do occur. Clues to a bacterial cause:

- Discharge is a deep yellow color.

- It has a more foul odor.

- Your child complains of pain or burning.

- The vagina is noticeably very red.

- Dark red pimples are spread around the area.

Vaginal Redness and Irritation

Some children will experience vaginal irritation from everyday factors, such as tight-fitting underpants or swimsuits, dirt, bath soaps,

DR. SEARS TIP
Help Your Child Be Comfortable While Being Examined

Vaginal discharge, irritation, and inflammation are a frequent nuisance in the growing infant, toddler, and child, and they necessitate an examination of the area. Here's how you can help your child feel comfortable. Try not to transfer vaginal-exam anxiety to your child. Let your child lie comfortably on your lap with her legs open in the diaper-changing position. Explain to your daughter in age-appropriate terms that the doctor is going to check her vagina and why. Put it in the context of her other body parts: "Your doctor will shine a light in your ears, count your teeth, open your mouth, feel your tummy, and check your vagina..." Perhaps have her bring a doll along "so the doctor can check your dolly too..."

diaper use in an older toddler, feces, or self-touching habits. These can lead to redness and pain, often without discharge. We address how to diagnose and soothe general vaginal irritation below.

Treating and Preventing Vaginal Infections and Irritation

Identify the trigger. Vaginal irritations and infections don't just happen, something causes them. The usual triggers are:

- antibiotics

- friction from tight-fitting clothing

- irritation from bubble baths, oils, and so on. (A lot of lotions, potions, and soaps that are put into bathwater can be irritating to sensitive vaginal tissue and cause "soap vulvitis.")

- Irritation from regular toilet paper. A few kids will be sensitive to the bleach or other chemicals in toilet paper. Try a chemical-free toilet paper from a health-food store.

- fecal irritation

- foreign bodies inserted in the vagina (A clue that a foreign body is stuck in the vagina is that the area will stink!)

- pinworms

Prevent the trigger. Once you identify the trigger, try to prevent it:

- Encourage your daughter to wear loose-fitting, cotton underwear and swimwear.

- Teach her to wipe from front to back to avoid getting rectal germs into the vagina.

- Instruct her not to put anything up into her vagina. Children explore and put things, such as crayons and toilet tissue, into many of their body openings (the ears, nose, and vagina).

- Avoid bubble baths and discourage your child from sitting in soapy water for more than ten minutes. If she's recovering from a vaginal infection, have her shower instead.

- Use probiotics following antibiotic therapy. If yeast symptoms worsen, apply an adult over-the-counter vaginal yeast cream once daily to the external vaginal area until better. Use a seven-day type of cream; the one- or three-day creams are too strong. Don't insert any cream into the vagina.

- If your daughter is going through a masturbation stage and you suspect this is the cause of the irritation, increase your surveillance (see Masturbation, page 390).

- Check for pinworms. (See Pinworms, page 431.)

- To soothe an itchy vagina, let her sit in warm bathwater (either plain water or with a few tablespoons of baking soda).

 **DR. SEARS TIP
Treat Both Ends**

If your infant gets recurrent vaginal yeast infections, suspect that it begins in the mouth as *oral thrush* (the name for oral yeast or candida infections). Treating one end will often help clear the other end. Recurrent oral thrush is also a common cause of candida diaper rash. (See Yeast Infections, page 542.)

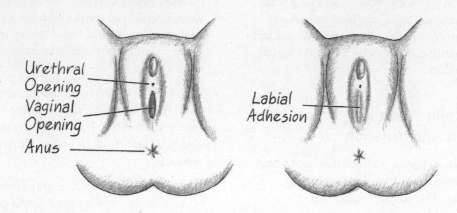

Labial Adhesions

You've brought your darling four-month-old in for a routine checkup, and you're so thankful that she's perfectly healthy. As your doctor is doing a head-to-toe checkup and examines the vaginal opening, he surprises you with "Her vagina seems to be closing up." This common and harmless quirk is called *labial adhesion.*

The cause. Leftover maternal estrogen keeps the cells lining the edges of the labia smooth in the very early months. By three to four months of age, two changes occur that trigger labial adhesions: The maternal estrogen effect wears off, and the constant irritation to the labia from rubbing on wet diapers sets up inflammation. Inflamed tissue, like scratches and cuts, grows together.

What to do. Unless the labial area is closed enough to obstruct urine flow, which is rare, labial adhesions are harmless. In most cases a child will begin exploring her own vagina and gradually and painlessly work apart any adhesions. Labia that remain stuck throughout childhood will usually separate during puberty

once the child's own female hormones cause the labia to mature. However, the labia occasionally remain firmly adhered and don't separate on their own. If there is little to no opening left, vaginal secretions and menstrual flow cannot come out. In such cases, a gynecologist must perform a separation procedure in the office. It is best to prevent labial adhesions in the first place (see page 59) or to gently separate any adhesions when they first appear during infancy if possible.

Depending on what the membrane looks like, the doctor will take one of several approaches: If the membrane is thin and see-through and only partially adhering to the labia, the doctor is likely to take the wait-and-see approach and simply follow the progression of the adhesion at each regularly scheduled checkup. Most pediatricians favor this approach because most of these labial adhesions resolve without medication or manual opening.

If the labia are more firmly adhered and almost completely closed, the doctor might prescribe an estrogen cream to soften up the adhesions. The doctor may then be able to separate any leftover adhesions using a metal tool.

It's a good idea to periodically check for these quirks during bathing and, if you notice an adhesion forming, mention it to your doctor at Baby's next regular checkup.

VITILIGO

Vitiligo is a painless, noncontagious skin condition characterized by patchy, ivory white areas of the skin. Although these patches may appear anywhere on the body, they are most common on the face, hands, arms, and legs, and appear bilaterally, meaning on both hands, both cheeks, both arms, or both legs. Vitiligo (from the Latin *viti* meaning "blemish" and *ligo* meaning "to cause") is believed to be an autoimmune quirk in which the body's own immune system attacks and weakens or destroys the pigment-producing cells of the skin called *melanocytes*. These white patches are more obvious in the summer months, when the surrounding skin tans, but the white patches don't.

How to Tell

Vitiligo is a cosmetic concern, not an infection. What happens to these patches varies greatly among children. Some patches fade or shrink with time; others stay the same for years; still others may get larger. Over time, some of the vitiligo patches will re-pigment on their own, eventually fading into a color similar to the surrounding skin. Vitiligo is often confused with eczema or fungal infections. Here's how to tell the difference.

Vitiligo patches:

- don't itch

- are more noticeable in the summer

- are symmetrical and bilateral patches (e.g., similar patches on both cheeks and both hands)

- have flat, irregular borders (fungal infections have raised or circular borders)

- are smooth (fungal infections and eczema are rough and scaly)

Vitiligo is generally not treated, especially in children, since many patches fade over time. If your teen has cosmetic concerns about these patches, consult a dermatologist. PUVA light therapy is sometimes effective.

VOMITING

Vomiting is always concerning for parents, but you can rest assured that it is usually harmless in the long run. Most kids can tolerate numerous episodes over several hours without getting dehydrated. Here's our guide to help you with your child's vomiting illness.

Common Causes

Stomach virus. Viruses are the most common cause of vomiting in children and adults. There are several different kinds (such as the flu, rotavirus, and others), but they all cause similar patterns of illness. They are contracted by contact with another sick person. These viruses usually come on suddenly, with fevers, aches, abdominal pain, and vomiting. Diarrhea may or may not follow. The vomiting can be treated, but there is no treatment for the illness itself. It just has to run its course. See page 278 for more on stomach viruses.

Food poisoning. Bacterial contamination of spoiled food is the second most common cause. Symptoms are similar to the stomach virus, but there is usually no fever or body aches, and diarrhea almost always follows. Symptoms can start anywhere from a few hours to a whole day after eating. Other clues that this may be food poisoning rather than a stomach virus are that the vomiting usually won't last more than twelve hours, you can think of a likely food culprit, and others who ate the same food are also ill. There is no treatment for food poisoning.

Infectious intestinal bacteria. This is a less common cause, but can be a more concerning one. There are several bacteria that cause this, including salmonella, shigella, campylobacter, and *E. coli*. They can be caught either by eating contaminated food (like food poisoning) or from contact with a sick person. Symptoms will vary, but usually include fever, vomiting, diarrhea (sometimes bloody), and abdominal pains. Some of these are treatable with antibiotics (see Diarrhea, page 277).

Throat and ear infections. Sometimes these routine infections can trigger vomiting. See pages 514 and 285 if you suspect these.

Carsickness. This can affect even young children. See page 211.

Uncommon Causes

Surgical emergencies. There are several intestinal problems that trigger vomiting, including intestinal obstruction and appendicitis. However, in these situations severe abdominal pain is the primary symptom. The vomiting is more secondary. We address these emergencies under Abdominal Pain, page 117.

Severe bladder or kidney infection. If accompanied by painful or frequent urination, fever, and lower to mid-back pain, vomiting can be a symptom of kidney infection. See page 194.

Meningitis. Vomiting along with fever, headaches, stiff neck, extreme irritability or lethargy, and light sensitivity should be evaluated right away. See page 393.

Medication overdose or poison ingestion. If you suspect your child may have ingested something harmful, call your doctor right away, or poison control at 1-800-222-1222.

Head injury. Vomiting can be a symptom of internal head injury. See page 351 if your child has had any trauma to the head.

Migraine headaches or abdominal migraines. Unexplained vomiting with abdominal pains and/or headaches may be a migraine. See page 396.

Brain tumor. Obviously this is very rare, but we're just trying to be thorough. Vomiting that gradually becomes more frequent over several weeks, along with headaches and deteriorating mental status, can be a sign of a tumor. In this case, there would be no other signs of obvious intestinal conditions such as abdominal pain or diarrhea.

Determining the Cause

Reading through the various causes may help you figure out what's going on. In general, vomiting with fever, abdominal pain, and diarrhea is some sort of intestinal illness. If there is no blood in the stools, then this is most probably an untreatable stomach virus. Bloody diarrhea may indicate an infectious condition that your pediatrician should evaluate. If your child has vomiting, pain, and diarrhea *without* fever, then this is probably food poisoning. The uncommon causes listed above are fairly self-explanatory; go to the more detailed explanations on the pages cited if you suspect one of these.

It isn't really necessary to determine the exact cause of vomiting on the first day of the illness. What's most important is to make sure there are no signs that it is one of the severe conditions listed above.

Keeping Your Child Hydrated

Don't panic. Kids can usually tolerate up to twelve hours of vomiting, without keeping any liquids down, before dehydration becomes a worry. Vomiting tends to go through stages. Supportive care will be different, depending on what stage your child is in.

Stage one: Repeated vomiting every five to thirty minutes. This first stage is the scariest for parents and kids. You feel so helpless because there's nothing you can do. There are no over-the-counter meds to try. Just keep your child upright, hold the bucket for him while he throws up, and wipe his face off when he's done. In between episodes just keep your child quiet. This first stage can last between one and four hours. Since this isn't enough time to cause dehydration, you don't even have to try to give your child liquids, which usually just come right back up anyway. If your infant or child begs to drink or to nurse at the breast, it's okay to oblige, even though it probably won't stay down.

Stage two: Vomiting slows to every one or two hours. Once the vomiting slows down, parents and kids can get a little rest between fits. It's okay to offer some sips of liquid during this time. Be careful though; too much too fast will just come right back up. A sip or two, or ice chips, every five or ten minutes is a good rule. This stage can last for as little as a few hours or as long as a day or two.

Stage three: Vomiting slows down more. Vomiting slows to only two to four times per day and eventually stops altogether. When things improve, it's okay to begin letting your child drink as much as he wants, as long as this doesn't trigger more frequent vomiting. Once he's been keeping liquids down for over twelve hours, go ahead and try some food if your child asks. Try something bland, such as crackers, bread, or soup. If he doesn't ask, his tummy probably isn't ready yet. Don't be too surprised if eating triggers vomiting again. Just wait it out and restrict him to liquids again.

What to drink. Kids need more than just water. They need sugar, salt, and electrolytes. An oral electrolyte drink from any drugstore is a good choice. Breast milk is perfect for the nursing baby. White grape juice or a sports drink diluted by half with water or a Popsicle also work. Don't use apple, pear, or cherry juice, as the sugar content may aggravate diarrhea.

Prescription Medications

Suppository meds can be prescribed by the doctor to slow down or stop the vomiting. These are especially useful during the first and second stages to help prevent dehydration. If your child is seen by the doctor during this time, he will likely prescribe one of these meds to be used every six hours as needed. Once your child is in stage three, it's probably better to allow occasional vomiting than to stay on the meds.

These medications will cause drowsiness, and there have been some cases of oversedation in kids under two years of age. They are used more cautiously with infants.

**DR. SEARS TIP
Be Prepared to Get
Through the Night**

If your child starts vomiting in the afternoon or evening, you may want to see or call the doctor to get a suppository prescription just in case the vomiting persists into the night.

When Not to Worry

In these common situations, you generally don't need to worry or seek medical care:

The first several hours. During stage one, with symptoms of a stomach virus, food poisoning, or intestinal infection as described above, you don't really need to see a doctor. So if vomiting hits in the middle of the night, it's usually okay to wait until morning to call the doctor.

Vomiting only a few times each day. Even if mild vomiting continues for two or three days, as long as the other symptoms are consistent with a routine intestinal virus or stomach flu, you don't really need to see a doctor.

Rebound vomiting. Some kids will appear to get better for a day or two, then vomiting starts all over. This is not uncommon.

Bloody streaks in the vomit. This can occur from minor soreness in the throat or the nose and isn't a worry. If there is more blood than just streaks, see the section below.

Vomiting caused by coughing. This isn't really an actual vomiting illness. See our cold and cough section, page 222, for more details.

When to Worry

Moderate to severe dehydration. This is always an indication to seek medical care. Mild dehydration is expected and not worrisome, but if vomiting goes on for more than six hours for an infant, twelve hours for a toddler, or sixteen hours for a child, you should call the doctor. See page 267 for a detailed description of how to tell if your child is dehydrated enough to call the doctor.

Vomiting with bloody diarrhea. This can indicate an infectious intestinal bacteria. This isn't a reason to rush to the emergency room or page the doctor overnight, but see the doctor when the office next opens. For more information, see page 277.

Vomiting blood. This can occur when blood vessels in the esophagus tear from the pressure of vomiting. If the blood is bright red and coming in large amounts, go to an emergency room right away.

Other serious signs. Any signs of surgical emergency, kidney infection, meningitis, poisoning, or head injury as discussed on page 536 should be evaluated in an emergency room if after hours or at the doctor's office right away.

WARTS

Warts are a very common infection of the skin that almost every child will deal with at some point in time. Warts are caused by viruses that get into the deep skin layers and cause the skin cells to harden and form a wart. Children are more likely to get warts than adults. They can appear on any part of the body.

Kinds of Warts

Common warts. Common warts are just that — the most common types of warts found in children. They usually appear on fingers, knees, hands, and elbows. They are generally small (less than a centimeter), raised, and often have black dots inside them.

Plantar warts. These are similar to common warts, but are found on the soles of the feet and can often grow larger than common warts. They may become uncomfortable because of their location on the soles of the feet.

Molluscum warts. These can appear anywhere on the body as small (about a quarter of an eraser head or less), firm blisters with tiny dimples in the center. See page 401 for more details.

Genital warts. These are discussed on page 469.

Are Warts Contagious?

Yes, but a child has to come into close and prolonged physical contact with the wart of another child. A wart can be passed from one area of the body to another. If the child picks at her wart, she is more likely to get a wart on another area of her body. Warts are not passed on by the casual contact of daily life.

Treatment

Warts almost always go away by themselves. However, this process can take as long as several years. Warts are often removed if they are causing discomfort (such as plantar warts) or if the wart continues to grow in size. There are several treatment options:

Over-the-counter (OTC) wart acids. These can be effective for smaller warts if applied consistently. However, they can take weeks or months to remove the wart. Talk to your pediatrician before using OTC treatments if the wart is present on the face or genitals.

Liquid nitrogen. This is the most common treatment used in doctors' offices. Liquid

 **DR. SEARS TIP
Duct Tape Fixes Anything**

A successful home remedy for warts that we have recommended to patients is the use of duct tape. This process often works, but it can take six weeks to three months. Talk to your pediatrician before beginning this regimen:

1. Soak the wart in warm water for ten to fifteen minutes, then file down the outer skin layers of the wart with an emery board.

2. After soaking and filing down, place a small square of duct tape over the wart; use a Band-Aid or paper tape to keep it in place. You can use a waterproof Band-Aid if your child bathes daily.

3. After three days, remove the duct tape and repeat step 1, soaking the wart in warm water for ten to fifteen minutes then filing down with an emery board.

4. Reapply duct tape as in step 2, and leave in place for several more days. Repeat this process for several weeks and the wart should slowly disappear.

Remember, this may take up to three months to be successful. Talk to your pediatrician if the wart is not going away or is getting larger despite treatment.

nitrogen freezes the wart and kills the virus inside the wart. After treatment, the wart usually falls off, or can be peeled off, within several days. For larger warts that invade deeper into the skin, two or three treatments with liquid nitrogen may be required. This procedure should be done carefully as the side effects include blistering of the surrounding skin and scarring of the area that is frozen.

Laser treatment. For warts that do not respond to freezing or that continue to return despite treatment with liquid nitrogen, laser treatment can be the next step. This should be done by a dermatologist trained in the use of laser.

Warts are more of a nuisance than anything else. See the doctor if the wart does not respond to OTC treatment or if the wart is on the face, near the fingernails, or in the genital area. Also, see the doctor right away if the wart appears to be getting infected.

WHOOPING COUGH (PERTUSSIS)

Whooping cough is a highly contagious disease caused by a type of bacteria known as *Bordetella pertussis,* which infects the respiratory tract. It is characterized by long periods of extremely violent and uncontrollable coughing spells. Whooping cough spreads as one infected person coughs or sneezes, releasing tiny droplets of saliva or mucus that contain the bacteria into the air. These tiny droplets can be inhaled by another person and lead to whooping cough. Outbreaks often occur within families or in school or daycare.

Symptoms

Whooping cough is serious because it produces a thick, copious mucus that plugs little airways and compromises breathing. This excess mucus causes the characteristic cough and whoop. The child coughs to dislodge the mucus plugs from his little airways. Coughing escalates into a fifteen- to thirty-second bout of increasingly forceful coughs, with each cough pushing the mucus higher so it can be coughed out or swallowed. At the end of the coughing spell, the child is so hungry for air that he quickly takes a catch-up breath, producing a whooping sound. Then the child rests and seems well for an hour or so. The mucus reaccumulates and the whooping cycle starts all over again. These episodes of violent coughs may last for six to twelve weeks. Other symptoms of whooping cough might include:

- low-grade fever

- runny nose

- vomiting after a severe coughing spell

 DR. SEARS TIP
Try the Sipping Solution

Feeding an infant or young child with whooping cough can be challenging. Obviously, it is important not to feed children during coughing spells. This can cause them to choke. Also, full tummies and frequent coughing jags are a recipe for vomiting. Feed between coughing episodes or soon after one. Try letting your child sip on a smoothie after a coughing episode. Smoothies are an easy-in/easy-out way of feeding; they enter the stomach easily and empty quickly.

- short-term loss of consciousness if the coughing spell is severe enough to cause a lack of oxygen to the brain

- diarrhea

- in infants, blue appearance in the face following a severe coughing spell

Diagnosis

Taking a swab inside the nose or in the back of the throat and sending it for a culture can confirm infection with *Bordetella pertussis*. It is not uncommon for a test to be negative when in fact a child is infected. If the doctor strongly suspects whooping cough, he may not test for it. Other blood tests and/or a chest X-ray may be performed if he believes they are necessary.

Treatment

What the doctor might prescribe. Whooping cough is difficult to treat, which is why we stress prevention through immunization. Because whooping cough is caused by a bacteria, antibiotics are usually prescribed. However, antibiotics are most effective when used early in the course of the illness. The later antibiotics are started, the less effective they will be. The doctor will usually prescribe an antibiotic even if your child has suffered from whooping cough for several weeks. This is done to possibly shorten the duration of the illness, make your child less contagious, and prevent a secondary infection. If a family member is diagnosed with whooping cough, the doctor may recommend that the entire family be treated with a course of antibiotics.

Whooping cough is most dangerous for infants and the elderly, but it is rarely fatal. Infants with whooping cough under six months old may need to be hospitalized for close supervision and respiratory support. Over-the-counter cough medications and cough suppressants are generally not very effective in helping the symptoms of whooping cough. These types of medications should not be used for children under four years of age and without a doctor's advice.

What you can do at home. In addition to antibiotics, home treatment is aimed at thinning the mucus so your child can more easily cough it up:

- Steam it. Read our "steam-cleaning" method of thinning bronchial secretions, page 20.

- Water it. Hydrate your child well to thin the mucus.

- Clap it. Called *chest physiotherapy*, your pediatrician will show you how to clap on your child's back to help dislodge the mucus plugs.

- Rest it. Be sure your child rests after a coughing fit. He needs to recharge for the next one.

- Don't always suppress it. Your child's cough is his best "internal medicine" for dislodging mucus plugs, which is why we advise

---

 DR. SEARS TIP
"A Spoonful of Honey..."

Recent studies have shown that honey is a safer and more effective cough reliever than the over-the-counter dextromethorphan. But do not use honey in children younger than one year.

---

parents to hold cough suppressants during the day. Suppressants can be used at night if your child is unable to sleep because of the cough, but talk to your doctor first. He may recommend an expectorant or cough loosener instead of a cough suppressant.

Prevention

The whooping cough vaccine is currently recommended for all infants. It is usually administered at two, four, six, and eighteen months of age, followed by a booster between four and six years of age. The vaccine is usually combined with a vaccine for diphtheria and tetanus in the DTaP vaccine (see our vaccine section for more information, page 43). Since the initiation of routine universal vaccinations for children, the rates of whooping cough have dramatically decreased.

However, over the past two decades, researchers have found an increase in whooping cough rates among adolescents and adults because the whooping cough vaccine loses its effectiveness over a four- to twelve-year period. This means that although the vaccine effectively protects infants and children, on reaching adolescence or young adulthood it may no longer be effective. A whooping cough booster shot, called Tdap, is now recommended for all children and adolescents between eleven and eighteen years of age. This helps protect adolescents and adults from outbreaks as well as infants and children from exposure to whooping cough. Talk to your pediatrician about whether your child or adolescent should have the booster.

Some other important preventive measures include proper hygiene techniques among families and, as mentioned above, your pediatrician may advise antibiotic treatment for the whole family. Because it is so important, we'll reiterate that those at highest risk are infants less than six months of age and the elderly.

It is now recommended that adults up to the age of sixty-five receive this one-time whooping cough booster (Tdap). This is especially important when a new infant is born into the home.

YEAST INFECTIONS

Yeast infections are usually caused by a certain kind of yeast known as *Candida albicans*. In this section, we will discuss the two main types of yeast infections in children, oral thrush and yeast diaper rash. See page 532 for vaginal yeast problems.

Oral Thrush

Oral thrush is a yeast infection of the mouth and throat and is common during the first year of life. This is because the yeast enjoy the warm, moist environment that breastfeeding and/or bottlefeeding provides. Thrush appears as a coating or white patches on the tongue, inside the mouth and cheeks, and even in the back of the throat. It usually has a curd-like consistency to it. If you can scrape off some of the coating, your child

 **DR. SEARS TIP
Boil the Bottle!**

If your infant is bottlefeeding, be sure to maintain good hygiene. The nipple on the bottle is a good breeding ground for candidal yeast. Boil both pacifiers and nipples in water regularly to help prevent yeast.

probably has thrush. Thrush is usually pain-less, but if severe it can cause some pain and irritation.

Treatment. Most cases of oral thrush respond very quickly to antifungal liquid med-ications. These are usually administered by squirting a little of the medication into the inside of each cheek three to four times a day, or as directed by your pediatrician.

DR. SEARS TIP
Treat Thrush Longer

Assuming your child's oral thrush is respond-ing to the liquid antifungal medication, we always tell parents to continue to use the medication for at least two to three days after the thrush is completely gone. Some parents stop a little too early, and the thrush comes right back.

Can oral thrush affect breastfeeding? Yes. Infants can pass oral thrush to the nipples of breastfeeding mothers. This can make the nip-ples very sore, itchy, and burning. It is very common for an infant and breastfeeding mother to pass the thrush back and forth.

If a nursing mother is complaining of irri-tated and sore nipples, we also treat the mother. We recommend dabbing a white vine-gar solution (one tablespoon vinegar in eight ounces of water) onto the nipples after each feeding, as well as an OTC antifungal cream three times daily. Occasionally, mothers need to take antifungal medications by mouth to eradicate the candida yeast on the nipples.

Other causes. Oral thrush usually ceases to be a problem once the breastfeeding and/or bottlefeeding stage passes. However, older children can sometimes be affected. Causes include:

- Antibiotic use. Taking antibiotics can kill off normal, healthy bacteria in the mouth and digestive tract. This can allow an over-growth of candidal yeast, leading to oral thrush. This usually goes away once the course of antibiotics is finished. NEVER stop your child's antibiotics before talking to the doctor.

- Inhaled or oral steroid use. Inhalers con-taining steroids and oral steroid medica-tions can also lead to oral thrush if used over a long period of time. If your child is on one of these medications and develops oral thrush, talk to your pediatrician. DO NOT stop these steroid medications with-out first talking to the doctor.

- Impaired immune systems. Children with immune-system disorders, such as leu-kemia and HIV, are more prone to yeast infections. This is because the body has a hard time fighting off overgrowths of the yeast.

DR. SEARS TIP
Beware When Your Child
Is on Antibiotics

We recommend taking probiotics (such as *Lactobacillus acidophilus* or bifidobacteria) while on antibiotics. This can prevent yeast overgrowth from occurring.

Yeast Diaper Rash

This is the second most commonly seen yeast problem among infants.

Causes. *Candida albicans,* the normal culprit in yeast diaper rash, loves the moist environment inside of Baby's diaper, especially the moist folds around Baby's groin, genitalia, and rectal area. We see this classic "diaper rash that just won't go away" often. Almost every infant will get some form of a yeast diaper rash, and some rashes can be much more severe than others.

DR. SEARS TIP
Yeast Clues

Yeast diaper rash has a very different appearance from a typical non-yeast diaper rash. Yeast diaper rashes are usually much more red, swollen, and inflamed. Certain spots may even start to crack and bleed. Redness usually occurs in the groin, genital, and rectal areas, and red dots often spread out from the main area of redness.

Treatment. Treatment depends on how severe the rash is. In mild cases, we usually recommend an over-the-counter antifungal ointment or cream with clotrimazole. Apply this cream three to four times a day. The below measures should also be taken:

- Change diapers frequently.

- Clean the diaper area very gently with water and mild soap. Rinse, then pat dry.

- Let your child go without a diaper as much as possible.

- Apply a white zinc oxide barrier cream in between applications of the antifungal ointment.

- Give your baby an oral probiotic twice daily in food or drink. This will help diminish the yeast.

Persistent yeast diaper rash. The above measures will usually clear up a mild case of yeast diaper rash. However, infants and children can suffer from more severe yeast rashes, especially when the rash is left untreated for weeks at a time. If your child has a more severe yeast rash, the doctor might prescribe a stronger, prescription-strength antifungal ointment or cream. Be sure to follow the doctor's instructions, and talk to her if the yeast diaper rash worsens or returns following prescription treatment.

DR. SEARS TIP
Diaper Rash

As with oral thrush, antibiotics can also lead to yeast diaper rash. DO NOT stop antibiotics if your child gets a yeast diaper rash unless instructed to do so by your doctor. Take the above measures to treat the diaper rash. Again, giving your child probiotic supplements (such *Lactobacillus acidophilus* or bifidobacteria) while he is on antibiotics may help prevent yeast diaper rash.

IV

Medicine Cabinet

Throughout this book, we've given many recommendations on various medications. In this final section of the book, we will provide you with more detailed information on how to give medications, use antibiotics appropriately and safely, and understand the use and dosing of the most common medications.

Most parents, understandably, don't like to give their children any medication unless it is necessary. We prefer to limit medication in our practice as much as we can. But sooner or later, most children will catch a cold that could use some cold medicine, or develop a rash that needs a medicated cream, or have an allergic reaction that requires relief. There are a host of illnesses that may need over-the-counter (OTC) or prescription treatments. Here is our guide to understanding the most common medications you may find yourself administering to your child. In many cases, we will offer dosing suggestions. However, our dosing charts are intended as a guideline only, to help you understand a typical dose for a child's age. Medications come and go, and dosing recommendations may change. We advise you to consult the product packaging for proper dosing information.

GIVING MEDICINES

Your pediatrician prescribes a medicine, but it's up to Dr. Mom or Dr. Dad to get it down the child. Here are some pointers we use at home and in our practice:

Know the instructions. Be sure you understand the doctor's instructions about giving the medicine. Ask questions, such as: *How much? How often? Before or after meals? Should I wake my child to give her medicine? What should we do if we inadvertently miss a dose?* After you've picked up the medicine at the pharmacy, if the instructions on the bottle differ from what the doctor or pharmacist has told you, or if you're confused about the dosage or instructions, call the doctor for clarification.

Record how it works. Record which medication, which flavor, and which form of medicine work best for your child. The next time the doctor prescribes a medicine, volunteer your experience. For example, "The last antibiotic [name of medicine] gave her horrible diarrhea, but the one before [name of medicine] didn't." Let the doctor know which form of medicine your child prefers. Some children prefer liquid, others prefer chewables, and older children can swallow capsules.

Disguise the medicine. Remember how Mary Poppins sang, "A spoonful of sugar helps the medicine go down"? A favorite in our practice is to use the "sprinkle it" method. If the medicine comes in capsule form, open up the capsule and sprinkle the medicine on your child's favorite food. By using capsules, you avoid the artificial colorings and sweeteners that are often added to children's liquid medicine to make them more palatable. If your child will not take a liquid medicine, crush the chewable tablet between two spoons. To make the medicine as palatable as possible, bury the crushed pill in a sandwich (jam it into jam, place it under peanut butter) and chase it with a glass of your child's favorite drink. Make sure the first few bites contain all the medicine.

Numb the tongue. Let your child suck on a Popsicle or drink a cold smoothie just before taking the medicine, or cool the medicine in the refrigerator first. Numbing the taste buds gives the medicine a fighting chance of making it past a child's sensitive tongue.

Make magic paste. While most babies prefer liquid, if in the past your child has spit out the liquid medicine, ask the doctor to prescribe the medicine in chewable or tablet form. Crush the tablet between two spoons and add a couple drops of water to make a thick paste. To bypass the tongue, apply a fingertipful of the paste to the inside of your child's cheek a few times until she swallows all the medicine.

Try the cheek-pocket technique. Here's a Sears family favorite that may require two adults until you get used to it: With your child cradled on your lap and leaning back slightly, cup your child's lower face with your hand and use the middle or index finger to pull out the corner of her mouth, making a pocket in her cheek. This holds the child's mouth open and head still, and the traction on your child's cheek keeps her from spitting the medicine back out. With your other hand, squirt the medicine into this cheek pocket a little at a time. Squirting the medicine into the cheek pocket with the child's head tilted back a bit allows the medicine to bypass the sensitive taste buds of the tongue and is more likely to be swallowed without a protest. Necessity is the mother of invention, or in this case the father. I (Dr. Bill) discovered this technique when Martha (queen medicine-giver in our family) left me alone at medicine time with our eighteen-month-old son.

Aim away from the tongue. Remember, the most sensitive taste buds are toward the front and center of your child's tongue. Using a calibrated medicine dropper, squirt the medicine into the *side* of your child's mouth between cheek and gum. Squirt it slowly and point it toward the cheek. If you squirt it too strongly against the back of the throat, you may stimulate gagging.

Try a spoon. If using a spoon, try the "upper lip sweep." To get all of the medicine off the spoon, sweep the bowl of the spoon against the inside of your child's upper lip as you are pulling the spoon out of the mouth.

Avoid choking. Be sure to give the medicine with your child sitting up or leaning back only slightly. In this position, your child is less likely to gag and spit up the medicine. If your child is lying down, have him lie on his side and ease the medicine into the cheek nearest the mattress.

Make the pill easier to swallow. Children have great difficulty swallowing tablets. Place

 DR. SEARS TIP
Don't "Sweeten" the Deal

Although you want to make the medicine as palatable as possible, never tell your child that medication is candy. That's a sure way to entice your child to explore the medicine cabinet. Also, don't tell a child that a medication will taste good when you know it won't. Giving her a second dose will be impossible.

the pill near the tip of your child's tongue. Have him take a drink of water, hold it in his mouth, and bend his head forward so that his chin touches his chest. Then have him lift his head up quickly as he swallows. The pill will rise to the top of the water toward the back of the tongue and wash down easily with the swallow.

Play medicine-taking games. Try the run-and-bite method. Put the medicine on a spoon. Have your child run at you from about five feet away and stop immediately in front of the spoonful of medicine. He takes the medicine and swallows it down fast with a water chaser and continues on his journey. As an extra incentive, place a favorite treat on a table just beyond the spoonful of medicine. Close the game with a cheerful "All done!"

ALLERGIC REACTIONS

Diphenhydramine (Benadryl is the most common brand name). This liquid, chewable, or tablet antihistamine is used to help any type of allergic reaction subside. The most common reason to use this is for hives (see page 370). It can also help with itching and

Diphenhydramine: Can be given every six hours as needed.

Children under 2 years of age — consult a doctor
2 and 3 years — 12.5 milligrams
4 and 5 years — 18.75 milligrams
6 to 11 years — 25 milligrams
12 years and older — 50 milligrams

swelling from rashes, insect bites and stings, and allergic food reactions. It can be used at any age, but you should consult with your pediatrician if you feel your child under four years of age needs a dose. It lasts for about six hours and may make a child drowsy. Never use diphenhydramine for the purposes of sedation; improper use can cause oversedation and may be harmful.

For a guide to severe allergic reactions, see page 130. For hives, see page 370. For antibiotic reactions, see page 551. For food allergies, see page 327.

ANTIBIOTICS

Antibiotics are the most prescribed medicine in our country, and probably the most overly prescribed medicine as well. Decades of antibiotic misuse have gotten us into trouble now with resistant bacteria. But despite their overuse, antibiotics are an important part of our modern health-care system. When used appropriately, they save lives and prevent unnecessary pain and suffering. Almost every child ends up needing them at some point. Here is our guide to understanding appropriate antibiotic use and minimizing side effects.

Deciding When an Antibiotic Is Needed

Deciding whether an antibiotic is warranted is one of the most challenging aspects of pediatrics. It's a balancing act between making sure a serious bacterial infection isn't left untreated and trying to limit antibiotic overuse. There are two situations where a doctor might prescribe an antibiotic:

Bacterial infection. If the doctor can see a severe infection in the eyes, ears, sinuses, throat, or skin, or hear infectious sounds in the lungs with a stethoscope, then the decision is easy: use an antibiotic, especially if the child is acting particularly ill. If the doctor detects a mild infection and the child is feeling okay, then a wait-and-see approach may be taken, with a plan for possible antibiotics if the infection worsens. This can be safely done with sinus and ear infections in particular.

Suspected bacterial infection. Sometimes a child is feeling quite ill with a fever for several days, but the doctor doesn't detect any obvious infection. He or she can't tell whether your child has an untreatable virus that will go away on its own or a more serious bacterial infection. In such cases many doctors will prescribe a "just-in-case" antibiotic to cover your child. If a child is acting unusually ill, the doctor may do some tests to determine if it's a virus or bacteria, and if bacterial how severe it is and how aggressive to be with antibiotic treatment.

Here's an insider's tip for parents when their child has a suspected bacterial infection but the doctor isn't sure. It's certainly easier to prescribe a just-in-case antibiotic; the wait-and-see approach requires a lot more judgment and is often more taxing to the parent and the doctor. If your pediatrician does wisely take a wait-and-see approach, be sure you understand his instructions on what to look for and when to call back. Here's where the parent-pediatrician partnership really shines. In order for this approach to be in the best interest of your child, the doctor is trusting you to be not only a keen observer of your child's changing signs and symptoms, but an accurate reporter who knows when to call or come back should your child's symptoms worsen.

How parents can help. Since you've been spending the past few days observing your child, and the doctor only has a few minutes, be sure to accurately articulate how sick you feel your child is. Is she being bothered by some symptoms on and off but generally acting like her typical self? Or is she more lethargic than usual and feeling down and out most of the time? Does a pain reliever/fever reducer or cold medication perk her up close to normal for several hours? Or do such medications seem to have little effect? These are important things your doctor needs to know, so be sure to pass this information along.

Avoid the antibiotic parade. A common, but unfortunate, situation that occurs when the first antibiotic doesn't seem to work is that a stronger one is then given. The child gets almost better but gets sick again after the strong antibiotic is finished. A third antibiotic is prescribed and seems to help, but another illness hits a short time after and once again it's antibiotic time. If your child is headed down the path of repeated antibiotics, make a special effort to boost her immune system (see page 33) and consider reasons why this may be occurring, such as allergies or inadequate hand washing.

DR. SEARS TIP
Don't Push Your Pediatrician

Occasionally a parent might think, Why did we make the effort to come to the doctor when she didn't prescribe a medication? It often takes more time and medical judgment *not* to prescribe an antibiotic. And more natural remedies may be safer for your child in the long run.

This commonly occurs with ear infections that haven't completely resolved from one course of antibiotics. If a child feels better, but some infection or ear fluid is still present, more antibiotics may not be needed.

How to Give Antibiotics

Here are some important guidelines to follow when your child is prescribed antibiotics:

- Make sure you ask the pharmacist if it should be refrigerated or not.

- Ask if it should be taken with meals or on an empty stomach (this varies between antibiotics).

- Any antibiotic can be mixed into a small serving of any type of food or liquid if needed to get it down (even if recommended on an empty stomach).

- Be sure to finish the prescription as written.

- If you forget a dose and don't remember until the next one is due, don't worry. Just move on with the next dose. If you remember sooner, give the missed dose and delay the next a few hours.

- If you spill some or find there isn't enough in the bottle to finish, you've taken at least 75 percent of the prescribed days, and your child is all better, don't bother getting more to finish.

- See our child-friendly tips on how to get the medicine down on page 547.

Spitting up or throwing up a dose. In most cases, this isn't considered a reaction to the antibiotic, but rather an aversion to the taste. If a child spits up a dose within fifteen minutes of taking it, go ahead and repeat. If longer than that, enough will have absorbed that a repeat dose isn't necessary. If your child throws up three or four doses, this may mean that brand is too irritating and an alternative is needed.

Treating Antibiotic Side Effects

Preventing antibiotic side effects. Antibiotics will kill off some of the healthy bacteria that live in the intestines, allowing more irritating yeast and bacteria to overgrow and cause diarrhea and diaper rash. Don't wait for this to happen before you act. Buy a probiotic (e.g., acidophilus) from a health-food store or pharmacy and give this daily (a few hours apart from the antibiotic doses) during the course and for a few weeks after. These healthy probiotic bacteria will help replace the good intestinal bacteria, fight off any bad intestinal germs, and prevent some uncomfortable side effects.

Diarrhea or stomach upset. The unwelcome germs that can overgrow in the intestines during antibiotic use are irritating to the intestines and can cause abdominal pain and diarrhea. If you haven't yet started probiotics,

do so now. You can also increase the BRAT diet foods (banana, rice, applesauce, toast) to help slow down the diarrhea. If the diarrhea becomes more bothersome than the infection for which the antibiotics are being taken in the first place, stop them and contact your doctor when the office next opens. A day or two off antibiotics is fine in most cases.

Diaper rash. This occurs because any diarrhea caused by the antibiotics can be acidic and irritating to the bottom. Plus, yeast overgrowth within the gut can spread out around the bottom or genital area and cause a yeast rash. See page 275 for information on how to distinguish between these two types of diaper rash. This bothersome effect can be minimized by using generous amounts of white zinc diaper cream. If yeast is suspected, an OTC antifungal cream called clotrimazole can be applied two to three times daily mixed in with the regular diaper cream or put on separately. Probiotics given by mouth can also help the rash resolve.

 DR. SEARS TIP Heads-Up for Breastfeeding Moms

If a breastfeeding mom takes antibiotics, enough can get into the breast milk and into Baby to cause yeast to grow in the baby's mouth or in the diaper area. This is especially true if a baby takes antibiotics directly. This yeast can then transfer from the baby's mouth onto Mom's breasts and cause a very uncomfortable breast yeast infection. You can preempt this by starting probiotic capsules for yourself and a powder or liquid for the baby. Don't wait until this happens to start probiotics. See page 542 for more on thrush while breastfeeding.

Oral thrush. Sometimes yeast will overgrow within the mouth and cause white patches to grow on the tongue, inside the cheeks, and behind the lips. This is easily prevented and treated with probiotics. If it persists, the doctor can prescribe a liquid yeast medication. See page 540 for more on thrush.

Allergic rash. A child can have an allergic reaction to any antibiotic at any time during, and for a couple weeks after, the course of treatment. Antibiotic rashes come in two forms:

- Hives. These itchy welts are one type of antibiotic reaction. See page 370 for more details on how to treat with diphenhydramine (Benadryl).

- Generic rash. Antibiotics can also cause a non-specific red, bumpy, or lacy diffuse rash on various parts of the body. This is also an allergic reaction, but just not as severe as hives. No treatment is necessary unless itchy, in which case treat it as if it is hives.

If your child is being treated specifically with amoxicillin or Augmentin for tonsillitis, and develops an allergic-looking rash, this actually may mean your child has mono. The mono virus reacts with these two antibiotics in a unique way that triggers a rash. It's not an allergy at all. If this happens, it's better for the doctor to get a blood test to see if your child actually has mono instead of just automatically labeling your child allergic to these antibiotics (which would forever leave your child labeled allergic to all penicillins). See page 402 for more details on mono.

If your child has a rash during a course of treatment, stop the antibiotics and contact your pediatrician when the office opens to see if another antibiotic should be taken. If your child is still fairly ill from the initial infection, and the doctor's office doesn't open within twenty-four hours, have the doctor paged to discuss an alternative antibiotic.

FEVER AND PAIN RELIEF

This is perhaps the biggest reason that you may find yourself giving your child medication. We put these two categories together because the medicines to treat them are the same:

Acetaminophen (Tylenol). This medication can be used at any age, from newborns through the elderly, for the relief of pain from any cause and for fever. It is available in liquids, chewables, tablets, and suppositories (brand name FeverAll).

Acetaminophen: Can be given every four hours as needed and is based on weight.

12 pounds — 80 milligrams
15 pounds — 100 milligrams
18 pounds — 120 milligrams
23 pounds — 160 milligrams
28 pounds — 200 milligrams
35 pounds — 240 milligrams
45 pounds — 300 milligrams
60 pounds — 400 milligrams
75 pounds and up — 500 milligrams
150 pounds and up (adults) — 1,000 milligrams

Ibuprofen (Motrin, Advil). This medicine works a little bit differently from acetaminophen, and it is used for the same indications for infants three months and older through the elderly. It comes as liquid, chewables, and tablets. One main difference with ibuprofen is that it is also an anti-inflammatory (besides relieving pain and fever), so it may work better than acetaminophen for problems such as menstrual cramps, muscle and joint aches, injuries involving swelling, and fevers and irritability from vaccinations.

Ibuprofen: Can be given every six hours and is based on weight.

15 pounds — 50 milligrams
18 pounds — 75 milligrams
23 pounds — 100 milligrams
28 pounds — 125 milligrams
35 pounds — 150 milligrams
45 pounds — 200 milligrams
60 pounds — 250 milligrams
75 pounds and up — 300 milligrams
150 pounds and up (adults) — 600 milligrams

For more information on when and how to treat fever, see page 317.

STOCKING YOUR MEDICINE CABINET

Most medicines can be easily purchased at a local drugstore or grocery store when you need to treat your child. However, you might want to keep certain ones on hand (so you don't have to run out to a store in the middle of the night). In addition, some treatments are not so easy to find; you might want to purchase some every couple of years so you can have them handy should an urgent need arise.

Here is our *must-have-on-hand* list:

- acetaminophen

- ibuprofen

- antibiotic ointment (for cuts)

- diphenhydramine (Benadryl) for allergic reactions (see page 370)

- cough and cold medicine (see page 222 for our guide to using these)

- vitamin C (see page 37 for immune-boosting instructions)

- echinacea (see page 37 for immune-boosting instructions)

- Sinupret (see page 38 for information on this natural sinus-support supplement)

- mullein garlic eardrops for those middle-of-the-night earaches (see page 283)

- hydrocortisone cream 1 percent for itchy or irritated rashes

- anti-itch solution (calamine or Itch-X) for insect bite relief

You may also want to keep a standard first-aid kit well stocked to handle common wounds and injuries:

- Band-Aids

- paper tape (for wrapping wounds)

- sterile gauze pads (to place over large open wounds)

- gauze roll

- sterile saline bottle (for flushing out wounds)

- butterfly bandages (to close minor open cuts)

- antiseptic solution (hydrogen peroxide or Betadine)

- Ace wraps (for sprains)

- tweezers

- space blanket (silver-colored, folds up very small) to use for warmth or in case of shock

- pair of sterile gloves

- instant cold packs

- scissors

- oral thermometer (plastic, non-mercury)

Acknowledgments

This comprehensive book would not be possible without the hard work and dedication of our publisher, Little, Brown and Company. Our special thanks to Tracy Behar: her masterful editing always makes us sound every bit as smart as we think we are. And a thank you to Christina Rodriguez for her work as well. Pamela Marshall and Susanna Brougham provided meticulous copyediting. To Terry Adams, warm thanks for many years of guidance (and many more to come!), and to Sabrina Callahan and Heather Fain for efforts in marketing and publicity. We would also like to express our appreciation for the Denise Marcil Agency; Denise, thank you so much for your input on this and all our other works over the decades. And, finally, thanks to the thousands of patients who have come through our office doors over the years. You have taught us and helped shape us into the doctors we are today.

Index

Italic page numbers refer to illustrations.

About the Authors

William Sears, MD, and Martha Sears, RN, are the authors of more than thirty bestselling books on parenting and the parents of eight children. They are the pediatric experts on whom American parents increasingly rely for advice and information on all aspects of pregnancy, birth, child care, and family nutrition. Dr. Bill received his pediatric training at Harvard Medical School's Children's Hospital and Toronto's Hospital for Sick Children. He has practiced pediatrics for more than thirty years, and is an associate clinical professor at the University of California, Irvine, School of Medicine. Martha Sears is a registered nurse, breastfeeding consultant, and parenting and health consultant. They live in Dana Point, California.

Robert W. Sears, MD, is a board-certified pediatrician in private practice in Southern California. Dr. Bob received his medical degree from Georgetown University and completed his pediatric training at Children's Hospital Los Angeles. He has co-authored six books in the Sears Parenting Library, including *The Baby Book* (revised edition). He is also the author of *The Vaccine Book* and *The Autism Book,* and co-author of *HappyBaby*. He lives with his wife and three boys, ages seventeen, fourteen, and eight, in Dana Point, California.

James Sears, MD, is a pediatrician and co-host of the hit show *The Doctors,* a spin-off of *Dr. Phil.* Dr. Jim received his medical degree from Saint Louis University School of Medicine and did his pediatric residency at Tod Children's Hospital in Youngstown, Ohio. He frequently speaks to parenting groups around the country about children's nutrition. He is the proud father of two children, ages seventeen and thirteen, and resides in Southern California.

Peter Sears, MD, FAAFP, is a board-certified physician specializing in family practice. Dr. Peter received his medical degree from Ross University School of Medicine. He completed his residency training at the University of Tennessee Medical Center in Knoxville, Tennessee. Dr. Peter currently lives and practices in Nashville, Tennessee, and sees patients in his clinic from infancy through adolescence and adulthood. He is co-author of *L.E.A.N. Kids* with Dr. William Sears. He is the proud father of a four-year-old son.

575